THE ORGANIC CHEMISTRY
OF DRUG SYNTHESIS

The Organic Chemistry of Drug Synthesis

Volume 1

DANIEL LEDNICER
Chemical Research
Mead Johnson & Co.
Evansville, Indiana

LESTER A. MITSCHER
The University of Kansas School of Pharmacy
Department of Medicinal Chemistry
Lawrence, Kansas

with a Glossary by **Philip F. vonVoigtlander**
The Upjohn Company

A WILEY-INTERSCIENCE PUBLICATION

JOHN WILEY & SONS

New York • Chichester • Brisbane • Toronto

Copyright © 1977 by John Wiley & Sons, Inc.

All rights reserved. Published simultaneously in Canada.

Reproduction or translation of any part of this work beyond that permitted by Sections 107 or 108 of the 1976 United States Copyright Act without the permission of the copyright owner is unlawful. Requests for permission or further information should be addressed to the Permissions Department, John Wiley & Sons, Inc.

Library of Congress Cataloging in Publication Data:

Lednicer, Daniel, 1929-
  The organic chemistry of drug synthesis.

  "A Wiley-Interscience publication."
  1. Chemistry, Medical and pharmaceutical.
2. Drugs. 3. Chemistry, Organic. I. Mitscher, Lester A., joint author. II. Title.

RS421.L423   615′.191   76-28387
ISBN 0-471-52141-8

Printed in the United States of America

10

To

Beryle and Betty

whose steadfastness made that which follows become real

The three princes of Serendip, Balakrama, Vijayo, and Rajahsigha, as they traveled "...were always making discoveries, by accident and sagacity, of things they were not in quest of..."*

*Horace Walpole, in a letter of January 28, 1754, as quoted in "The Three Princes of Serendip," by E. J. Hodges, Atheneum, N.Y., 1964

Preface

There exists today an abundance of excellent texts covering the
various aspects of organic chemistry. The student of medicinal
chemistry can choose among any of a number of first-rate exposi-
tions of that field. The reader who is primarily interested in
the synthesis of some particular class of medicinal agents, however, will often find that he must consult either the original
literature or some specialized review article. The same quandary
faces the student who wishes to become acquainted with the biologic activity characteristic of some class of organic compounds.
There thus seemed to be a place for a book that would cover specifically the chemical manipulations involved in the synthesis of
medicinal agents. A book then was intended that would supplement
both the available medicinal and organic chemistry texts.

Comprehensive coverage of both the preparation and biologic
activity of all organic compounds reported in the literature to
show such activity would lead to a truly enormous treatise. In
order to keep this book within bounds, we deliberately restricted
our coverage to medicinal agents that have been assigned *generic
names*. This means that at some time during the development of a
drug, the sponsoring laboratory has felt the agent to have sufficient promise to apply to the USAN Council or its equivalent
abroad for the granting of such a name. By far, the majority of
the compounds in this volume denoted by generic names are marketed as drugs; some compounds, however, have either gotten only
as far as clinical trial and failed, or are as yet in early pre-
marketing stages. We have not excluded the former since these
are often closely related to drugs in clinical practice and thus
serve as further illustration of molecular manipulation. We have
further kept the book fairly current insofar as drugs available
for sale in the United States are concerned. The informed reader
will note that this book is not nearly as current when it comes
to drugs available only outside this country—our own version of

the drug lag.

In order to sustain the chemical focus of the book, we departed in organization from the traditional texts in medicinal chemistry. The current volume is organized by structural classes rather than in terms of pharmacologic activities. This seems to allow for more natural treatment of the chemistry of many classes of compounds, such as the phenothiazines which form the nucleus for more than a single class of drugs. This framework has admittedly led to some seemingly arbitrary classifications. The sulfonamides, for example, are all regarded as derivatives of *p*-aminobenzenesulfonamide even though this is sometimes the smallest moiety in a given sulfa drug; should these be classed as sulfonamides or as a derivative of the appropriate heterocycle? In this case at least, since the biologic activity is well known to be associated with the sulfonamide portion—the pharmacophoric group—the compounds are kept together. Occasionally the material itself demanded a departure from a purely structural approach. The line of reasoning that leads from morphine to the 4-phenylpiperidines is so clear—if unhistoric—as to demand exposition in an integral chapter. The chronologically oriented chapter on the development of the local anesthetics is included specifically to give the reader some appreciation of one of the first approaches to drug development.

We hope it is clear from the outset that the syntheses outlined in this book represent only those published in the literature. In many cases this can be assumed to bear little relation to the processes used in actually producing the drugs on commercial scale. The latter are usually developed after it is certain the drug will be actually marketed. As in the case of all large-scale organic syntheses, they are changed from the bench-scale preparations in order to take into account such factors as economics and safety. Details of these are not usually readily available.

Again in the interest of conciseness, the discussion of the pharmacology of the various drugs was cut to the bone. The activity is usually indicated by only a short general phrase. Comparisons among closely related analogs as to differences in efficacy or side effects are usually avoided. Such discussion more properly belongs in a specialized text on clinical pharmacology. Since we do not presume that the reader is acquainted with biologic or medical terms, a glossary of the more common terms used in the book has been included following the last chapter. This glossary is intended more to provide simple definitions than in-depth pharmacologic discussion. We urge the reader interested in further study of such entries to consult any of the excellent reference works in medicinal chemistry, such as Burger's "Medicinal

Chemistry" or Rushig and Ehrhard's "Arzneimittel."

This book assumes a good working knowledge of the more common organic reactions and a rudimentary knowledge of biology. We hope it will be of interest to all organic chemists curious about therapeutic agents, how these were developed, the synthetic operations used in their preparation, and the types of structures that have proven useful as drugs. We hope further that this long look at what has gone before may provide food for thought not only to the practicing medicinal chemist but also to the organic chemist engaged in research in pure synthetic chemistry.

Finally, we would like to express our most sincere appreciation to Ms. Carolyn Jarchow of The Upjohn Company. Among the press of daily responsibilities she not only found time for typing this manuscript, but provided the mass of structural drawings as well.

Daniel Lednicer   Kalamazoo, Michigan
Lester A. Mitscher   Lawrence, Kansas

October 1975

Contents

xiii

THE ORGANIC CHEMISTRY
OF DRUG SYNTHESIS

CHAPTER 1

Introduction

Medicinal chemistry, like truth, defies ready definition. The practicing organic chemist as a rule knows operationally what is, or more often what is not, medicinal chemistry. He would be hard pressed, however, to set down on paper a rigorous definition of that discipline.

Organic chemistry and medicinal chemistry share a venerable common history. Many of the founders of organic chemistry had an intense interest not only in molecules from nature but also in the effects of synthetic compounds on living systems. One need mention in this connection only Emil Fischer's work in carbohydrates and proteins and Paul Ehrlich's pioneering work on chemotherapy. With the development of a series of efficacious synthetic medicinal agents, a body of lore evolved concerning the molecular modifications that would most likely lead to biologically active molecules. Almost of necessity, then, this specialized knowledge engendered the discipline that came to be known as medicinal chemistry. The operational manipulations were still those or organic chemistry, as indeed were the molecules being modified; the emphasis of the work was subtly changed, however, from that of classic organic chemistry. The overriding goal became the creation of molecules that would alter some process in a living system. Tangentially, then, we approach an organic chemist's working definition of medicinal chemistry:

> The use of synthetic organic chemistry to create molecules that will alter in a useful way some disease process in a living system.

The use of drugs to treat disease antedates modern science by a good many millenia. Every culture sooner or later developed its own pharmacopeia. These compendia of natural products and

1

extracts were interesting collections of many substances, most
of which were at best useless, but include a residue of drugs
with indisputable biologic activity. Opium, hashish, cocaine,
and caffeine all derive from these ancient sources. It was
natural therefore that medicinal chemistry at its birth concentrated on medicinal agents related to natural products. Despite
some early successes, this area remained essentially quiescent
until the development of more sophisticated synthetic methods
made the preparation of more complex molecules feasible.

A second broad source for biologically active molecules
came out of the biochemical investigation on hormonal substances.
This work led to the isolation of such substances as thyroxin,
epinephrine, the steroids, and most recently the prostaglandins.
Synthetic work that took the structure of epinephrine as its
starting point resulted in the development of a host of drugs
useful as, respectively, central nervous system stimulants, antiappetite agents, and blood-pressure-lowering compounds. The
original indication for the preparation of steroid drugs seemed
to be for use in replacement therapy for cases of insufficiency.
A combination of clever synthetic work and serendipitous biology led to a drug that bids fair to revolutionize the sexual
ethic in Western society—the Pill. Analogous manipulation of
the cortisone molecule has yielded a series of extremely potent
antiinflammatory agents. More recently this process has been
repeated with the prostaglandins. In this case, the introduction of the first prostaglandin into medical practice—as an
abortifacient agent—came within a mere dozen years of the identification of these elusive and unstable hormonal agents.

The third, and to date, perhaps the most important source
of new structures for drugs, comes from the synthetic efforts of
the medicinal chemist combined with the various biologic screens
operated by his colleague, the pharmacologist. Prompted either
by some pet structural theory or some dimly perceived structural
features present in biologically active compounds described in
the literature, medicinal chemists have frequently prepared
structurally novel compounds. More often than not, the results
of testing these merely added to the world's enormous mass of
negative data. Sometimes, however, these compounds turned out
to have biologic activity, although not necessarily that which
was intended. Such a finding then started the arduous and ex-
citing search for the structural features that optimize activity
at the expense of side effects. (It can be stated baldly that
the drug without side effects has yet to be devised.) If all
went well—which it does for only about one in five thousand compounds synthesized—the compound eventually reached the marketplace as a drug with a generic name.

Since this is a profit-oriented world, research programs
are sometimes started in order to prepare a variation on a competitor's drug. Although at first sight it is an activity to be
viewed askance, this endeavor has often met with unexpectedly
fruitful results. Small variations on the phenothiazine antihistamines—prompted perhaps by motivation such as the above—led
to the first drugs available for treatment of schizophrenia.
Modification of the central heterocyclic ring then gave a series
of drugs effective for the treatment of depression—the tricyclic
antidepressants.
     For the past few years, however, there has been a hiatus in
the pace of discovery of novel medicinal agents. It has been
postulated by some that the field has now slowed down due to the
limitations of the almost strictly empirical approach that has
been applied to date to drug development. It is possible, too,
that the higher standards of efficacy and safety that a new drug
must meet today, combined with the enormously increased costs of
clinical trials, have acted to keep all but the most promising
new drugs off the market.
     No discussion of drug development is complete without men-
tion of the serious efforts being applied towards rational drug
development. The availability of sophisticated new methods has
made it possible to describe the structure of biologically active compounds in such detail as to include the molecular orbital structure. New recognition of the effect of such physical
properties as lipid-water distribution on biologic activity has
come from the work of Hansch. Ready access to computers has
led to many studies on the correlation of these physical properties and biologic activity. Since this field is so young, it
has yet to make its mark on drug development.
     In sum, then, the sources for the inspiration that have led
to the development of drugs have been many and varied. In all
of these, however, the process involved synthetic organic chemistry at some important early stage. This book explores the
chemistry that has actually been used to prepare the organic
compounds that eventually became drugs. Since this is done from
the viewpoint of organic chemistry, the book—except for the
first historical chapter—is organized on a structural rather
than a pharmacologic framework. This book is intended as a
supplement rather than a substitute for the current texts in
medicinal chemistry. The reader is thus urged to consult the
latter when he finds the admittedly cursory discussions of biologic activity to be found below inadequate.

CHAPTER 2

A Case Study in
Molecular Manipulation:
The Local Anesthetics

Man's use of drugs predates by at least several millenia the development of any systematic study of therapeutics or pharmacology. The inquisitive nature of Homo sapiens led him to ingest
will-nilly various plants found in his environment. Those which
produced either pleasant or apparently therapeutic effects were
incorporated into his culture. Those which produced toxic effects were relegated to use in hunting or warfare or in satisfy-
ing his other notable characteristic—belligerence. Thus, various
parts of the world have seen the use of such plant products as
opium, hashish, cocaine, and alcohol as part of the ritual of
life. To this day, new alkaloids with effects on the central
nervous system are being discovered as a result of their use by
Amazonian tribes.

The growth of the exact sciences in the nineteenth century
led to chemical and pharmacologic investigation of these various
plant products. This work usually involved isolation and attempts at structural determination of the active principles from
the extracts. Since many of these organic compounds have fairly
complex structures and the extant methods of structure determination were limited by imperfections in organic theory as well
as by the lack of spectroscopic methods, these were often not
correctly identified for many years. The partial structures
that were obtained did, however, suggest that the active compounds were not easily attainable by total synthesis, given the
methods then available. Initial efforts at the preparation of
synthetic versions of the active compounds at that time usually
consisted in the preparation of structural fragments that
embodied various known features of the natural product. This
process of stripping down the molecule had the advantage not

only of defining that part of the molecule necessary for biologic activity but also provided molecules ammenable to commercial preparation by total synthesis. One should hasten to add that this approach was only successful in certain instances.

The line of research that led from the isolation of cocaine to the development of the local anesthetics is perhaps a classic example of the molecular dissection approach to medicinal chemistry. It had been known from the time of the Conquistadores that the Incas of the Andean Altoplano chewed the leaves of the coca bush (Erythroxylon coca) in order to combat fatigue and deaden the pangs of hunger. Wohler discovered the local deadening of pain produced by dilute solution of the alkaloid, cocaine, obtained from extracts of the leaves;[1] the first rational recorded use of the extracts in medicine was as a local anesthetic for opthalmic surgery. It was early determined that hydrolysis of cocaine affords benzoic acid, methanol, and a nonsaponifiable fragment dubbed ecgonine (2).[2]

Oxidation of ecgonine (2) by means of chromium trioxide was found to afford a keto acid (3). This was formulated as shown based on the fact that the compound undergoes ready thermal decarboxylation to tropinone (4).[3-5] The latter had been obtained earlier from degradative studies in connection with the structural determination of atropine (5) and its structure established independently.[6-8] Confirmation for the structure came from the finding that carbonation of the enolate of tropinone does in fact lead back to ecgonine.[9] Reduction, esterification with methanol followed by benzoylation then affords cocaine.

Although the gross structure was known by the turn of the century, the stereochemistry was not fully elucidated until some fifty years later. In essence, the relative steric position of the acid and hydroxyl functions was established by acyl migration from oxygen to nitrogen and back. Thus, Curtius reaction on benzoylecgonine *(6)* affords amine, *7*, in which the new amine group can be assumed to have the same stereochemistry as the precursor, carboxyl. That this is *cis* to the acyl group can be inferred from the finding that treatment of *7* with base gives the amide *(8)*; this reverts to the ester with acid.[10]

6   7

                                                    8

Degradation of cocaine by means of cyanogen bromide leads to the well-known demethylation-*N*-cyanation reaction. Hydrolysis of the *N*-cyano function affords the carbamate *(10)*. Treatment of that carbamate with sodium methoxide leads to formation of the cyclic acyl urea *(11)*, demonstrating the *cis* relation of the carboxyl group and the nitrogen bridge in cocaine.[11,12] Finally, correlation of ecgoninic acid *(12)*, an oxidation product of ecgonine with L-glutamic acid, showed the absolute configuration of cocaine to be 2(R)-carbomethoxy-3(S)-benzoyloxy-1(R)tropane.

The bulk of the work on analogs of cocaine was aimed at compounds that would maximize the local anesthetic component of the biologic activity of that compound. Although pain is essential to alert sentient organisms to injury, there are situations in which this reaction can be inconvenient and deleterious. One need bring to mind only the many forms of minor surgery in which the procedure is made more convenient for both the physician and patient by the fact that the area under attack has been treated so as to cease transmission of the pain signal. Although the

9

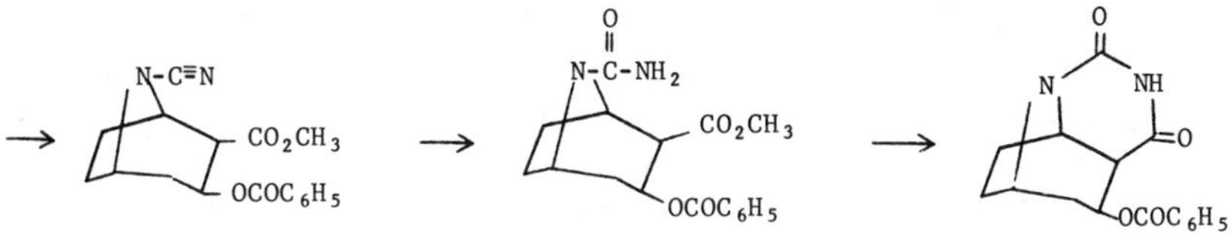

10

11

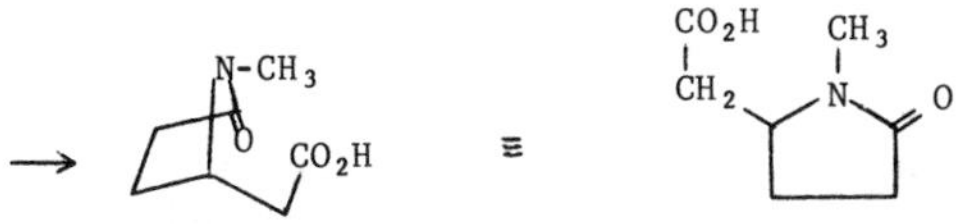

12

molecular mode of action of this class of drugs is as yet un-
clear, it is known that these agents in some way specifically
bind to a component in nerve axons so as to interrupt nervous
conduction. The fact that these drugs are usually administered
subcutaneously or topically means that their locus of action
tends to be restricted to the vicinity of the site of administration. Several local anesthetics show some vasoconstrictor action; this serves to inhibit diffusion from the injection site
and further localize the affected area. Local anesthetics are
sometimes injected directly into the lower section of the spine
so as to block sensation in areas below the injection. This
technique, known as spinal anesthesia or "saddle block," was at
one time used extensively in childbirth.

  Reduction of tropanone affords the alcohol epitropanol (13),
epimeric with the alcohol obtained on hydrolysis of atropine.
The finding that the benzoyl ester, *tropacocaine (14)*, possessed
local anesthetic activity showed that the carbomethoxy group was
not required for activity.[14]

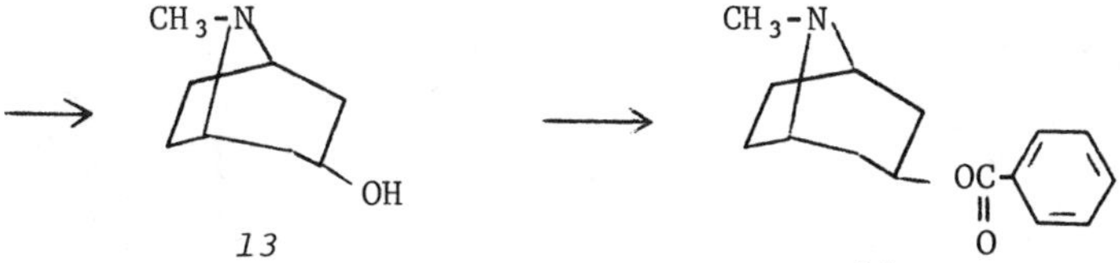

13

14

The bicyclic tropane ring of cocaine of course presented
serious synthetic difficulties. In one attempt to find an appropriate substitute for this structural unit, a piperidine was
prepared that contained methyl groups at the point of attachment
of the deleted ring. Condensation of acetone with ammonia affords the piperidone, 17. Isophorone (15) may well be an intermediate in this process; conjugate addition of ammonia would
then give the aminoketone, 16. Further aldol reaction followed
by ammonolysis would afford the observed product. Hydrogenation
of the piperidone (18) followed then by reaction with benzoyl
chloride gives the ester, 19. Ethanolysis of the nitrile (20)
affords alpha-eucaine (21),[15] an effective, albeit somewhat
toxic, local anesthetic.
        Condensation of the intermediate, 16, with acetaldehyde
rather than acetone gives the piperidone containing one less
methyl group (22). Reduction of the ketone with sodium amalgam

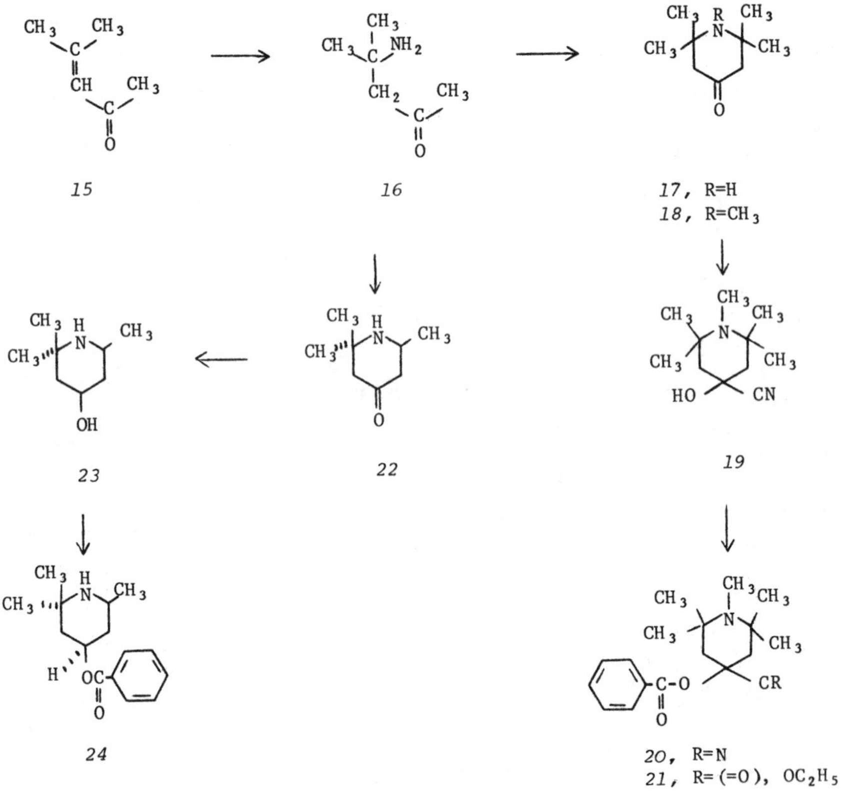

15

16

17, R=H
18, R=CH$_3$

23

22

19

24

20, R=N
21, R= (=O), OC$_2$H$_5$

affords largely the equatorial alcohol *(23)*. Esterification by means of benzoyl chloride gives *beta-eucaine (24)*,[16,17] an effective local anesthetic.

The observation that very significant parts of the cocaine molecule could be deleted from synthetic analogs without loss of biologic activity led to the search for the minimal structural feature consistent with activity. This exercise, sometimes referred to as molecular dissection, not only led to great simplification of the structure of local anesthetics but resulted finally in the preparation of active molecules that bear only the remotest structural relation to the prototype, *cocaine*.

1. ESTERS OF AMINOBENZOIC ACIDS AND ALKANOLAMINES

a. Derivatives of Ethanolamine

A chance observation made some time prior to the full structural elucidation of *cocaine* in fact led to one of the more important classes of local anesthetics. It was found that the simple ethyl ester of p-aminobenzoic acid, *benzocaine (25)*,[18] showed activity as a local anesthetic. It is of interest to note that this drug, first introduced in 1903, is still in use today. Once the structure of cocaine was established, the presence of an alkanolamine moiety in cocaine prompted medicinal chemists to prepare esters of aminobenzoic acids with acyclic alkanolamines. Formula *26* represents the putative relationship of the target substances with cocaine.

Preparation of the prototype in this series, *procaine (31)*,[19] starts with the oxidation of p-nitrotoluene *(27)* to the corresponding benzoic acid *(28)*. This is then converted to the acid chloride *(29)*; reaction of the halide with diethylaminoethanol affords the so-called basic ester *(30)*. Reduction by any of a series of standard methods (e.g., iron and mineral acid, catalytic reduction) affords *procaine (31)*.[19]

The ready acceptance of *procaine* in the clinic as a local

$$O_2N-\langle\bigcirc\rangle-CH_3 \longrightarrow O_2N-\langle\bigcirc\rangle-COR \longrightarrow O_2N-\langle\bigcirc\rangle-CO_2CH_2CH_2N\begin{smallmatrix}C_2H_5\\C_2H_5\end{smallmatrix}$$

27   28, R=OH   30
                                 29, R=Cl

$$H_2N-\langle\bigcirc\rangle-CO_2CH_2CH_2N\begin{smallmatrix}C_2H_5\\C_2H_5\end{smallmatrix}$$

31

anesthetic led to the preparation of an enormous number of analogs based on this relatively simple structure. The chemistry
involved in this work tends to be relatively simple by today's
standards and is passed over quickly. It was soon found that
the esterification reaction could be performed directly on an
appropriate derivative of the aminobenzoic acid itself. Thus,
ester interchange of an ester of *p*-aminobenzoic acid *(32)* with
diethylaminoethanol leads to the desired basic ester. (The reaction is driven to completion by removal of the liberated lower
alcohol by distillation.) In an alternate approach, the sodium
salt of the acid *(32a)* is alkylated to the ester by means of 2-
chlorotriethylamine. Compounds containing alkoxy groups tend to
be prepared from the hydroxylated nitrobenzoic acids. Thus, for
example, alkylation of *33* with propyl bromide in the presence of
sodium carbonate affords the ester-ether, *34*. Hydrolysis of the
ester followed by esterification of the acid chloride by means
of diethylaminoethanol gives the intermediate, *35*. Reduction of
the nitro group gives *propoxycaine (36)*.[20] Reductive alkylation
of the *N,N*-dimethyl analog of procaine *(37)* with butyraldehyde
affords the corresponding *N*-butyl analog, *tetracaine (38)*.[21]

Table 1 lists some additional simple analogs of procaine
attainable by variations of the methods outlined above. *Paraethoxycaine* is of particular note in that it demonstrates that

$$H_2N-\langle\bigcirc\rangle-CO_2R \longrightarrow \underset{\sim}{31} \longleftarrow H_2N-\langle\bigcirc\rangle-CO_2Na + ClCH_2CH_2N\begin{smallmatrix}C_2H_5\\C_2H_5\end{smallmatrix}$$

32   32a

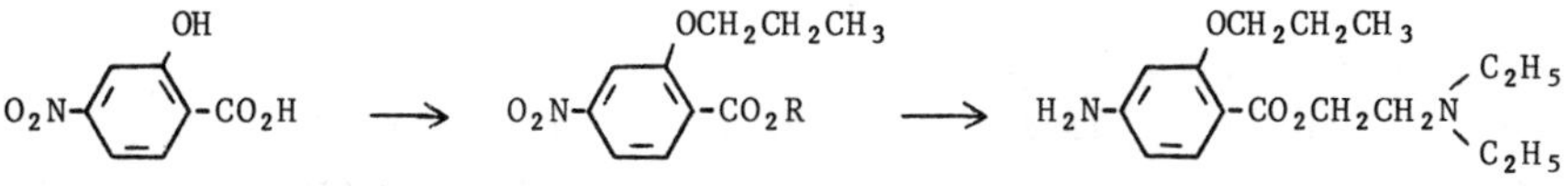

$$33 \quad \rightarrow \quad 34, \ R=CH_2CH_2CH_3 \quad \rightarrow \quad 36$$
$$35, \ R=CH_2CH_2N\text{-}C_2H_5 / C_2H_5$$

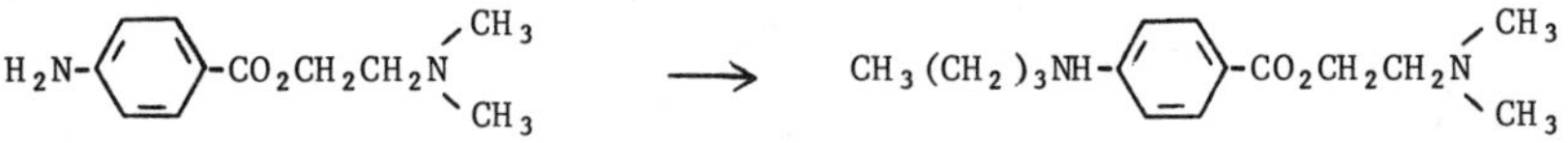

$$37 \quad \rightarrow \quad 38$$

not only do these compounds exhibit low order of positional specificity for activity, but functional groups may even be interchanged at will (e.g., ethoxy for amino).

Table 1

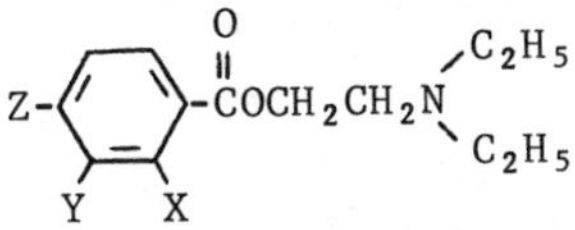

X	Y	Z	Generic Name	Reference
OH	H	NH_2	*Hydroxyprocaine*	22
Cl	H	NH_2	*Chloroprocaine*	23
H	$O(CH_2)_3CH_3$	NH_2	*Ambucaine*	24
$O(CH_2)_3CH_3$	NH_2	H	*Metabutoxycaine*	25
H	NH_2	$O(CH_2)_2CH_3$	*Proparacaine*	26
H	H	OC_2H_5	*Paraethoxycaine*	27

b. Modification of the Basic Ester Side Chain

The structure of the side chain carrying the aliphatic basic nitrogen atom shows the same lack of structural demand for biologic activity as does the exact nature of the substitution pattern in the aromatic ring.
    Thus, acylation of 3(N,N-dibutylamino)propanol (39) with p-
nitrobenzoyl chloride affords the intermediate, 40. Reduction
of the nitro group gives butacaine (41),[28] an agent equipotent
as cocaine as a topical anesthetic.

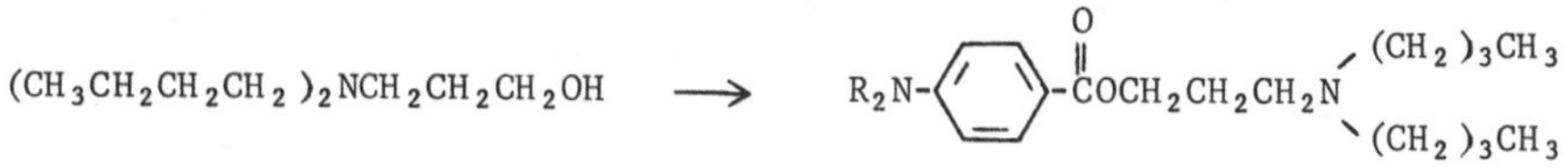

$$(CH_3CH_2CH_2CH_2)_2NCH_2CH_2CH_2OH \longrightarrow R_2N-\langle\rangle-\overset{\overset{O}{\|}}{C}OCH_2CH_2CH_2N\overset{\diagup(CH_2)_3CH_3}{\diagdown(CH_2)_3CH_3}$$

39

40, R=O
41, R=H

    Incorporation of extensive branching in the side chain sim-
ilarly does not decrease pharmacologic activity. Reductive alkylation of aminoalcohol, 42, with isobutyraldehyde affords the
amine, 43. Acylation of the amine with benzoyl chloride probably goes initially to the amide (44). The acid catalysis used
in the reaction leads to an N to O acyl migration to afford isobucaine (45).[29]

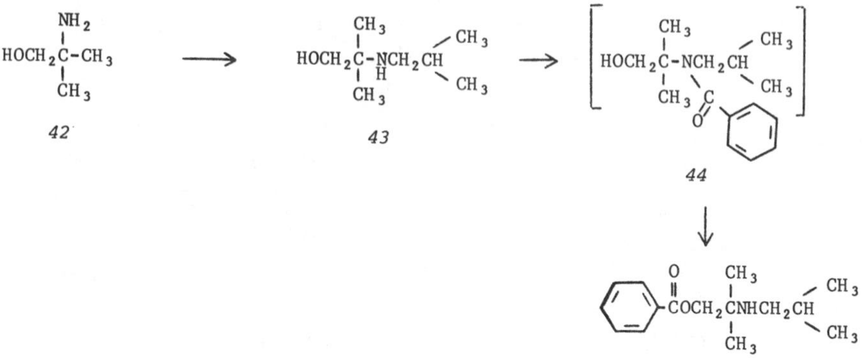

42   43   44

45

    In an analogous sequence, reductive alkylation of aminoal-
cohol, 46, with cyclohexanone affords the secondary amine (47).
Acylation with benzoyl chloride affords hexylcaine (48)[30] in a
reaction that may again involve acyl migration.
    Inclusion of the basic side chain nitrogen atom in a hetero-

cyclic ring is apparently consistent with activity. Condensation of α-picoline with formaldehyde affords the alcohol, *49*. Treatment of this with sodium in alcohol leads to reduction of the aromatic ring and formation of the corresponding piperidine *(50)*. Acylation with the acid chloride from anthranilic acid followed by exposure to acid affords *piridocaine (51)*.[31]

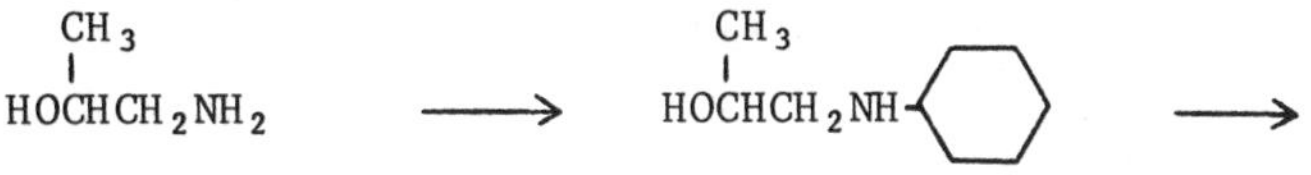

46 *47*

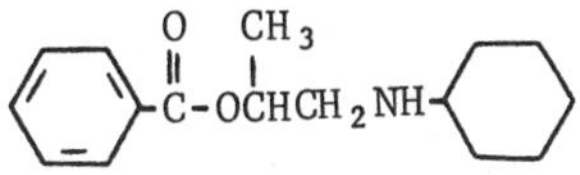

48

Benzoylation of 3-chloropropan-1-ol affords the haloester, *52*. Condensation of this intermediate with the reduction product of α-picoline *(53)* affords the local anesthetic, *piperocaine (54)*.[32]

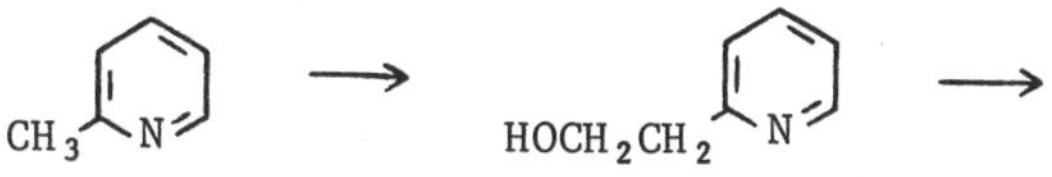

49

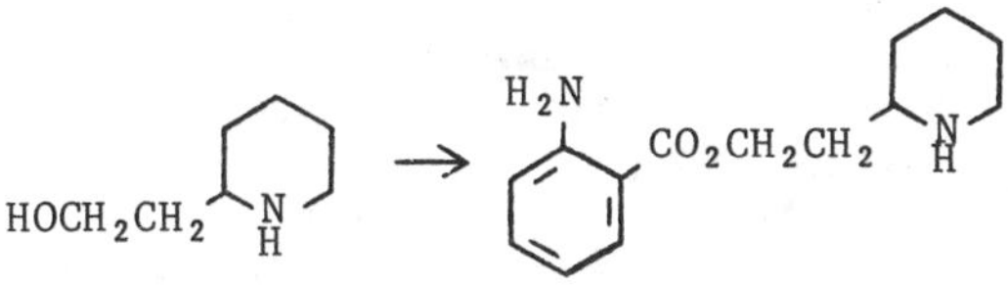

50 *51*

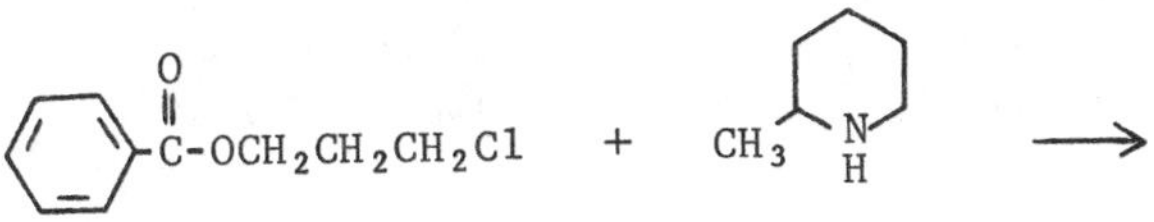

52 *53*

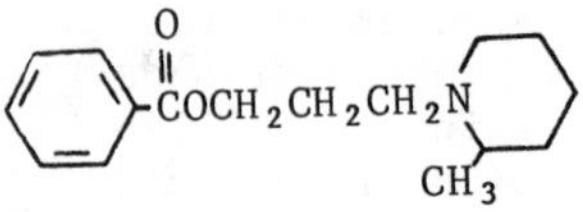

$$\text{54}$$

In a variation of the scheme above, alkylation of p-hydroxy-benzoic acid with cyclohexyl iodide affords the cyclohexyl ether, *55*. (Under alkaline reaction conditions, the ester formed concurrently does not survive the reaction.) Acylation of the acid chloride obtained from *55* with the preformed side chain *(56)* gives *cyclomethycaine (57)*.[33]

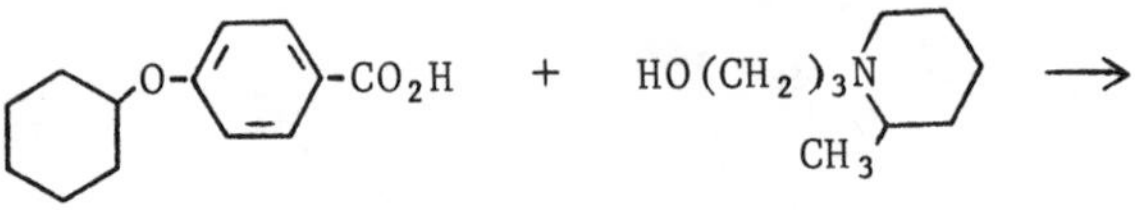

$$\text{55} \qquad \text{56}$$

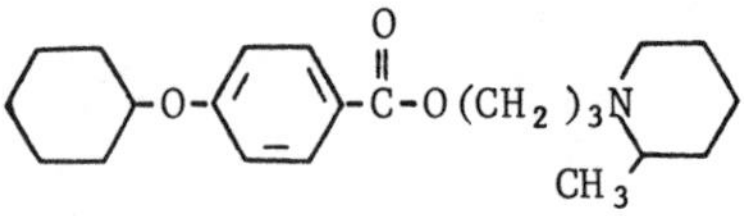

$$\text{57}$$

2. AMIDES AND ANILIDES

The common thread in the local anesthetics discussed thus far has been the presence of an aromatic acid connected to an aliphatic side chain by an ester linkage. It is well known in medicinal chemistry that such ester functions are readily cleaved by a large group of enzymes (esterases) ubiquitously present in the body. In the hope of increasing the half-life of the local anesthetics, an amide bond was used as replacement for the ester. There was obtained an agent, *procainamide (58)*, that indeed still showed local anesthetic activity. In addition, however, this drug proved to have a direct depressant effect on the cardiac ventricular muscle. As such, the drug found use in the clinic as an agent for the treatment of cardiac arrhythmias. It should be noted that it has since been largely supplanted by the anilides discussed below.

Research aimed at the preparation of antipyretic agents re-

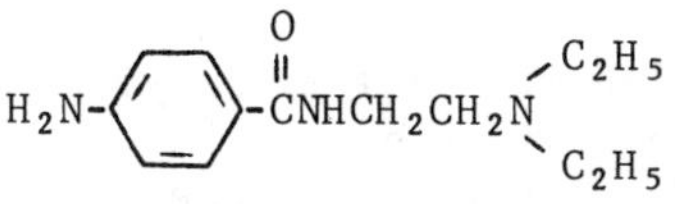

$$H_2N-\langle\!\!\!\bigcirc\!\!\!\rangle-\overset{O}{\overset{\|}{C}}NHCH_2CH_2N\overset{C_2H_5}{\underset{C_2H_5}{\big\langle}}$$

58

lated to quinine adventitiously led to the preparation of an ex-
traordinarily potent albeit rather toxic local anesthetic. Acylation of isatin (59) affords 60. Treatment of the product (60)
with sodium hydroxide affords the substituted quinolone, 62. The
transformation may be rationalized by assuming the first step to
involve cleavage of the lactam bond to afford an intermediate
such as 61. Aldol condensation of the ketone carbonyl with the
amide methyl group leads to the observed product (62). Such rearrangements are known as Pfitzinger reactions. Treatment with
phosphorus pentachloride serves both to form the acid chloride
and to introduce the nuclear halogen (63) (via the enol form of
the quinolone). Condensation of the acid chloride with N,N-di-
ethyl ethylenediamine gives the corresponding amide (64). Displacement of the ring halogen with the sodium salt from n-butanol
completes the synthesis of *dibucaine* (65).[34]

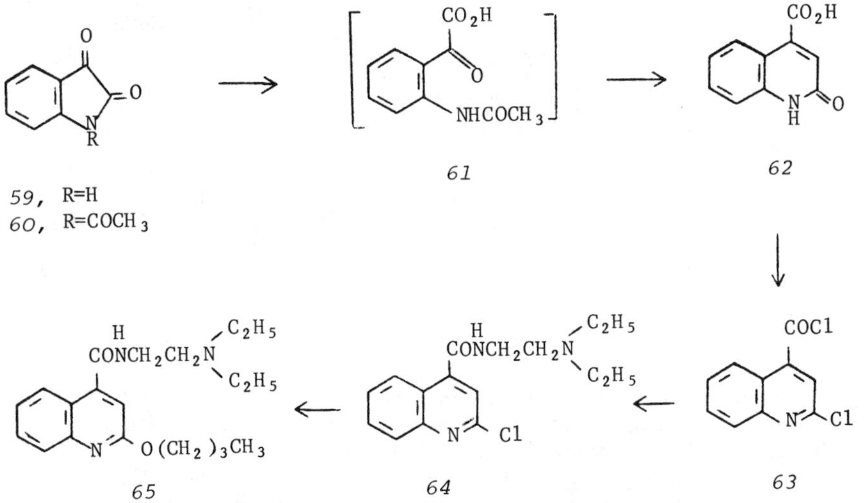

59, R=H
60, R=COCH₃

61

62

65

64

63

Continued synthetic work in the general area of anesthetic
amides revealed the interesting fact that the amide function can
be reversed. That is, compounds were at least equally effective
in which the amide nitrogen was attached to the aromatic ring
and the carbonyl group was part of the side chain.

Preparation of the first of these anilides begins with the acylation of 2,6-xylidine with chloroacetyl chloride to give chloroamide *(64)*. Displacement of the halogen by means of diethylamine affords *lidocaine (65)*.[35] Use of pyrrolidine as the nucleophile in the last step affords *pyrrocaine (66)*.[36] The amide functionality in *lidocaine* as well as the steric hindrance caused by the presence of two ortho groups render this agent unusually resistant to degradation by enzymatic hydrolysis. This, in conjunction with its rapid onset of action, has led to widespread use of this drug for the establishment of nerve blocks prior to surgery. It should be added that *lidocaine* is finding increasing use as an antiarrhythmic agent, probably as a consequence of its depressant effect on the ventricular cardiac muscle.

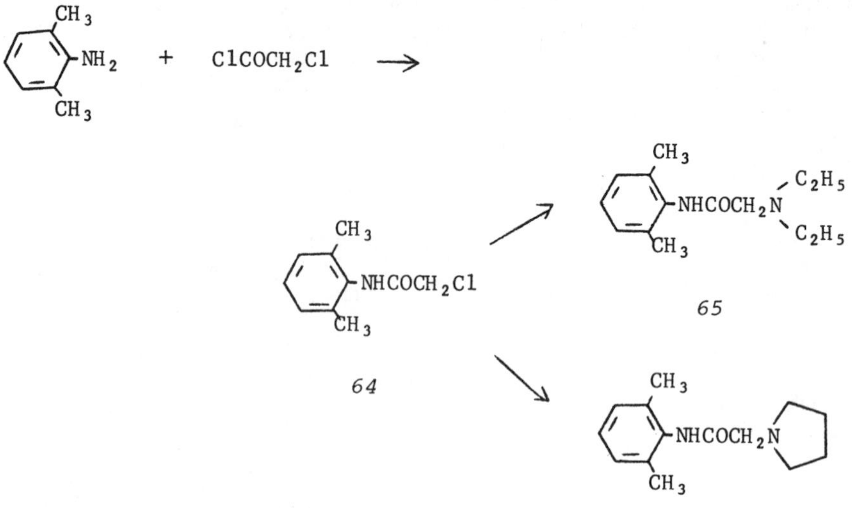

In this small subseries, too, the basic nitrogen atom can be included in a ring. Condensation of pyridine-2-carboxylic acid with ethyl chloroformate in the presence of base affords the mixed anhydride *(67)*, an activated form of the acid equivalent in some ways to an acid chloride. Reaction of this anhydride with 2,6-xylidine gives the corresponding amide. Alkylation of the pyridine nitrogen with methyl iodide affords the pyridinium salt *(69)*. Catalytic hydrogenation of this salt leads to reduction of the heterocyclic ring (which has lost some aromatic character by the presence of the charged nitrogen). There is thus obtained *mepivacaine (71).*[37] In much the same vein, alkylation of the intermediate, *68*, with butyl iodide (to *70*) followed by catalytic reduction leads to *bupivacaine (72).*[38]

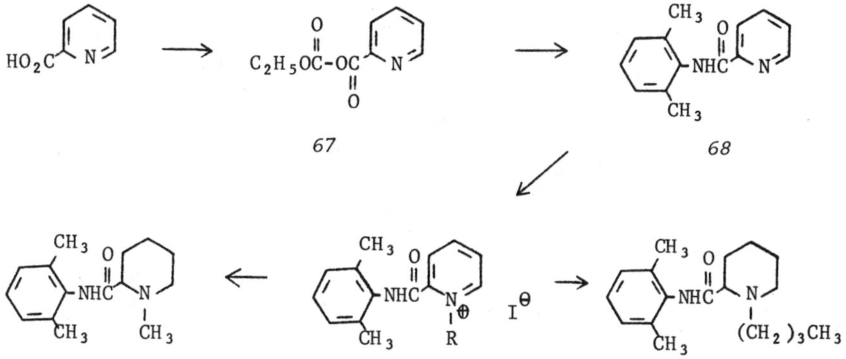

67

68

71

69, R=CH$_3$
70, R=(CH$_2$)$_3$CH$_3$

72

Acylation of *ortho*-toluidine with 2-bromopropionyl bromide affords the haloamide *(73)*. Displacement of the halogen by means of butylamine affords *prilocaine (74).*[39]

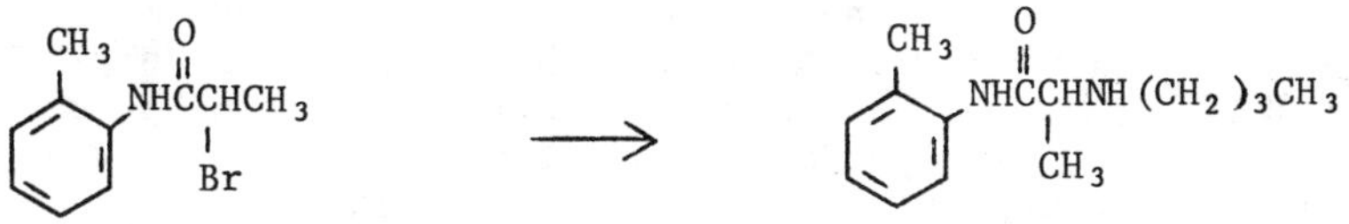

73

74

Replacement of one of the aromatic methyl groups in *lidocaine* by a carboxylic ester proves consistent with pharmacologic activity. The product, *tolycaine (76),*[40] is obtained from the anthranilic ester, *75,* by the same two-step scheme as the prototype drug.

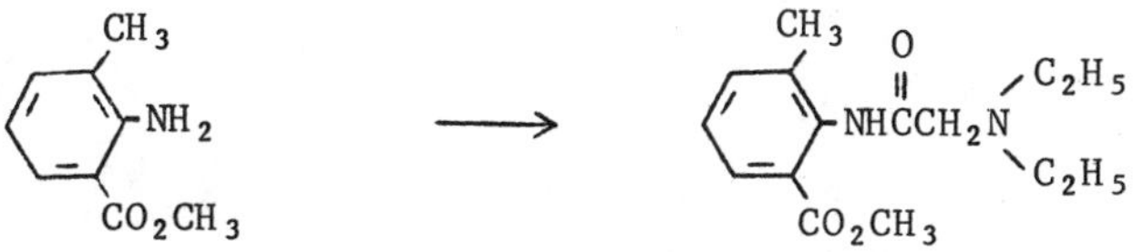

75

76

3. MISCELLANEOUS STRUCTURES

As shown above, the attachment of the aromatic ring to the carbon
chain bearing the basic nitrogen may be accomplished through an
ester or an amide configured in either direction. A simple ether
linkage fulfills this function in yet another compound that exhibits local anesthetic activity. Thus, alkylation of the mono
potassium salt of hydroquinone with butyl bromide affords the
ether *(77)*; alkylation of this with *N*-(3-chloropropyl)morpholine
affords *pramoxine (78)*.[41]

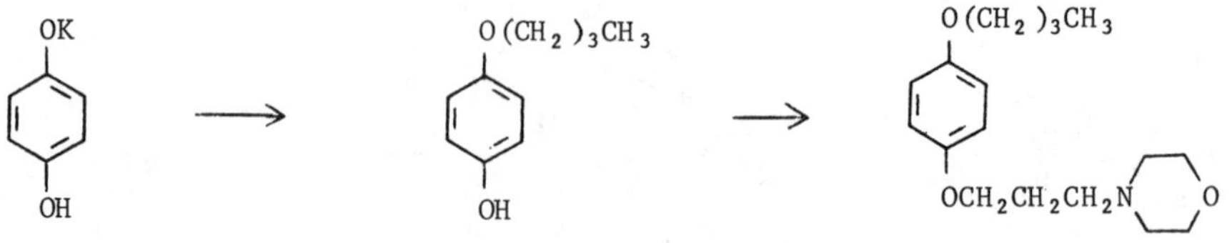

OK   O(CH$_2$)$_3$CH$_3$ O(CH$_2$)$_3$CH$_3$

$\longrightarrow$ $\longrightarrow$

OH   OH   OCH$_2$CH$_2$CH$_2$N O

                             77   *78*

   One of the more complex local anthetics in fact comprises a
basic ether of a bicyclic heterocyclic molecule. Condensation of
1-nitropentane with acid aldehyde, *79*, affords the phthalide, *81*,
no doubt via the hydroxy acid, *80*. Reduction of the nitro group
via catalytic hydrogenation leads to the amine *(82)*.[42] Treatment of that amine with sodium hydroxide leads to ring opening of
the lactone ring to the intermediary amino acid, *83*. This cyclizes spontaneously to the lactam so that the product isolated
from the reaction mixture is in fact the isoquinoline derivative
(84). Dehydration by means of strong acid affords the isocar-
brostyril *(85)*.[43] Phosphorus oxychloride converts the oxygen
function to the corresponding chloride *(85)* via the enol form.
Displacement of halogen with the sodium salt from 2-dimethyl-
aminoethanol affords *dimethisoquin (87)*.[44]
   Carbamates in some ways incorporate features of both esters
and amides in the same function. Reaction of the piperidine
bearing the diol side chain *(88)* with phenyl isocyanate affords
the *bis*-carbamate. This product, *diperodon (89)*,[44,45] has found
some use as a local anesthetic.

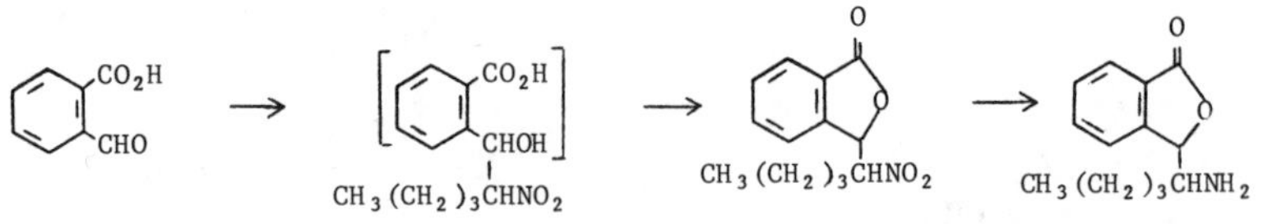

CO$_2$H $\rightarrow$ CO$_2$H $\rightarrow$ $\rightarrow$

CHO   CHOH

                  CH$_3$(CH$_2$)$_3$CHNO$_2$ CH$_3$(CH$_2$)$_3$CHNO$_2$ CH$_3$(CH$_2$)$_3$CHNH$_2$

79

                  80   *81*   *82*

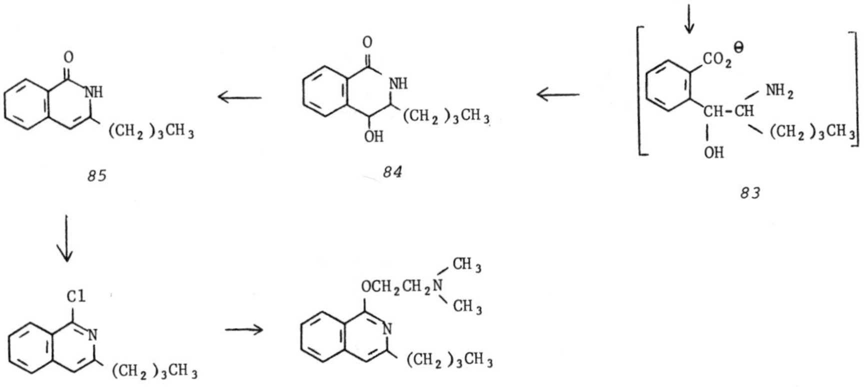

The low structural specificity in the local anesthetic series is perhaps best illustrated by *phenacaine (91)*, a local anesthetic that lacks not only the traditional ester or amide function but the basic aliphatic nitrogen as well. First prepared at
the turn of the century, a more recent synthesis starts by condensation of *p*-ethoxyaniline with ethyl orthoacetate to afford
the imino ether *(90)*. Reaction of that intermediate with a second mole of the aniline results in a net displacement of ethanol,
probably by an addition-elimination scheme. There is thus obtained the amidine, *91, phenacaine.*[46]

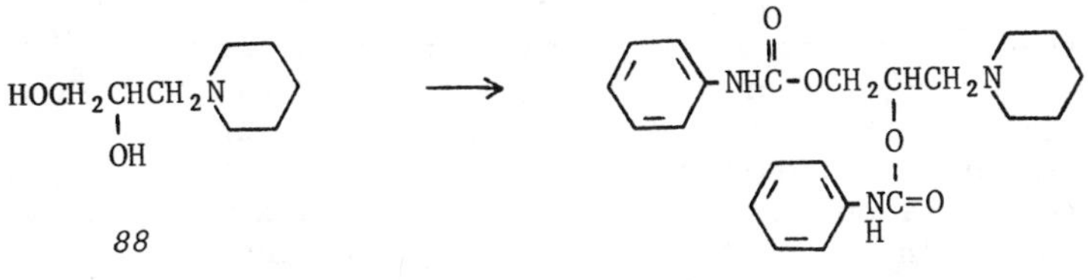

The story outlined above illustrates well the course frequently taken in drug development. Although the lead for the
local anesthetics came from a naturally occurring compound, the
sequence is much the same when the initial active compound is uncovered by some random screening process. Initial synthetic
work usually tends to concentrate on some analytic process aimed
at defining the portions of the lead molecule necessary for biologic activity. Further effort often ensues in order to minimize
some side effect, reduce toxicity, or provide better oral activity. The further analogs thus provided often lead to a rede-

$$C_2H_5O-\langle\text{—}\rangle-NH_2 \longrightarrow C_2H_5O-\langle\text{—}\rangle-N=C\begin{smallmatrix}OC_2H_5\\ \\CH_3\end{smallmatrix} \longrightarrow$$

90

$$C_2H_5O-\langle\text{—}\rangle-N=C\begin{smallmatrix}H\\N-\langle\text{—}\rangle-OC_2H_5\\CH_3\end{smallmatrix}$$

91

finition of the minimal active structure. Once the structure of some new drug is made public, commercial considerations enter. Much work is then devoted by companies other than that which did the original work in order to develop some analog that will gain them a proprietary position in that field. Although often excoriated by the consumer minded, this so-called molecular manipulation has in fact often resulted in significant advances in therapy. At least several instances are noted later in this book in which the drug of choice was in fact produced some time after the lead compound had appeared, by workers at a rival concern.

The low structural requirements for local anesthetic activity do not maintain in all classes of drugs. Structural requirements for biologic activity in fact follow a full continuum from those cases in which addition of a single carbon atom serves to abolish activity to the case of the local anesthetics that tolerate quite drastic alterations.

This observation perhaps arises out of the mechanism by which drugs exert their biologic effects. A substantial number of medicinal agents owe their action to more or less direct interaction with specific biopolymers known as receptors. Many of these receptors normally serve as targets for molecules produced for natural functioning of the organism. Drugs thus act either by substituting for the natural hormone or by competing with it for receptor sites (agonist or antagonist activity). Thus, the activities of such drugs that include the steroids and prostaglandins tend to exhibit great sensitivity to structural changes.

At the other end of the continuum there exist drugs that act by some as yet undefined general mechanisms. Much work is currently devoted to study of the fine physiochemical structure of medicinal agents in this class. Considerable progress has been achieved towards a better understanding of the effects of biologic activity of such factors as water-lipid partition co-efficients, molecular orbital relationships, and tertiary structure. It is thus not inconceivable that a set of compounds that bears little similarity to the eye of the organic chemist are in fact quite similar when redefined in the appropriate physical chemical terms.

REFERENCES

1. F. Wohler, Ann., 121, 372 (1862).
2. W. Lossen, Ann., 133, 351 (1865).
3. R. Willstatter and W. Muller, Chem. Ber., 31, 1202 (1898).
4. C. Liebermann, Chem. Ber., 23, 2518 (1890).
5. R. Willstatter and A. Bode, Chem. Ber., 34, 519 (1901).
6. R. Willstatter, Chem. Ber., 31, 1534 (1898).
7. G. Merling, Chem. Ber., 24, 3108 (1891).
8. R. Willstatter, Chem. Ber., 29, 393 (1896).
9. R. Willstatter and A. Bode, Chem. Ber., 34, 1457 (1901).
10. G. Fodor, Nature, 170, 278 (1952).
11. K. Hess, A. Eichel, and C. Uibrig, Chem. Ber., 50, 351 (1917).
12. G. Fodor, O. Kovacs, and I. Weisz, Nature, 174, 141 (1954).
13. E. Hardegger and H. Oh, Helv. Chim. Acta, 38, 312 (1955).
14. H. A. D. Jowett and F. L. Pyman, J. Chem. Soc., 95, 1020 (1909).
15. C. Harries, Ann., 328, 322 (1903).
16. G. Meiling, Chem. Ber., 6, 173 (1896).
17. H. King, J. Chem. Soc., 125, 41 (1924).
18. H. Salkowski, Chem. Ber., 28, 1917 (1895).
19. A. Einhorn and E. Uhlfelder, Ann., 371, 125 (1909).
20. R. O. Clinton and S. Claskowski, U. S. Patent 2,689,248 (1954).
21. O. Eisler, U. S. Patent 1,889,645 (1932).
22. W. Grimme and H. Schmitz, Chem. Ber., 84, 734 (1917).
23. H. C. Marks and M. I. Rubin, U. S. Patent 2,460,139 (1949).
24. J. Buchi, E. Stunzi, M. Flurg, R. Hirt, P. Labhart, and L. Ragaz, Helv. Chim. Acta, 34, 1002 (1951).
25. Anon., British Patent 728,527 (1955).
26. R. D. Clinton, U. J. Salvador, S. C. Laskowski, and M. W. Ison, J. Amer. Chem. Soc., 74, 592 (1952).
27. W. G. Christiansen and S. E. Harris, U. S. Patent 2,404,691 (1946).
28. W. B. Burnett, R. L. Jenkens, C. H. Peet, E. E. Dreger, and R. Adams, J. Amer. Chem. Soc., 59, 2248 (1937).

29. J. R. Reasenberg and S. D. Goldberg, *J. Amer. Chem. Soc.,* *67*, 933 (1945).

30. A. C. Cope and E. M. Hancock, *J. Amer. Chem. Soc., 66*, 1453 (1944).

31. L. A. Walter and R. J. Fosbinder, *J. Amer. Chem. Soc., 61*, 1713 (1939).

32. S. M. McElvain, U. S. Patent 1,784,903 (1930).

33. S. M. McElvain and T. P. Carney, *J. Amer. Chem. Soc., 68*, 2592 (1946).

34. K. Miescher, *Helv. Chim. Acta, 15*, 163 (1932).

35. N. F. Lofgren and B. J. Lundquist, U. S. Patent 2,441,498 (1948).

36. N. Lofgren, C. Tegner, and B. Takman, *Acta Chem. Scand., 11*, 1724 (1957).

37. H. Rinderknecht, *Helv. Chim. Acta, 42*, 1324 (1959).

38. Anon., British Patent 869,978 (1959).

39. N. Lofgren and C. Tegner, *Acta Chem. Scand., 14*, 486 (1960).

40. R. Hiltmann, F. Mietzsch, and W. Wirth, U. S. Patent 2,291,077 (1960).

41. J. W. Wilson, C. L. Zirkle, E. L. Anderson, J. J. Stehle, and G. E. Ullyott, *J. Org. Chem., 16*, 792 (1951).

42. J. W. Wilson and E. L. Anderson, *J. Org. Chem., 16*, 800 (1951).

43. J. W. Wilson, N. D. Dawson, W. Brooks, and G. E. Ullyott, *J. Amer. Chem. Soc., 71*, 937 (1949).

44. T. H. Rider, *J. Amer. Chem. Soc., 52*, 2115 (1930).

45. M. S. Raasch and W. R. Brode, *J. Amer. Chem. Soc., 64*, 1112 (1942).

46. R. H. DeWolfe, *J. Org. Chem., 27*, 490 (1962).

CHAPTER 3

Monocyclic Alicyclic Compounds

As the preceding section correctly suggests, aromatic rings a-
bound in compounds that show biologic activity. The reasons for
this are many; the role of the pi electrons in some form of
charge transfer complex ranks among the more important. There
are few monocyclic alicyclic compounds known that are used as
medicinal agents.

The relatively few older agents in this class tend to be analogs of aromatic compounds in which that ring has been reduced
and perhaps contracted as well. The fact that these retain activity suggests that the ring plays a largely steric role in the
biologic activity in these agents.

This past decade, however, has seen the elucidation of a potent class of biologically active compounds that have in common
a cyclopentane ring. It is to these, the prostaglandins, that we
address ourselves first.

1.   PROSTAGLANDINS

The previous chapter traced the evolution of a biologically active compound isolated from plant material—cocaine—into an extensive series of drugs by chemical dissection of that molecule. A-
nother frequently applied approach to drug development depends on
the identification and study of the organic compounds that regu-
late most of the functions of mammalian organisms: the hormones,
neurotransmitters, and humoral factors. Although many of these
factors are high-molecular-weight polypeptides, a significant
number of these substances are relatively simple organic compounds of molecular weight below 600, and therefore accessible by
synthesis using common laboratory methods. In the usual course
of events, the existence of a humoral factor is first inferred
from some pharmacologic observation. Isolation of the active

principle is often accomplished with the aid of some bioassay
that involves the original pharmacology such as, for example, the
contraction of an excised muscle strip in an organ bath. Put
simply, in this way, during the isolation process, the fraction
to be kept is distinguished from those to be discarded. Structure determination follows the isolation of the regulating factor
as a pure compound; once a time-consuming process, the advent of
modern instrumental methods has greatly shortened the time of
this last step. The sensitivity of the newer methods has further
drastically reduced the sample size required for structural a-
ssignment. The quantities of hormones available from mammalian
sources tend to be on the diminutive side. A thorough study of
the pharmacology of a newly isolated humoral substance usually
relies on the availability of significant quantities of that compound; the ingenuity of the synthetic organic chemist has usually
stepped in to fill this demand by preparation of the agent in
question by either partial or total synthesis. The further
pharmacology thus made possible often has a feedback effect on
the direction of synthetic programs. Thus, the data from animal
testing may suggest the need for a less readily metabolized analog, an antagonist, a compound that shows a split among the
several activities of the prototype, or perhaps simply one that
is active by mouth. All these reasons have, in fact, served as
goals for such analog programs. The chemical scheme of organization of this volume leads us to postpone the discussion of the
best-known example of this approach, the steroids, to a later
chapter. Instead, the development of the most recent class of
drugs to be developed from mammalian leads is discussed first.

The observation that human seminal fluid contains a humoral
principle that causes both smooth muscle contraction and vaso-
constriction was made independently by Goldblatt and von Euler
in the mid-1930s. The latter was able to show that this principle was a lipid-soluble substance different from any of the
other substances known at the time; the name prostaglandins was
given these substances after their putative source, the prostate
gland. (Subsequent work showed that much higher levels of these
compounds can be obtained from the seminal vesicles; vesiculo-
glandin might thus have been a more appropriate and euphonious
name.) The ready degradation of these substances and the lack
of many of today's techniques for effecting separation of complex mixtures thwarted further development of the lead at that
time.

The observation lay dormant until the 1950s when Bergstrom
and his colleagues in Sweden, in some elegant work, were able to
isolate two of the prostaglandins in pure form (PGE_1, $PGF_1\alpha$).
Spectral methods for structure determination, too, had made giant

strides in the intervening two decades. The structural assignment of the prostaglandins did not lag far behind their isolation.[1]

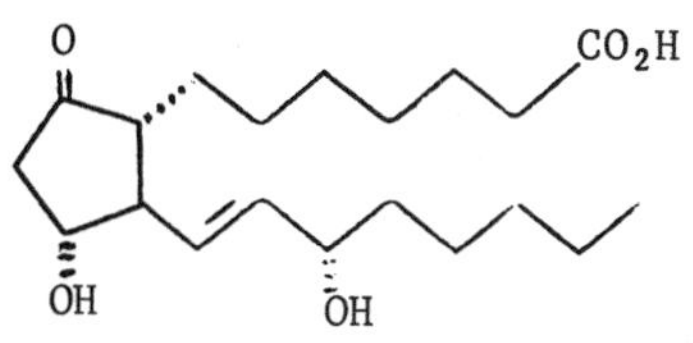

PGE$_1$

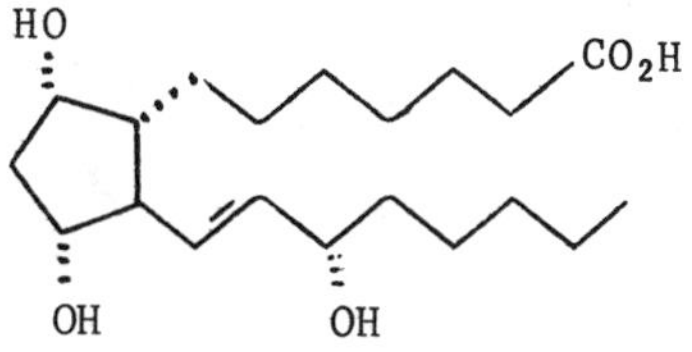

PGF$_1\alpha$

PGE$_1$ and PGF$_1\alpha$ were in fact only the first of an impressive
series of prostaglandins found to occur in various tissues in
the animal kingdom. It was in fact determined quite early that
these compounds are by no means restricted to the accessory sex
glands or for that matter to males; prostaglandins have been
detected in trace quantities in a host of tissues in mammals of
both sexes. The nomenclature of the naturally occurring compounds and certain derivatives followed the usage of the Swedish
workers. The prefix is followed by a letter designating the
state of oxidation of the cyclopentane ring: A denotes the conjugated enone, obtained by direct dehydration; B represents the
enone in which the double bond has migrated to the more highly
substituted position; E denotes the hydroxy ketone; F denotes
the diol. (PG-C, D, G, and H have been described as well but are
beyond the scope of this chapter.) The numeral subscript refers
to the number of double bonds in the side chain: 1 is always a
trans-olefin at 13,14; 2 contains a cis double bond at 5,6 in
addition to that of a PG$_1$, while a PG$_3$ contains the first two as
well as a third olefin (cis) at 17,18. Like many natural products that contain chiral centers, prostaglandins occur in optically active form; the absolute configuration has been determined to be as depicted above. The convention has been adopted
that α denotes a substituent below the plane of the ring and β
above. The letter α in PGF$_1\alpha$ thus refers to the configuration
of the alcohol group at 9. Structures of PGA$_2$ and PGB$_3$ are
shown by way of illustration. More highly substituted prostaglandins obtained by total synthesis are named as derivatives of
the parent hydrocarbon, prostanoic acid (5); the α and β nota-
tion is again used to denote stereochemistry.
    The extreme potency of the prostaglandins in a variety of
pharmacologic test systems was apparent even in the absence of
good sources of supply of these compounds. Although ubiquitous

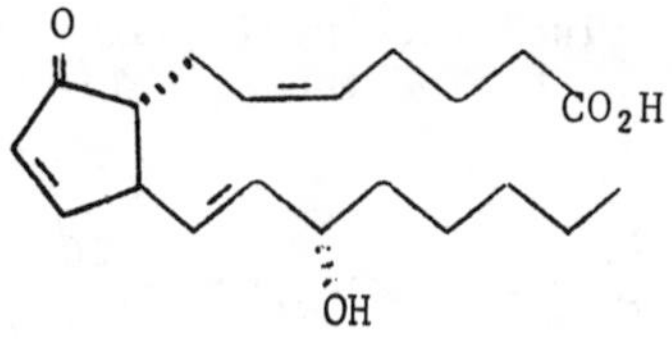

PGA$_2$ 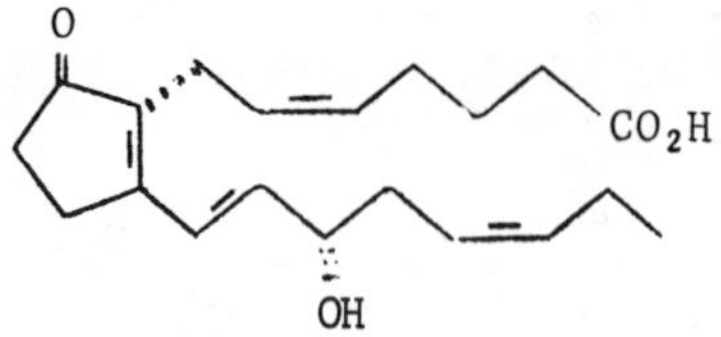   PGB$_3$

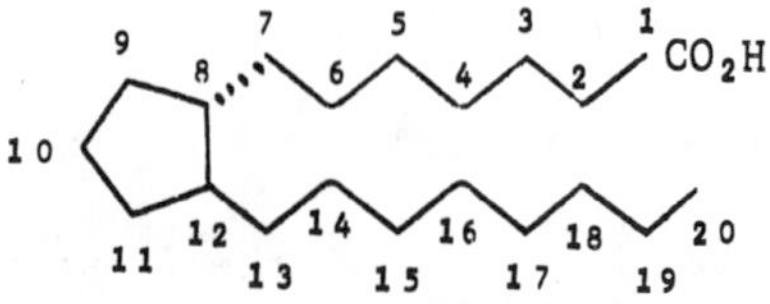

5

in the animal kingdom, they occur in concentrations too low to make their isolation by extraction an attractive proposition. It was soon found that the biologic precursors of prostaglandins are the essential fatty acids. This finding was in fact applied in obtaining the first supplies of prostaglandins from sources other than extraction of tissue.[2] Thus, for example, mixture of PGE$_1$ and PGF$_1\alpha$ is obtained from *in vitro* enzymic conversion of 8,11, 14-eicosatrienoic acid *(6)* by sheep seminal vessicles. There is good evidence that the cyclization occurs by direct attack of molecular oxygen via an internal peroxide such as *6a*.

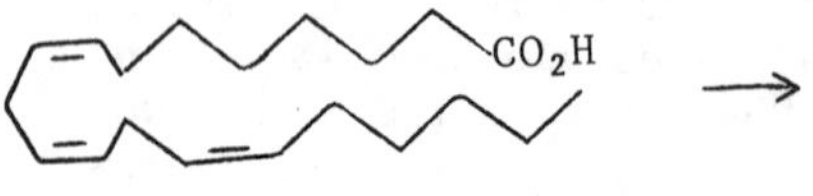

6

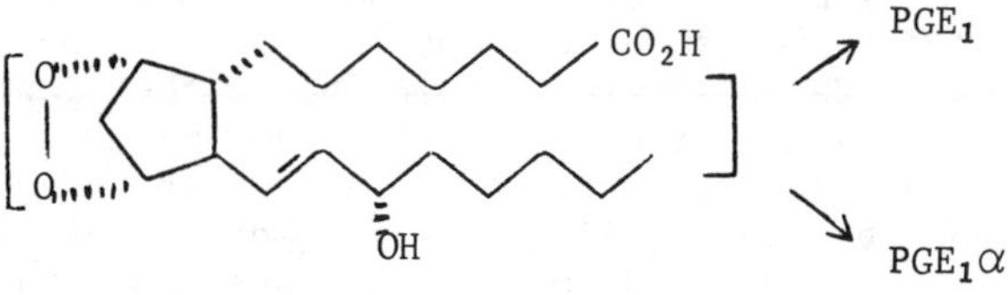

6a

Further pharmacologic investigation made possible by these sources of prostaglandins identified many areas in which the drugs might have useful activity. These, to name only a few, included interruption of pregnancy and treatment of hypertension, ulcers, and possibly asthma. At the same time, two of the key problems of this class of agents were uncovered: the very rapid metabolism of prostaglandins and the associated low oral activity as well as the complex set of biologic activities displayed by each of the naturally occurring compounds. Practical syntheses were therefore needed in order both to prepare materials for further study in sizeable quantity and also to permit the preparation of analogs in order to overcome the shortcomings of the natural products. Work towards the solution of this problem constituted one of the intensive areas of synthetic organic chemistry in the past decade. Many very elegant total synthesis have been developed for both the prostaglandins and their analogs. The limitation of space confines our attention to only three of these with apologies to the chemists whose work has been omitted; the reader is referred to a recent review for a summary of alternate routes.[3]

The intense activity in this field—it has been estimated that as many as a thousand analogs have been prepared to date—promises a number of drugs in the near future. At this writing, two prostaglandins are available for use by the clinician. Both these compounds, *dinoprost* (7, PGF$_2\alpha$) and *dinoprostone* (8, PGE$_2$), are used for the termination of pregnancy in the second trimester.

7   8

The gross molecular structure of the prostaglandins presents two problems at first sight. The first of these is the presence of the five-membered ring; although a veritable host of reactions are at hand for the construction of cyclohexanes, the menu for cyclopentanes is relatively limited. The problem of stereochemistry is superimposed on this. Neglecting for the moment the geometry of the double bonds, the four chiral centers mean the gross structure 8 has 16 isomers; 7 has 32 isomers.

In one of their solutions to the problem, Corey and his coworkers solved the first problem by starting with a preconstructed cyclopentane; the stereochemistry was steered by deriving the oxygen atoms from a rigid bicyclic molecule. Alkylation of

the anion of cyclopentadiene with chloromethyl ether affords diene, *10*. Special precautions must be taken in this reaction to
avoid the thermal and base-catalyzed migration of the double
bonds to the more stable position adjacent the alkyl group.
Diels-Alder addition of the latent ketene, 2-chloroacrylonitrile,
gives the adduct, *11*, as a mixture of isomers. Treatment of this
with base presumably first gives the cyanohydrin; this hydrolyzes
to the intermediate, *12*, under the reaction conditions. In an
alternate approach, *10* is condensed with 2-chloroacryloyl chloride to give *13*. This compound is then treated with sodium azide
to give first the acid azide. This rearranges to the isocyanate,
15, on heating. This last hydrolyzes to *12* under very mild conditions.[4]

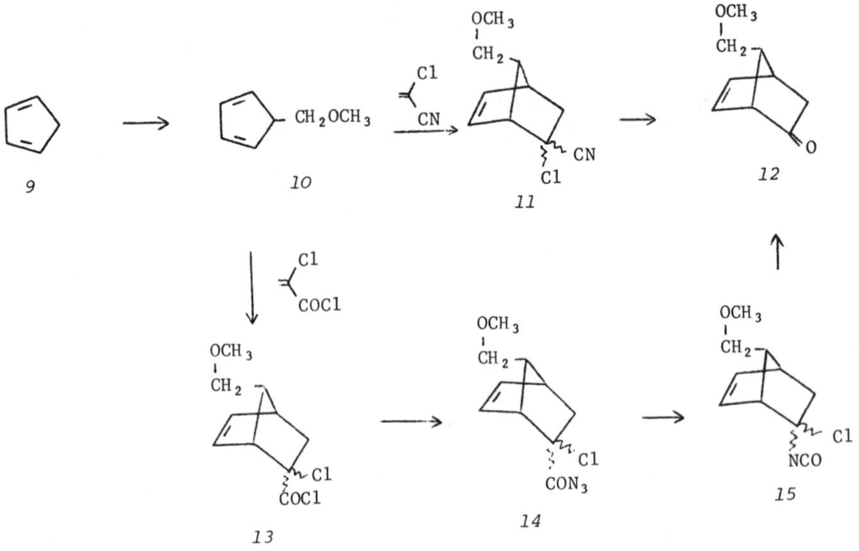

Oxidation of the ketone, *12*, under Bayer-Villiger conditions
(peracid) rearranges the carbonyl group to the corresponding lactone without affecting the isolated double bond *(16)*. Saponification of the lactone gives the hydroxy acid, *17*. When this
last is treated with an iodine:iodide mixture in base, there is
obtained the iodolactone, *18*. It should be noted that this reaction is of necessity both regio- and stereospecific; addition to
the other face of the ring is sterically prohibited, while addition to the other side of the double bond would afford a more
strained ring system. Acetylation followed by reductive removal
of iodine with tributyltin hydride gives the key intermediate,

19. This molecule now carries both oxygens of future prostaglandin as well as the anchors for the side chains, all in the proper relative configuration. In subsequent work, hydroxyacid, *17*, was resolved into its optical isomers; that corresponding to the configuration of natural prostaglandins was carried through the scheme below to give optically active *19* and eventually chiral PGs.[5]

The methyl ether in *19* is then cleaved by treatment with boron tribromide; oxidation of the primary alcohol thus obtained (*20*) with a pyridine:chromium trioxide complex known as Collins reagent affords aldehyde, *21*. This is condensed without prior purification with the ylide obtained from the phosphonate, *22*. There is thus obtained the intermediate, *23*, which now incorporates one of the requisite side chains two hydrogen atoms removed from the natural configuration. In the original work, the side chain ketone at *15* was reduced with zinc borohydride to give mixtures of α and β alcohols.[6] In a later modification, *23* is deacetylated and condensed with biphenylisocyanate. Reduction of the ketourethane is accomplished with the extremely bulk alkylborane, *26*. The bulk of the large substituent at 11 in combination with the steric demands of the reagent ensure the formation of a large preponderance of the desired 15α hydroxyl compound. Removal of the urethane (lithium hydroxide) followed by reclosure of the lactone with ethyl chloroformate gives *25*.[7]

Reaction of *25* with dihydropyran serves to protect the hydroxyls by converting these to the tetrahydropyranyl ethers (THP). Reduction of the lactone thus protected with diisobutyl aluminum hydride at -78° affords the corresponding lactol *(27)*. Condensation of the lactol with the ylide from phosphonium salt, *29*, proceeds, presumably via the small amount of hydroxyaldehyde in equilibrium with the lactol, to yield the intermediate, *28*. The Wittig reaction must be carried out under "salt-free" conditions in order to insure the *cis* geometry of the double bond at 5,6. Removal of the protecting groups affords *dinoprost (7)*. Careful oxidation of *28* prior to removal of the protecting groups leads *dinoprostone (8)*.[6,7]

This synthetic scheme is well suited to the preparation of other prostaglandins or for that matter analogs. The use of a suitably unsaturated ylide for the reaction with *21* leads eventually to PGE$_3$ and PGF$_{3\alpha}$.[8] Since the key intermediate, *21*, contains the bulk of the functionality that distinguishes prostaglandins, analogs can, in principle at least, be readily prepared by using variously modified ylides at the synthetic branching points, *21* and *27*.

The synthetic route to the prostaglandins developed by Kelly and his colleagues at Upjohn similarly depends on a rigid polycyclic framework for establishment of the stereochemistry. The synthesis differs significantly from that above in that a rearrangement step is used to attain the stage comparable to *23*.

Epoxidation of norbornene was found some time prior to this work not to stop at the monoepoxide step. Instead, this intermediate goes on to rearrange to the bicyclic aldehyde, *31*.[9]

Ketalization of the aldehyde with neopentyl glycol *(32)* followed by reaction with dichloroketene gives the 2+2 cycloadduct, *33*. The halogen is then removed by reduction with zinc

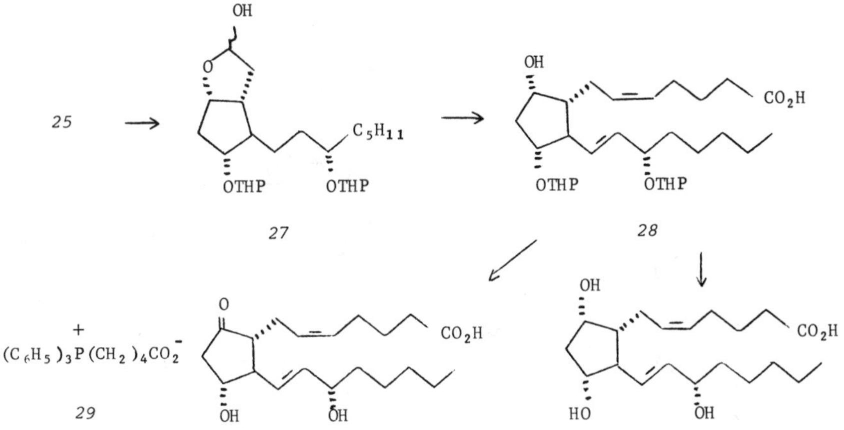

in ammonium chloride. Reaction of the cyclobutanone, which of
course occurs in both the R and S forms, with 1-ephedrine *(35)*
affords the oxazolidone, *36*, as a pair of diastereomers (R1 and
S1). The higher melting of these is then separated by crystallization; chromatography of this isomer over silica affords directly optically active *37* of the same absolute configuration as
the target molecule.[10] Bayer-Villiger oxidation followed by deketalization affords lactone aldehyde, *38*. This is then reacted
in a Wittig condensation with the ylide from hexyltriphenylphos-
phonium bromide to give *39*.

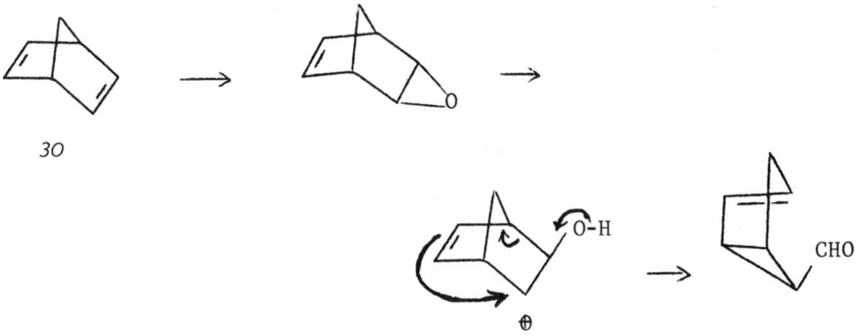

  Opening of the cyclopropyl ring by the cyclopropylcarbinyl-
homoallyl arrangement, a scheme developed earlier for prosta-

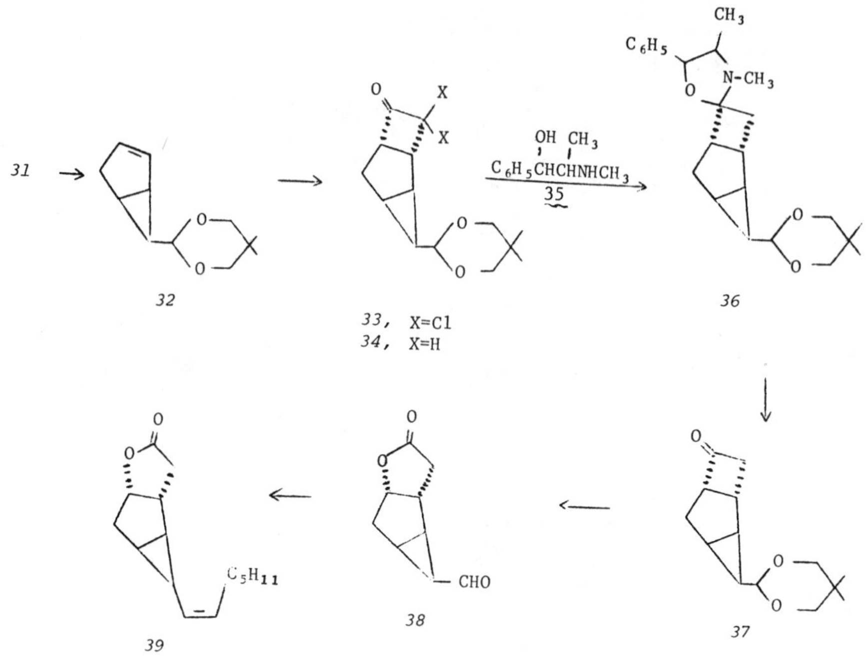

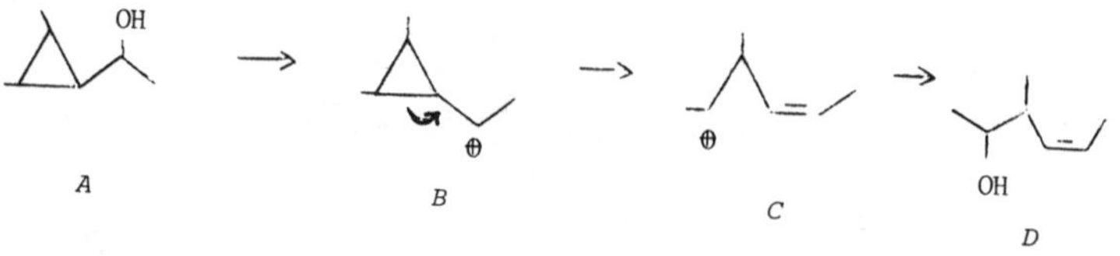

glandin synthesis,[11] is one of the key steps in the present route
as well. A generalized mechanistic scheme for this reaction,
well known in simpler systems, is depicted above (A to D).
Regio- and stereoselectivity are maintained by the demands of orbital overlap.

Epoxidation of the olefin, 36, affords 40. Solvolysis of
the latter in dry formic acid gives a mixture of the desired product, 42 (both α and β hydroxyl at 15), as well as a mixture of
the glycols (41). Solvolytic recycling of the mixture in the
same medium affords eventually about a 45% yield of the product,

43,[12] identical to intermediate 25 in the synthesis discussed
earlier. It should be noted that this synthesis, too, is well
suited for the preparation of analogs, since it presents a synthetic branch point at 38 in addition to that which occurs later.
Intermediate 43, when subjected to the required further steps,
gives dinoprostone, or alternately, dinoprost.

    Drugs of particularly complex structure are often prepared
commercially by partial synthesis from some abundant, structurally related, natural product obtained from plants. The majority
of steroid drugs are in fact prepared in just this way. Prostaglandins are unique in that no prostanoid compounds have yet
been found in plants, a perhaps surprising finding in view of the
wide distribution of essential fatty acids in plant materials.
The unexpected source of starting material for partial synthesis
of these agents was the sea. The isolation of 15(R)-PGA$_2$ and its
acetate (44) from the lowly sea whip,[13] Plexura homomalla, one of
the so-called soft corals, made an approach to prostaglandins
from natural products possible.
    In a process developed by the group at Upjohn, acetate 44 is
first treated with basic hydrogen peroxide. These conditions,
known to be selective for epoxidation of the double bonds of e-
nones, afford the epoxide, 45, as well as some of the β isomer.
Reductive opening of the oxirane with aluminum amalgam leads to
the hydroxyketone (46); regiospecificity is probably attained by
the greater reactivity of the bond α to the ketone towards heter-
olysis. This compound is then converted to its trimethylsilyl
ether; reduction of the ketone by means of sodium borohydride
followed by hydrolysis of the acetate triol gives 47 accompanied
by a small amount of the 9β isomer. Oxidation of 41 with 2,3-
dichlorodicyanoquinone interestingly proceeds selectively at the
allylic alcohol at 15 to give the corresponding side chain ketone, 48. Reduction of the ketone—as the bis-trimethylsilyl e-
ther—affords largely the 15α hydroxy compound (7). In effect
then, this sequence (47→7) serves as a means of inverting the

configuration at 15 from that found in the sea to that required
for *dinoprost (7)*.

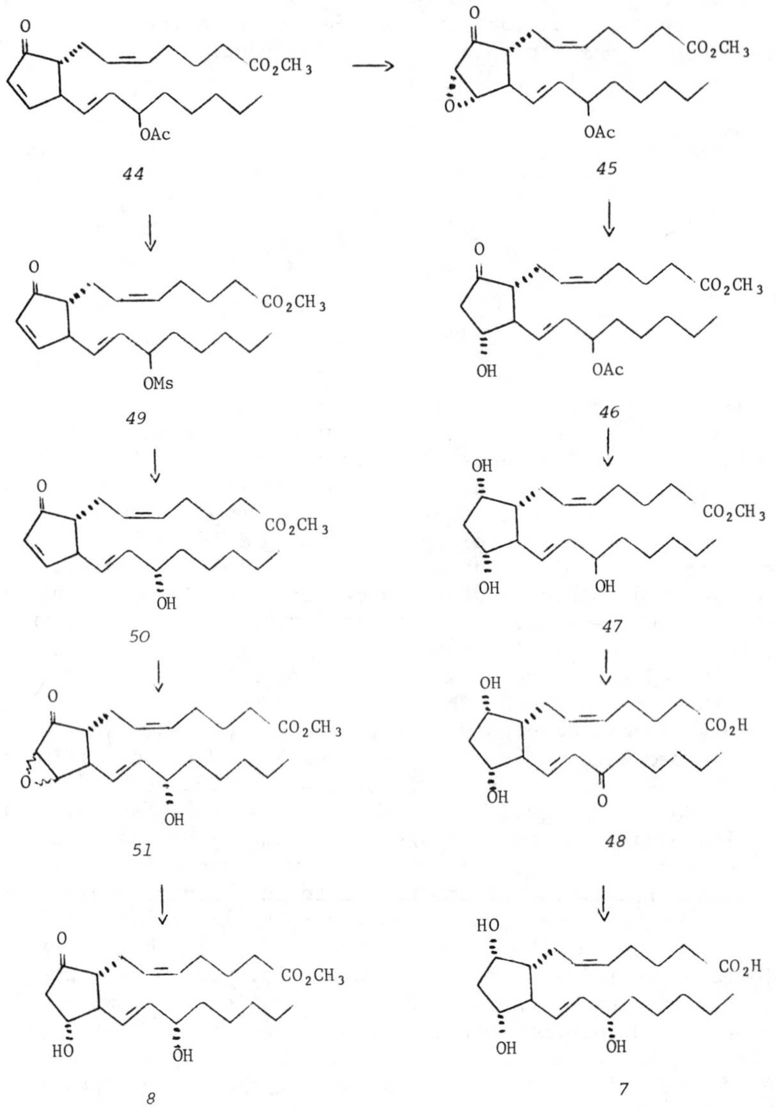

In a variation on this scheme, the 15 acetate is first saponified and the resulting alcohol converted to the methanesul-
fonate (49). Solvolysis in acetone results in what in essence is
an SN_1 displacement and thus affords a 1:1 mixture of 15α and 15β
isomers. The former is isolated to afford the desired product
with the mammalian configuration at 15 (50). Application of the
epoxidation scheme mentioned above (44 to 46) leads to dinoprostone (8).

Subsequent further investigation of the coral divulged the
interesting fact that colonies from some locations yield the analog of 44 in which the configuration at 15 is exclusively (S).[15]
This natural product is simply the acetate of 50. Conversion of
this to dinoprostone devolves on hydration of the double bond at
10,11. Hydrolysis by means of esterases present in the coral effects both deacetylation and removal of the methyl ester. The
latter is restored by mild means with methyl iodide on the salt
of the acid. The resulting hydroxyester (50) is then epoxidized
(51, basic hydrogen peroxide) and reduced (aluminum amalgam) to
give 8.[16]

2. MISCELLANEOUS ALICYCLIC COMPOUNDS

The simplification of the local anesthetic pharmacophore of cocaine to an aryl substituted ester of ethanolamine has been described previously. Atropine (52) is a structurally closely related natural product whose main biologic action depends on inhibition of the parasympathetic nervous system. Among its many
other actions, the compound exerts useful spasmolytic effects.
It was therefore of some interest to so modify the molecule as to
maximize this particular activity at the expense of the side effects. In much the same vein as the work on cocaine, the structural requirements for the desired activity had at one time been
whittled down to embrace in essence an α-substituted phenylacetic
acid ester of ethanolamine (53).

52

53

A further simplification of the requirements for activity
came from the preparation of two spasmolytic agents that completely lack the aromatic ring. Thus, double alkylation of phenylacetonitrile *(54)* with 1,5-dibromopentane leads to the corresponding
cyclohexane *(55)*. This intermediate is then saponified and the
resulting acid *(56)* esterified with *N,N*-diethylethanolamine.
Catalytic reduction of the aromatic ring affords *dicyclonine*
(51).[17]

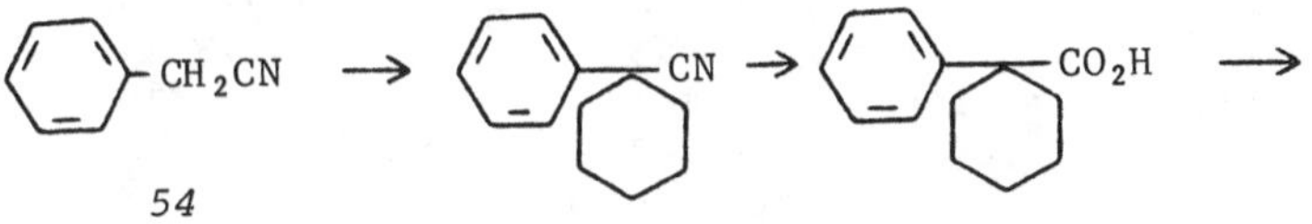

54   55   56

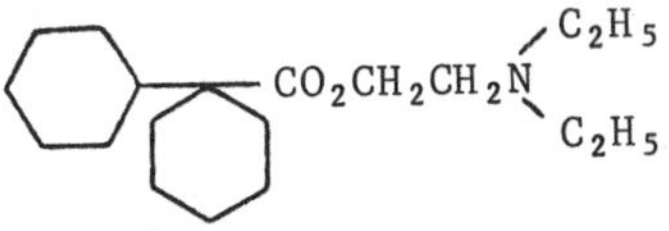

57

An interesting variation of this theme starts with the α-
chlorination of dicyclohexylketone *(58)*. Treatment of the halogenated intermediate with base leads to the acid, *60*, by the
Favorski rearrangement. Esterification of the acid with 2(1-
pyrolidino)ethanol yields *dihexyrevine (61)*.[18] Both this agent
and its earlier congener are recommended for use in GI spasms.

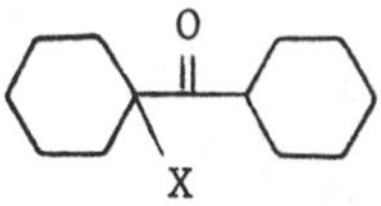

58, X=H
59, X=Cl

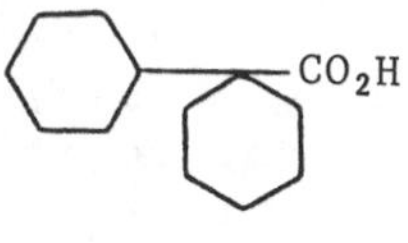

60

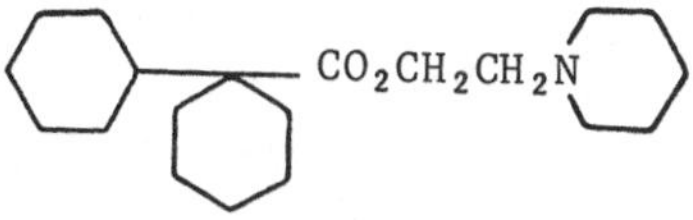

61

Amphetamine *(62)* is an agent closely related to the biogenic amines involved in various processes of the central nervous system. As such it is a drug with a multitude of activities; its main clinical use is as a central stimulant. This very activity, in fact, stands in the way of exploitation of the drug's activity as a local vasoconstricting agent, and thus constriction of mucous membranes. Preparation of the fully saturated analog *(64)* by catalytic reduction of *methamphetamine (63)* affords a compound that retains the desired activity with some reduction in side effect.[19] The product, *propylhexedrine (64)*, is used as a nasal decongestant.

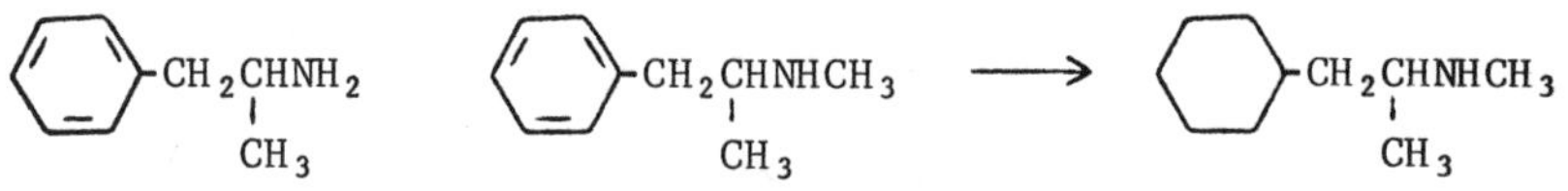

62   63   64

Further indication that the carbocyclic ring in this series serves a largely steric function comes from the finding that a five-membered ring analog, *cyclopentamine (69)*, is also biologically active. Condensation of cyclopentanone with cyanoacetic acid in a modified Knoevnagel reaction followed by decarboxylation affords the unsatured nitrile, *65*. Reduction of the double bond and subsequent reaction of the product *(66)* with methylmagnesium halide leads to the methyl ketone, *67*. This affords the desired product *(69)* on reductive amination with methylamine.[20]

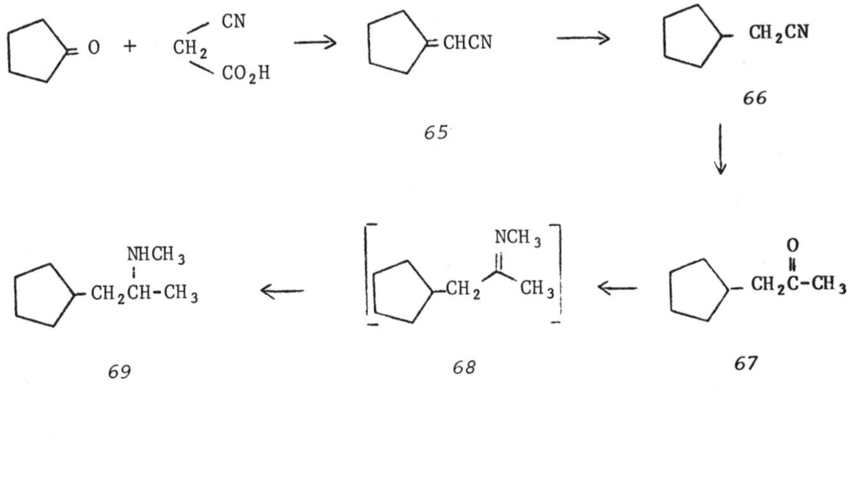

65   66

69   68   67

Although chemically related to the above cycloalkylamines, *pentethylcyclanone (71)* is stated to have antitussive activity. The compound is prepared rather simply by alkylation of the anion *(70a)* of the self-condensation product of cyclopentanone *(70)* with *N*-(2-chloroethyl)-morpholine.[21]

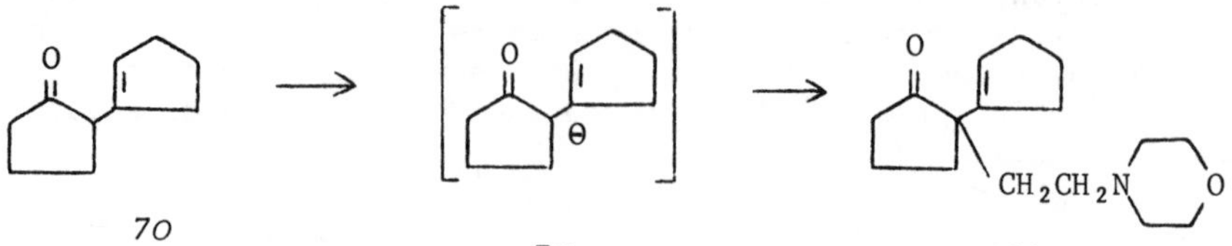

The hypnotic activity of ethanol is too well known to need comment. It is an interesting sidelight that this is a property shared with a number of other alcohols of relatively low molecular weight. Activity in fact increases with lipid solubility. This is probably due to better absorption and, with branching on the carbinol carbon, perhaps decreased metabolic destruction. Conversion of a hypnotic alcohol to its carbamate often serves to impart sedative properties to the agent. Thus, reaction of the product of ethynylation of cyclohexanone *(72)* with phosgene followed by ammonia gives the sedative-hypnotic, *meparfynol (74)*[22]; reaction with allophanyl chloride gives directly the sedative-hypnotic, *clocental (25)*.[23]

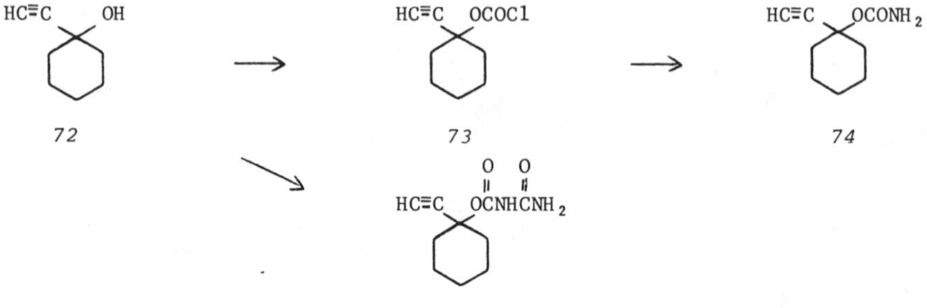

REFERENCES

1. S. Abrahamsson, S. Bergstrom, and B. Samuelsson, *Proc. Chem. Soc., 1962*, 332.

2. (a) E. G. Daniels and J. E. Pike, "Prostaglandin Symposium of the Worcester Foundation for Expt. Biol.," P. W. Ramwell and J. E. Shaw (Eds.), Interscience, N. Y. (1963); (b) D. A. van Dorp, R. K. Beerthuis, D. H. Nutgren, and H. VonKeman, *Nature, Lond.*, *203*, 839 (1964).

3. U. Axen, J. E. Pike, and W. P. Schneider, *Total Synthesis of Prostaglandins, Synthesis*, Vol. 1, J. W. ApSimon (Ed.), Wiley, N. Y., 1973.

4. E. J. Corey, T. Ravindranathan, and S. Terashima, *J. Amer. Chem. Soc.*, *93*, 4326 (1971).

5. E. J. Corey, T. K. Schaaf, W. Huber, V. Koelliker, and N. M. Weinshenker, *J. Amer. Chem. Soc.*, *92*, 397 (1970).

6. E. J. Corey, N. M. Weinshenker, T. K. Schaaf, and W. Huber, *J. Amer. Chem. Soc.*, *91*, 5675 (1969).

7. E. J. Corey, K. Becker, and R. V. Varma, *J. Amer. Chem. Soc.*, *94*, 8616 (1972).

8. E. J. Corey, H. Shirahama, H. Yamamoto, S. Terashima, A. Venkateswarlo, and T. K. Schaaf, *J. Amer. Chem. Soc.*, *93*, 1491 (1971).

9. J. Meinwald, S. S. Labana, and M. S. Chade, *J. Amer. Chem. Soc.*, *85*, 582 (1963).

10. R. C. Kelly and V. Van Rheenen, *Tetrahedron Lett.*, 1709 (1973).

11. G. Just, Ch. Simonovitch, F. H. Lincoln, W. P. Schneider, U. Axen, G. B. Spero, and J. E. Pike, *J. Amer. Chem. Soc.*, *91*, 5364 (1969).

12. R. C. Kelly, V. VanRheenen, I. Schletter, and M. D. Pillai, *J. Amer. Chem. Soc.*, *95*, 2746 (1973).

13. A. J. Weinheimer and R. L. Spraggins, *Tetrahedron Lett.*, 5185 (1969).

14. G. L. Bundy, F. H. Lincoln, N. A. Nelson, J. E. Pike, and W. P. Schneider, *Ann. N. Y. Acad. Sci.*, *180*, 76 (1971).

15. W. P. Schneider, R. D. Hamton, and L. E. Rhuland, *J. Amer. Chem. Soc.*, *94*, 2122 (1972).

16. G. L. Bundy, W. P. Schneider, F. H. Lincoln, and J. E. Pike, *J. Amer. Chem. Soc.*, *94*, 2124 (1972).

17. C. H. Tilford, M. G. VanCampen, and R. S. Shelton, *J. Amer. Chem. Soc.*, *69*, 3902 (1947).

18. M. Kopp and B. Tchoubar, *Bull. Soc. Chim. France*, 84 (1952).

19. B. L. Zemitz, E. B. Macks, and M. L. Moore, *J. Amer. Chem. Soc.*, *69*, 1117 (1947).

20. E. Rohrman, U. S. Patent 2,520,015 (1950).

21. H. Veberwasser, German Patent 1,059,901 (1959).

22. K. Junkmann and H. Pfeiffer, U. S. Patent 2,816,910 (1957).

23. W. Grimene and H. Emde, German Patent 959,485 (1957).

CHAPTER 4

Benzyl and Benzhydryl Derivatives

The previous chapter pointed up the relative paucity of useful medicinal agents to be found among simple monocyclic alicyclic compounds. Current intensive research on the prostaglandins may, of course, change that in the future. It is well known, however, that the chances of finding a biologically active molecule increase dramatically with the incorporation into the structure of one or more aromatic or heteroaromatic rings. This common observation has been ascribed to many of the known properties of these rings, such as their rigid planarity, the ability of the pi cloud to enter into charge-transfer complexes, or the polarizability of the same cloud, to name only a few. Much effort is currently devoted to theoretical studies bearing on these points.

As will be seen, the arylaliphatic compounds represent one of the larger structural classes of drugs; these compounds show therapeutic activity in a widely divergent series of pathologic states. Discovery of activity in this series has tended to be largely empirical. The description of a novel active structure usually heralded the preparation of a flood of analogs, by the originator in order to improve the therapeutic ratio and by his competitor in order to gain some proprietary patent position. Some of the more imaginative analog programs were sometimes rewarded by the finding of novel structures with unanticipated biologic activities.

1. AGENTS BASED ON BENZYL AND BENZHYDRYL AMINES AND ALCOHOLS

    a. Compounds Related to Benzhydrol

Many of the more debilitating symptoms of allergic states such as rashes, rhinitis, and runny eyes, are thought to be due to hist-

amine released as the end product of a lengthy chain of biochemical reactions that begins with the interaction of the allergen
with some antibody. Although this process is known in some detail, attempts to intervene therapeutically in a rational manner
have not thus far been successful. It has been known for some
time, however, that a fairly large class of organic compounds
would alleviate many of the symptoms of allergic reactions.
Since there was some evidence that these compounds owe their action to interference with the action of histamine, this class has
earned the soubriquet "antihistamines." This class of drugs is
further characterized by a spectrum of side effects which occur
to a greater or lesser degree in various members. These include
antispasmodic action, sedative action, analgesia, and antiemetic
effects. The side effects of some of these agents are sufficiently pronounced so that the compounds are prescribed for that effect proper. Antihistamines, for example, are used as the sedative-hypnotic component in some over-the-counter sleeping pills.

The prototype of the antihistamines based on benzhydrol,
diphenhydramine (3), is familiar to many today under the trade
name Benadryl®. Light-induced bromination of diphenylmethane affords benzhydryl bromide *(2)*. This is then allowed to react with
dimethylaminoethanol to give the desired ether.[1] Although no
mechanistic studies have been reported, it is not unlikely that
the bromine undergoes SN_1 solvolysis in the reaction medium; the
carbonium ion then simply picks up the alcohol. It might be noted in passing that the theophyline salt of *4* is familiar to many
travelers as a motion sickness remedy under the trade name
Dramamine®.

Several analogs bearing different substituents on the aromatic rings are accessible by essentially the same route. The
appropriate benzhydrol *(4)* is first prepared by reaction of an

1   2   3

arylmagnesium halide with a benzaldehyde (economics probably dic-
tates which reagent shall bear the substituent). Reaction of the
alcohol with thionyl chloride gives the benzhydryl chloride *(5)*.
This last is converted to the amino ether *(6)* with dimethylaminoethanol as above. The anisyl derivative *(6a), medrylamine*,[2] is

used largely as an antihistamine, as is the *p*-bromo analog, *bro-modiphenhydramine (6b)*.[3] The *o*-tolyl compound, *orphenadrine (6c)*,[4] exhibits diminished antihistaminic properties at the expense of antispasmodic activity. It has found some use in control of the symptoms of Parkinson's disease. We shall meet this type of activity, referred to for simplicity as antiparkinson activity, again.

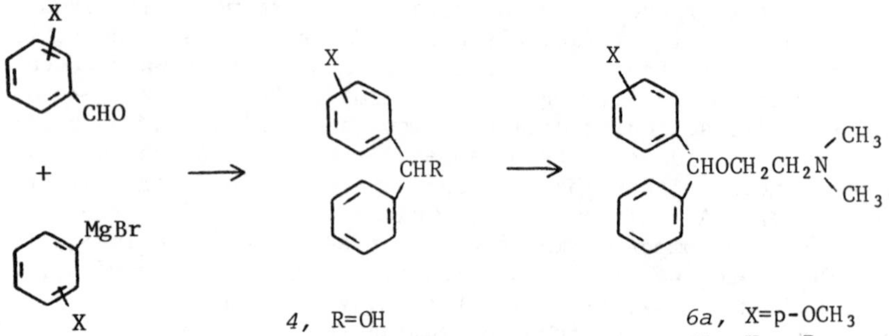

4,	R=OH
5a,	R=Cl; X=p-OCH$_3$
5b,	R=Cl; X=p-Br
5c,	R=Cl; X=o-CH$_3$
5d,	R=Cl; X=p-Cl

6a,	X=p-OCH$_3$
6b,	X=p-Br
6c,	X=o-CH$_3$

Oxygen to nitrogen spacing apparently is not too critical for retention of activity. Thus, inclusion of the nitrogen atom in either a five- or six-membered ring affords active compounds. Alkylation of benzhydryl bromide *(2)* with 4-hydroxy-1-methylpiperidine affords the potent antihistamine, *diphenylpyraline (7)*.[5] Similarly, alkylation of the *p*-chloro benzhydryl halide *(5d)* with 3-hydroxy-1-methylpyrrodiline gives *pyroxamine (8)*.

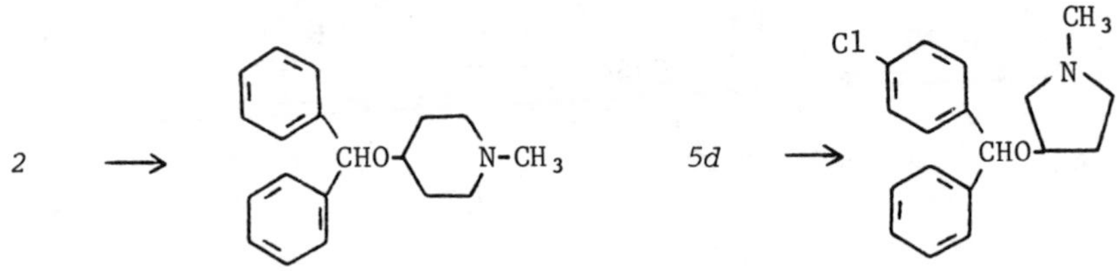

Inclusion of a second nitrogen atom in the side chain seemingly increases the spasmolytic effect of the benzhydrol derivatives. Alkylation of the benzdryl chloride *(9)* with the sodium salt obtained from N-(2-hydroxyethyl)-piperazine affords the basic ether *(10)*. Alkylation of this intermediate with α-chloro-o-xylene gives *chlorbenzoxamine (11)*.[6]

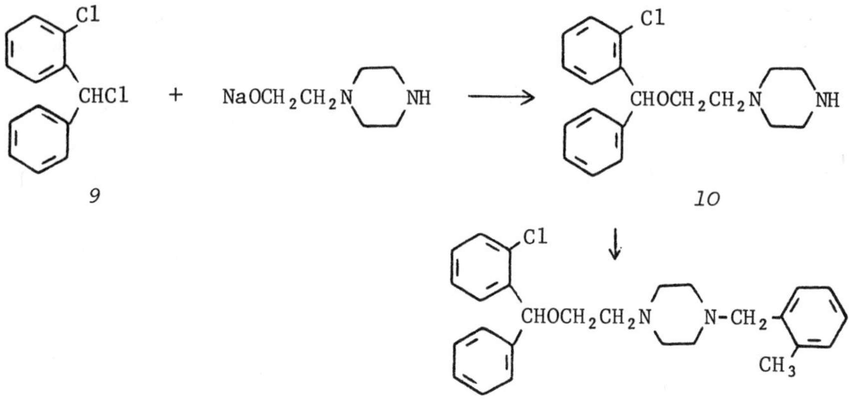

When the additional nitrogen atom is included in one of the aromatic rings, on the other hand, there is obtained a compound with antihistaminic properties. Reaction of the Grignard reagent from 4-chlorobromobenzene with pyridine-2-aldehyde gives the benzhydrol analog *(12)*. The alcohol is then converted to its sodium salt by means of sodium, and this salt is alkylated with N-(2-chloroethyl)dimethylamine. *Carbinoxamine (13)* is thus obtained.[7,8]

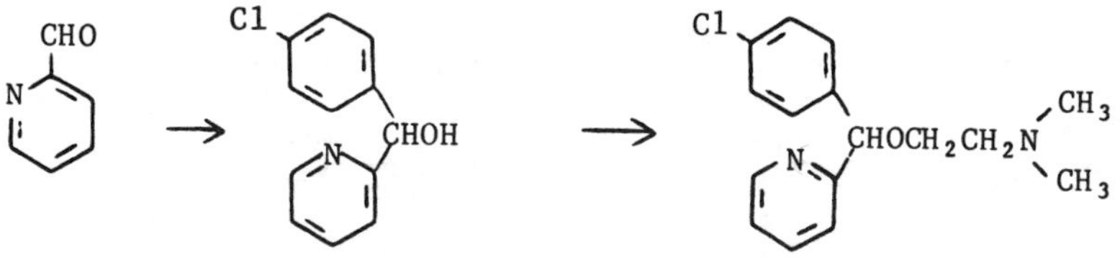

The oxygen atom in these molecules can in many cases be dispensed with as well; substitution of sulfur for nitrogen affords a molecule whose salient biologic properties are those of a sedative and tranquilizer. Friedel-Crafts acylation of the *n*-butyl ether of thiophenol with benzoyl chloride gives the corresponding benzophenone. Reduction of the ketone *(15)* followed by

treatment with thionyl chloride affords the benzhydryl chloride
(16). Displacement of the halogen with thiourea gives, by reaction of the last at its most nucleophilic center, the isothio-
uronium salt, *17*. Hydrolysis of the salt leads to the sulfur
analog of a benzhydrol *(18)*. Alkylation of the sodium salt of
this last with N-(2-chloroethyl)dimethylamine affords *captodiamine*
(19).[9]

The substitution of the lone proton on the benzhydryl carbon
by a methyl group again affords compounds with antihistamine activity. Reaction of an appropriate acetophenone *(21)* with phenylmagnesium bromide affords the desired tertiary alcohols *(22)*.

14   15, X=OH   17
          16, X=Cl

19   18

Alkylation of these as their sodium salts with the ubiquitous N-
(2-chloroethyl)dimethylamine affords the desired antihistamines.
There are thus obtained, respectively, *mephenhydramine (23a)*,[10]
chlorphenoxamine (23b),[11] and *mebrophenhydramine (23c)*.[12] Alkylation of the tertiary alcohol, *22b*, with the pyrrolidine derivative, *24*, affords *meclastine (25)*.[13] In much the same vein, reaction of 2-acetylpyridine with phenylmagnesium bromide gives the
tertiary alcohol, *27*. Alkylation in the usual way leads to the
potent antihistamine, *doxylamine (28)*.[14]

Performance of an imaginary 1,2-shift on the benzhydrol antihistamines, that is, attachment of the side chain directly to the
benzhydryl carbon while leaving the hydroxyl group intact, affords
a series of molecules with markedly altered biologic activities.
As a class, these agents tend to be devoid of antihistaminic activity, while they retain some of the sedative and antiparkinson

activity. It should be noted that these agents are of only minor importance in drug therapy today.

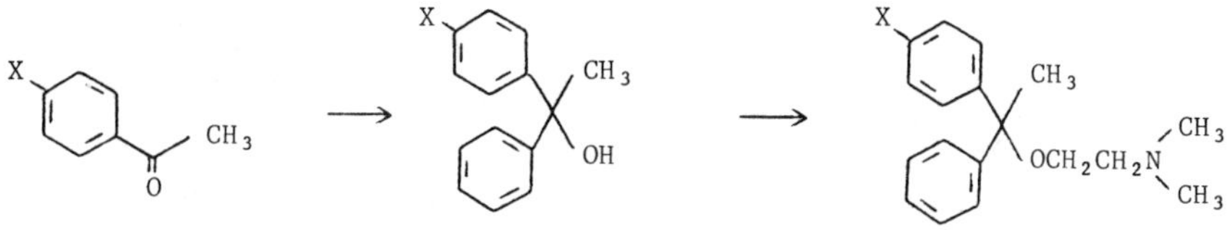

21a, X=H
21b, X=Cl
21c, X=Br

22a, X=H
22b, X=Cl
22c, X=Br

23a, X=H
23b, X=Cl
23c, X=Br

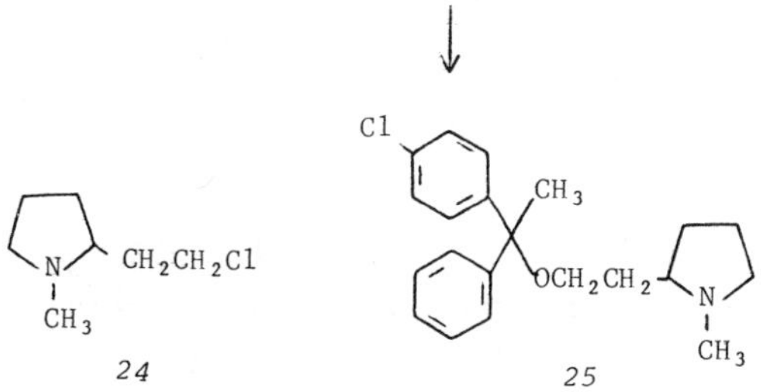

24

25

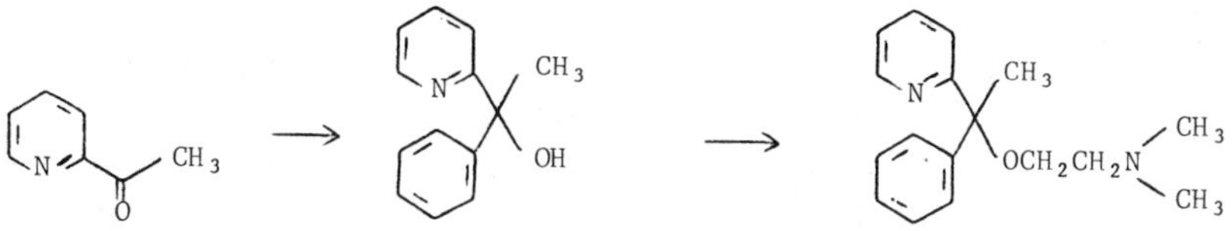

26

27

28

The prototype, *diphenidol (30)*, is used as an antiemetic This agent is obtained in one step from the reaction of the Grignard reagent of halide, *29*, with benzophenone.[15] The lower homolog, *32*, is effective chiefly as a muscle relaxant and antiparkinson agent. Conjugate addition of piperidine to ethyl acrylate gives the amino ester *(31)*. Condensation of this with phenylmagnesium bromide affords *pirindol (32)*.[16]

Introduction of branching in the side chain is apparently consistent with retention of the antiparkinson activity. Bromination of propiophenone gives the brominated ketone, *33*. Dis-

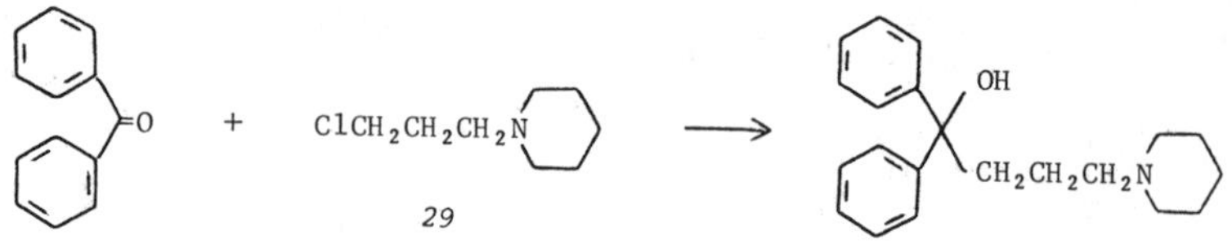

placement of halogen with piperidine leads to the aminoketone
(34). Condensation of the last with phenylmagnesium bromide affords the spasmolytic agent, *diphepanol (35)*.[17]

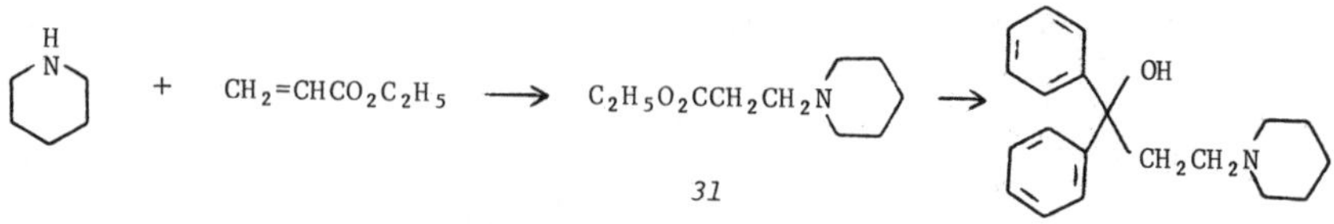

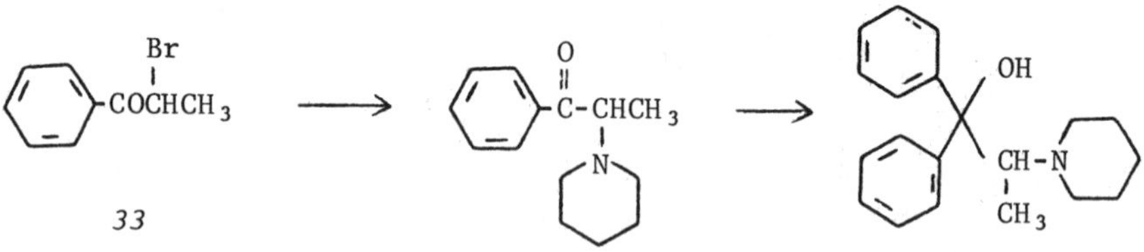

Condensation of the anion obtained on reaction of acetonitrile with sodium amide, with *o*-chlorobenzophenone *(36)*, affords
the hydroxynitrile, *37*. Catalytic reduction leads to the corresponding amino alcohol (note that the benzhydryl alcohol is not
hydrogenolyzed). Reductive alkylation with formaldehyde and hydrogen in the presence of Raney nickel gives the antitussive a-
gent, *chlorphedianol (39)*.[18]
Cyclization of the side chain onto the nitrogen atom leads
to compounds with sedative and tranquilizing activity. The lack
of structural specificity, that is, the fact that both positional
isomers *(41,43)* show the same activity, is notable. Thus, condensation of the Grignard reagent from 2-bromopyridine with benzophenone affords the tertiary carbinol, *40*. Catalytic reduction

in acetic acid leads to selective hydrogenation of the heterocyclic ring and formation of *azacyclonol (41)*.[19] The analogous sequence using an organometallic derived from 4-bromopyridine gives
pipradol (43).[20]

Substitution of an alicyclic ring for one of the aromatic
rings in the amino alcohols such as *32* or *39* produces a series of
useful antispasmodic agents that have found some use in the treatment of the symptoms of Parkinson's disease. Mannich reaction of
acetophenone with formaldehyde and piperidine affords the aminoketone, *44a*. Reaction of the ketone with cyclohexylmagnesium

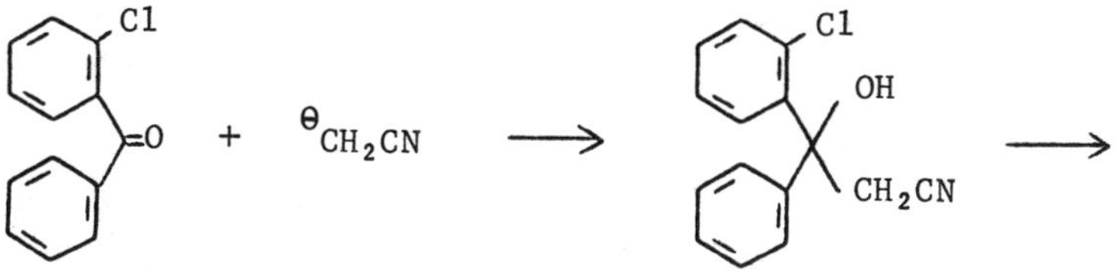

36   37

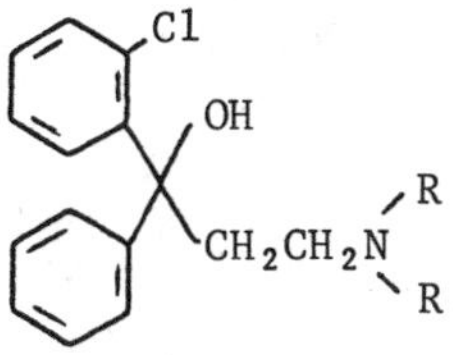

38, R=H
39, R=CH$_3$

bromide leads to *trihexyphenidil (45)*[21]; alternately, condensation with the Grignard reagent from cyclopentyl bromide affords
cycrimine (46).[22] Reaction of the aminoketone, *44a*, with the
Grignard reagent from the bicyclic halide, *47* (from addition of
hydrogen bromide to norbornadiene), affords *biperidin (48)*.[23]

In much the same vein, the Mannich product from acetophenone
with formaldehyde and pyrrolidine *(44b)* affords *procyclidine (49)*
on reaction with cyclohexylmagnesium bromide. In an interesting
variation, the ketone is first reacted with phenylmagnesium bromide. Catalytic hydrogenation of the carbinol *(50)* thus obtained
can be stopped after the reduction of only one aromatic ring.[24]

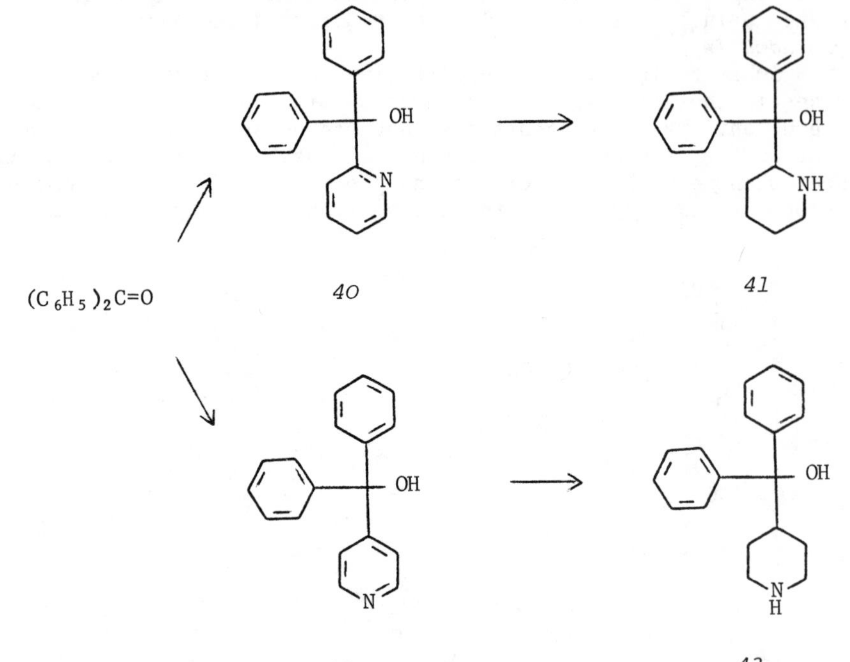

$(C_6H_5)_2C=O$

40

41

42

43

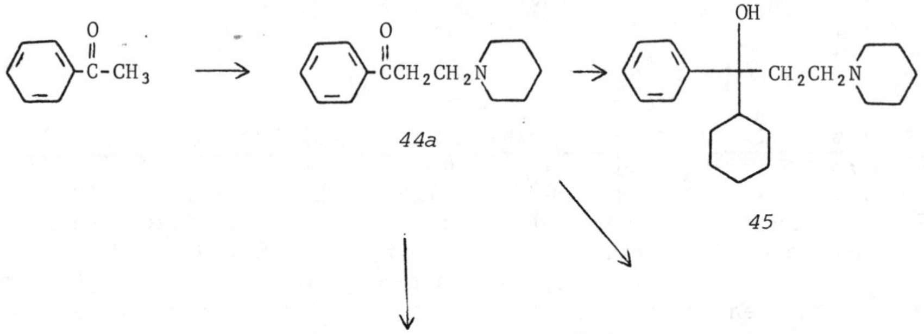

44a

45

44a

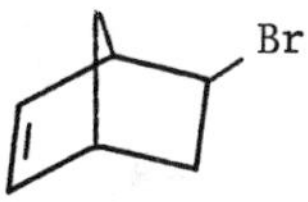

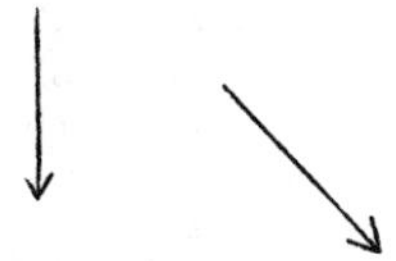

47

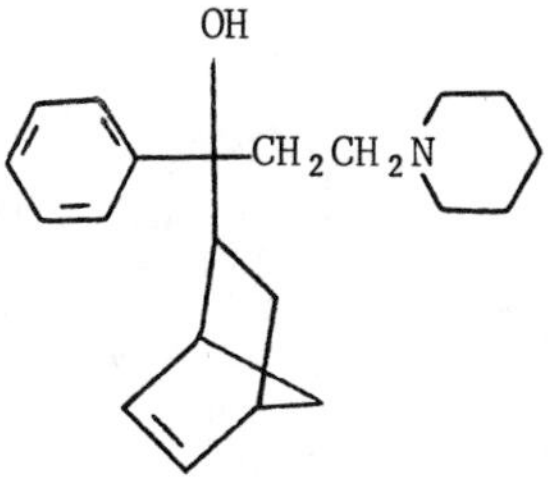

48

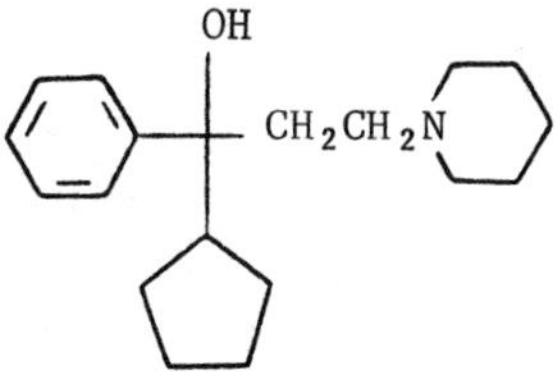

46

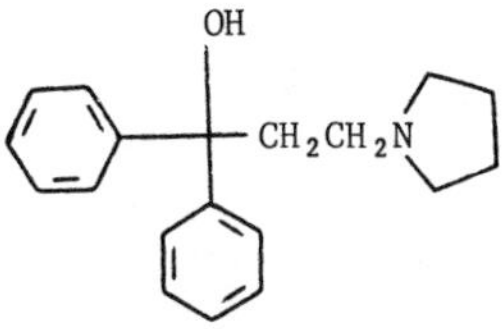

50

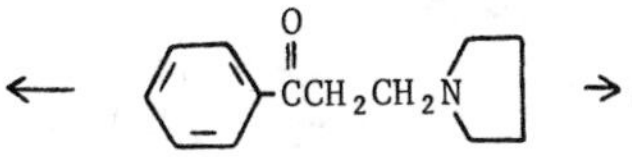

44b

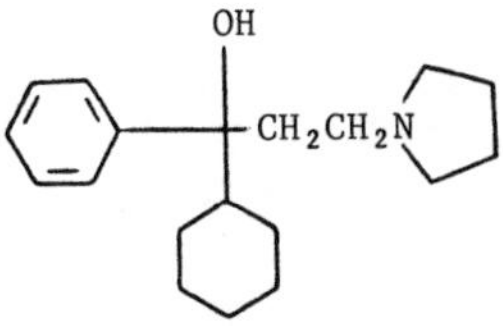

49

Relatively small modifications of the structures of the a-
bove spasmolytic agents produce a dramatic change in biologic activity. Incorporation of a methylene between the aromatic ring
and the quaternary center, methylation of the side chain, and
finally esterification of the alcohol yields *propoxyphene*. This
agent, under the trade name of Darvon® (now available as a generic
drug), has been in very wide use as an analgesic agent for the
treatment of mild pain. Mannich reaction of propiophenone with
formaldehyde and dimethylamine affords the corresponding aminoketone *(51)*. Reaction of the ketone with benzylmagnesium bromide

gives the amino alcohol *(52)*. It is of note that this intermediate fails to show analgesic activity in animal assays. Esterification of the alcohol by means of propionic anhydride affords
the propionate *(53)*.[25] The presence of two chiral centers in
this molecule means, of course, that the compound will exist as
two racemic pairs. The biologic activity has been found to be
associated with the α isomer. Resolution of that isomer into its
optical antipodes showed the *d* isomer to be the active analgesic;
this is now denoted as *propoxyphene (d,53)*. The *l* isomer is almost devoid of analgesic activity; the compound does, however,
show useful antitussive activity and is named *levopropoxyphene*
(1,53).[26]

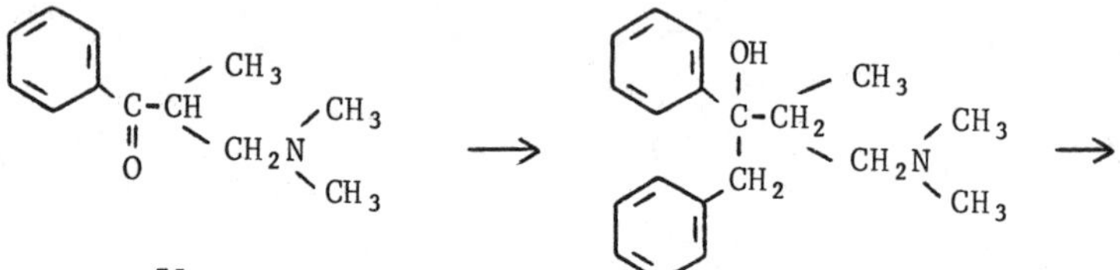

51   52

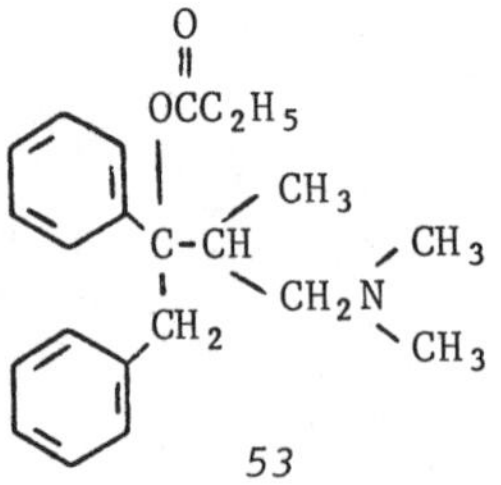

53

b. Compounds Related to Benzylamine

Further illustration for the lack of structural specificity required for antihistaminic activity comes from the finding that
ethylenediamines carrying both a benzylamine and an additional
aromatic substituent on one of the nitrogens afford a series of
useful therapeutic agents. Alkylation of benzylaniline with *N*-
(2-chlorethyl)dimethylamine affords *phenbenzamine (54)*.[27] Treatment of the secondary amine with *N*-(2-chloroethyl)pyrrolidine affords the antihistamine, *histapyrrodine (55)*.[28]
     As in the case of the benzhydryl ethers, inclusion of the

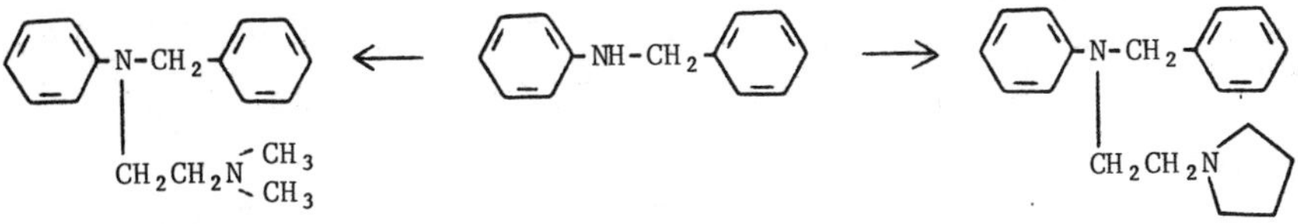

nitrogen atom in a ring is consistent with activity. Thus, condensation of N-methyl-4-piperidone with aniline yields the corresponding Shiff base. Reduction followed by alkylation of the
secondary amine (57) with benzyl chloride by means of sodium a-
mide affords bamipine (58).[29]

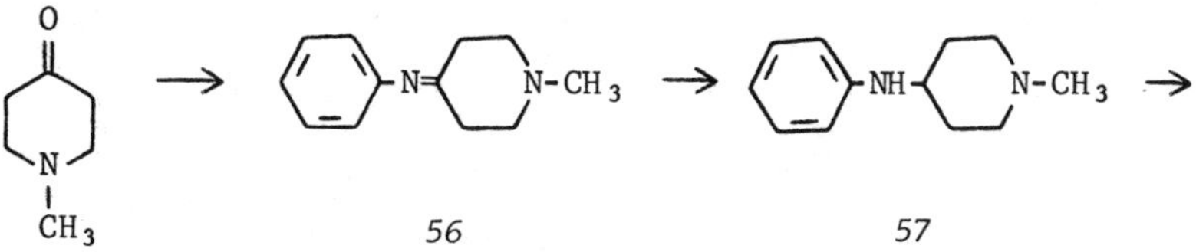

Substitution of a 2-pyridyl residue for the phenyl attached
directly to nitrogen affords a series of potent antihistamines.
Preparation of these compounds, too, is accomplished by a series
of alkylation reactions. It is further probable that the order
of the reaction can be readily interchanged. Thus, alkylation
of 2-aminopyridine with the chloroethyldimethylamine side chain
leads to the diamine, 59. Alkylation with benzyl chloride affords tripelenamine (60); reaction with p-methoxybenzyl chloride
leads to pyrilamine (61).[30]
     In a variation on this approach, p-chlorobenzaldehyde is
first condensed with 2-aminopyridine. Reduction of the resulting
Shiff base (62) affords the corresponding secondary amine. Alkylation with the usual side chain affords the antihistamine, chlorpyramine (64).[31]

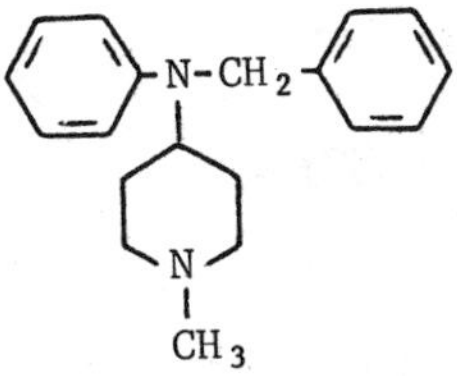

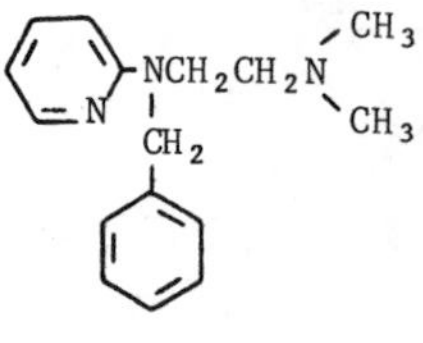

59

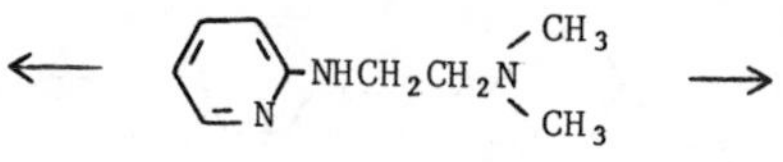

60

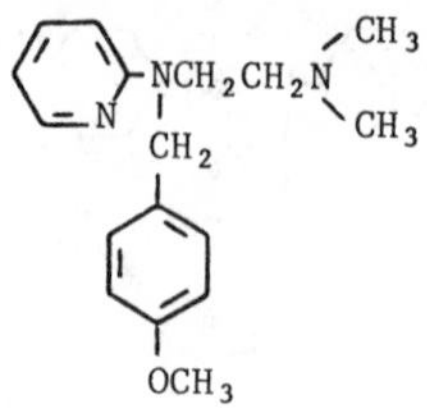

61

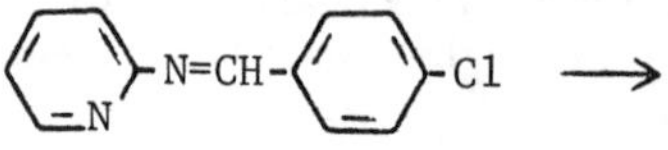

62

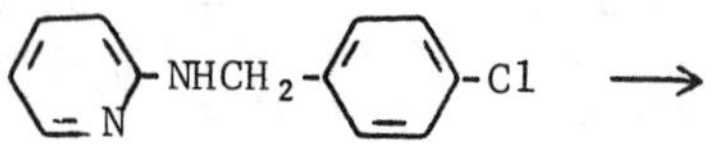

63

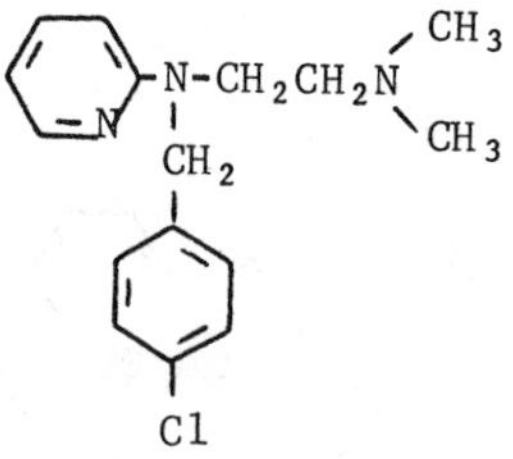

64

Aromatic rings containing more than one hetero atom also yield active antihistamines. Alkylation of 2-aminopyrimidine (65) with p-methoxybenzyl chloride gives the corresponding secondary amine (66). Alkylation with the usual chloroamine affords thonzylamine (67).[32] Application of the same sequence to 2-aminothiazole (68) affords zolamine (70).

The isosteric relationship of benzene and thiophene has often led medicinal chemists to substitute the sulfur containing heterocycle for benzene drugs in biologically active molecules. That this relationship has some foundation in fact is attested by the observation that the resulting analogs often possess full biologic activity. Alkylation of the diamine, 71 (obtained from aniline and the chloroethylamine), with 2-chloromethylthiophene affords the antihistamine methaphenylene (72).[33] The correspond-

65 66 67

68 69 70

ing agent containing the cyclic side chain is obtained by alkylation on the secondary amine, *57*, with the same halide; *methaphencycline (73)*[34] is thus obtained.

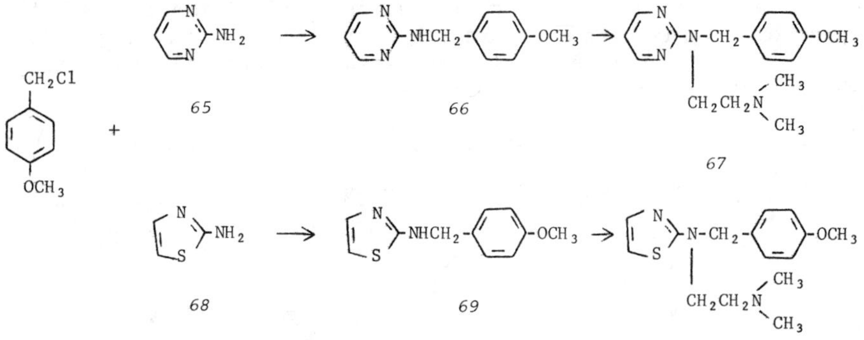

Interestingly, replacement of both benzene rings of the prototype molecule *(54)* by heterocyclic rings is not only consistent with activity, but yields two of the more potent antihistamines.

71 72

57 73

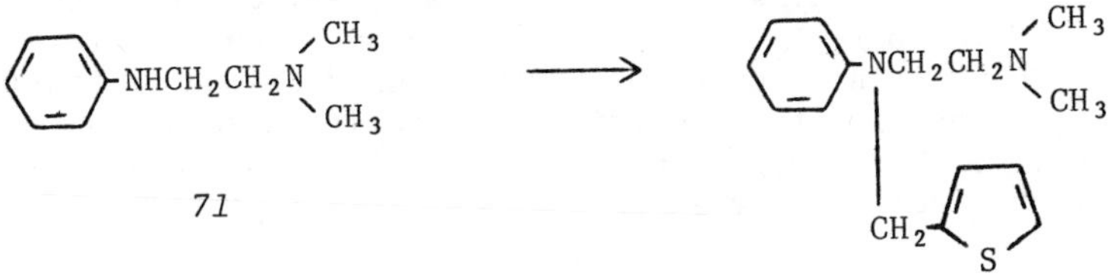

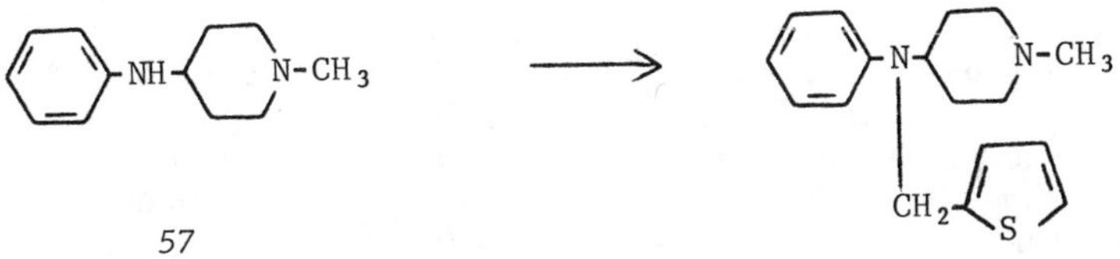

Resorting to alkylation chemistry again, 2-aminopyridine is condensed with the usual side chain halide to give diamine, *74*. Alkylation of this with 2-chloromethylthiophene gives *methapyrilene
(75)*.[35] Reaction with 2-chloromethyl-5-chlorothiophene affords
the potent antihistamine *chlorothen (76)*.[35]

Appropriately substituted benzylamines have provided a number of drugs useful in the treatment of high blood pressure. The
fact that pharmacologic studies have shown these agents to act by
very different mechanisms makes it likely that the benzylamine
nucleus plays at best a small role in the biologic action of
these compounds. Rather, these compounds are thought to owe
their activity to the particular functionality (pharmacophoric
group). The observation that a similar group often has the same
activity when attached to a quite different amine bears out this
suspicion. Thus, alkylation of benzylmethylamine with propargyl
bromide affords *pargyline (77)*.[36] This drug, developed initially
as an antidepressant, acting by monamine oxidase inhibition (MAO
inhibition, see aromatic hydrazines for fuller discussion), was
found to lower blood pressure in hypertensive individuals by
some as yet undefined mechanism.

Blood pressure is under the control of the autonomic
(sometimes called the involuntary or reflex) nervous system.
That is, the pressure is adjusted automatically in response to
signals from various baroreceptors. Control of abnormally high
pressure can, at least in theory, be achieved by interfering with
the chain of transmission of the neural signals that lead to ele-
vation of pressure. Initial success in control of hypertension
was met with the ganglionic blocking agents which in effect in-

terrupted all neuronal signals. Since many other bodily functions are under autonomic control, this mode of therapy had a
significant number of side effects. The next development, the
peripheral sympathetic blocking agents, acts further down the
chain of control and thus shows more specificity for blood pressure response. Many of the sympathetic responses are mediated at
the last stage by reaction of a neurotransmitter amine such as
norepinephrine (see below) with a receptor site on the tissue
that is to give the response. Sophisticated pharmacologic study
has led to the classification of these as α and β sympathetic receptors (the details are beyond the scope of this book). Drugs
are now available whose effects can be explained by the assump-
tion of blockade of either α or β receptors. The goal of work in
this field is, of course, to find drugs that will block specifically either α or β receptors in only the cardiovascular system.

Quaternization of o-bromo-N,N-dimethylbenzylamine with the
p-toluene-sulfonate of ethanol affords *bretylium tosylate (78)*,[37]
an antihypertensive agent acting by peripheral sympathetic blockade.

The guanidine function has proven particularly useful in
providing antihypertensives that act by peripheral sympathetic
blockade. Several such compounds that contain a quite different
hydrocarbon moiety are met later *(guanadrel, guanethidine, guancycline, debrisoquin)*. Reaction of benzylamine with methyl isothiocyanate gives the corresponding thiourea *(79)*. Methylation
affords the product of alkylation at the most nucleophilic center, the thioenol ether *(80)*. Displacement of the thiomethyl
group by methylamine (probably by an addition elimination process) affords *bethanidine (81)*.[38]

Reaction of dibenzylamine with ethylene oxide affords the
amino alcohol, *82*. Treatment of that product with thionyl chloride gives the α-sympathetic blocking agent, *dibenamine (83)*.[39]
Condensation of phenol with propylene chlorohydrin *(84)* gives the
alcohol, *85*. Reaction with thionyl chloride affords the chloride
(86). Use of the halide to alkylate ethanolamine affords the secondary amine *(87)*. Alkylation of this last with benzyl chloride
(88) followed by conversion of the hydroxyl to chloride by means
of thionyl chloride completes the preparation of *phenoxybenzamine
(89)*.[40] This agent, too, is an antihypertensive drug that owes
its action to blockade of the α-sympathetic receptors. The blockade induced by these drugs is of unusually long duration (the β-
haloamine function is known to be a good alkylating agent for
many polypeptides). This very long duration of action and a certain lack of specificity for the cardiovascular system has diminished the usefulness of these agents.

The more familiar method of inducing surgical anesthethesia

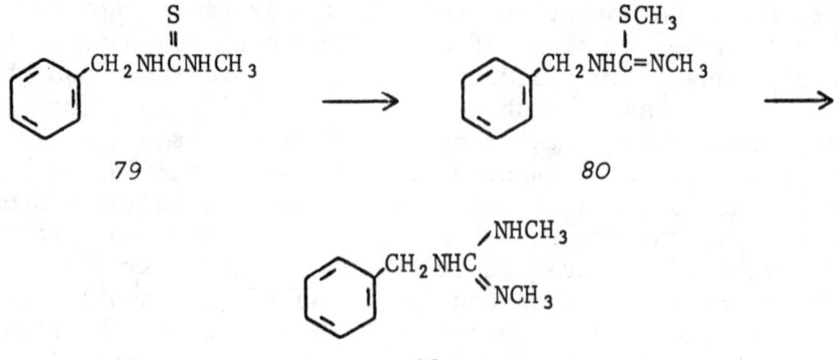

79

80

81

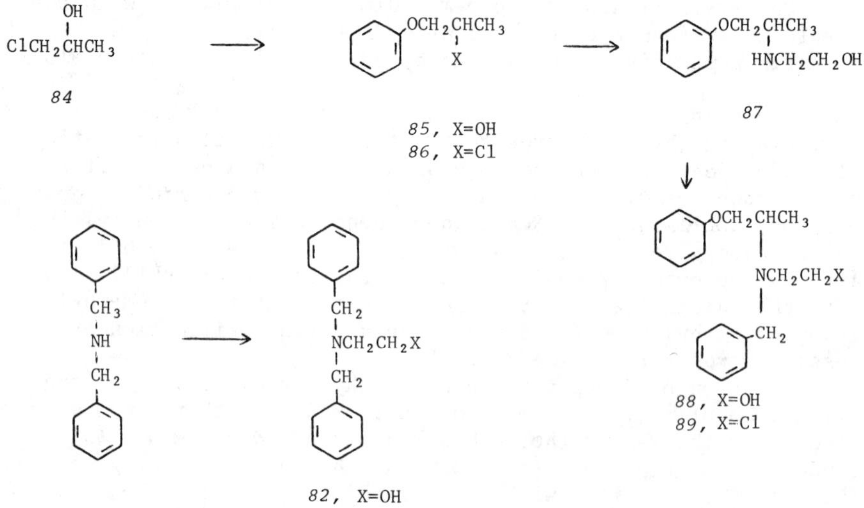

84

85, X=OH
86, X=Cl

87

82, X=OH
83, X=Cl

88, X=OH
89, X=Cl

is by the administration of low molecular compounds such as ether or chloroform by inhalation. Such anesthesia can, however, also be achieved by parenteral administration of a quite different set of agents. Two of these can be regarded as derivatives of benzylamine. Reaction of cyclohexanone with piperidine hydrochloride and potassium cyanide affords the aminonitrile, *90*; this intermediate is, at least formally, the analog of a cyanohydrin with piperidine taking the place of water in the reaction sequence. *Phencyclidine*[41] *(91)* can be obtained by reaction of that amino-

nitrile with phenylmagnesium bromide. Although the overall sequence suggests displacement of cyanide ion, there is some evidence from related systems to suggest that the actual reaction
pathway involves preionization of *90* to the ternary imine *(92)*,
followed by addition of the organometallic reagent.

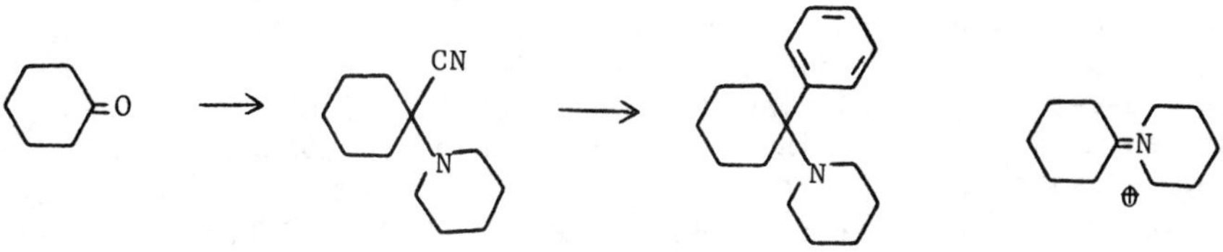

Preparation of the oxygenated analog, *ketamine*, proceeds by
a quite different route. Addition of cyclopentylmagnesium bromide to *o*-chlorobenzonitrile gives the ketone, *93*. Bromination
of the ketone affords *94*. Reaction of that intermediate with
aqueous methylamine affords the imino alcohol *(95)* obtained by
hydrolysis of the halogen and transformation of the ketone to the
imine (though not necessarily in that order). Thermolysis of the
imine hydrochloride leads one of the cyclopentane bonds to undergo a 1,2 shift to the adjacent unsaturated center and thus ring
enlargement. Loss of a proton with ketonization gives the parenteral general anesthetic agent *ketamine (96)*.[42]

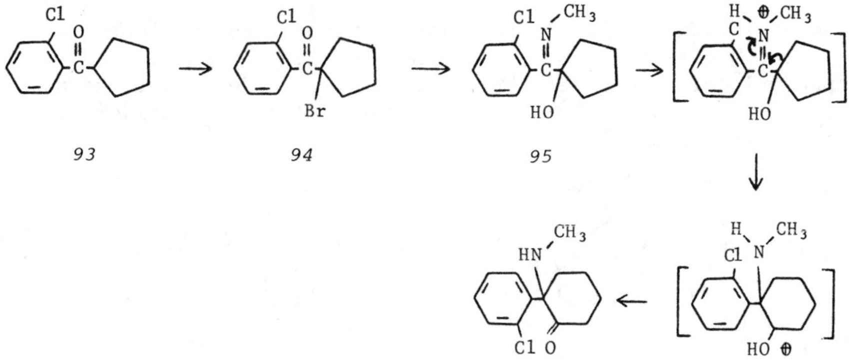

c. Compounds Related to Benzhydrylamine

As previously shown, derivatives of benzhydrol have provided a
large number of useful antihistaminic agents. Continued delving
into the structural requirement for activity revealed that the
oxygen atom could, in fact, be replaced by nitrogen. It is of
note that the nitrogen atom remote from the benzhydryl carbon is
included in a piperazine ring in these drugs. Much of this chemistry is rendered possible by the various techniques that have
been developed for placing differing substitution on the two nitrogen atoms. Piperazine can, for example, be monoacetylated
(a); alkylation of the remaining nitrogen followed by deacylation
allows a different alkyl group to be placed at the remaining heteroatom.

    Reaction of benzhydryl chloride with *N*-methylpiperazine (b)
gives *cyclizine (97)*[43]; analogous reaction with *p*-chlorobenzhy-
dryl chloride *(5d)* affords *chlorocyclizine (98)*.[43]

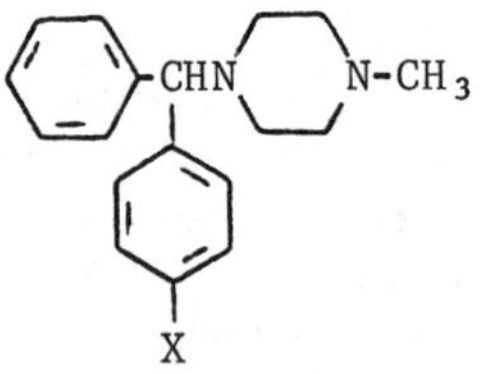

97, X=H
98, X=Cl

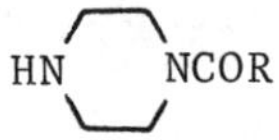

(a)

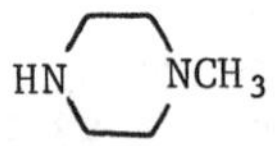

(b)

    Acylation of the monosubstituted piperazine, *99* (obtainable
by the protection-deprotection scheme outlined above), with
cinnamoyl chloride gives the corresponding amide *(100)*. Reduction of the carbonyl by means of lithium aluminum hydride affords
cinnarizine (101).[44]

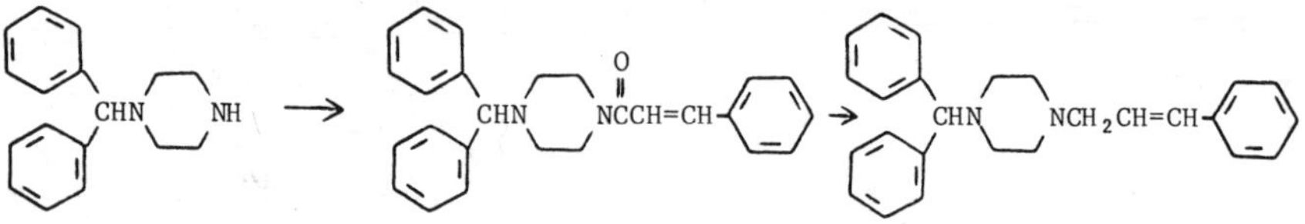

99   100   101

    Alkylation of the *p*-chloro analog *(102)* of the monosubsti-
tuted piperazine with *m*-methylbenzyl chloride *(103)* yields the

antihistamine *meclizine (105)*[45]; reaction of *102* with *p*-tertiary-butylbenzyl chloride *(104)* gives *buclizine (106)*.[45] Alkylation of the terminal nitrogen with hydrophilic side chains derived from polyethylene glycols affords compounds in which the sedative properties inherent in antihistamines are accentuated. Thus, alkylation of *102* with the chloro derivative of diethylene glycol *(107)* affords the sedative *hydroxyzine (108)*[46]; in the same vein, alkylation with the derivative of triethylene glycol *(109)* gives *hydrochlorobenzethylamine (110)*.[47]

103

104

$ClCH_2CH_2O(CH_2CH_2O)_nH$

107, n=1
109, n=2

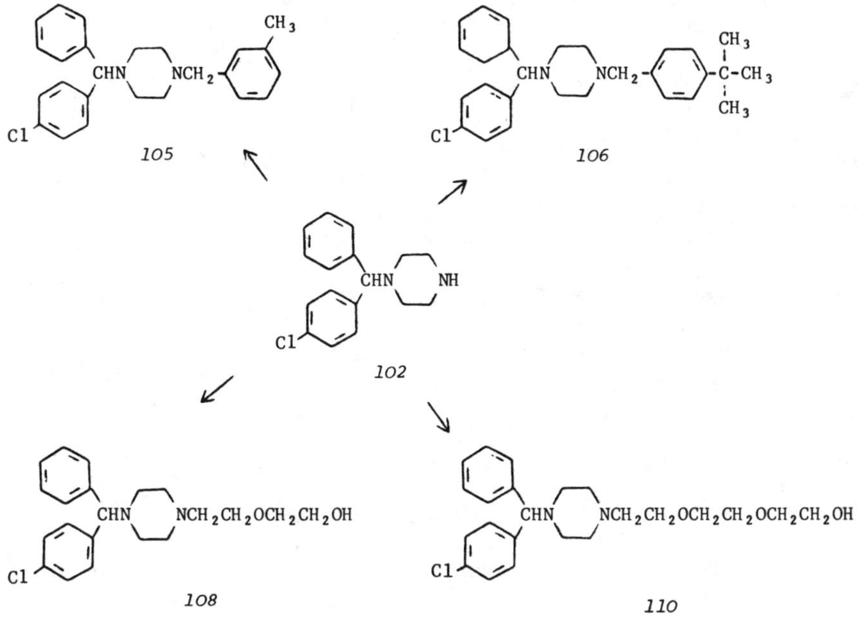

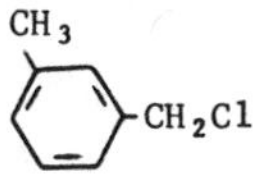

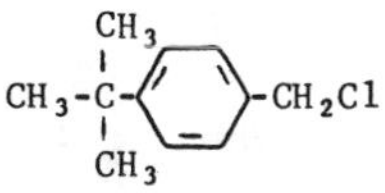

REFERENCES

1.   G. Rieveschl, Jr., U. S. Patent 2,421,714 (1947).
2.   H. Morren, U. S. Patent 2,668,856 (1954).
3.   G. Rieveschl, Jr., U. S. Patent 2,257,963 (1950).
4.   A. F. Harms and W. T. Nauta, J. Med. Chem., 2, 57 (1960).
5.   L. H. Knox and R. Kapp, U. S. Patent 2,479,843 (1949).
6.   H. G. Morren, R. Denayer, R. Linz, H. Strubbe, and S. Trolin, Ind. Chim. Belg., 22, 429 (1957).
7.   C. H. Tilford and R. S. Shelton, U. S. Patent 2,606,195 (1952).
8.   A. P. Swain, U. S. Patent 2,800,485 (1957).
9.   O. H. Hubner and P. V. Petersen, U. S. Patent 2,830,088 (1958).
10. M. Protiva and J. Jilek, Chem. Listy, 43, 257 (1949).
11. H. Arnold, N. Brock, E. Kuhas, and D. Lorenz, Arzneimittel Forsch., 4, 189 (1954).
12. L. Novak and M. Protiva, Coll. Czech. Chem. Commun., 24, 3966 (1959).
13. Anon., British Patent 942,152 (1963).
14. N. Sperber, D. Papa, E. Schwenk, and M. Sherlock, J. Amer. Chem. Soc., 71, 887 (1949).
15. K. Miescher and A. Marxer, U. S. Patent 2,411,664 (1946).
16. D. W. Adamson, British Patent 624,118 (1949).
17. L. Stein and E. Lindner, U. S. Patent 2,827,460 (1958).
18. R. Lorenz and H. Henecka, U. S. Patent 3,031,377 (1962).
19. C. H. Tilford, R. S. Shelton, and M. G. VanCampen, J. Amer. Chem. Soc., 70, 4001 (1948).
20. E. L. Schumann, M. G. VanCampen, and R. C. Pogge, U. S. Patent 2,804,422 (1957).
21. J. J. Denton, W. B. Neier, and V. A. Lawson, J. Amer. Chem. Soc., 71, 2053 (1949).
22. J. J. Denton, H. P. Schedl, V. A. Lawson, and W. B. Neier, J. Amer. Chem. Soc., 72, 3795 (1950).
23. W. Klavehn, U. S. Patent 2,789,110 (1957).
24. D. W. Adamson, P. A. Barrett, and S. Wilkinson, J. Chem. Soc., 52 (1951).
25. R. A. Pohland and H. R. Sullivan, J. Amer. Chem. Soc., 75, 4458 (1953).
26. R. A. Pohland and H. R. Sullivan, J. Amer. Chem. Soc., 77, 3400 (1955).
27. L. P. Kyrides and F. B. Zienty, U. S. Patent 2,634,293 (1953).
28. H. Hopff and C. S. Schuster, U. S. Patent 2,623,880 (1952).
29. R. Kallischnigg, U. S. Patent 2,683,714 (1954).
30. C. P. Huttrer, C. Djerassi, W. L. Beears, R. L. Mayer, and

C. R. Scholz, *J. Amer. Chem. Soc.*, *68*, 1999 (1946),
31. R. F. Phillips and E. M. Cates, U. S. Patent 2,607,778 (1952).
32. H. L. Friedman and A. V. Tolstouhov, U. S. Patent 2,465,865 (1949).
33. F. Leonard and U. V. Solmssen, *J. Amer. Chem. Soc.*, *70*, 2066 (1948).
34. A. Stoll and J. P. Bourguin, U. S. Patent 2,717,251 (1955),
35. R. C. Clapp, J. H. Clark, J. R. Vaughan, J. P. English, and G. W. Anderson, *J. Amer. Chem. Soc.*, *69*, 1549 (1947),
36. W. B. Martin, U. S. Patent 3,155,584 (1964),
37. F. C. Copp and D. Stephenson, U. S. Patent 3,038,004 (1962).
38. E. Walton and G. K. Ruffell, British Patent 973,882 (1964),
39. E. Rabald and H. Dimroth, German Patent 824,208 (1951).
40. J. F. Kerwin and G. E. Ullyott, U. S. Patent 2,599,000 (1952).
41. E. F. Godefroi, V. H. Maddox, H. Woods, and R. F. Parcell, U. S. Patent 3,097,136 (1963).
42. C. L. Stevens, I. L. Keundt, M. E. Munk, and M. D. Pillai, *J. Org. Chem.*, *30*, 2967 (1965).
43. R. Baltzly, R. DuBrevil, W. S. Ide, and E. B. Lorz, *J. Org. Chem.*, *14*, 775 (1949).
44. P. A. J. Janssen, U. S. Patent 2,882,271 (1959).
45. H. Morren, U. S. Patent 2,709,169 (1955).
46. H. Morren, U. S. Patent 2,899,436 (1959).
47. H. Morren, British Patent 817,231 (1959).

CHAPTER 5

Phenethyl and Phenylpropylamines

By the turn of the century the theory of chemical mediation of physiologic responses had gained some currency. There ensued in some laboratories an intense search for endogenous chemical modifiers of bodily responses. The first such agent to be isolated from mammalian tissue was the ubiquitous hormone, epinephrine—at that time known as adrenaline. This compound has played an important role in pharmacology as well as in medicinal chemistry. In the former, a study of this molecule has gone far towards elucidating the operation of the sympathetic nervous system. At the same time, chemistry based on the phenethylamine portion of epinephrine has served as a prototype for subsequent researches built around the theme of modifying an endogenous hormone in order both to modulate its biologic effects and to provide hormone antagonists. Current work on blockers of the β receptors in the sympathetic nervous system in order to provide drugs for treatment of diseases of the cardiovascular system suggests that the final word in this story remains to be written.

Breathing, heart action, control of blood pressure, glandular secretions, and related involuntary actions aimed at maintaining the organism are all under control of the autonomic nervous system which consists of the sympathetic (adrenergic) and parasympathetic (cholinergic) components. Signals that originate in the brain terminate at neurosecretory cells that release on neural stimulation a small amount of a specific hormone. In the case of the cholinergic system, this agent is acetylcholine. Of more direct concern, stimulation of a nerve in the adrenergic system results in release of norepinephrine. This amine, released at the appropriate site, interacts with a receptor on the target tissue; this interaction brings about the observed physiologic response (e.g., contraction of an involuntary muscle). This chain of action has been recently further detailed: norepinephrine is thought to stimulate the enzyme adenyl cyclase which in turn

causes formation of 3',5'-cyclic adenyl phosphate (3',5' cAMP).
This last may be the true intracellular messenger molecule.
      Epinephrine itself does find some use in clinical medicine.
The drug is used in order to increase blood pressure in cases of
circulatory collapse, and to relax the bronchial muscle in acute
asthma and in anaphylactic reactions. These activities follow
directly from the agent's physiologic role. The biogenetic precursor of epinephrine, norepinephrine, has activity in its own
right as a mediator of sympathetic nerve action. (An apocryphal
story has it that the term *nor* is derived from a label seen on a
bottle of a key primary amine in a laboratory in Germany: *N* ohne
R). This agent, too, is used to increase blood pressure.
      Friedel-Crafts acylation of catechol with chloroacetyl chlo-
ride gives the α-haloacetophenone *(2)*. Displacement of halogen
by methylamine *(3)* followed by catalytic reduction gives the
amino alcohol *(4)*. Resolution as the tartrate salt affords the
(-) isomer, *epinephrine (4)*. Substitution of ammonia as the base
in this sequence gives *norepinephrine*. Isolation of the (-) isomer affords *levarterenol (5)*.[1] Reaction of the same halide with
isopropylamine followed by reduction leads to *isoproterenol (6)*.
This agent, used as the racemate, is employed largely for its
effect in relieving bronchial spasms in asthmatics. It might be
noted in passing that *isoproterenol* occupies an important role in
pharmacology in the classification of sympathetic receptors.
      Removal of one of the aromatic hydroxyl groups gives an
agent similar to epinephrine in its effects but with longer dura-

tion of action. The largest use of this drug, however, depends
on its vasoconstricting action; *phenylephrine* is used extensively
as a nasal decongestant due to its ability to constrict the blood
vessels in mucous tissue on local application. In one published

synthesis, the benzyl ether of *m*-hydroxybenzaldehyde is subjected
to Reformatski reaction with ethyl bromacetate to give the hydroxyester *(8)*. Treatment with hydrazine leads to the hydrazide *(9)*.
This last is then rearranged to the intermediate isocyanate by
means of nitrous acid; intramolecular addition of the hydroxyl
group gives the oxazolidone *(11)*. The presence of an acyl group
on nitrogen avoids some of the difficulties often encountered in
attempts to monomethylate amines. In this case, the reaction is
accomplished by means of sodium hydride and methyl iodide. Treatment with strong acid cleaves both the heterocycle, which is in
effect a cyclic carbonate, and the benzyl ether. *Phenylephrine*
(13)[2] is thus obtained.

The isomer of *isoproterenol* in which both aromatic hydroxyl
groups are situated meta to the side chain also exhibits bronchiodilating activity. Oxidation of 3,5-dimethoxyacetophenone by
means of selenium dioxide affords the glyoxal derivative *(15)*.
Treatment of the aldehyde with isopropylamine in the presence of

hydrogen and Raney nickel leads to the amino alcohol *(16)*. (The
sequence probably proceeds by first addition of the amine to the
aldehyde. Reduction of either the carbinolamine or the Shiff
base derived therefrom gives an aminoketone; reduction of the ketone will afford the amino alcohol.) Removal of the ethereal
methyl groups by means of hydrogen bromide gives *metaproterenol*
(17).[3]

Condensation of the substituted phenethyl bromide, *18*, with
piperazine can be stopped at the monosubstituted amine *(19)*. Reaction of this amine with propiophenone and formaldehyde in a
Mannich reaction affords *eprazinone (20)*,[4] an antitussive agent.
Substitution of an aromatic heterocycle directly onto the

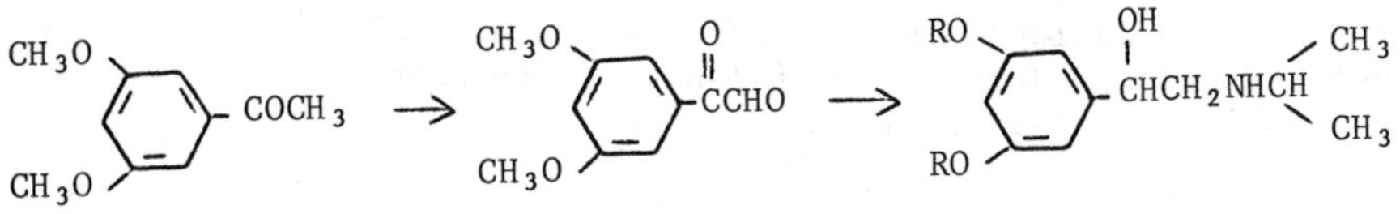

14 → 15 → 16, R=CH$_3$
                17, R=H

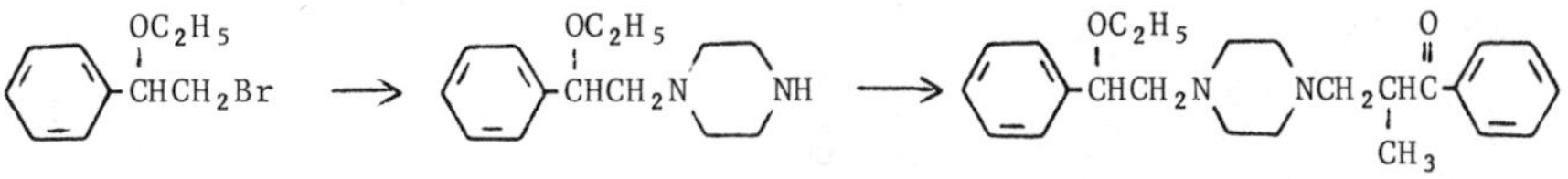

18 → 19 → 20

nitrogen of these amino alcohols markedly changes the activity of these compounds. Thus, the compound substituted by a 2-pyridyl group, *phenyramidol (21)*, finds use largely as a muscle relaxant. This agent is obtained by reaction of the anion from 2-aminopyridine with styrene oxide.[5]

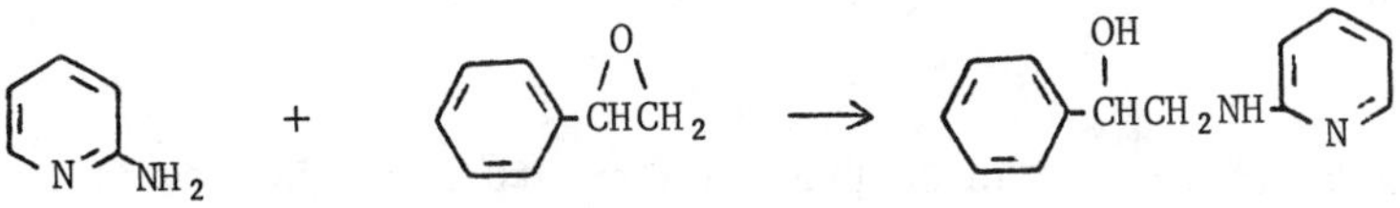

21

Replacement of the aromatic hydroxyl groups in isopreterenol by chlorine again causes a marked shift in biologic activity. This agent, *dichloroisoproterenol (25)*, was found to be an antagonist rather than agonist towards the β-sympathetic receptors. Although this first of a long series of so-called β blockers had limited practical utility, it pointed the way to the development of drugs with many applications in the control of some of the complications of heart disease such as arythmia, angina, and lately possibly hypertension. It is thought that these agents act by antagonizing the effects of endogenous epinephrine by competing with the latter for receptor sites.

Preparation of the prototype starts with the radical side chain bromination of dichloroacetophenone to give the bromoketone *(23)*. The carbonyl group is then reduced by means of sodium borohydride; displacement of halogen by means of isopropylamine

affords *dichloroisoproterenol (25)*.[6] Starting with 2-acetylnaph-
thalene, an analogous scheme affords *pronethanol (27)*, while the
methanesulfonyl derivative of *p*-aminoacetophenone *(28)* leads to
the β-blocker *soltalol (29)*.

22, X=H   24   25
23, X=Br

26   27

28   29

Alkylation on the carbon atom remote from the aromatic ring
affords a further series of useful medicinal agents. Although
these are by an large no longer frank sympathetic agonists, they
retain sufficient properties of the parent compounds to find use
as central nervous system stimulants, bronchiodilators, and when
appropriately modified, appetite-suppressing agents. The first
of these compounds, interestingly, derives from ancient Chinese
folk medicine. For millenia, the stems of various species of
Ephedra had been in use in China as mild stimulants. Investigation of the plant revealed the active compound to be the alkaloid,
ephedrine (31), whose structure proved to be remarkably close to
that of epinephrine (absolute configuration shown). In an interesting synthesis[7] of this agent, benzaldehyde is first fermented
with glucose and yeast. There results the addition of acetate in
a reaction similar to an acyloin condensation. As in almost all
enzymatically catalyzed reactions, the newly formed chiral center
is introduced stereospecifically—as it happens, in the desired
sense. Reductive amination is then employed to introduce the
nitrogen atom. If we assume for the moment that the Shiff base

is an intermediate in this reaction, this molecule can be depicted as in either A or B. It should be noted that each of these
contains an interaction between the hydroxyl and another medium-
sized group. In the case of A, however, this interaction is
mitigated by the possibility of chelation. The stereochemistry
of *ephedrine (31)* is in fact that obtained by reduction of A.

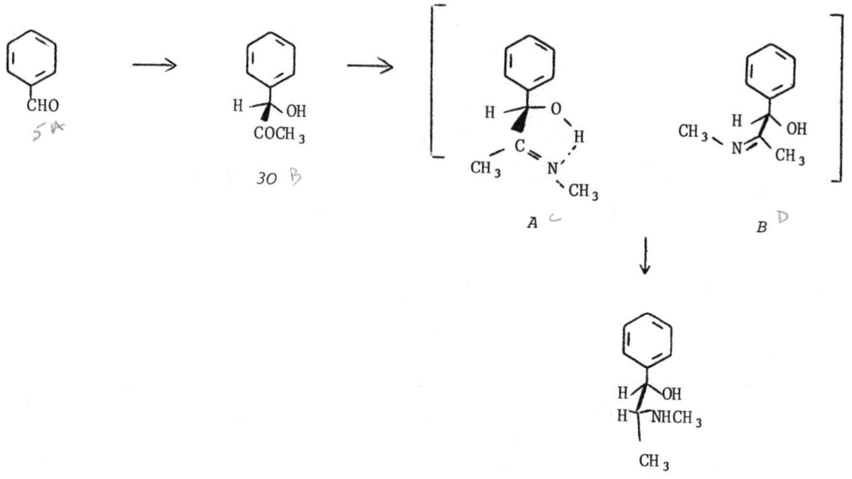

Mannich condensation of the primary amine corresponding to
ephedrine *(32)* with formaldehyde and *m*-methoxyacetophenone yields
oxyfedrine (33)[8]; this agent retains the vasodilating activity of
ephedrine and is in fact denoted a coronary vasodilating agent.

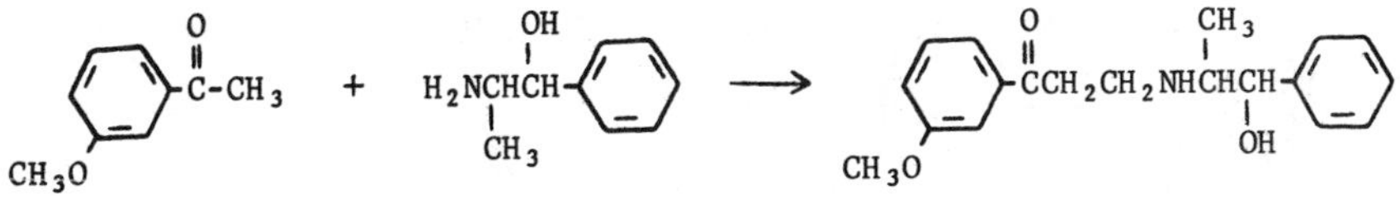

Addition of a hydroxyl group to the aromatic ring of ephedrine as well as changing the substitution on nitrogen leads to a
compound whose main activity is to raise blood pressure. Thus,
formation of the Shiff base of the *m*-hydroxy analog of *30* with
benzylamine *(34)*, followed by catalytic reduction, yields *metaraminol (35)*. When optically active hydroxyketone is employed in

the synthesis, steric induction again obtains; the drug is thus obtained directly as the (-) isomer.

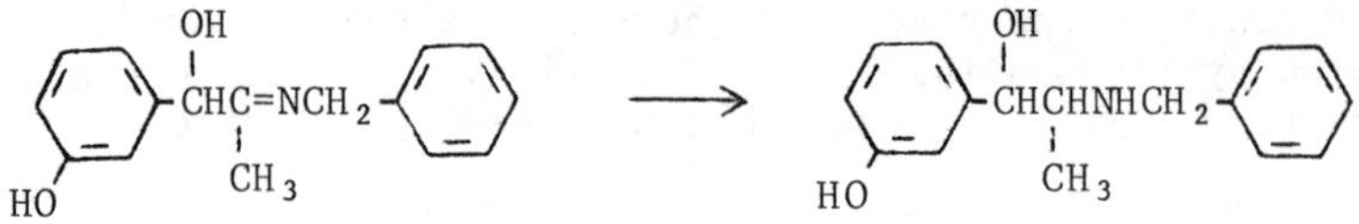

34   35

The homolog of epinephrine in this series is a potent vaso-constrictor. Reaction of 3,4-dimethoxypropiophenone with butyl nitrite leads to nitrosation at the α position *(36)*. Stepwise reduction of the nitrosoketone leads to the amino alcohol *(37)*. Removal of the methyl ether affords racemic *38*. Resolution of this last followed by separation of the (-) isomer gives *levonordefrine (38)*.[9]

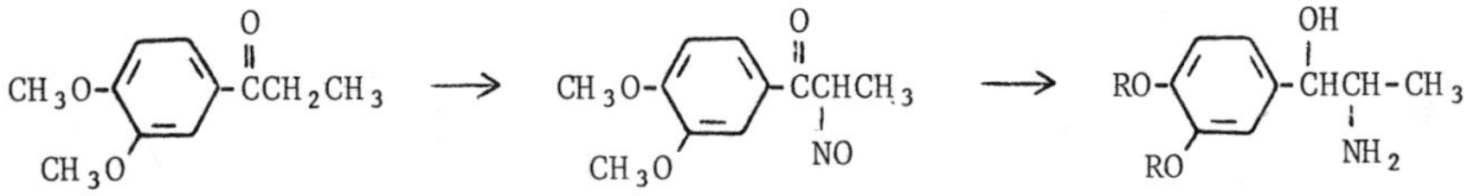

36

37, R=H
38, R=CH$_3$

A closely related compound bearing oxygen substitution at the 2 and 5 positions shows activity as a β-sympathetic blocking agent. Acylation of the dimethyl ether of hydroquinone with propionic anhydride gives the ketone *39*. This is then brominated to *40*. Displacement by halogen by tertiary butylamine *(41)* followed by reduction of the carbonyl group gives the amino alcohol. It is of note that the product, *butoxamine (42)*, is obtained exclusively as its erythro isomer.[10]

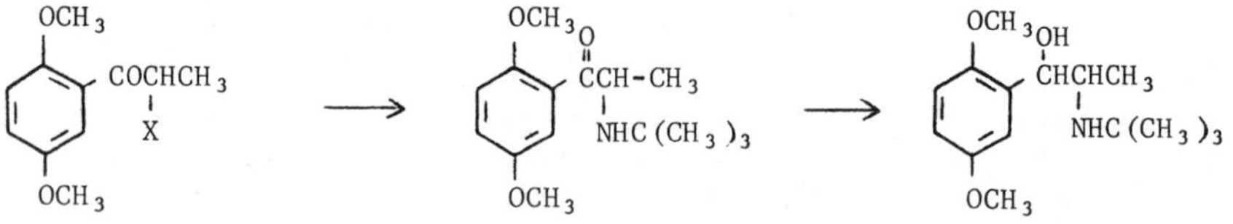

39, X=H
40, X=Br

41

42

Incorporation of a hydroxyl group at the para position of ephedrine in addition to alkylation of nitrogen with a somewhat more complex side chain gives a drug whose main action is that of a peripheral vasodilator. Reductive amination of phenoxyacetone *(43)* (obtained from sodium phenoxide and chloroacetone) with ammonia and hydrogen affords amine, *44.* Syntheses of the remaining fragment starts with the benzylation of p-hydroxypropiophenone *(45).* Bromination of the product gives *47.* Displacement of halogen by amine, *44,* leads to the aminoketone, *48.* The benzyl group is then removed by hydrogenolysis (note that the carbonyl is apparently untouched by this reaction). Reduction of the carbonyl group by means of sodium borohydride affords *isoxsuprine (50).*[11] The analog, *51,* in which the ether oxygen is replaced by methylene, has much the same activity as *50.* This compound, *nylidrin (51),* is obtainable by reduction of the Shiff base from p-hydroxyephedrine and 4-phenyl-2-butanone.

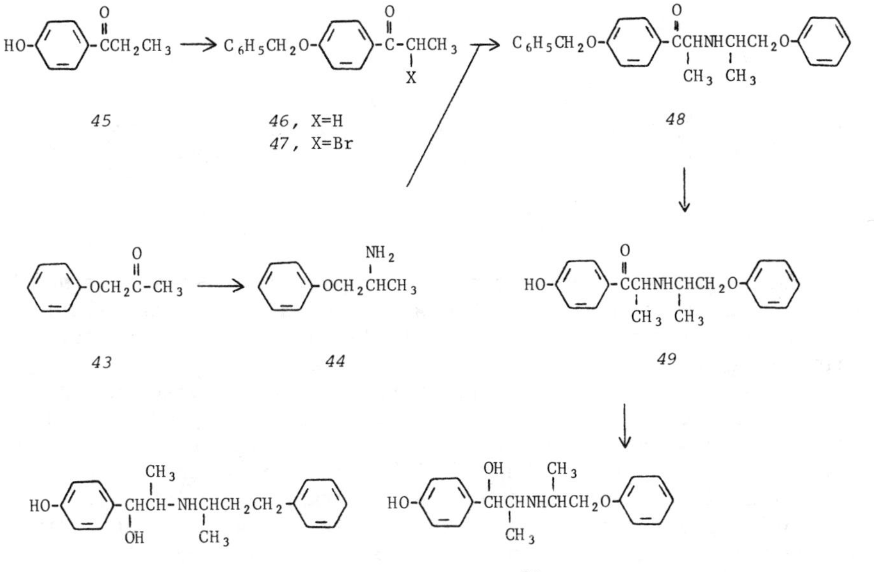

Omission of the side chain hydroxyl group from molecules based on epinephrine or ephedrine does not abolish the sympathomimetic activity of the resulting compounds. Many of these agents exert a considerable stimulant action on the central nervous system. As such, drugs in this class have been widely used—and abused—as agents to combat fatigue and drowsiness. These are the classical "pep pills." Many of these drugs, in addition, show decided activity in suppressing appetite. Much work has gone into structural modifications aimed at splitting the central nervous system stimulant activity from the antiappetite effect. This action, referred to an anorexic activity, is highly desirable in drugs aimed at combatting obesity.

The prototype, *amphetamine (52)*, is obtained by reductive amination of phenylacetone by means of ammonia and hydrogen.[12] Isolation of the (+) isomer by resolution gives *dextroamphetamine*, a somewhat more potent stimulant than the racemate.

Reduction of phenylacetone in the presence of methylamine rather than ammonia gives *methamphetamine (53)*, an agent similar in action to the primary amine. Alkylation of *53* with benzyl chloride affords the analog, *benzphetamine (54)*.[12]

Incorporation of a metatrifluoromethyl group often has a potentiating effect on the activity of drugs acting on the central nervous system. The preparation of the amphetamine analog bearing this substituent begins with formation of the oxime of *m*-trifluoromethylphenylacetone *(56)*. Catalytic reduction of that oxime gives the corresponding primary amine, *57*. Acylation of the amine with acetic anhydride *(58)*, followed by metal hydride reduction, affords *fenfluramine (58)*.[14]

Extension of the alkyl group on the carbon bearing the amine changes the pharmacologic profile. Reductive amination of *1*-phenylbutanone-2 *(60)* with pyrrolidine in formic acid gives *prolitane (61)*,[15] a central nervous system stimulant agent with antidepressant properties.

Incorporation of a phenolic hydroxyl group greatly attenu-

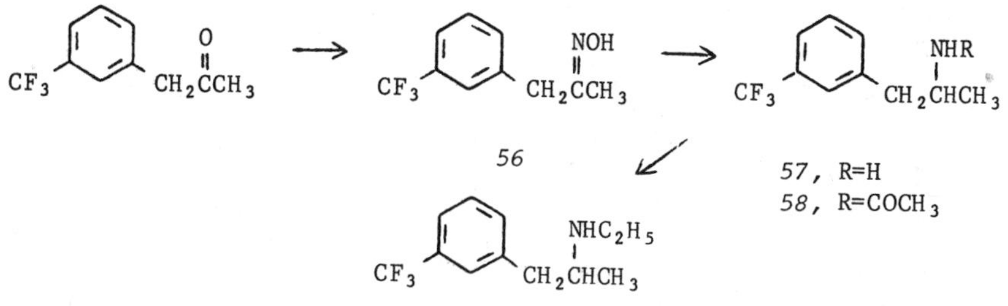

56

57, R=H
58, R=COCH₃

59

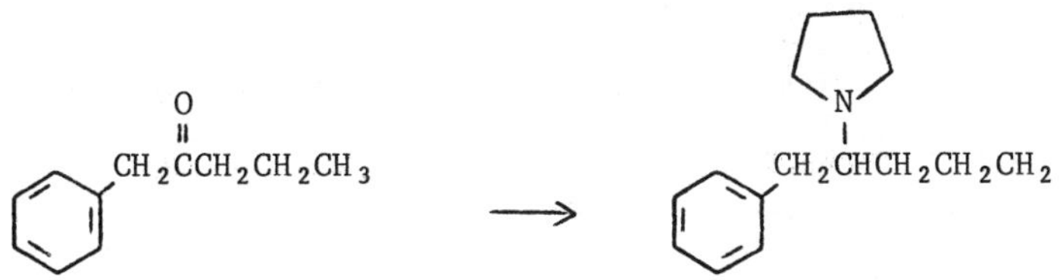

60

61

ates the CNS activity in the amphetamine series; there is obtained instead an agent that finds use in conjunction with atropine in opthalmology as a drug for dilating the pupil of the eye (midriatic). Condensation of anisaldehyde with nitroethane gives the nitrostyrene (62). Treatment with hydrogen chloride in the presence of iron hydrolyzes this enol nitro compound to the corresponding phenyl acetone (63). This last is then converted to the primary amine (64) by way of the oxime. Removal of the ethereal methyl group with strong acid gives *hydroxyamphetamine (65)*.[16]

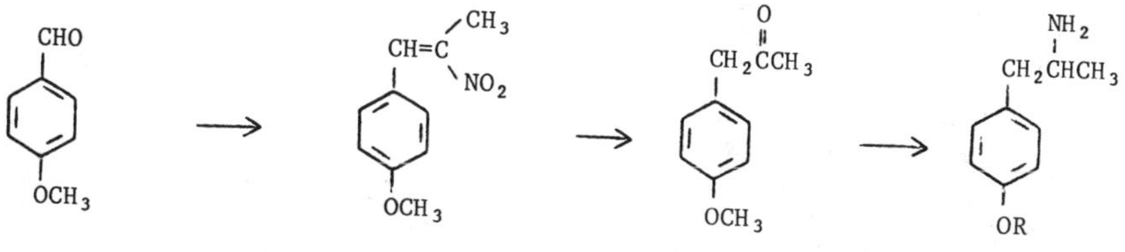

62

63

64, R=CH₃
65, R=H

Primary amines are often rapidly inactivited *in vitro* by one of several pathways for metabolic degration. One of the more

important of these—oxidative deamination—begins by oxidation of
the amine to the corresponding Shiff base. Amphetamine derivatives bearing alkyl groups of the α position should therefore
have longer duration of action by virtue of the lack of hydrogen
at the oxidizable position. The synthesis reported for one such
agent starts with the Friedel-Crafts acylation of benzene with
isobutyryl chloride to give ketone (66). Alkylation of the anion
of this ketone with benzyl chloride gives 67. Nonenolizable
ketones are known to cleave on treatment with strong base. Thus,
exposure of 67 to sodium amide gives the scision product, amide
68. Hoffmann degradation of the amide (68) by means of sodium
hypochlorite gives phentermine (69),[16] an agent used to control
obesity by suppression of appetite. Methylation of the primary
amine via its benzal derivative (70) affords mephentermine (71).[16]
Reaction of the methylated compound with chloroacetyl chloride
yields the halogenated amide, 72. Use of this compound to effect
a double alkylation on ethanolamine affords oxoethazine (73).[17]
This apparently small change alters the activity of the end product to that of a local anesthetic.

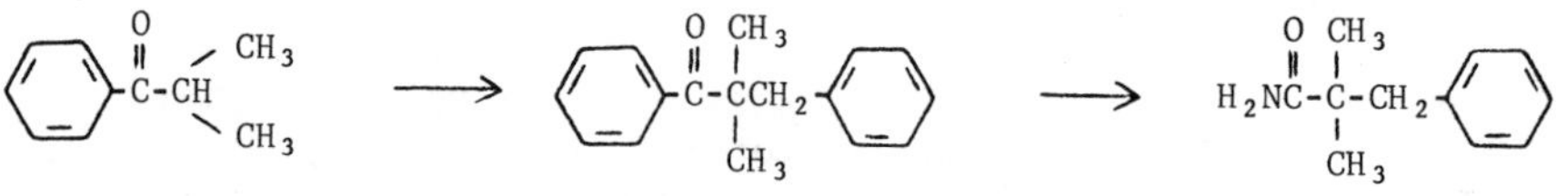

66

67

68

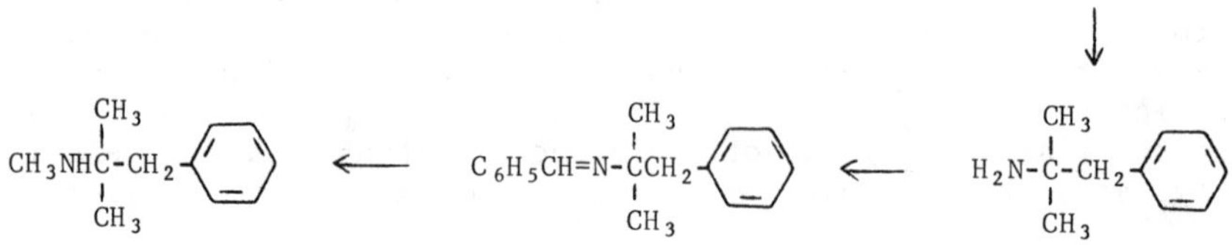

71

70

69

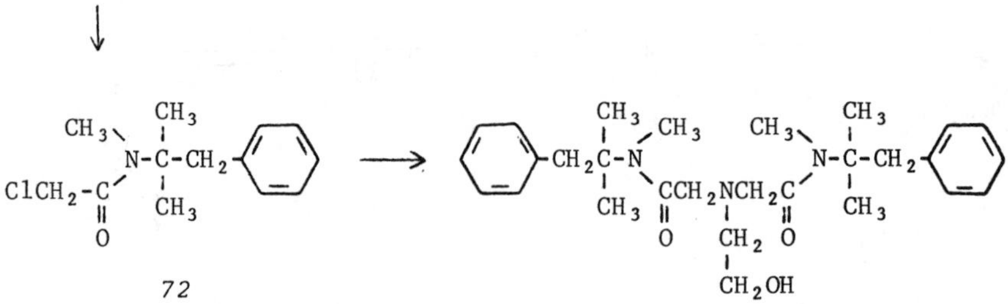

72

73

The p-chloro analog of *phentermine* has much the same activity as the parent compound, with perhaps a somewhat decreased activity on the central nervous system. Alkylation of p-chlorobenzyl chloride with the carbanion obtained from treatment of 2-nitropropane with strong base affords the compound containing the required carbon skeleton (74). Catalytic reduction of the nitro group yields *chlorphentermine* (75).[18]

$$
\begin{array}{c}
CH_3 \\
| \\
O_2N\text{-}CH \\
| \\
CH_3
\end{array}
\quad + \quad
ClCH_2\text{-}\!\!\bigcirc\!\!\text{-}Cl
\quad \longrightarrow \quad
\begin{array}{c}
CH_3 \\
| \\
O_2N\text{-}C\text{-}CH_2\text{-}\!\!\bigcirc\!\!\text{-}Cl \\
| \\
CH_3
\end{array}
\quad \longrightarrow \quad
\begin{array}{c}
CH_3 \\
| \\
H_2N\text{-}C\text{-}CH_2\text{-}\!\!\bigcirc\!\!\text{-}Cl \\
| \\
CH_3
\end{array}
$$

$$\qquad\qquad\qquad\qquad\qquad\qquad\qquad 74 \qquad\qquad\qquad\qquad\qquad 75$$

Incorporation of the phenethyl moiety into a carbocyclic ring was at first sight compatible with amphetamine-like activity. Clinical experience with one of these agents, *tranylcypromine (79)*, revealed the interesting fact that this drug in fact possessed considerable activity as a monamine oxidase inhibitor and as such was useful in the treatment of depression. Decomposition of ethyl diazoacetate in the presence of styrene affords a mixture of cyclopropanes in which the *trans* isomer predominates. Saponification gives acid 77. Conversion to the acid chloride followed by treatment with sodium azide leads to the isocyanate, *78*, via Curtius rearrangement. Saponification of *78* affords *tranylcypromine (79)*.[19]

$$
\bigcirc\!\!\text{-}CH\text{=}CH_2 \quad + \quad N_2CHCO_2C_2H_5 \quad \longrightarrow \quad \bigcirc\!\!\!-\!\!\triangledown^{\text{\tiny ...}CO_2R} \quad \longrightarrow \quad \bigcirc\!\!\!-\!\!\triangledown^{\text{\tiny ...}NCO}
$$

$$\qquad\qquad\qquad\qquad\qquad\qquad\qquad\qquad 76,\ R=C_2H_5 \qquad\qquad\qquad 78$$
$$\qquad\qquad\qquad\qquad\qquad\qquad\qquad\qquad 77,\ R=H$$

$$\downarrow$$

$$\bigcirc\!\!\!-\!\!\triangledown^{\text{\tiny ...}NH_2}$$

$$\qquad\qquad\qquad\qquad\qquad\qquad 79$$

A somewhat more complex application of this notion is represented by the CNS stimulant *fencamfine (83)*. Diels-Alder addition of cyclopentadiene and nitrostyrene affords the norbornene
derivative, *80*. Catalytic hydrogenation reduces both the remaining double bond and the nitro group *(81)*.[20] Condensation with
acetaldehyde gives the corresponding imine *(82)*; a second reduction step completes the synthesis of *fencamfine (83)*.[21]

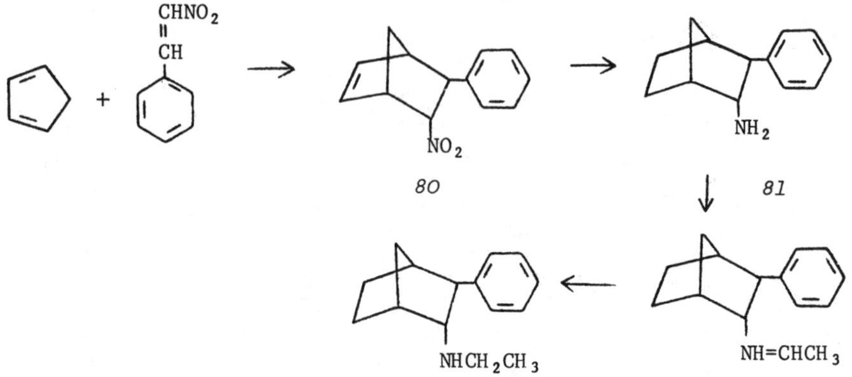

In the discussion of benzylamines, we have met medicinal
agents that owe their activity to some particular functionality
almost without reference to the structure of the rest of the
molecule. The hydrazine group is one such function in that it
frequently confers monamine oxidase-inhibiting activity to molecules containing that group. Such agents frequently find use as
antidepressants. Thus, reduction of the hydrazone of phenyl-
acetaldehyde *(84)* affords the antidepressant *phenelzine (85)*.
Similar treatment of the derivative of phenylacetone *(86)* gives
pheniprazine (87).[22]

84, R=H   85, R=H
86, R=CH₃   87, R=CH₃

Yet another example of a so-called pharmacophoric group is the biguanide functionality, a grouping associated with oral anti-diabetic activity (see the section on sulfonylureas for a fuller discussion of this activity). Condensation of 2-phenethylamine with dicyanamide affords directly the orally active hypoglycemic agent *phenformin (88)*.[23]

88

The structural constraints of the present chapter have suf-ficient breadth to allow inclusion of an antibiotic whose basic structural element is the phenethylamine moiety. The biologic activity, it need hardly be said, has little in common with the foregoing drugs. *Chloramphenicol*, the first of the broad-spectrum antibiotics, was initially isolated from cultures of various *Streptomyces* strains. Structural determination revealed the drug to be one of the simpler molecules among the antibiotics. This very simplicity made the agent amenable to preparation by total synthesis both in the laboratory and on commercial scale. The first published synthesis of *chloramphenicol*[24] establishes the carbon skeleton and the bulk of the functionality in the very first step. Thus, base-catalyzed condensation of benzaldehyde with nitroethanol affords the aldol product *(89)* as a mixture of stereoisomers. Catalytic reduction of the total mixture gives the aminodiol, *90*. At this point the threo isomer is separated and resolved into the optical isomers; the (-) isomer is then elabo-rated further. Acylation by means of dichloroacetyl chloride followed by treatment with base to remove o-acylated products affords the amide *(91)*. Acetylation by means of acetic anhydride protects the hydroxyl groups towards the conditions of the next step as their acetates *(92)*. The array of functionality present in this molecule is surprisingly stable to strong acid; nitration proceeds in a straightforward manner to afford the compound con-taining the nitro group in the para position. Treatment of this intermediate *(93)* with base removes the ester acetate groups to afford finally *chloramphenicol (94)*.

The apparently loose structural requirements for antihista-minic agents have already been alluded to. Thus, active compounds are obtained almost regardless of the nature of the atom that con-nects the side chain with the benzhydryl moiety. In fact, a methylene group, too, can also serve as the bridging group. Re-action of the aminoester, *95* (obtained by Michael addition of

$$\underset{}{\text{C}_6\text{H}_5}\text{-CHO} \quad + \quad \underset{\text{CH}_2\text{CH}_2\text{OH}}{\overset{\text{NO}_2}{|}} \quad \longrightarrow \quad \underset{}{\text{C}_6\text{H}_5}\text{-}\underset{\underset{\text{NO}_2}{|}}{\overset{\text{OH}}{\underset{|}{\text{CH}}}}\text{CHCH}_2\text{OH} \quad \longrightarrow \quad \underset{}{\text{C}_6\text{H}_5}\text{-}\underset{\underset{\text{NH}_2}{|}}{\overset{\text{OH}}{\underset{|}{\text{CH}}}}\text{CHCH}_2\text{OH}$$

$$\qquad\qquad\qquad\qquad\qquad\qquad\qquad\qquad\qquad\qquad\qquad 89 \qquad\qquad\qquad\qquad\qquad\qquad\qquad\qquad 90$$

$$\text{O}_2\text{N-}\underset{\underset{\text{NHCOCHCl}_2}{|}}{\overset{\overset{\text{OCOCH}_3}{|}}{\text{CHCHCH}_2\text{OCOCH}_3}} \quad \longleftarrow \quad \underset{\underset{\text{NHCOCHCl}_2}{|}}{\overset{\overset{\text{OCOCH}_3}{|}}{\text{CHCHCH}_2\text{OCOCH}_3}} \quad \longleftarrow \quad \underset{\underset{\text{NHCOCHCl}_2}{|}}{\overset{\overset{\text{OH}}{|}}{\text{CHCHCH}_2\text{OH}}}$$

$$\qquad\qquad 93 \qquad\qquad\qquad\qquad\qquad\qquad 92 \qquad\qquad\qquad\qquad\qquad\qquad 91$$

$$\text{O}_2\text{N-}\underset{\underset{\text{NHCOCHCl}_2}{|}}{\overset{\overset{\text{OH}}{|}}{\text{CHCHCH}_2\text{OH}}}$$

$$\qquad 94$$

piperidine to ethyl acrylate), with an excess of phenylmagnesium bromide gives the aminocarbinol, *96*. Hydrogenolysis of the *bis* benzylic hydroxyl group affords the antihistamine *fenpiprane* (*97*).[25]

$$\text{C}_2\text{H}_5\text{O}_2\text{CCH}_2\text{CH}_2\text{N} \quad \longrightarrow \quad (\text{C}_6\text{H}_5)_2\text{C}(\text{OH})\text{CH}_2\text{CH}_2\text{N} \quad \longrightarrow \quad (\text{C}_6\text{H}_5)_2\text{CHCH}_2\text{CH}_2\text{N}$$

$$\qquad 95 \qquad\qquad\qquad\qquad\qquad\qquad 96 \qquad\qquad\qquad\qquad\qquad\qquad 97$$

   Substitution of an amphetamine-like moiety on the nitrogen atom of this molecule markedly alters biologic activity; the product, *prenylamine* (*102*), exhibits coronary vasodilator activity. Knoevnagel condensation of benzaldehyde with malononitrile gives the unsaturated cyanoester (*98*). The second phenyl group is introduced by means of conjugate addition of phenylmagnesium bromide (*99*). Hydrolysis followed by decarboxylation affords the nitrile (*100*). Reduction of the nitrile to the corresponding amine (*101*) followed by alkylation with 2-chloro-1-phenylpropane yields *prenylamine* (*102*).[26]

   Substitution of a pyridyl ring for one of the benzene rings

of these agents gives compounds with somewhat enhanced activity, as in the case of the oxygen- and nitrogen-bridged antihistamines. Starting materials for the preparation of these agents are the same diarylcarbinols used to prepare the hetero-bridged compounds. These *(103)* are first converted to the respective chlorides *(104)* by treatment with thionyl chloride. Catalytic reduction gives

98 *99* *100*

102 *101*

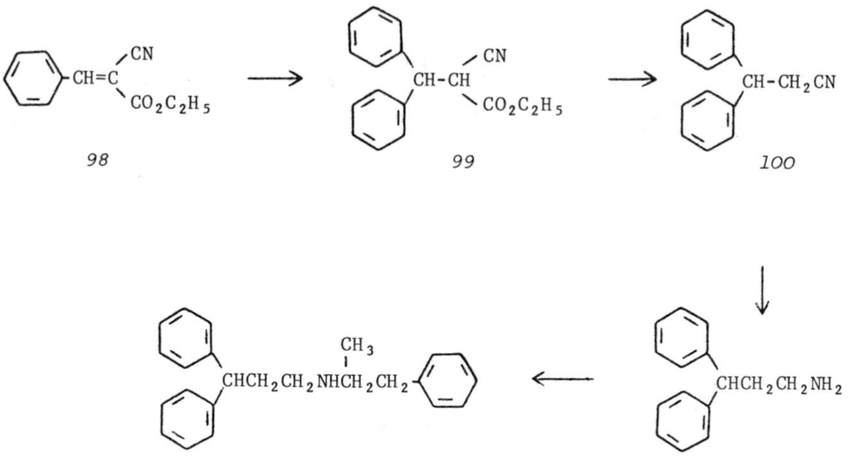

the diarylmethanes *(105)*. The protons on the methylene group of these compounds are sufficiently acidic to be removed by strong bases such as sodium amide or butyl lithium. Alkylation of the resulting carbanion with *N*-(2-chloroethyl)dimethylamine affords, respectively, *pheniramine (106)*,[27] *chlorpheniramine (107)*,[27] or *brompheniramine (108)*. Resolution of the two halogenated antihistamines revealed that the antihistaminic activity was associated with the (+) isomer; these are denoted *dexchlorpheniramine (+107)* and *dexbrompheniramine (+108)*.

103, X=H,Cl,Br
Y=OH
104, X=H,Cl,Br
Y=Cl

105, X=H,Cl,Br

106, X=H
107, X=Cl
108, X=Br

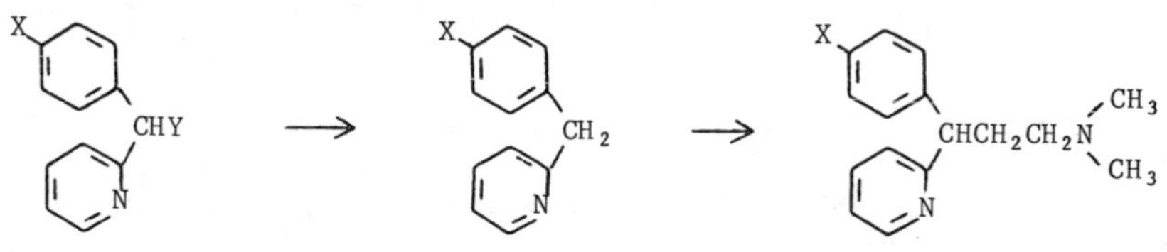

The presence of unsaturation in the side chain is also compatible with antihistaminic activity. Mannich condensation of p-chloroacetophenone with formaldehyde and pyrollidine affords the amino ketone, 109. Reaction with an organometallic reagent from 2-bromopyridine gives 110. Dehydration leads to triprolidine (111).[28]

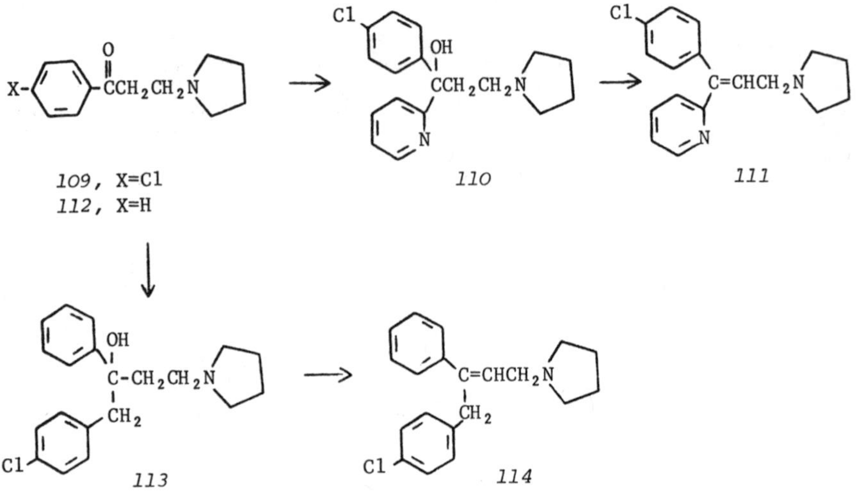

109, X=Cl
112, X=H

110

111

113

114

Reaction of the Mannich product (112) from acetophenone itself with the Grignard reagent from p-chlorobenzyl chloride gives the carbinol, 113. Dehydration in this case gives the antihistamine pyrrobutamine (114).[29] It is not immediately clear why dehydration does not occur in the other sense so as to afford the energetically more favored stilbene.

As a class, analgesics tend to be built around portions of the morphine molecule that, as a minimum, incorporate a piperidine ring. The detailed discussion of the chemistry and biologic activity of these compounds is therefore incorporated in that particular section of this volume. Biologic activity, however, cannot be always neatly categorized; there exists a series of narcotic analgesics whose structure and chemistry more nearly fit those of the phenylpropylamines than those of the morphine analogs. The curious reader is asked to skip to that section for a fuller discussion of the rationale for what follows. Suffice it to say for the present that extensive dissection of the morphine molecule evolved the so-called morphine rule. This holds that the structural elements necessary for analgesic activity are represented by the partial structure below.

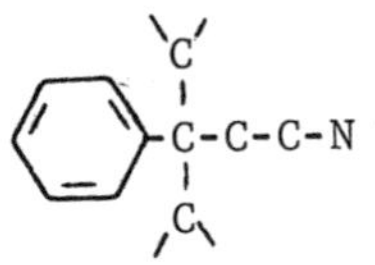

The first of the analgesic agents to incorporate the structural elements of this rule in an acyclic compound, *methadone*
(119), was developed in Germany during the Second World War.
Details as to structure and synthesis were available to the outside world immediately following the end of hostilities only in
the form of intelligence reports. Repetition of the putative
synthesis revealed that ambiguity existed as to the structure of
the final product. The key step, alkylation of the anion obtained
from diphenylacetonitrile with *N*-(2-chloropropyl)-dimethylamine,
in fact affords a pair of isomeric amines. One of these can be
imagined to arise by straightforward displacement of halogen by
the carbanion *(115)*. The isomeric amine is thought to arise by
internal cyclization of the haloamine to the aziridinium salt
(117) prior to alkylation. Attack on this charged species by the
carbanion at the center most susceptible to nucleophilic displacement will afford the isomeric amine *(116)*. Reaction of the abnor-
mal alkylation product *(116)* with ethylmagnesium bromide affords,
after hydrolysis of the intermediate imine, the compound that
turned out to be *methadone (119)*.[30] Similar treatment of the
expected alkylation product gives *isomethadone (118)*.[30]

Synthesis of the intermediate aminonitrile for *methadone* by
a régiospecific route served to confirm the structure. Alkylation of diphenylacetonitrile with 1-chloro-2-propanol affords the
alcohol, *120*, free of isomeric products (although it is possible
here, too, to imagine cyclization of the halide prior to alkylation). The hydroxyl is then converted to the bromide *(121)* by

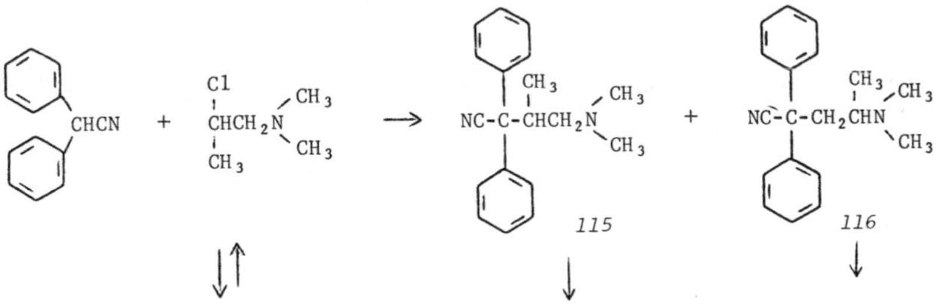

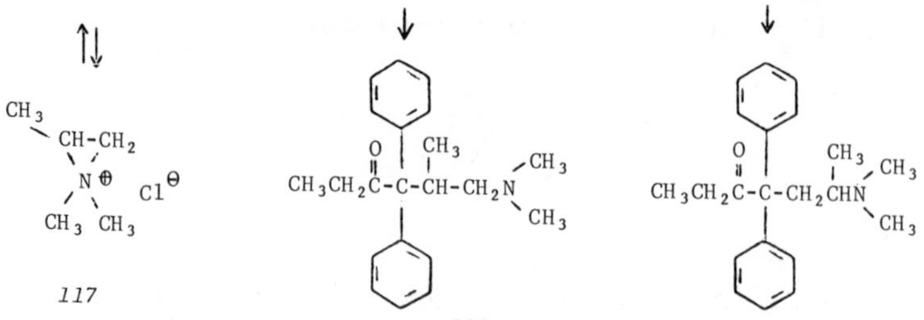

117

118

119

means of phosphorus tribromide. Displacement of halogen by means of dimethylamine completes the synthesis of an amine identical to 116.[31,32] In much the same vein, displacement of halogen on 121 with morpholine gives the amine, 122. Elaboration of the nitrile to the ketone affords the analgesic, *phenadoxone (123)*.[33] This same scheme, starting with displacement of halogen by piperidine, gives *dipipanone (125)*.[34]

Omission of the side chain methyl group also leads to an active analgesic, the potency of which is somewhat less than half that of the parent. Alkylation of the familiar nitrile with N-(2-chloroethyl)dimethylamine gives the amine, 126. Reaction with

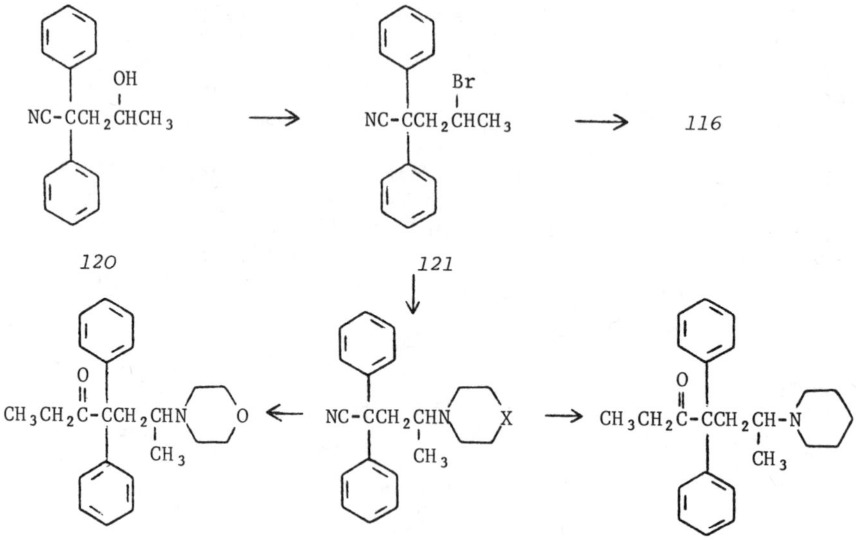

120

121

116

123

122, X=O
124, X=CH$_2$

125

ethyl Grignard reagent leads to *normethadone (127).*[35]

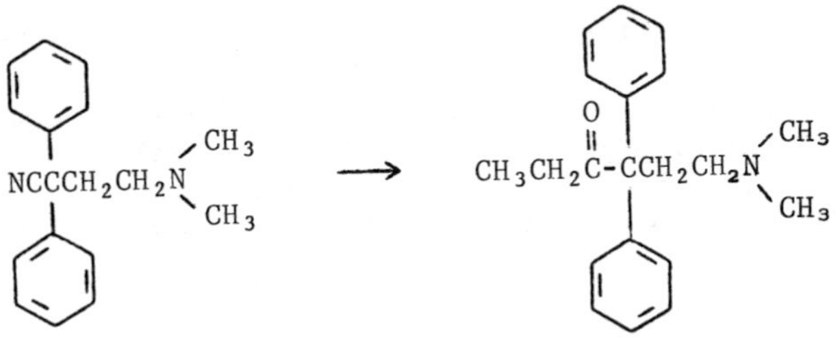

126   127

Modification of the ketonic side chain is also consistent with retention of analgesic activity. Thus, reduction of *methadone* with lithium aluminum hydride affords the alcohol, *128* (apparently as a single diastereomer). Acetylation gives *acetylmethadol (129).*[36]

Hydrolysis of the nitrile in *130* (obtained by an alkylation analogous to that used to prepare *126*) affords the acid, *131.* Esterification with ethanol affords the analgesic agent, *norpipanone (132).*[35]

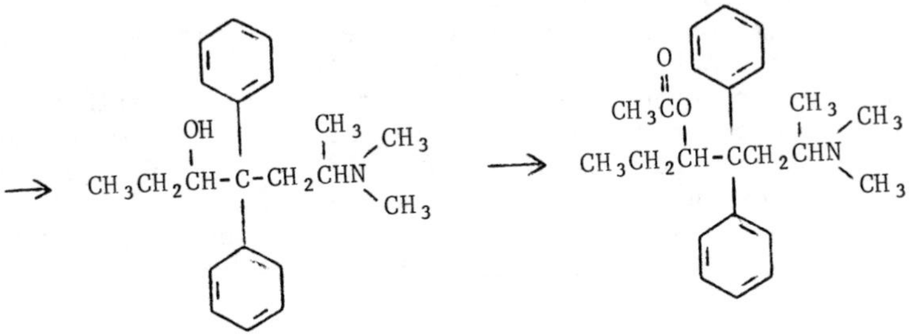

128   129

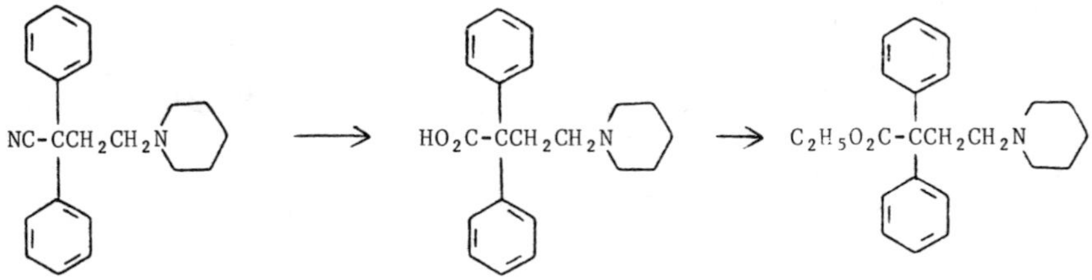

130   131   132

Replacement of the ketone by an amide leads to increased potency. Hydrolysis of nitrile, *133* (obtained by alkylation of diphenylacetonitrile with the morpholine analog of the chloroamine used in the original preparation of *methadone*), affords acid, *134*. Conversion to the acid chloride followed by reaction with pyrrolidine affords *racemoramide (135)*.[37] Separation of the (+) isomer by optical resolution gives *dextromoramide*, an analgesic an order of magnitude more potent than *methadone*.

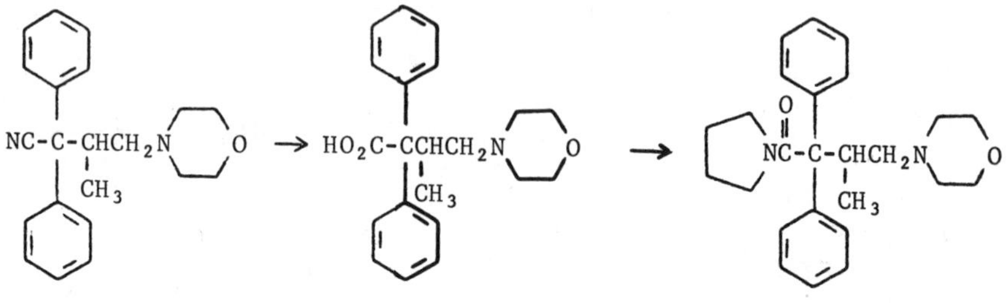

NC-C-CHCH2N
O
CH3
HO2C-CCHCH2N
O
CH3
O
NC-C-CHCH2N
O
CH3

133 *134* *135*

Replacement of one of the phenyl groups by an alkyl group of similar bulk, on the other hand, alters the biologic activity in this series. Alkylation of phenylacetonitrile with isopropyl bromide affords the substituted nitrile, *136*. Treatment of the anion prepared from *136* with strong base with 2-dimethylamino-1-chloropropane gives *isoaminile (137)*.[38] It is of note that alkylation of this halide, isomeric with that used in the early *methadone* synthesis, is apparently unaccompanied by isomer formation. *Isoaminile* is an agent with antitussive activity.

CH2CN
CH3
CH3
CH
CHCN
CH3
CH3
CH
CH3
NC-CCH2CHN
CH3
CH3

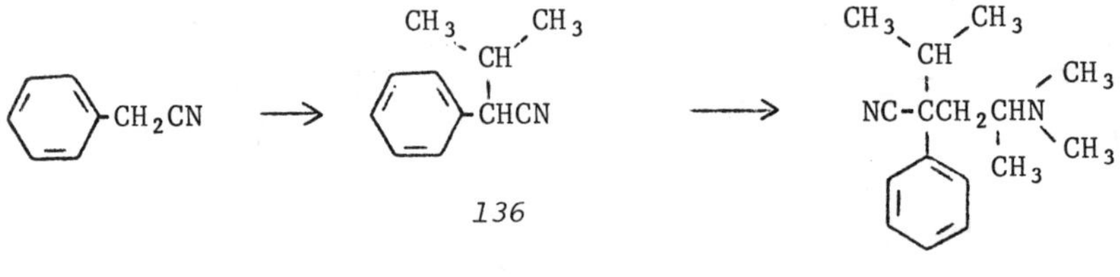

136

137

REFERENCES

1. H. Loewe, *Arzneimittel Forsch.*, *4*, 586 (1954).
2. E. D. Bergman and M. Sulzbacher, *J. Org. Chem.*, *16*, 84 (1951).
3. Anon. Belgian Patent 611,502 (1961).
4. M. Constantin, J. F. Pognat, and G. Streichenbrecher, *Arnzeimittel Forsch.*, *24*, 1793 (1974).
5. A. P. Gray, D. E. Heitmeier, and E. E. Spinner, *J. Amer. Chem. Soc.*, *81*, 4351 (1959).
6. J. Mills, U. S. Patent 2,938,921 (1960).
7. G. P. Menshikov and M. M. Rubenstein, *J. Gen. Chem. U. S. S. R.*, *13*, 801 (1943).
8. K. Thiele, U. S. Patent 3,225,095 (1965).
9. W. H. Hartung, J. C. Munch, E. Miller, and F. Crossley, *J. Amer. Chem. Soc.*, *53*, 4149 (1939).
10. Anon. Netherlands Patent Application 6,407,885 (1963).
11. H. D. Moed and J. VanDijk, *Rec. Trav. Chim. Pays Bas*, *75*, 1215 (1956).
12. W. H. Hartung and J. C. Munch, *J. Amer. Chem. Soc.*, *53*, 1875 (1931).
13. R. V. Heinzelman and B. D. Aspergren, U. S. Patent 2,789,138 (1957).
14. L. Bereyi, P. Hugon, J. C. LeDouarec, and H. Schmitt, French Patent M1658 (1963).
15. E. Seeger and A. Kottler, German Patent 1,093,799 (1960).
16. L. L. Abell, W. R. Bruce, and J. Seifter, U. S. Patent 2,590,079 (1952).
17. J. Seifter, R. S. Hanslick, and M. E. Freed, U. S. Patent 2,780,646 (1957).
18. G. G. Bachman, H. B. Haas, and G. O. Platau, *J. Amer. Chem. Soc.*, *76*, 3972 (1954).
19. A. Burger and W. L. Yost, *J. Amer. Chem. Soc.*, *70*, 2198 (1948).
20. G. I. Poos, J. Kleis, R. R. Wittekind, and J. Roseneau, *J. Org. Chem.*, *26*, 4898 (1961).
21. J. Thesing, G. Seitz, R. Hotory, and S. Sommer, German Patent 1,110,159 (1961).
22. J. H. Biel, A. E. Drukker, T. F. Mitchell, E. P. Sprengler, P. A. Nunfer, A. C. Conway, and A. Horita, *J. Amer. Chem. Soc.*, *81*, 2805 (1959).
23. S. L. Shapiro, V. A. Parrino, and L. Freedman, *J. Amer. Chem. Soc.*, *81*, 2220 (1959).
24. J. Controulis, M. C. Rebstock, and H. M. Crooks., Jr., *J. Amer. Chem. Soc.*, *71*, 2463 (1949).
25. A. W. Ruddy and J. S. Buckley, *J. Amer. Chem. Soc.*, *72*, 718

(1950).

26. G. Erhart, *Arch. Pharm.*, *295*, 196 (1962).

27. N. Sperber and D. Papa, U. S. Patent 2,567,245 (1951).

28. D. W. Adamson, P. A. Barrett, J. W. Billinghurst, and T. S. G. Jones, *J. Chem. Soc.*, 312 (1958).

29. J. Mills, U. S. Patent 2,655,509 (1953).

30. E. M. Schultz, C. M. Robb, and J. M. Sprague, *J. Amer. Chem. Soc.*, *69*, 188 (1947).

31. E. M. Schultz, C. M. Robb, and J. M. Sprague, *J. Amer. Chem. Soc.*, *69*, 2454 (1947).

32. N. R. Easton, J. H. Gardner, and J. R. Stevens, *J. Amer. Chem. Soc.*, *69*, 2941 (1947).

33. M. Bockmuhl and G. Erhart, *Ann.*, *561*, 52 (1948).

34. P. Ofner and E. Walton, *J. Chem. Soc.*, 2158 (1950).

35. D. J. Dupre, J. Elks, B. A. Hems, K. N. Speyer, and R. M. Evans, *J. Chem. Soc.*, 500 (1949).

36. M. E. Speeter, W. M. Byrd, L. C. Cheney, and S. S. Binkley, *J. Amer. Chem. Soc.*, *71*, 57 (1949).

37. P. A. J. Janssen, *J. Amer. Chem. Soc.*, *78*, 3862 (1956).

38. W. Stuhmer and S. Funke, U. S. Patent 2,934,557 (1960).

CHAPTER 6

Arylacetic and
Arylpropionic Acids

Organic compounds that share some feature of structure or functionality often exhibit similar biologic effects. Thus, although
the arylalkylamines differ in pharmacologic profile, their effects
tend to be those which are mediated via the autonomic or central
nervous system. The arylacetic and arylpropionic acids by contrast show no such common targets. It is of note in this connection that, unlike the corresponding amines, these acids find few
structural counterparts among endogenous mammalian hormones.

As every sufferer of a toothache knows, inflammation and pain
often go together. Specific drugs are available to treat each of
these; the steroid antiinflammatory agents will deal very specifically with inflammation, while the narcotic analgesics will go
far towards obviating pain. There is often, however, an under-
standable reluctance to rely on such potent drugs for treatment
of trivial, though annoying, inflammation and pain. One of the
oldest drugs in the modern armamentarium, *aspirin*, interestingly
enough, is effective in the treatment of both inflammation and
minor pain (in the words of the immortal ads: minor aches, neu-
ralgia, and neuritis). A recently discovered use of this drug
ironically pointed out one of its major shortcomings. *Aspirin*
can be used with some effect for the treatment of the pain and
inflammation attendant to arthritis. Its low potency, however,
necessitates its administration in gram quantities. Many individuals unfortunately find that their stomachs are intolerant of
such large quantities of *aspirin*. While the steroids are quite
effective for treatment of arthritis, clinicians usually prefer
to reserve these drugs for more serious cases because of the
potential side effects. An interesting sidelight is the observation that most of the known antiinflammatory drugs, steroids or
not, show a tendency to exacerbate existing stomach ulcers and
perhaps even precipitate these. There exists, therefore, a real
place in medicine for a more potent aspirin-like compound with

reduced side effects.
     Acetylation of isopropylbenzene gives the corresponding ace-
tophenone (2). Wilgerodt oxidation of the ketone leads to the
corresponding acetic acid, ibufenac (3),[1] an antiinflammatory
agent with somewhat greater potency than aspirin. In one of several processes for the preparation of the methylated analog (5),
the acetophenone is converted to its cyanohydrin (4). Heating
with hydrogen iodide and red phosphorus reduces the benzylic
hydroxyl while simultaneously effecting hydrolysis of the nitrile.
There is thus obtained ibuprofen (5),[1] an agent with about twice
the potency of the prototype (3).

     Friedel-Crafts acylation of biphenyl with acetyl chloride
gives the ketone (6). Rearrangement to the acetic acid is again
achieved by means of the Wilgerodt reaction. Esterification
followed by alkylation of the anion obtained by treatment of the
ester (7) with strong base with ethyl iodide affords the alkylated
intermediate (8). Saponification gives the analgesic namoxyrate
(9). An analogous scheme applied to the 3-fluorobiphenyl derivative (10) affords first the acetic ester (11). In order to circumvent the complications often involved in achieving monoalkylation of such compounds, the ester is first converted to the malonate (12) by means of sodium ethoxide and ethyl carbonate. Alkylation of 12 can, in fact, afford only the monoethyl compound (13).
Acid hydrolysis of the esters with concomitant decarboxylation
gives the potent antiinflammatory agent, flubiprofen (14).[2]
     In a similar scheme, acylation of 2-methoxynaphthalene gives
ketone, 15. This is then converted to the acetic acid by the
Wilgerodt reaction. Esterification, alkylation of the carbanion
(sodium hydride; methyl iodide), and finally saponification
affords naproxen (17).[3] The intense current effort on nonsteroid
antiinflammatory agents and acrylacetic acids in particular make

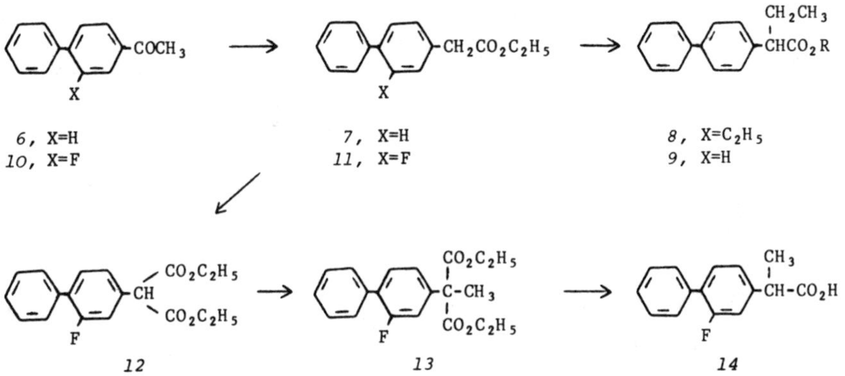

6, X=H
10, X=F

7, X=H
11, X=F

8, X=C$_2$H$_5$
9, X=H

12

13

14

it probable that the above are but the forerunners of an extensive
series of clinical agents.

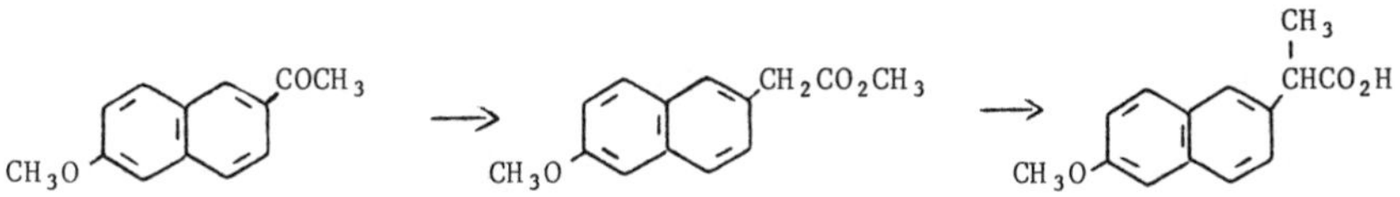

15

16

17

A compound closely related to *naproxen* has radically different pharmacologic properties; *methallenestril (23)* is in fact a
synthetic estrogen. At the time clinicians first started to fore-
see a use for compounds with estrogenic effects, naturally occurring compounds such as estrone or estradiol were all but unavail-
able in any quantity. Many groups thus undertook a systematic
search for simplified structures that would possess the desired
hormonal property. One such approach was based on the known
estrogenic activity of doisynolic acid *(18)*, a degradation product from alkali fusion of estrone.[4] Condensation of the substituted propionaphthone *(19)* with the brominated isobutyrate ester
(20) in a Reformatski reaction gives a hydroxyester *(21)* whose
carbon skeleton mimics that of the degradation product. Saponification followed by dehydration gives the unsaturated acid *(22)*.
Hydrogenation completes the synthesis of *methallenestril (23)*.[5]
Attachment of a group containing a basic nitrogen atom to
the phenylacetic acid side chain affords a drug that has found
use as a mild stimulant. (Careful examination of the structure

19 *20* *21* *22* *23* *18*

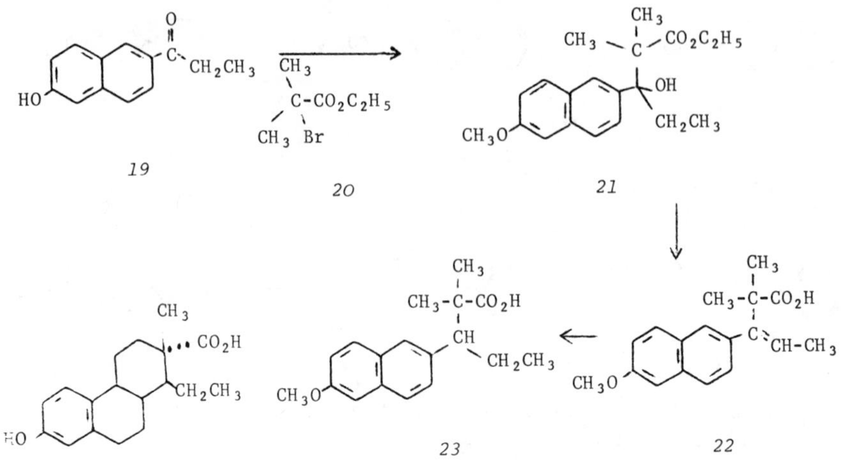

will reveal a structural fragment related to amphetamine.) This drug, *methyl phenidate*, has gained some fame under the trade name of Ritalin® for its paradoxical use as a means for controlling hyperkinetic children. Alkylation of the carbanion obtained from phenylacetonitrile with 2-chloropyridine gives the diarylacetonitrile *(24)*. Treatment with sulfuric acid gives partial hydrolysis to the amide *(25)*. Reflux in methanol affords the corresponding ester *(26)*. Catalytic hydrogenation over platinum results in reduction of the heterocyclic ring to afford *methyl phenidate (27)*.[6]

24

25, $R=NH_2$
26, $R=OCH_3$

27

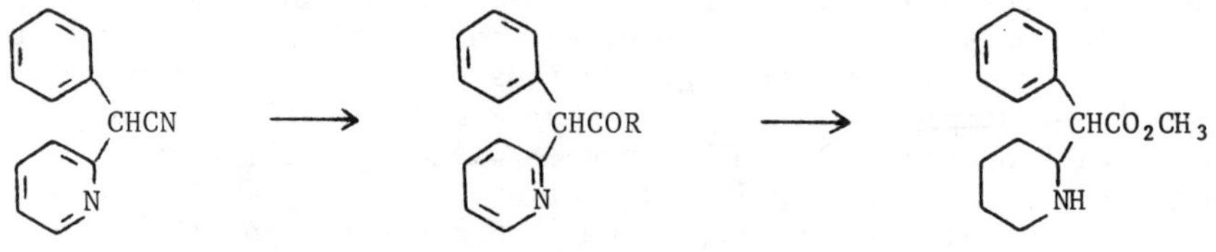

Incorporation of the benzylic carbon of phenylacetic acid into a cyclohexane ring affords an agent whose activity is closely related to that of the narcotic analgesics. This activity is particularly noteworthy for the fact that this structure repre-

sents a departure from the "morphine rule" cited earlier. Formation of the dimethylamine enamine from crotonaldehyde affords the
basically substituted butadiene (28). Diels-Alder condensation
with the unsaturated ester (29) gives a pair of isomeric 1:1
adducts in the ratio of 3:1. The predominant product (30) is
that which results from that transition state that involves the
fewest steric interactions (A). [The transition state to form
the minor isomer (B) involves interaction of the relatively bulky
phenyl and dimethylamino group, while the same intermediate towards the major product involves the smaller carbethoxy group in
the same interaction.] The major product, *tilidine* (30),[7] is an
analgesic effective against severe pain.

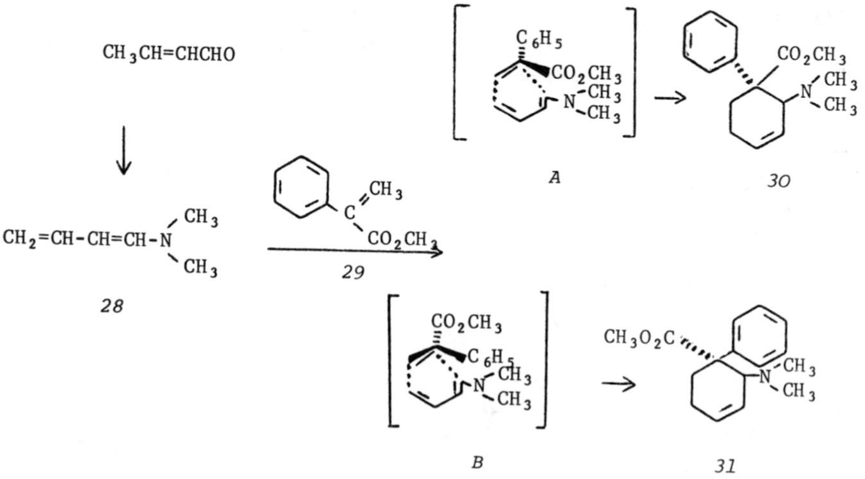

The natural product, *atropine* (32), can be regarded as a
highly substituted ester of phenylacetic acid and an amino alcohol. Although the agent is used clinically, chiefly as a midriatic agent, the molecule possesses a host of other biologic activities. The drug has antispasmodic, bronchiodilating, and antisecretory activity. Atropine thus provided an attractive starting point for efforts to synthesize agents that would show some
of the above actions.

In fact, esters of amino alcohols and 2,2-disubstituted
phenylacetic acids show useful antitussive activity; the mechanism of action may include bronchiodilation. Double alkylation
of the anion of phenylacetonitrile with 1,4-dibromobutane gives
the cyclopentane-substituted derivative (33). Saponification

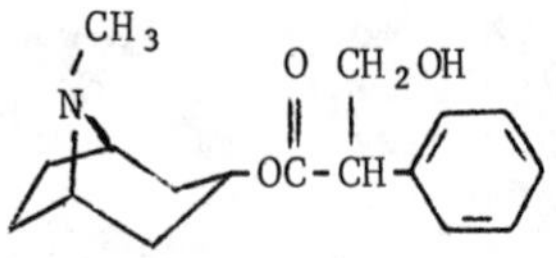

32

followed by treatment with thionyl chloride affords the acid
chloride (35). Condensation with diethylaminoethanol gives car-
amiphene (36).[8] Displacement of one of the halogens of β,β-di-
chloroethyl ether by means of the sodium salt from 34 gives the
haloester (37). The action of dimethylamine on this intermediate
affords carbetapentane (39).[9] Alkylation of phenylacetonitrile
with an excess of ethyl iodide gives the substituted nitrile (39).
A sequence similar to that used in going from 34 to 38 gives the
antitussive, oxeladine (40).[10]

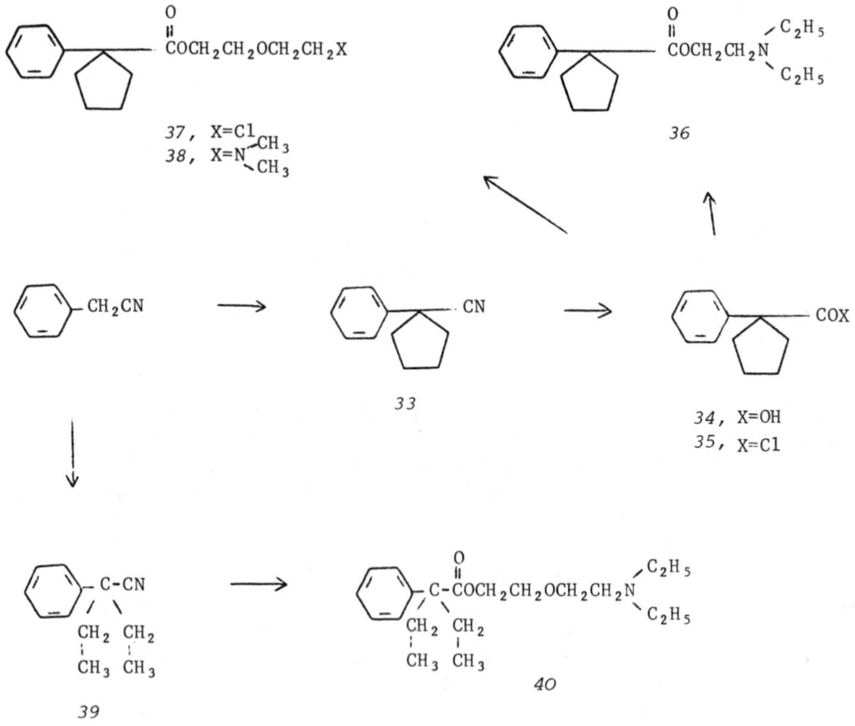

37, X=Cl
38, X=N$<$CH$_3$ CH$_3$

36

33

34, X=OH
35, X=Cl

39

40

Esters of diphenylacetic acids with derivatives of ethanolamine show mainly the antispasmodic component of the atropine
complex of biologic activities. As such they find use in treatment of the resolution of various spastic conditions such as, for
example, gastrointestinal spasms. The prototype in this series,
adiphenine (47), is obtained by treatment of diphenyl acetyl chloride with diethylaminoethanol. A somewhat more complex basic
side chain is accessible by an interesting rearrangement. Reductive amination of furfural *(42)* results in reduction of the heterocyclic ring as well and formation of the aminomethyltetrahydro-
furan *(43)*. Treatment of this ether with hydrogen bromide in
acetic acid leads to the hydroxypiperidine *(45)*, possibly by the
intermediacy of a carbonium ion such as 44. Acylation of the
alcohol with diphenylacetyl chloride gives *piperidolate (46)*.[11]

The presence of an additional alkyl group on the benzylic
carbon is consistent with antispasmodic activity in this series.
Alkylation of ethyl diphenyl acetate by means of sodium amide and
methyl iodide followed by saponification gives the acid, *49*.
Esterification with diethylaminoethanol affords *aprophen (50)*.[12]

The second aromatic ring can, interestingly, be replaced by
a cycloalkyl group. Thus, treatment of diethyl phenylmalonate
with 1,2-dibromocyclopentane in the presence of strong base
affords the cyclopentenyl derivative *(52)*. [The fact that the
olefin ends up in the relatively unfavored position suggests that
the initial step in this reaction may be elimination of hydrogen

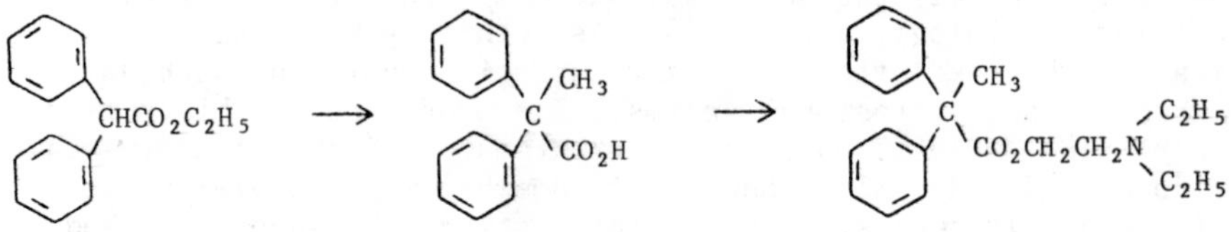

48   49   50

bromide to give the allylic halide (53); this last would suffer
displacement to lead to the observed olefin.] Hydrolysis of the
ester groups with concomitant decarboxylation gives the phenylacetic acid (54). Esterification of the acid with 2-(N-pyrroli-
dino)ethanol via its acid chloride affords the antispasmodic
agent cyclopyrazolate (55).[13]

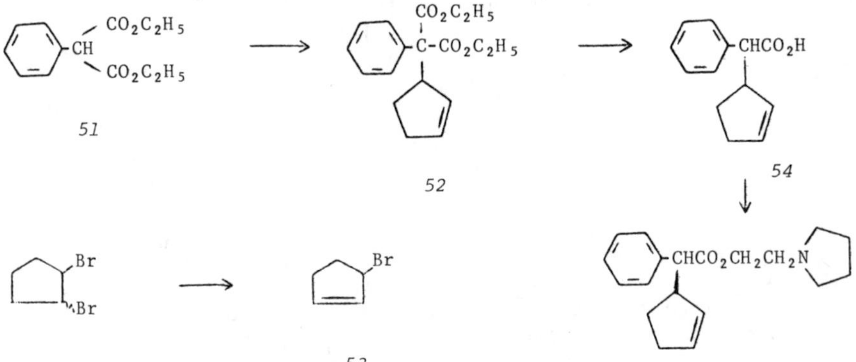

51

52

54

53

55

Treatment of the sodium salt of phenylacetic acid with iso-
propylmagnesium bromide affords the so-called Ivanov reagent, a
formally doubly charged species whose anionic moiety is often
formulated as 56. This dianion undergoes aldol condensation with
cyclopentanone to give the corresponding hydroxyacid (57). Alkylation of the salt of the acid with N-(2-chloroethyl)dimethylamine
gives cyclopentolate (58).[14] This agent has atropine-like activity with the midriatic component predominating.

A rather more complex amino alcohol side chain is accessible
by a variation of the Mannich reaction. Taking advantage of the
acidic proton in acetylenes, propargyl acetate (61) is condensed
with formaldehyde and dimethylamine to give the acetylated amino

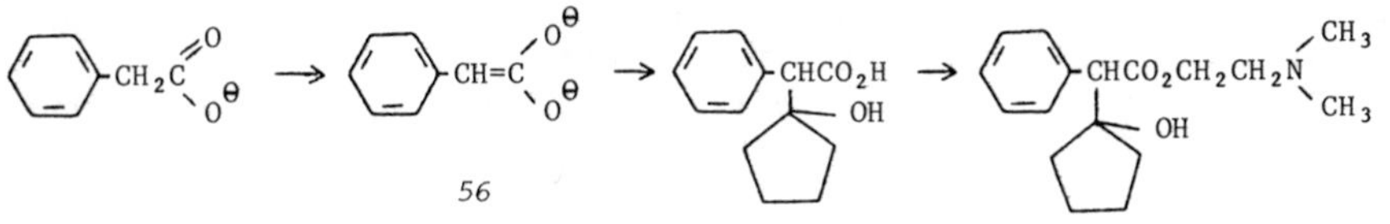

56

57   58

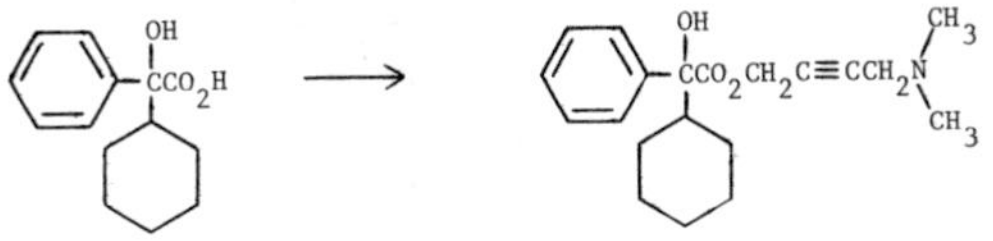

59   60

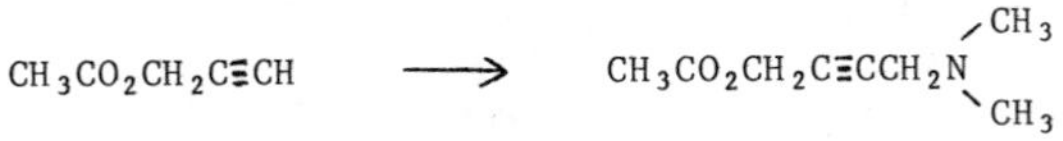

$CH_3CO_2CH_2C\equiv CH \longrightarrow CH_3CO_2CH_2C\equiv CCH_2N\begin{smallmatrix}CH_3\\CH_3\end{smallmatrix}$

61   62

alcohol *(62)*. Ester interchange of this with the product from partial hydrogenation of benzilic acid *(59)*, gives the anti-spasmodic agent, *oxybutynin (60)*.[15]

Incorporation of a hydroxyl group directly onto the benzylic carbon of the diphenylacetic acid again changes the pharmacologic profile of the compound; although the drug retains the anticho-linergic activity of atropine, its main use has been in the treatment of anxiety and tension. Oxidation of benzoin *(63)* with potassium bromate leads to benzilic acid *(64)* by the well-known rearrangement of the intermediate, benzil. Esterification by means of diethylaminoethanol affords *benactizine (65)*.[16]

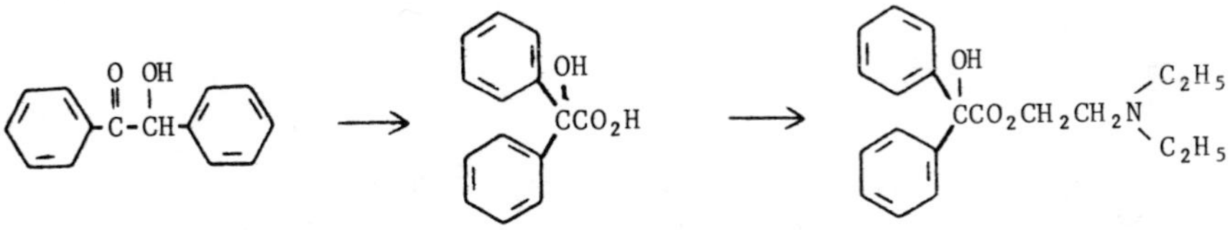

63   64   65

Peripheral vascular disease, often one of the sequelia of atherosclerosis, is characterized by markedly decreased circula-

tion in the extremities. The course of the disease is frequently
punctuated by acute episodes in which the blood vessels undergo
spastic closure. One of the few nonnitrogen-containing phenylacetic acid derivatives to show antispasmodic activity has found
some use in the treatment of this disease. The drug, *cyclandelate (67)*,[17] is obtained by esterification of mandelic acid *(66)*
with 3,5,5-trimethylcyclohexanol.

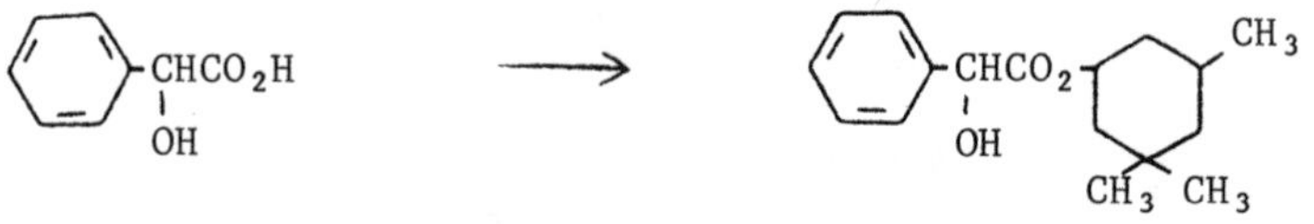

66   67

The placement of a nitrogen atom directly on the benzilic
carbon atom is apparently consistent with antispasmodic activity.
Esterification of 2(*N*-piperidyl)ethanol by means of chloroacyl
chloride *(68)* gives the basic ester *(69)*. Displacement of the
remaining halogen by piperidine gives *dipiproverin (70)*.[18]

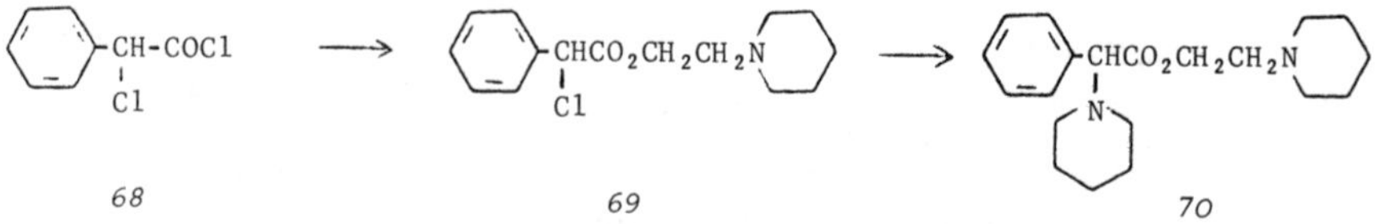

68   69   70

Antispasmodic activity, interestingly, is maintained even in
the face of the deletion of the ethanolamine ester side chain.
Reaction of anisaldehyde with potassium cyanide and dibutylamine
hydrochloride affords the corresponding α-aminonitrile *(72)* (a
functionality analogous to a cyanohydrin). Treatment with sulfuric acid hydrolyzes the nitrile to the amide to yield *ambucetamide (73)*.[19]

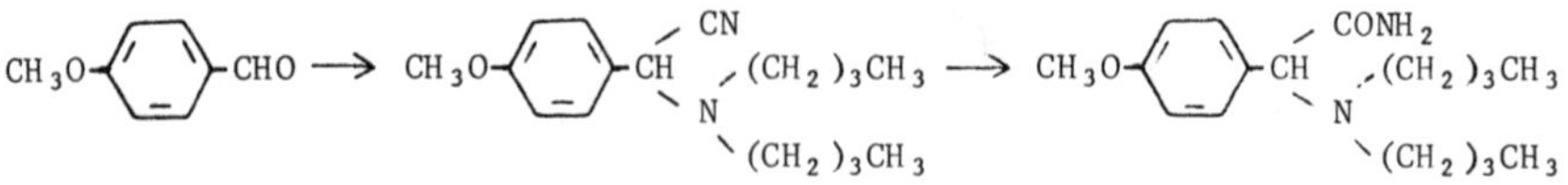

71   72   73

The activity of acylureas as hypnotic and anticonvulsant
agents is dealt with in some detail later. This is again one of
the cases in which the functionality rather than structure deter-
mines pharmacologic activity. Thus, acylation of urea with
phenylacetyl chloride gives the anticonvulsant agent, *phenacemide*
(74).[20]

$$\text{—CH}_2\text{COCl} \quad + \quad \text{H}_2\text{NCONH}_2 \quad \longrightarrow \quad \text{—CH}_2\overset{\overset{\text{O}}{\|}}{\text{C}}\text{NH}\overset{\overset{\text{O}}{\|}}{\text{C}}\text{NH}_2$$

74

It will be recalled that both epinephrine and norepinephrine
are pressor agents, that is, they cause an increase in blood
pressure. It would therefore be expected that antagonists to
these endogenous pressor amines might have a useful effect on
hypertension. One approach to this problem consists in the preparation of compounds that interfere with biosynthesis of these
amines by the administration of false substrates that would be
unable to go through the final steps of biogenesis. A crucial
step in the biosynthetic scheme for formation of norepinephrine
consists in the decarboxylation of DOPA (dihydroxyphenylalanine,
75) to dopamine *(76)*. (Side chain hydroxylation completes the
scheme.) Substitution at the carbon adjacent the carboxyl group
should hinder this reaction. Reaction of the substituted phenylacetone *(77)* with ammonium chloride and potassium cyanide affords
the corresponding α-aminonitrile *(78)*. The L isomer is then
separated from the racemate by means of the camphorsulfonic acid
salt. (The unwanted D isomer can then be subjected to basic
hydrolysis to give back starting ketone that can be then recy-
cled.) Treatment of the L isomer with concentrated sulfuric acid
at the same time effects hydrolysis of the nitrile to the acid
and cleavage of the remaining methyl ether. There is thus obtained *methyldopa (79)*.[21] While this drug has in fact found considerable use as an antihypertensive agent, there is evidence to
indicate that the mechanism of action may be considerably more
involved than a simple block of pressor amine synthesis.

The thyroid gland, located in the base of the neck, exerts
a key role on growth and metabolism. In contrast with that of
some of the other endocrine glands, this control is effected
through a pair of relatively simple molecules, *thyroxine*, and
its close congener, *triiodothyronine*. Cases of thyroid deficiency (hypothyroidism) are common enough to warrant the production

CH_3O-⟨ring, HO⟩-CH_2COCH_3 → CH_3O-⟨ring, HO⟩-$CH_2\overset{NC}{\underset{}{C}}\overset{NH_2}{\underset{}{}}CH_3$ → HO-⟨ring, HO⟩-$CH_2\overset{NH_2}{\underset{CH_3}{C}}CO_2H$

77   78   79

HO-⟨ring, HO⟩-$CH_2\overset{NH_2}{CH}CO_2H$ → HO-⟨ring, HO⟩-$CH_2CH_2NH_2$

75   76

of these hormones commercially. In contrast to the steroid hormones, thyroxine and its analogs have few, if any, applications beyond replacement therapy. Since the structure of the hormone is constant among most mammals, crude extracts of thyroid glands from slaughterhouses constitute an important form of drug for treatment of deficiencies. The pure hormones are used in medicine as well; these in turn are obtained both by total synthesis and purification of extracts from animal sources.

One published synthesis starts by the formation of the benzenesulfonate of phenol, 77. This compound, it should be noted, is particularly suited for nucleophilic aromatic substitution, since the benzenesulfonate is activated by the ortho nitro, as well as the para carbonyl group. In fact, treatment of 77 with the anion from the monomethyl ether of hydroquinone gives the diphenyl ether (79). Azlactones such as 80 have proven of great utility in synthesis, since the parent amino acid is cyclized into a form that masks both the amino and carboxyl groups. The reactivity of the methylene group is enhanced by the adjacent imine. Condensation of the aldehyde group of 79 with 80 by means of sodium acetate and acetic anhydride affords 81. When the condensation product is exposed to sodium methoxide, this reagent attacks the carbonyl group of the azlactone; the ring is thus opened to form the ester enamide (82). Reduction of this product with Raney nickel selectively reduces the aromatic nitro group to the corresponding amine (83). This amine is then transformed to an iodo group by diazotization and treatment of the diazonium salt with iodine-sodium iodide. Catalytic hydrogenation over platinum reduces the enamine double bond; hydrolysis of this ester-amide gives the amino acid *(86)*. The aromatic methyl ether in the remote ring is then cleaved by means of hydroiodic acid *(80)* to afford the key diodo intermediate *(87)*. The L form of this amino acid is isolated by optical resolution for further elaboration to the thyroid hormones. In the course of synthetic work on the thyroid hormones, a series of specialized reactions have been developed for the direct introduction of iodine ortho to phenolic groups. Thus, treatment of the diiodo compound with either the sodium salt of N-iodo-p-toluenesulfonamide or a mixture of iodine and sodium iodide in aqueous dimethylamine affords L-triiodothyronine,[22] which goes by the generic name of *liothyronine (88)*. This compound, interestingly, is more active as a thyroid hormone than *thyroxine* itself. Treatment of intermediate *(87)* with an excess of one of the iodinating reagents gives *levothyroxine (89)*.[22] Preparation of the diiodo derivative from the D form of the intermediate, *87*, gives *dextrothyroxine*, a compound with much reduced thyroid activity that has been used for the treatment of elevated cholesterol levels.

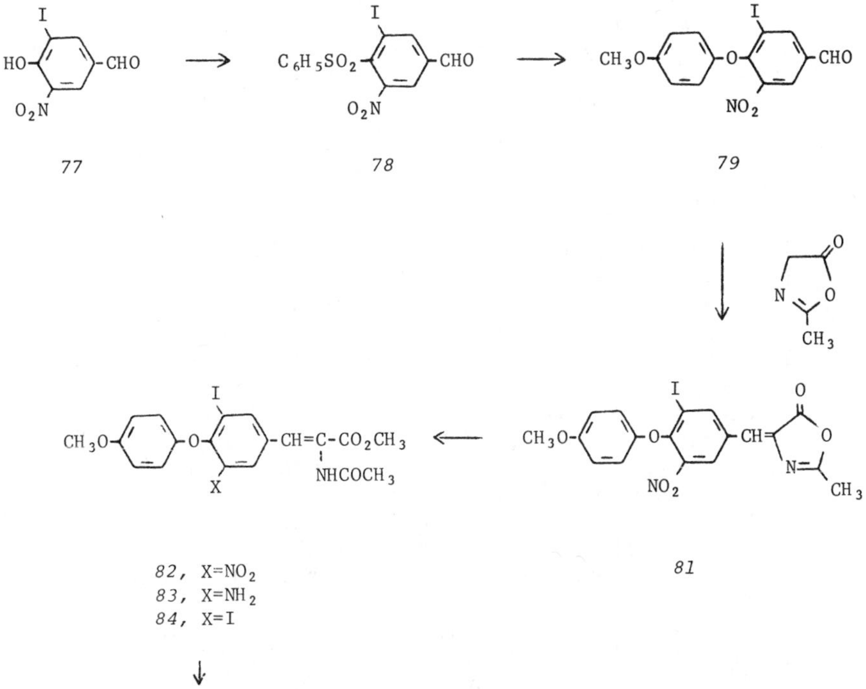

77   78   79

82, X=NO$_2$
83, X=NH$_2$
84, X=I

81

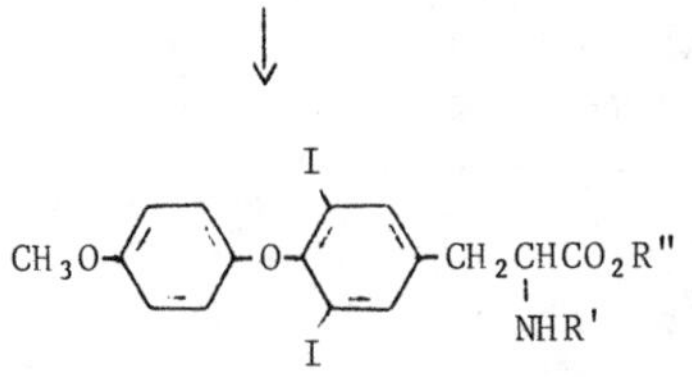

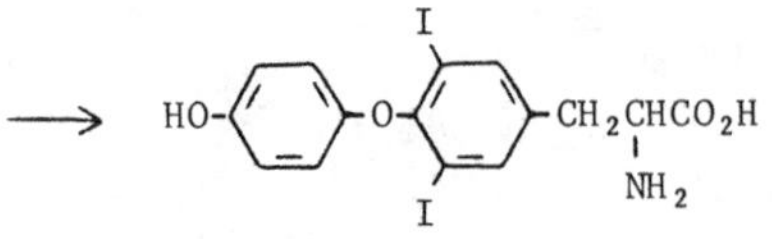

85, R'=COCH₃; R"=CH₃
86, R'=R"=H

87

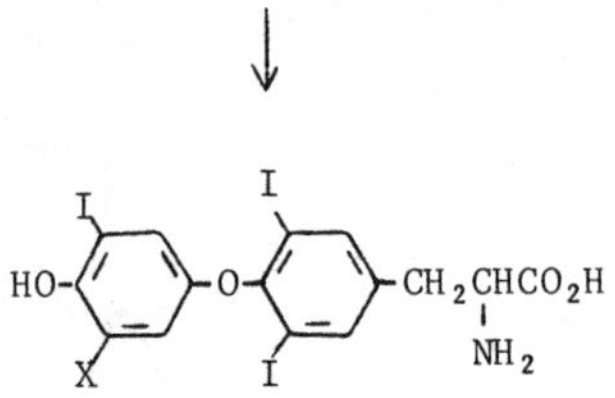

88, X=H
89, X=I

REFERENCES

1. J. S. Nicholson and S. S. Adams, U. S. Patent 3,228,831 (1966).
2. S. S. Adams, J. Bernard, J. S. Nicholson, and A. B. Blancafort, U. S. Patent 3,755,427 (1973).
3. I. T. Harrison, B. Lewis, P. Nelson, W. Rooks, A. Roszkowski, A. Tomalonis, and J. H. Fried, *J. Med. Chem., 13*, 203 (1970).
4. K. Miescher, *Helv. Chim. Acta, 27*, 1727 (1944).
5. A. Horeau and J. Jacques, *Compt. Rend., 224*, 862 (1947).
6. L. Panizzon, *Helv. Chim. Acta, 27*, 1748 (1944).
7. G. Satzinger, *Ann., 728*, 64 (1962).
8. H. Martin and F. Hafliger, U. S. Patent 2,404,588 (1946).
9. Anon., British Patent 753,799 (1956).
10. V. Petrow, O. Stephenson, and A. M. Wild, U. S. Patent 2,885,404 (1959).
11. J. H. Biel, H. L. Friedman, H. A. Leiser, and E. P. Sprengler, *J. Amer. Chem. Soc., 74*, 1485 (1952).
12. H. E. Zaugg and B. W. Horrom, *J. Amer. Chem. Soc., 72*, 3004

(1950).

13. H. G. Kolloff, J. H. Hunter, E. H. Woodruff, and R. B. Moffett, *J. Amer. Chem. Soc.*, *70*, 3862 (1948).

14. G. R. Treves, U. S. Patent 2,554,511 (1951).

15. Anon., British Patent 940,540 (1963).

16. F. F. Blicke and C. E. Maxwell, *J. Amer. Chem. Soc.*, *64*, 428 (1942).

17. N. Brock, E. Kuhas, and D. Lorenz, *Arzneimittel Forsch.*, *2*, 165 (1952).

18. H. Najer, P. Chabrier, and R. Guidicelli, *Bull. Soc. Chim. (Fr.)*, 335 (1958).

19. P. A. J. Janssen, *J. Amer. Chem. Soc.*, *76*, 6192 (1959).

20. M. A. Spielman, A. O. Geiszler, and W. J. Close, *J. Amer. Chem. Soc.*, *70*, 4189 (1948).

21. D. Reinhold, R. A. Firestone, W. A. Gaines, J. Chemerda, and M. Sletzinger, *J. Org. Chem.*, *33*, 1209 (1968).

22. H. Nahm and W. Siedel, *Chem. Ber.*, *96*, 1 (1963).

CHAPTER 7

Arylethylenes and Their Reduction Products

The isolation of the estrogens, the so-called female sex hormones, occasioned intensive work on the endocrine activity of this series of endogenous compounds. This was hampered in no small way by the minute quantities in which these hormones occur in nature as well as by the lack of sources of these agents other than isolation from mammals. However, enough data was accumulated to indicate that such agents had great potential for the treatment of the various dysfunctions that result from deficient levels of estrogens. Initial attempts to prepare these compounds by total synthesis were hindered by the fact that the structure of the estrogens had been only partly solved. It was known, however, that steroids consisted of a tetracyclic nucleus, and in the estrogens such as, for example, estrone (1), one of these rings was present as an aromatic phenol. The demonstration that the phenathrene derivative, 2,[2] showed estrogenic activity in experimental animals encouraged further departures from the vaguely realized steroid nucleus in the search for estrogenic agents. The great variety of structures that have by now been shown to exhibit estrogenic activity[2] leads to the suspicion that the estrogen receptor may be unusually nonspecific compared to receptors for other steroid hormones.

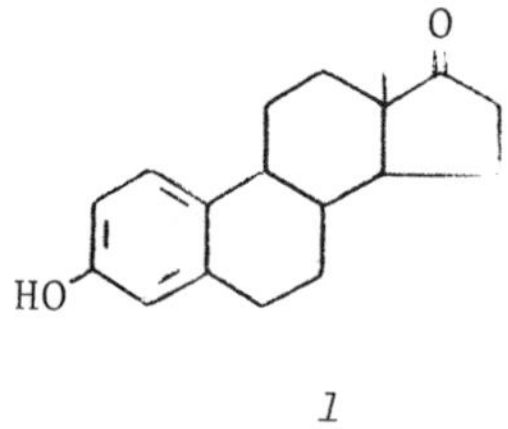

1

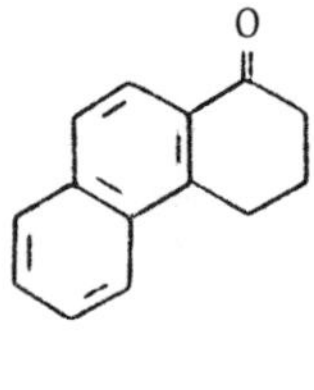

2

One of the first of the synthetic estrogens devoid of the
steroid nucleus, *diethylstilbestrol (7)*, is still fairly widely
used today. Although initially employed for cases of estrogen
deficiency, the drug has found utility in such diverse uses as in
the fattening of cattle and the recently approved indication as a
"morning-after" contraceptive. The initial synthesis for this
agent involves first the alkylation of desoxyanisoin *(3)* with
ethyl iodide by means of strong base *(4)*. Reaction of the product with ethylmagnesium bromide gives the corresponding alcohol
(5). Dehydration under acidic conditions affords largely the
trans olefin *(6)* accompanied by a minor amount of the *cis* isomer.
Cleavage of the methyl ether groups in the *trans* isomer to the
phenol completes the synthesis of *diethylstilbestrol (7)*.[3] It is
of note that the molecule can be coiled so as to assume the shape
of a steroid.   (The aromatic rings assume the functions of the
terminal rings, while each of the ethyl groups provides bulk
corresponding to the remaining alicyclic rings.)

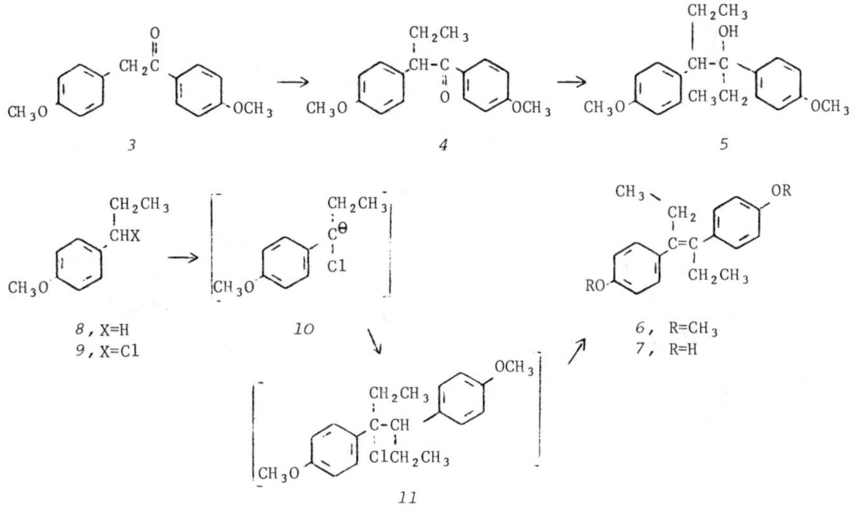

An interesting alternate synthesis for this agent starts
with the chlorination of the benzylic carbon of *8* by means of *N*-
chlorosuccinimide. Treatment of the chloro compound *(9)* with
sodium amide in liquid ammonia serves to remove remaining proton
on that carbon. This carbanion *(10)* then performs an alkylation
reaction on unreacted starting chloride. The product of this.
alkylation *(11)* still contains a fairly acidic benzylic proton;

removal of this proton leads to beta elimination of hydrogen chloride and formation of the stilbestrol intermediate in a single step (6).[4]

Catalytic reduction of diethylstilbestrol proceeds stereospecifically (see Newman projections below) to afford the meso isomer, hexestrol (12).[5] This synthetic estrogen is said to produce fewer side effects than the parent molecule. The meso form is more potent than the DL isomer. An alternate synthesis of this drug involves the cobaltous chloride-catalyzed coupling of the Grignard reagent from 13 with the analogous benzilic chloro compound (9). Demethylation of the product (14) gives hexestrol.[6] The higher melting point of the meso form allows its separation from the DL by-product formed in this reaction by recrystallization.

$$7 \longrightarrow$$

CH$_3$-CH
CH-CH
CH$_2$
CH$_3$
RO ... OR

$$\longleftarrow 9 +$$

CH$_2$CH$_3$
Br-CH
OCH$_3$

12, R=H
14, R=OCH$_3$

13

CH$_3$CH$_2$ ... H ... OH
CH$_2$CH$_3$
H
HO

7

$$\longrightarrow$$

CH$_3$CH$_2$ ... H ... OH
CH$_2$CH$_3$
H
HO

12

Self-condensation of the substituted propiophenone, 15, by the pinacol reaction proceeds to give the glycol, 16, as the meso isomer. (If it is assumed that the transition state for this reaction resembles product, this stereoselectivity can be rationalized on the grounds of steric interaction; compare A, which leads to the observed product, with B.) Dehydration under very specialized conditions (acetyl chloride, acetic anhydride) affords the bisstyrene-type diene (17). Removal of the acyl groups by means of base affords the synthetic estrogen, dien-

estrol (18).[7]

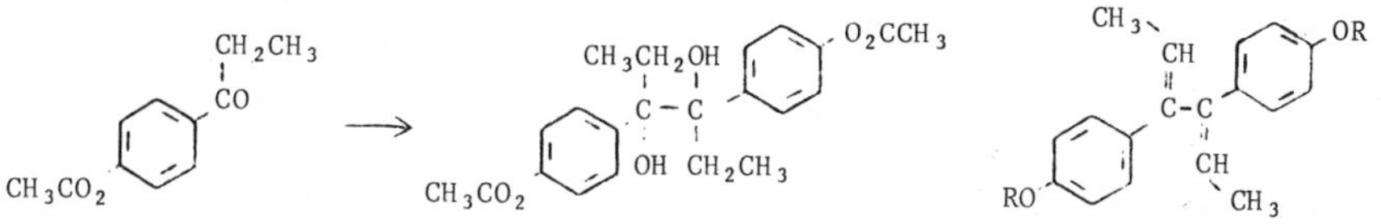

15   16   17, R=CH₃CO
                            18, R=H

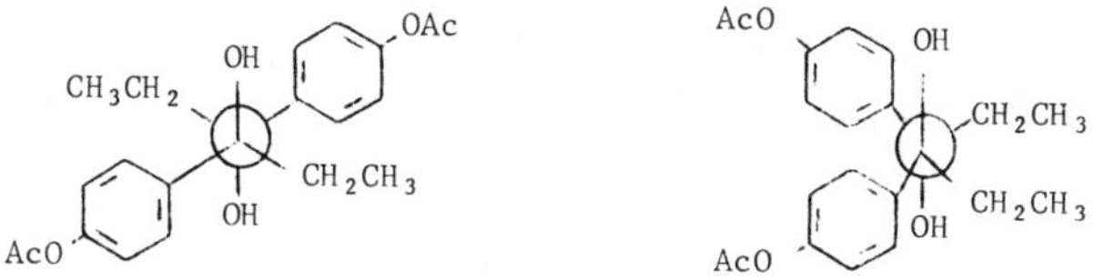

A   B

Insertion of an additional carbon atom between the two aromatic rings, interestingly, does not diminish estrogenic activity.
Aldol condensation of anisaldehyde with p-methoxybutyrophenone
(19) gives the substituted chalcone *(20)*. A second ethyl group
is then introduced into the molecule by conjugate addition of
ethylmagnesium bromide *(21)*. Reaction of the saturated ketone
with methylmagnesium bromide leads to the carbinol *(22)*. Dehydration followed by catalytic reduction completes construction of
the carbon skeleton. Cleavage of the aromatic ether groups by
means of hydrogen bromide affords the synthetic estrogen, *benzestrol (24)*.[8]

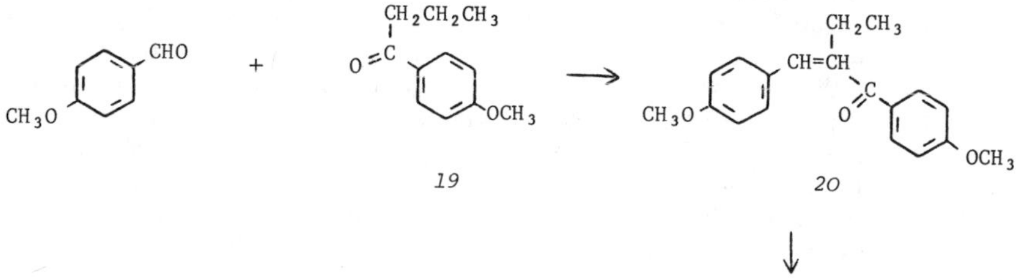

19   20

CH$_3$O—⟨benzene ring⟩—CHCH-C(CH$_3$)(OH)(CH$_2$CH$_3$)—⟨benzene ring⟩—OCH$_3$ with CH$_2$CH$_3$

22   ←   21

CH$_3$O—⟨benzene ring⟩—CH-CH-C(=O)(CH$_2$CH$_3$)—⟨benzene ring⟩—OCH$_3$ with CH$_2$CH$_3$

RO—⟨benzene ring⟩—CH-CH-CH(CH$_3$)(CH$_2$CH$_3$)—⟨benzene ring⟩—OR with CH$_2$CH$_3$

23, R= CH$_3$
24, R=H

The observation that one of the ethyl groups in stilbestrol
can be replaced by an aromatic ring and the other by halogen with
full retention of biologic activity illustrates the structural
latitude in this series of drugs.   Reaction of 4,4'-dimethoxy-
benzophenone (25) (obtained by Friedel-Crafts acylation of ani-
sole by p-methoxybenzoylchloride) with the Grignard reagent from
p-methoxybenzyl chloride affords the alcohol (26).   Acid-catalyzed
dehydration gives the corresponding ethylene (27).   Chlorination
of the vinyl carbon by either chlorine in carbon tetrachloride or
N-chlorosuccinimide affords the estrogen, chlortrianisene (28).[9]
    Alkylation of one of the phenolic groups of the triarylethyl-
ene synthetic estrogens with an alkyl group terminating in basic
nitrogen causes a fundamental change in biologic activity.   First,
the intrinsic activity of the compound is markedly reduced.   Unlike the pure estrogens, which show increasing biologic responses
with increasing doses, the resulting agents, called impeded estrogens, show a low maximal response regardless of dose.   More important is the finding that these agents will antagonize many of
the effects of concurrently administered pure estrogens.   Agents
of this class are therefore sometimes called estrogen antagonists.
At one time estrogen antagonists seemed to hold much promise as
contraceptive agents, since these compounds are remarkably effective in inhibiting pregnancy in the laboratory rat.   Further in-

vestigation showed that this effect was not manifested in higher
species since these, unlike the rat, are not exquisitely sensitive to estrogen levels for conception. The first of these
agents, ironically, has found use as a drug for treatment of in-
fertility. Ovulation is triggered in women by a series of hormones secreted by the pituitary gland. The estrogen antagonists
are known to suppress this secretion. Once administration of the
drug is stopped, the gland rebounds with the outpouring of very
large amounts of pituitary hormones, triggering ovulation.

Alkylation of 4-hydroxybenzophenone by means of base with 2-
chlorotriethylamine affords the so-called basic ether (29). In a
sequence analogous to the preparation of 28, the ketone is first
reacted with benzylmagnesium chloride (30). Dehydration (31) and
chlorination complete the synthesis of clomiphene (32).[10] It is
of note that the commercial product is in fact a mixture of the
two geometrical isomers. These have been separated and seem to
differ in some degree in their endocrine properties.

Substitution of thiophene rings for the benzene rings and a
slight modification in the carbon skeleton leads to a marked
alteration in pharmacologic activity. The agents obtained by
these modifications are apparently devoid of endocrine activity;
instead, the compounds possess analgesic activity. Possibly as
a result of some side effects, their use is restricted to veterinary practice. Michael addition of dimethylamine to ethyl cro-
tonate gives the aminoester (33). Condensation with the lithium
reagent from 2-bromothiophene leads to addition of two equivalents of the organometalic (34). Dehydration yields dimethyl-

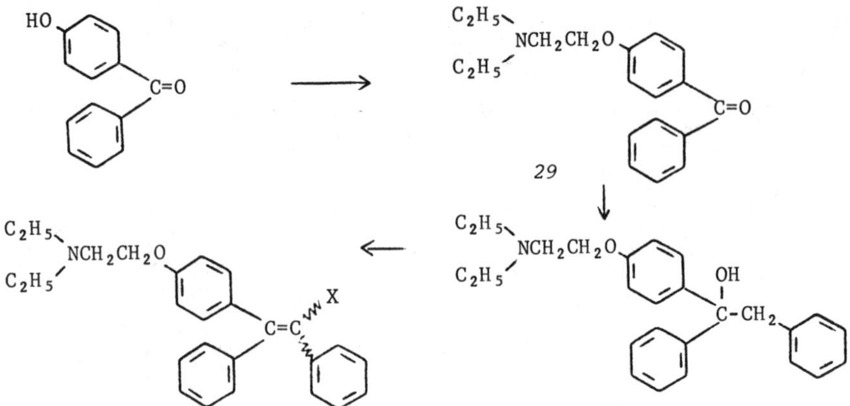

31, X=H
32, X=Cl

thiambutene (35).[11] The same scheme starting with the diethylamine adduct *(36)* affords the analog, *diethylthiambutene (38).*[11]

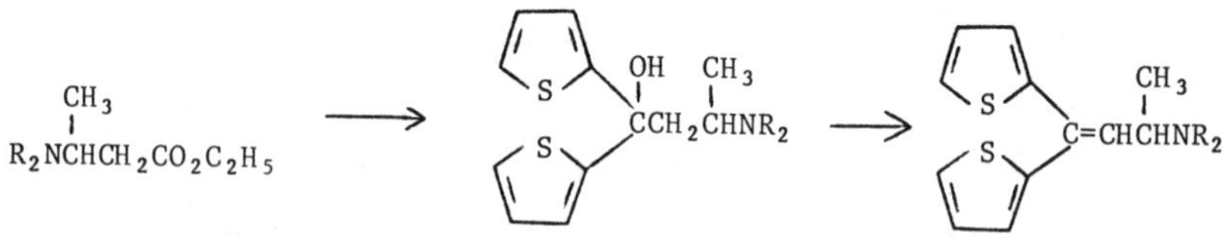

33, R=CH$_3$ 34, R=CH$_3$ 35, R=CH$_3$
36, R=C$_2$H$_5$ 37, R=C$_2$H$_5$ 38, R=C$_2$H$_5$

REFERENCES

1. J. W. Cook, E. C. Dodds, and C. L. Hewett, *Nature, 131*, 56
    (1933).
2. See, for example, D. Lednicer in *Contraception; The Chemical
    Control of Fertility*, (D. Lednicer, Ed.), Marcel Dekker,
    N. Y., 1969, p. 197.
3. E. C. Dodds, L. Goldberg, W. Lawson, and R. Robinson, *Nature,
    142*, 34 (1938).

4. M. S. Kharasch and M. Kleinman, *J. Amer. Chem. Soc.*, *65*, 11
    (1943).
5. N. R. Campbell, E. C. Dodds, and W. Lawson, *Nature*, *142*,
    1121 (1938).
6. M. S. Kharasch and M. Kleinman, *J. Amer. Chem. Soc.*, *65*, 491
    (1943).
7. E. C. Dodds, L. Goldberg, W. Lawson, and R. Robinson, *Proc.
    Roy. Soc. (Lond.) B127*, 148 (1939).
8. A. H. Stuart, A. J. Shukis, R. C. Tallman, C. McCann, and G.
    R. Treves, *J. Amer. Chem. Soc.*, *68*, 729 (1946).
9. R. S. Shelton and M. G. VanCampen, U. S. Patent 2,430,891
    (1947).
10. R. E. Allen, F. Palapoli, and E. L. Schumann, U. S. Patent
    2,914,563 (1959).
11. D. W. Adamson, *J. Chem. Soc.*, 885 (1950).

CHAPTER 8

Monocyclic Aromatic Compounds

Although medicinal agents discussed in previous chapters often contained benzene rings, these were usually at some remove from the pharmacologically significant functionality. In a number of those agents, furthermore, the aromatic ring provided only steric bulk, as evidenced by the fact that in at least some cases reduction of the ring still provided active molecules. The compounds in the present section carry the functionality directly on the benzene ring. There is good evidence that the aromatic character of this ring plays an important role in their drug action.

1. BENZOIC ACIDS

The introduction of the salicylates into therapy begins with the identification more than a century and a half ago of the substance in the bark of willow trees *(Salix sp.)*, the glycoside salicin, *1*, which was responsible for the antipyretic action of extracts known since antiquity. Degradation by chemical and enzymatic means of *1* gave glucose and salicyl alcohol *(2)*. Further work on this natural product showed that salicylic acid *(3)*, prepared by oxidation of the alcohol, had analgesic, antipyretic, and antiinflammatory activity in its own right. Salicylic acid itself, however, proved too irritating to mucous membranes to be used as such. Its acetyl ester, prepared by any of the standard ways, overcomes the irritation sufficiently for the drug to be used orally. This, of course, is now familiar to all as *aspirin* *(4)*.

One of the first prodrugs, *aspirin*, is cleaved to the active agent, salcylic acid, in the liver as well as various other tissues. Despite the advent of numerous newer agents for the alleviation of the pain and inflammation characteristic of inflammatory diseases, *aspirin* remains the most widely used drug for this

108

purpose. The safety of *aspirin* and the fact that it is available
without prescription also makes it one of the most widely used
drugs for self-medication. It has been estimated that some 35
tons are consumed daily in the United States alone.

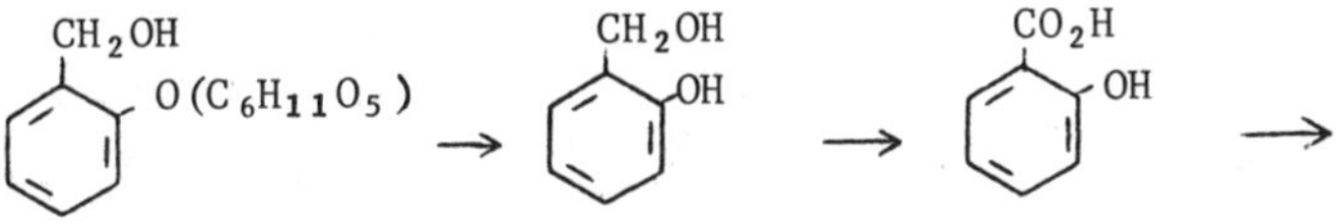

The popularity of *aspirin* has led to the preparation of a
host of relatively simple derivatives in the hope of finding a
drug that would be either superior in action or better tolerated.
Salicylamide (5), for example, is sometimes prescribed for patients allergic to *aspirin*. It should be noted, however, that
this agent is not as active as the parent compound as an antiinflammatory or analgesic agent. This may be related to the fact
that *salicylamide* does not undergo conversion to salicylic acid
in the body.

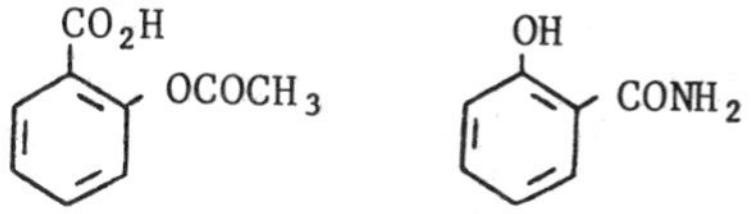

Substitution of an amino group into the molecule affords an
agent with antibacterial activity. Although seldom used alone,
para-aminosalicylic acid (PAS, 7) has been employed as an adjunct
to *streptomycin* and *isoniazid* in treatment of tuberculosis.
(There is evidence the drug acts as an antimetabolite for the
para-aminobenzoic acid required for bacterial metabolism.) One
of the more recent of the many preparations for this drug involves carboxylation of meta-aminophenol *(6)* by means of ammonium
carbonate under high pressure.[1]

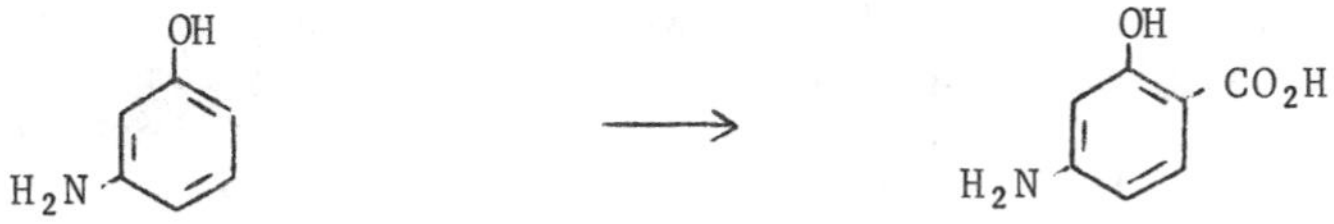

Further substitution of benzoic acid leads to a drug with antiemetic activity. Alkylation of the sodium salt of p-hydroxybenzaldehyde *(8)* with 2-dimethylaminoethyl chloride affords the so-called basic ether *(9)*. Reductive amination of the aldehyde in the presence of ammonia gives diamine, *10*. Acylation of that product with 3,4,5-trimethoxybenzoyl chloride affords *trimethobenzamide (11)*.[2]

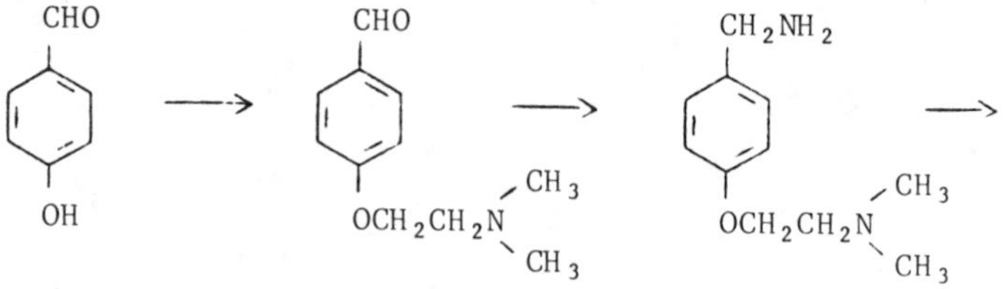

8   *9*   *10*

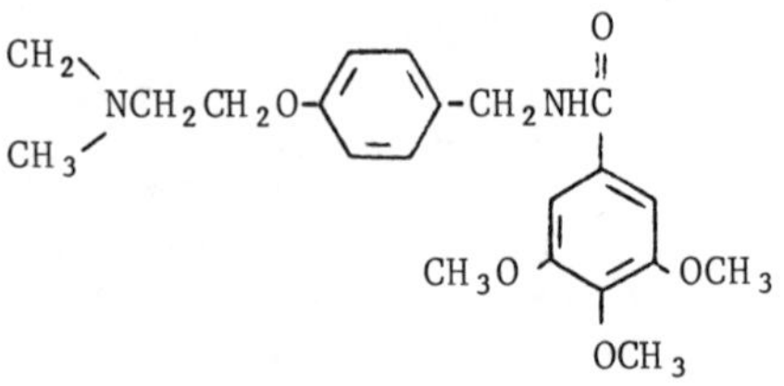

11

2. ANTHRANILLIC ACIDS

The relatively low potency of *aspirin* in overcoming the symptoms of inflammatory diseases has led to a continuing search for new antiinflammatory agents. Although many more potent agents have been introduced to clinical practice, most of these elicit some side effects that limit their use. Derivatives of *N*-aryl anthranillic acids have provided a series of quite effective antiinflammatory drugs, the so-called fenamic acids.

Ullman condensation of *m*-trifluoromethylaniline *(13)* with *o*-iodobenzoic acid in the presence of copper-bronze affords *flufenamic acid (14)*.[3] An analogous reaction of *o*-chlorobenzoic acid with 2,3-dimethylaniline *(15)* gives *mefenamic acid (16)*;[4] *meclofenamic acid (18)* is obtained by Ullman condensation employing 2,6-dichloro-3-methylaniline *(17)*.

12a, R'=I
12b, R'=Cl

13, X=Y=H;Z=CF$_3$
15, X=H;Y=Z=CH$_3$
17, X=Y=Cl;Z=CH$_3$

14, X=Y=H;Z=CF$_3$
16, X=H;Y=Z=CH$_3$
18, X=Y=Cl;Z=CH$_3$

3. ANILINES

Although aniline was found to possess peripheral analgesic activity more than a century ago, its use in medicine was precluded by the toxic manifestations produced by that compound. Metabolic oxidation of this amine gives largely phenylhydroxylamine (19). This compound, which is known to convert hemoglobin to the form that is incapable of binding oxygen, methemoglobin, is thought to be responsible for the toxicity of aniline. Paradoxically, another product of metabolic hydroxylation, p-aminophenol, again shows analgesic activity; this compound, too, however, shows too narrow a therapeutic ratio for use as a drug. Formation of derivatives of aniline that circumvent hydroxylation on nitrogen has provided a number of useful peripheral analgesics.

Thus, acetylation of aniline affords acetanilide (20), an analgesic widely used in proprietary headache remedies. A similar transformation on p-aminophenol gives the analgesic, acetaminophen (21). It is of interest that the latter is also formed in vivo on administration of 21. An interesting preparation of this drug involves Schmidt rearrangement of the hydrazone (24) from p-hydroxyacetophenone.[5]

The duration of action of acetaminophen is limited by the formation of water-soluble derivatives of the phenol (glucuronide and sulfate) that are then excreted via the kidney. Protection of the phenol as an ether inhibits such inactivation without diminishing biologic activity. Acetylation of p-ethoxyaniline[6] affords the widely used peripheral analgesic, phenacetin (25). This drug is quite frequently found in headache remedies in combination with aspirin and caffeine (APC®, PAC®). Although the aniline derivatives show analgetic potency comparable to aspirin, they apparently have no effect on inflammation.

Physostigmine (36) is actually a complex fused heterocycle rather than a simple derivative of aniline. The drug is men-

NH$_2$ → NH$_2$ (OH) → NHCOCH$_3$ (OH) $\longleftarrow$ X=C-CH$_3$ (OH)

21

22, X=O
23, X=NNH$_2$

NHOH

19

NHCOCH$_3$

20

NH$_2$ OC$_2$H$_5$

24

→ NHCOCH$_3$ OC$_2$H$_5$

25

tioned at this particular point because analysis of the structure
eventually led to a simple aniline derivative with much the same
activity as the natural product. The alkaloid was first isolated
from the ordeal bean *(Physostigma venenosum)* of West Africa (so
named by its use by witch doctors in a trial process analogous to
the trial by fire used in other cultures). Pharmacologic investigation showed the drug to be of value in the treatment of glaucoma
by reducing intraocular pressure when applied topically to the
eye. One of the more recent total syntheses of this compound
starts by aldol condensation of the substituted acetophenone, *26*,
with ethyl cyanoacetate *(27)*. Conjugate addition of hydrogen cyanide to the product followed by hydrolysis and decarboxylation of
the resulting acid affords the dinitrile, *28b*. Catalytic reduction of the nitrile affords diamine, *29*; this is converted to the
bis-*N*-methyl derivative by the Decker monoalkylation procedure
(30). Treatment of that intermediate with hydrogen iodide effects
removal of the phenolic methyl ether groups to yield hydroquinone,
31. Oxidation of *31* with potassium ferricyanide possibly involves
first formation of the benzoquinone *(32)*; Shiff base formation
with the amine would then give *33*. Aromatization of that intermediate would then afford the iminium salt, *34*; addition of the
second amine to this leads to the observed reaction product, *35*.

Reaction of the phenol with methyl isocyanate then gives *physostigmine (36)*.[7]

The relative inaccessibility of *physostigmine* led to molecular dissection studies to define the parts of the molecule necessary for activity. A surprisingly simple derivative of *m*-hydroxyaniline, *neostigmine (40)*, proved to have the same activity as the complex heterocyclic molecule. In addition, this drug has found use as a cholinsterase inhibitor in pathologic conditions such as myasthenia gravis, marked by insufficient muscle tone. Reaction of *m*-dimethylaminophenol *(37)* with phosgene affords tne carbamoyl chloride, *38*. Treatment with dimethylamine gives the

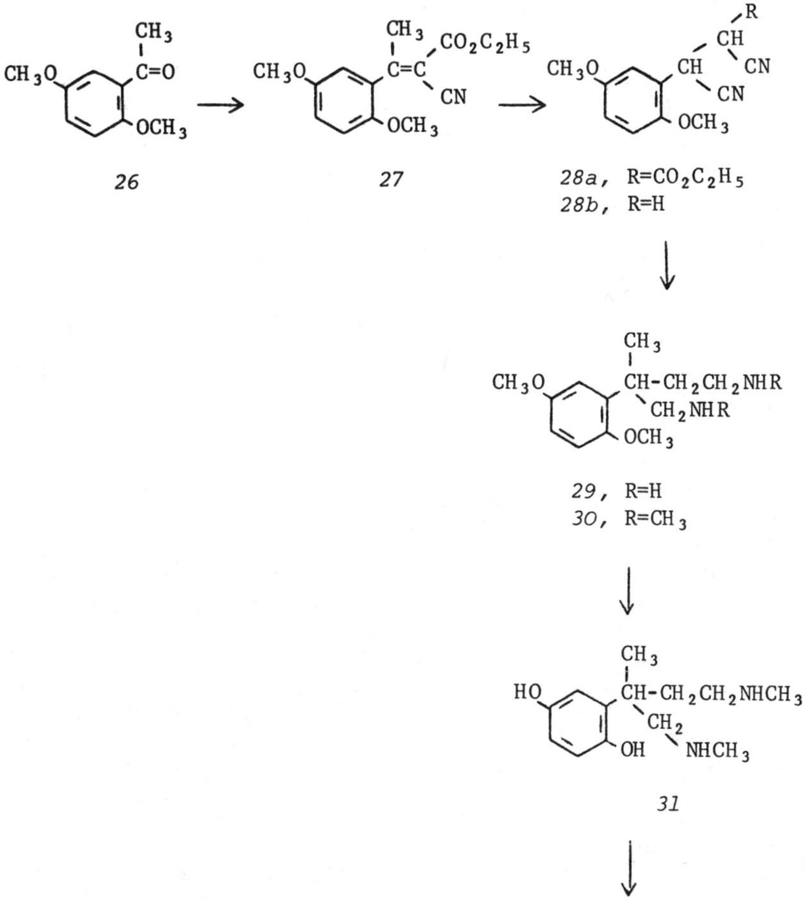

26   27   28a, R=CO$_2$C$_2$H$_5$
                                                       28b, R=H

29, R=H
30, R=CH$_3$

31

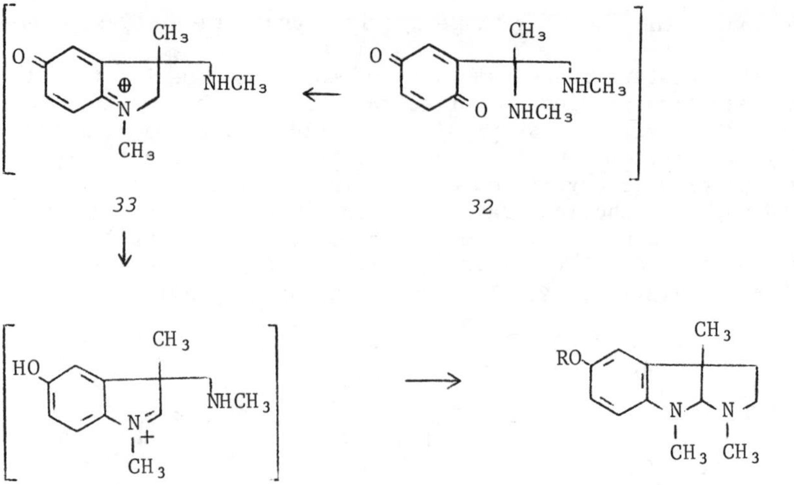

33   ←   32

↓

34   35, R=H
                                      36, R=CONHCH3

corresponding carbamate *(39)*. Quaternization with bromomethane
affords *neostigmine (40)*.[8]

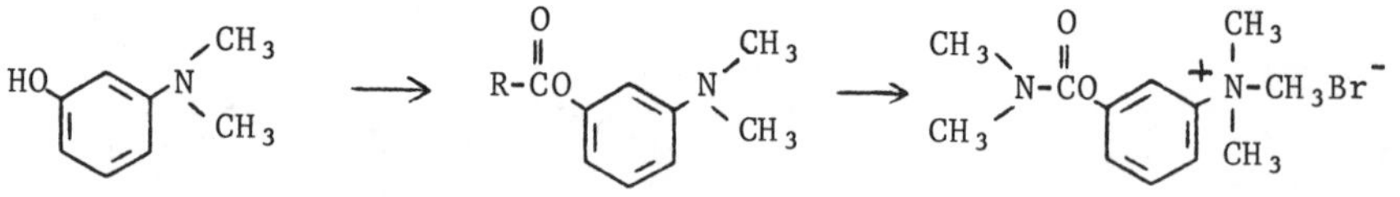

37   38, R=Cl   40
                   39, R=N⟨CH3
                          CH3

        The great diversity of forms characteristic of the life cy-
cle of the causative agent of malaria—the *plasmodia*—has led to
the development of a series of chemically distant drugs for com-
bating the organism at different stages. During an intense effort
aimed at the development of antimalaria drugs in the 1940s, it
was found that sulfonamides containing a pyrimidine ring had some
activity against *plasmodia* at an early stage in the life cycle.
The analog program on pyrimidines included some open-chain versions of this heterocycle as well. These last, the biguanides,
were found to be quite active in their own right. (It was subsequently established that these compounds undergo oxidative
cyclization to dihydropyrimidines in the body to give the actual
antimalarial—see *cycloguanyl*).

Alkylation of isopropylamine with cyanogen bromide affords the intermediate, *41*. Condensation of this with *p*-chlorophenyl-guanidine (*42*, obtainable, for example by reaction of the aniline with S-methylthiourea) affords directly *chlorguanide* or *paludrine* (*42*).[9,10] The same sequence starting with *m*-chloroaniline leads to the biguanide, *44*; chlorination in acetic acid gives *chlorpro-guanil* (*45*),[11] a compound with a somewhat longer duration of action.

4.   DERIVATIVES OF PHENOLS

The low structural specificity of the antihistamines has already been noted. It is perhaps not too surprising, therefore, to find that attachment of the basic side chain directly onto one of the aromatic rings affords active compounds. In an unusual reaction reminiscent of the Claisen rearrangement, benzyl chloride affords the substituted phenol, *46*, on heating with phenol itself. Alkyl-ation of *46* with 2-dimethylaminoethyl chloride gives *phenyltolox-amine (47)*.[12] Alkylation of that same intermediate (*46*) with 1-bromo-2-chloropropane, leads to *48*. Use of that halide to alkyl-ate piperidine gives the antihistamine, *pirexyl (49)*.[13]

The basic ether of a rather more complex phenol, interesting-ly, exhibits α-sympathetic blocking rather than antihistaminic activity. Nitrosation of the phenol derived from *p*-cymene *(50)* gives the expected nitroso derivative *(51)*. Reduction *(52)* followed by acylation gives the acetamide, *53*. Alkylation of the phenol with 2-dimethylaminoethyl chloride gives the correspond-ing basic ether *(54)*. Hydrolysis of the amide gives the free

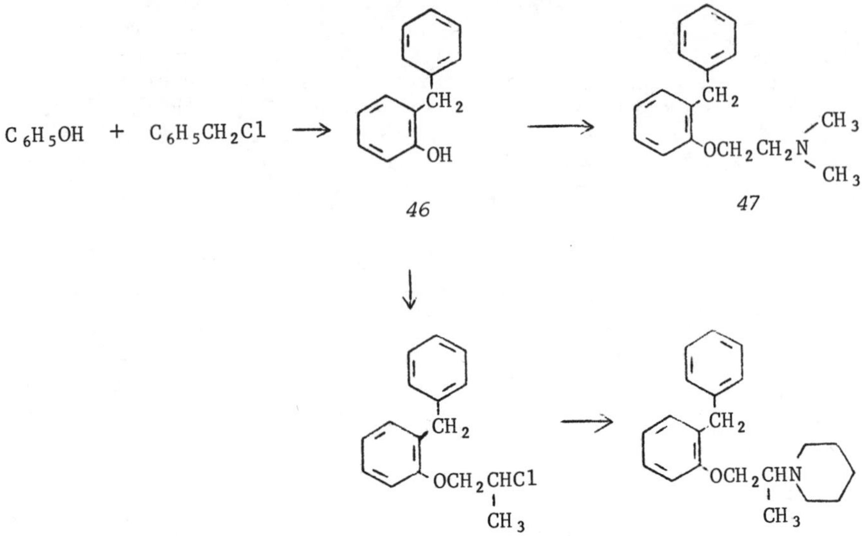

C_6H_5OH + $C_6H_5CH_2Cl$ $\longrightarrow$

46

47

48

49

amine *(55)*; this aniline is then converted to the phenol *(56)*
via the diazonium salt. Acylation of that product affords *moxy-sylyt (57)*.[14]

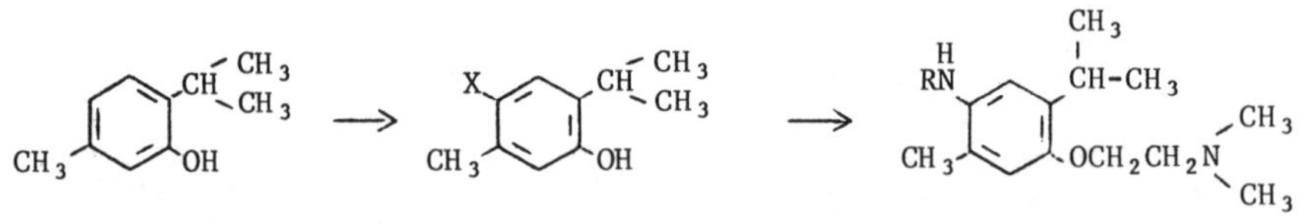

50

51, X=NO
52, X=NH$_2$
53, X=NHCOCH$_3$

54, R=COCH$_3$
55, R=H

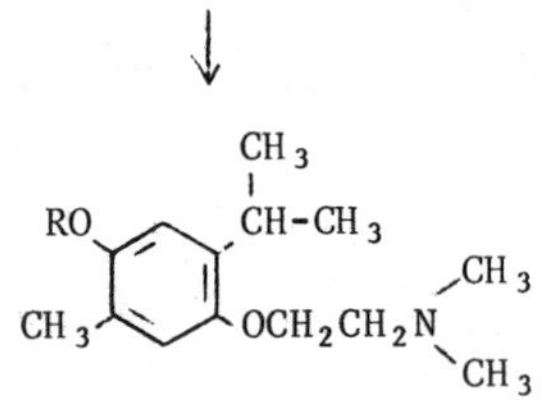

56, X=H
57, X=COCH$_3$

The guanidine function, when attached to an appropriate lipo-philic function, often yields compounds that exhibit antihyper-tensive activity by means of their peripheral sympathetic block-ing effects. Attachment of an aromatic ring via a phenolic ether seems to fulfill these structural requirements. Alkylation of 2,6-dichlorophenol with bromochloroethane leads to the interme-diate, 58. Alkylation of hydrazine with that halide gives 59. Reaction of the hydrazine with S-methylthiourea affords the guani-dine, *guanoclor* (60).[15]

58, R=Cl
59, R=NHNH$_2$

60

As noted previously (see Chapter 5), modification of the substitution pattern on the aromatic ring and on nitrogen com-pounds related to epinephrine affords medicinal agents that show β-sympathetic blocking activity. Such agents have an important place in the treatment of many of the manifestations of diseases of the cardiovascular system such as, for example, arrhythmias, angina, and even hypertension. Interposition of oxygen between the propanolamine side chain and the aromatic ring has proven fully compatible with this activity.

Reaction of epichlorohydrin with 1-naphthol affords the glycidic ether (61). Opening of the oxirane ring with isopropyl-amine gives racemic *propranolol* (62),[16,17] the only β-blocker available for sale in the United States. It is of note that the *l* isomer is some 60 to 80 times more potent than its epimer.

An analogous sequence on the allyl ether of catechol (63) leads to *oxyprenolol* (64); in the same vein, *ortho*-allylphenol (65) affords *alprenolol* (66).[19]

61

62

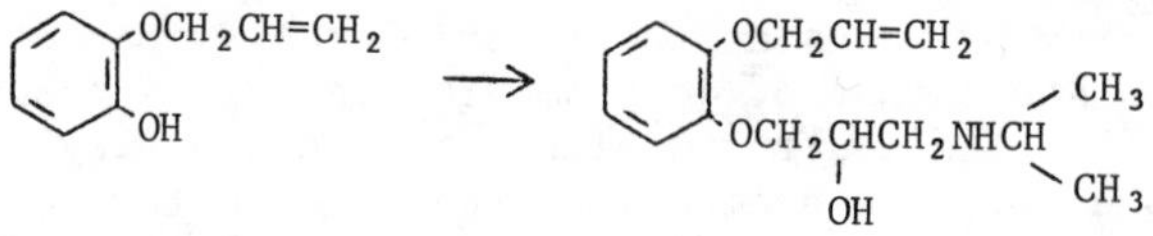

63 → 64

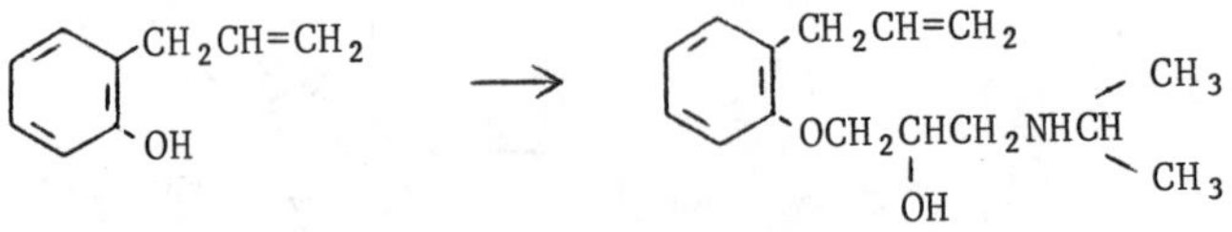

65 → 66

Terminally O-arylated glycerols and their derivatives have yielded a number of useful skeletal muscle relaxants that possess some sedative properties. Thus, alkylation of *o*-cresol with 1-chloropropan-2,3-diol affords *mephenesin (67)*. Treatment of the glycol with phosgene selectively forms the terminal carbamoyl chloride; reaction of that with ammonia gives *mephenesin carbamate (68)*.[19] An analogous scheme starting with catechol monomethyl ether *(69)* gives the sedative often included in cough syrups, *guaiaphenesin (70)*;[19] conversion to the carbamate affords *methocarbamol (71)*.[20] Application of the three-step sequence to *p*-chlorophenol affords *chlorphenesin carbamate (72)*.[21]

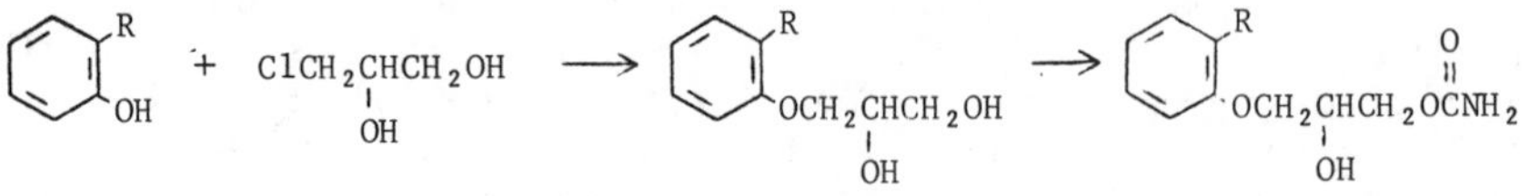

69, R=OCH$_3$

67, R=CH$_3$
70, R=OCH$_3$

68, R=CH$_3$
71, R=OCH$_3$

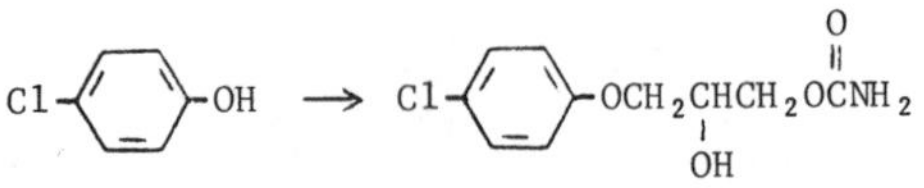

72

Reaction of the glycol, *70*, affords an oxazolidinone rather than the expected carbamate *(71)* on fusion with urea. It has been postulated that the urea is in fact the first product formed. This compound then undergoes O to N migration with loss of carbon dioxide; reaction of the amino alcohol with the isocyanic acid known to result from thermal decomposition of urea affords the observed product, *mephenoxolone (74)*[22]; this compound shows activity quite similar to that of the carbamate. An analogous reaction on the glyceryl ether, *75*, affords *metaxalone (76)*.[22]

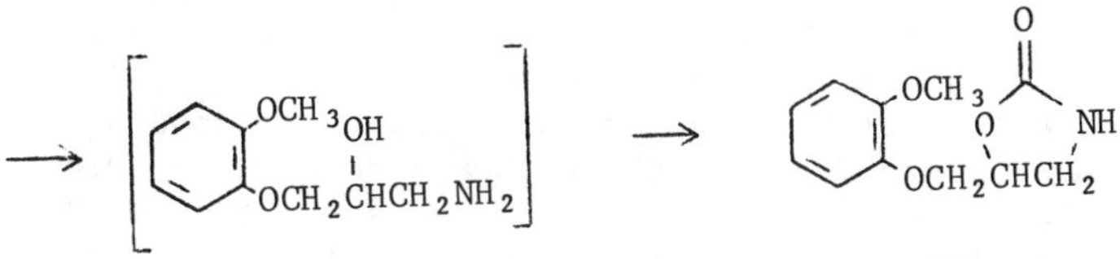

Epidemiologic studies have established a firm association between elevated blood lipids and atherosclerosis. Although the normalization of such elevated lipids would seem a desirable goal, there is as yet no evidence to show whether this has any effect on the course of the disease. One of the more effective agents available for lowering elevated triglyceride levels is a compound that more closely resembles a plant hormone than a medicinal agent. The drug may be prepared, albeit in low yield, by straightforward alkylation of phenol with ethyl isobutyrate. A more interesting method involves reaction of the phenol with chloroform and acetone to afford the acid, *77a*. Esterification with ethanol gives *clofibrate (77b)*.[23]

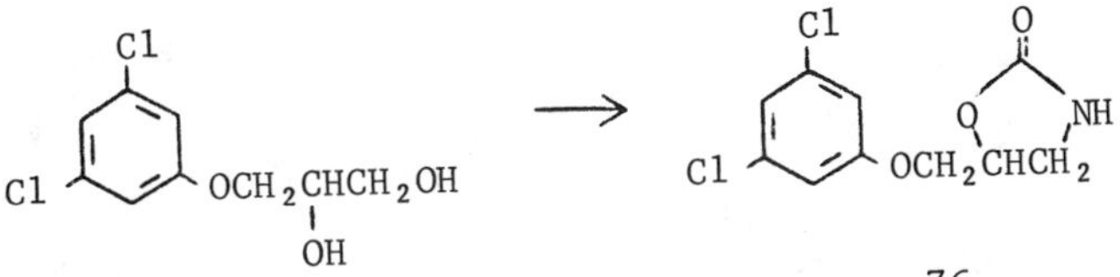

A fuller discussion of diuretic compounds will be found later in this section. Suffice to say that the majority of these

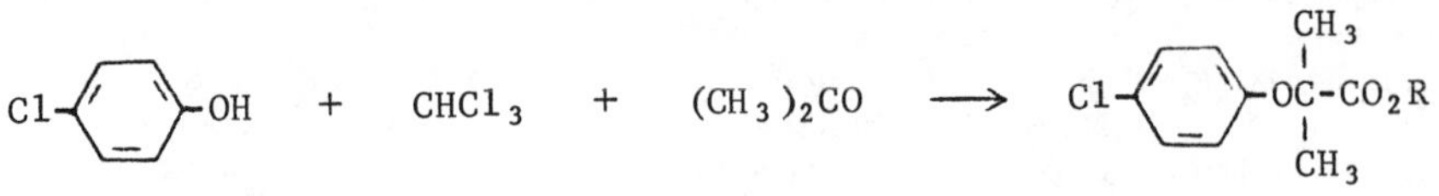

77a, R=H
77b, R=C$_2$H$_5$

agents contain one or more sulfonamide groups. *Ethacrynic acid
(81)* thus stands by itself structurally as a diuretic. Alkylation of 2,3-dichlorophenol by means of ethyl bromoacetate followed by saponification of the product gives the acid, *78*. Acylation with butyryl chloride leads to the corresponding ketone
(79). Mannich reaction to the carbonyl group with formaldehyde
and dimethylamine leads to amine, *80*. Elimination of dimethylamine by means of base affords *ethacrynic acid (81)*.[24]

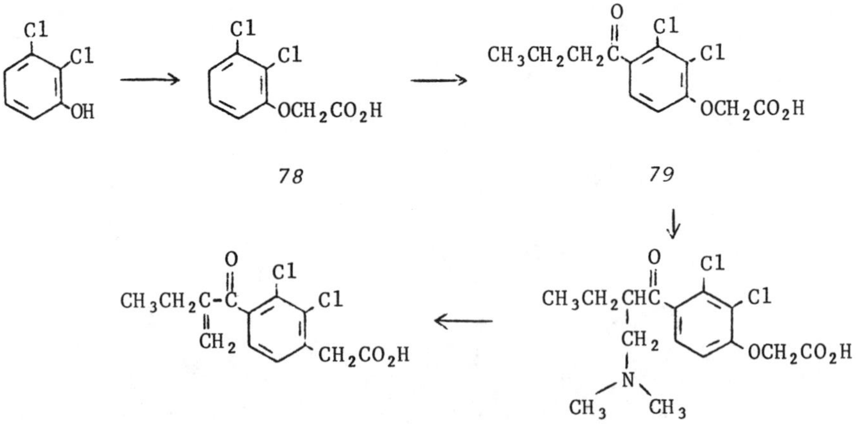

78

79

81

80

5. DERIVATIVES OF ARYLSULFONIC ACIDS

a. Sulfanilamides

Rather early in the evolution of bacteriology it was noted that
these single-celled organisms readily stain with organic dye molecules. An elaborate classification scheme can in fact be de-

vised for bacteria based on their behavior to various dyes. Some
effort, most notably on the part of Paul Ehrlich, was devoted to
finding dyes that would bind to bacteria without affecting mammalian cells. It was hoped that in this way a dye could be devised that was toxic to the microbe without affecting the mammalian host—in effect an antibiotic. This concept seemed to have
finally borne fruit some forty years after the initial work with
the introduction of the dye *protonsil (82)* as an effective antibacterial agent.[25]

Careful metabolic work on this drug by a group of French
workers showed that the agent was in fact cleaved to *sulfanilamide (83)* and the amine, *84, in vivo*. Testing of the two fragments revealed that the activity of the drug resided entirely in
the *sulfanilamide* fragment. That compound in fact showed full
activity when administered alone *in vitro* or *in vivo*.[26]

$$H_2N-\!\!\!\bigcirc\!\!\!-N=N-\!\!\!\bigcirc\!\!\!-SO_2NH_2 \;\longrightarrow\; H_2N-\!\!\!\bigcirc\!\!\!-SO_2NH_2 \;+\; H_2N-\!\!\!\bigcirc\!\!\!-NH_2$$

NH$_2$		NH$_2$
82	*83*	*84*

Dihydropteroic acid *(85)* is an intermediate to the formation
of the folic acid necessary for intermediary metabolism in both
bacteria and man. In bacteria this intermediate is produced by
enzymatic condensation of the pteridine, *86*, with para-aminobenzoic acid *(87)*. It has been shown convincingly that sulfanilamide and its various derivatives act as a false substrate in
place of the enzymatic reaction; that is, the sulfonamide blocks
the reaction by occupying the site intended for the benzoic acid.
The lack of folic acid then results in the death of the micro-
organism. Mammals, on the other hand, cannot synthesize folic
acid; instead, this compound must be ingested preformed in the
form of a vitamin. Inhibition of the reaction to form folic acid
is thus without effect on these higher organisms.

$$HO_2C-\!\!\!\bigcirc\!\!\!-NH_2 \;+\; HOCH_2-\cdots \;\longrightarrow$$

87   *86*

$$\text{HO}_2\text{C} - \text{C}_6\text{H}_4 - \overset{\text{H}}{\text{N}}\text{CH}_2 - \cdots \rightarrow \text{folic acid}$$

85

Both the dramatic effectiveness and shortcomings of this first antibiotic spurred the preparation of more than 5000 analogs. Although great improvements were eventually realized, the class as a whole suffers from a relatively narrow antibacterial spectrum, comparatively low potency, and rapid development of resistant organisms. An unexpected bonus from the clinical trials carried out on new experimental sulfa drugs was the development of entirely new classes of drugs. In essence, each of these followed from discovery of an apparent side effect by acute clinical observation. Thus, the finding that the sulfonyl urea analogs resulted in lowered blood sugar led to the oral antidiabetic agents. In this way, there were also discovered structural modifications that endowed this class of compounds with diuretic activity and uricosuric activity. A later section in the book details how the findings from the sulfonamide derivatives were developed and elaborated into molecules that bear little resemblance to the humble progenitor, *sulfanilamide*.

Besides the shortcomings noted above, some of the early sulfa drugs were poorly soluble in water. Since the drugs are excreted largely unchanged in the urine, crystals of the compounds sometimes formed in the kidneys and urine with attendant discomfort and tissue damage. Considerable attention was therefore devoted to preparation of agents with better solubility characteristics.

The drugs are available by one of two fairly straightforward routes. Chlorosulfonation of acetanilide gives the corresponding sulfonyl chloride (88); reaction with the appropriate amine gives the intermediate, 89. Hydrolysis in either acid or base leads to the sulfanilamide (90).

$$\text{CH}_3\overset{\text{O}}{\underset{\text{H}}{\text{CN}}} - \text{C}_6\text{H}_5 \longrightarrow \text{CH}_3\overset{\text{O}}{\underset{\text{H}}{\text{CN}}} - \text{C}_6\text{H}_4 - \text{SO}_2\text{Cl} \longrightarrow \text{RN} \overset{\text{H}}{} - \text{C}_6\text{H}_4 - \text{SO}_2\text{NHR}'$$

88

89, R=COCH$_3$
90, R=H

In the alternate approach, the amide formation is performed on *para*-nitrobenzenesulfonyl chloride *(91)*. Reduction by either chemical or catalytic methods affords directly the desired product *(90)*.

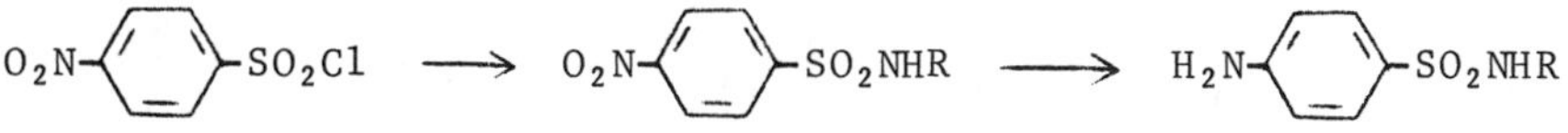

$$O_2N-\langle\bigcirc\rangle-SO_2Cl \longrightarrow O_2N-\langle\bigcirc\rangle-SO_2NHR \longrightarrow H_2N-\langle\bigcirc\rangle-SO_2NHR$$

                91   92   90

Since the chemistry involved in the synthesis of these agents is self-evident, they are listed without comment in Table 1 below. The preparation of selected more complex basic residues is detailed in the section that follows.

Table 1.   Derivatives of Sulfanilamide

$$H_2N-\langle\bigcirc\rangle-SO_2NHR$$

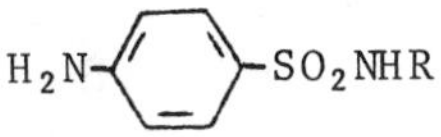

Compound Number	Generic Name	R	Reference
90	*Sulfanilamide*	H	
93	*Sulfacetamide*	$-COCH_3$	27
94	*Sulfaproxylene*	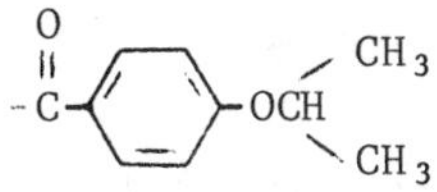 $-\overset{\overset{O}{\|\|}}{C}-\langle\bigcirc\rangle-OCH\overset{\diagup CH_3}{\diagdown CH_3}$	28
95	*Sulfacarbamide*	$-\overset{}{\underset{\|\|}{C}}NH_2$ O	29
96	*Sulfathiourea*	$-\overset{}{\underset{\|\|}{C}}NH_2$ S	30
97	*Sulfaguanidine*	$\overset{NH}{\overset{\|\|}{-C-NH_2}}$	31

Table 1, continued

98	Sulfisoxazole		32
99	Sulfamoxole		33
100	Sulfaphenazole		34
101	Sulfasomizole		35
102	Sulfathiazole		36
103	Sulfapyridine		37
104	Sulfachloropyridazine		38
105	Sulfamethoxypyridazine		39
106	Sulfadiazine		31
107	Sulfamerazine		40

Table 1, continued

108	Sulfadimidine	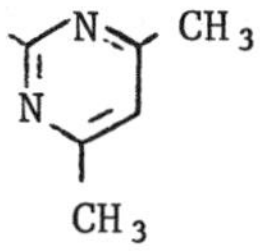	41
109	Sulfaisodimidine	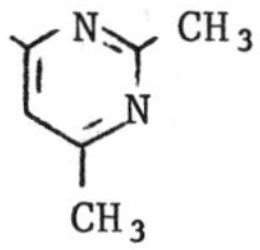	42
110	Glymidine	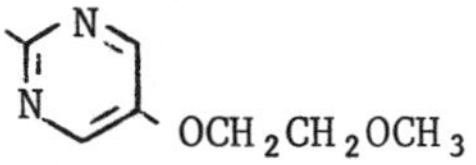	43
111	Sulfameter	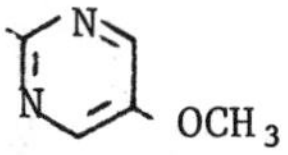	44
112	Sulfadimethoxine	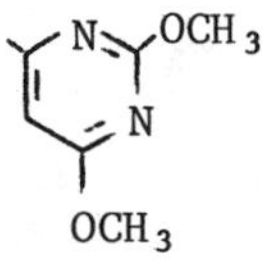	45
113	Sulformethoxine	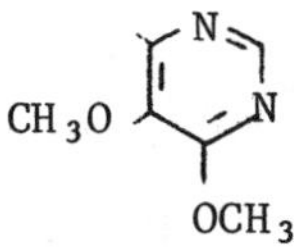	46
114	Sulfalene	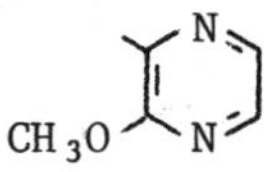	47
115	Sulfamethizole	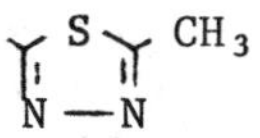	48
116	Sulfaethidole	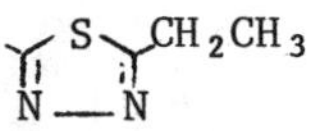	49
117	Glyprothiazole	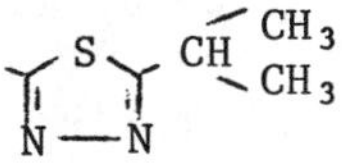	49

Table 1, continued

| 118 | Glybuthiazole | $\begin{array}{c} CH_3 \\ | \\ S \quad C-CH_3 \\ | \\ N-N \quad CH_3 \end{array}$ | 50 |

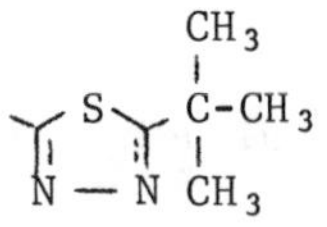

Claisen condensation of propionitrile with ethyl acetate in the presence of sodium ethoxide gives the cyanobutanone, *119*. This presumably forms oxime, *120*, on reaction with hydroxylamine; that intermediate is not isolated as it cyclizes spontaneously to the isoxazole, *121*. Acylation of the isoxazole with the sulfonyl chloride, *88*, affords *sulfisoxazole (98)* after removal of the acetyl group.

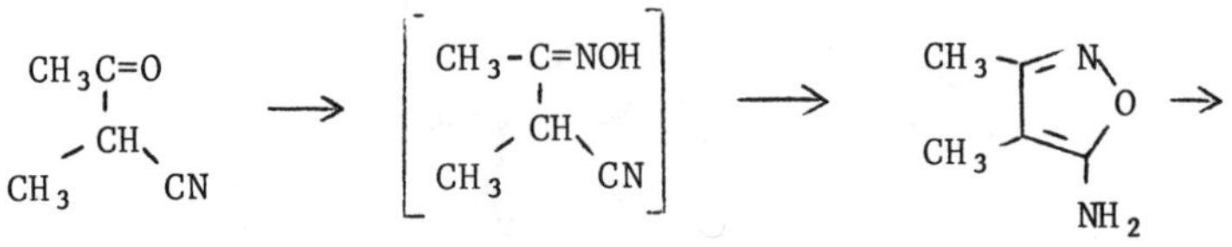

      119   120   121

The aminothiazole, *123*, required for preparation of *sulfathiazole (102)*, one of the older sulfonamides still in use, is available directly from the reaction of 1,2-dichloroethoxyethane with thiourea. The intermediate, *122*, is not observed, as elimination of ethanol is spontaneous under the reaction conditions.

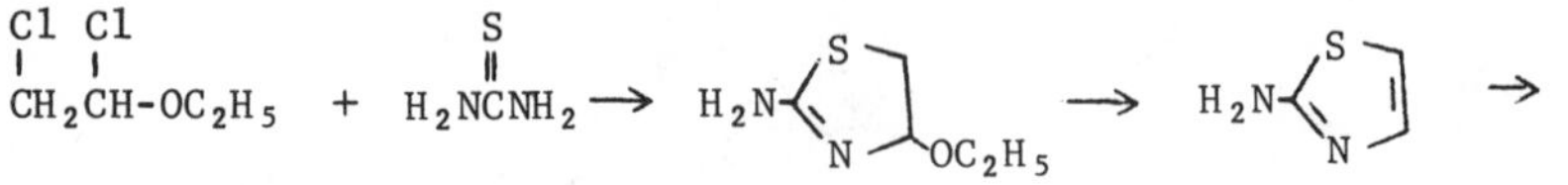

                      122   123

Acylation of thiosemicarbazide with propionyl chloride, interestingly, does not stop at the acylated product *(124)*. Instead, this intermediate cyclizes to the thiadiazole, *125*, under the reaction conditions. Hydrolysis then affords the heterocyclic amine, *126*. Acylation by *88* followed by removal of the acetyl group affords *sulfaethidole (116)*; variation of the acid chloride used in the preparation of the heterocycle leads to *117* and *118*.

The heterocyclic moiety of a sulfonamide need not be pre-

$$\text{CH}_3\text{CH}_2\overset{\overset{\text{O}}{\|}}{\text{C}}\text{Cl} \quad + \quad \text{H}_2\text{N-C}\overset{\nearrow\text{NH}_2\text{NH}_2}{\underset{\searrow\text{S}}{}} \quad \rightarrow$$

$$\left[\text{CH}_3\text{CH}_2\overset{\overset{\text{O}}{\|}}{\text{C}}-\overset{\text{H}}{\text{N}}-\text{C}\overset{\nearrow\text{NH}_2\text{NH}_2}{\underset{\searrow\text{S}}{}} \quad \underset{\text{O}}{\overset{\diagup\text{CCH}_2\text{CH}_3}{}}\right] \quad \rightarrow \quad \underset{\underset{\text{H}}{\text{RN}}}{}\overset{\text{N}-\text{N}}{\underset{\text{S}}{}}\text{CH}_2\text{CH}_3$$

$$124 \qquad\qquad\qquad\qquad 125, \text{ R=COCH}_2\text{CH}_3$$
$$126, \text{ R=H}$$

formed before attachment of the sulfonamide fragment. In an interesting variation on the above sequence, the semicarbazide of acetaldehyde (127) is acylated with the sulfonyl chloride, 88. Oxidation of the intermediate leads the semicarbazone to cyclize to a thiadiazole (129). Deacetylation affords the *sulfamethizole* (115).

$$88 \quad + \quad \text{H}_2\text{N}\overset{\overset{\text{S}}{\|}}{\text{C}}\overset{\text{H}}{\text{N}}\text{HN=CCH}_3 \quad \rightarrow \quad \text{CH}_3\overset{\overset{\text{O}}{\|}}{\text{C}}\overset{\text{H}}{\text{N}}-\underset{}{\bigcirc}-\text{SO}_2\overset{\text{H}}{\text{N}}-\text{C}\overset{\nearrow\text{NHN}}{\underset{\searrow\text{S}}{}}\overset{}{\text{C}}\text{-CH}_3$$

$$127 \qquad\qquad\qquad\qquad 128$$

$$\downarrow$$

$$\underset{\text{RN}}{\overset{\text{H}}{}}-\underset{}{\bigcirc}-\text{SO}_2\overset{\text{H}}{\text{N}}\overset{\text{N}-\text{N}}{\underset{\text{S}}{}}\text{CH}_3$$

$$129, \quad \text{R=CH}_3\text{CO}$$
$$115, \quad \text{R=H}$$

It may be speculated that one spur to the synthesis of the numerous pyrimidine-substituted sulfonamides was the known efficacy of *sulfaguanidine*; an aminopyrimidine does, of course, contain a good part of the guanidine functionality. One of the classical preparations of 2-aminopyrimidine starts with the condensation of guanidine with formylacetic ester (130) to give the pyrimidone, 131 (shown as the keto tautomer). Reaction with phosphorus oxychloride converts the oxygen to chlorine (132) via

the enol. Catalytic hydrogenation affords the desired amine
(133). This is then taken on to *sulfadiazine (106)* in the usual
way.

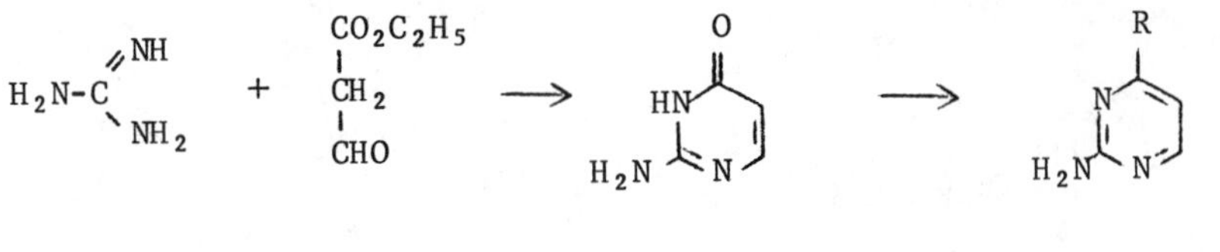

130   131   132, R=Cl
                                                      133, R=H

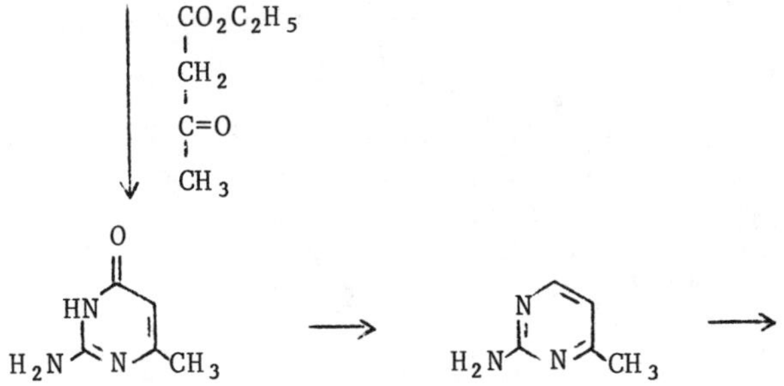

134   135   107

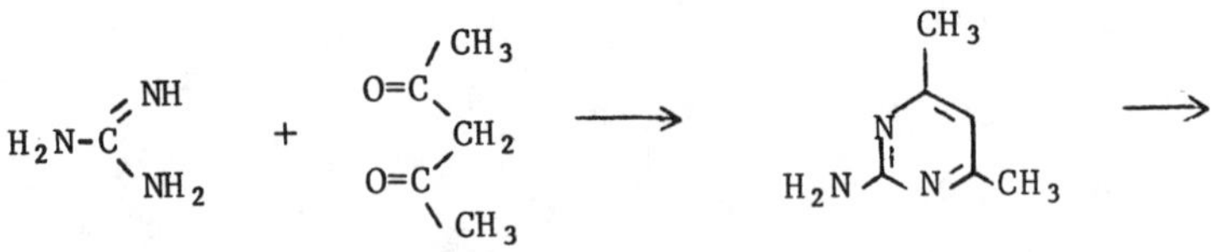

136

This sequence is equally applicable to keto esters. Thus,
condensation of guanidine with ethyl acetoacetate gives the
pyrimidone, *134*. Elaboration as above gives the pyrimidine, *135*;
acylation with the sulfonyl chloride *(88)* followed by hydrolysis
yields *sulfamerazine (107)*. Reaction of guanidine with beta
dicarbonyl compounds gives the pyrimidine directly. Condensation
of the base with acetonyl acetone affords the starting amine for
sulfadimidine (108).

A somewhat different approach is used to prepare the compounds containing the amine at the 4 position. Condensation of
the amidine from acetonitrile *(138)* with the enol ether from
formylacetonitrile *(137)* leads to the requisite pyrimidine *(139)*.

Since the ring nitrogen at 3 is now comparable in reactivity to
the amine at 4, acylation with one equivalent of *88* gives a mixture of products. The desired product, *sulfaisodimidine (109)*,
can be obtained by acylation with an excess of the sulfonyl chloride *(140)* followed by alkaline hydrolysis. The rate of saponification of the sulfonamide group attached to the ring nitrogen is
sufficiently greater to cause it to be lost selectively.

$$CHOC_2H_5$$
$$CH$$
$$CN$$

137   *138*   *139*

140, $Ar=p-CH_3CNHC_6H_4$

Inclusion of oxygen on the pyrimidine ring has been found
empirically to increase the effective serum half-lives.
Villsmeier reaction on the dimethylacetal of methoxyacetaldehyde
(141) with phosgene and dimethylformamide affords the acrolein
derivative, *142*. Condensation of this with guanidine gives the
pyrimidine, *143*. (The enamine can be viewed as a latent aldehyde-
the dimethylamino group is probably lost in the course of an addition elimination reaction with one of the guanidine groups.) This
pyrimidine serves as starting material for *sulfameter (111)*.

$$CH_3OCH_2CH$$

141   *142*   *143*

The preparation of *sulfadimethoxine (112)* takes advantage of
the observation that inclusion of electron-releasing substituents
on a pyrimidine ring activates halogen attached to the ring towards nucleophilic aromatic substitution. Preparation of the
required starting material begins by conversion of barbituric
acid *(144)* to the trihalide *(145)* by means of phosphorus oxychloride. Treatment with two equivalents of sodium methoxide effects
displacement of only two of the halogens *(146)*. Reaction of that
intermediate with the sodium salt from *sulfanilamide (93)* effects
replacement of the remaining chlorine to give *sulfadimethoxine*
(112).

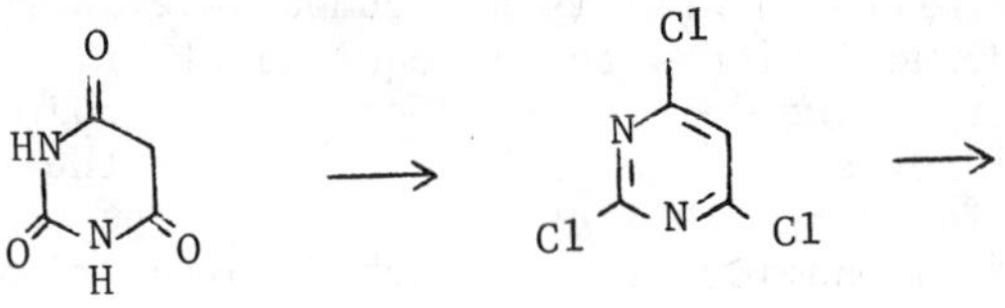

144   145

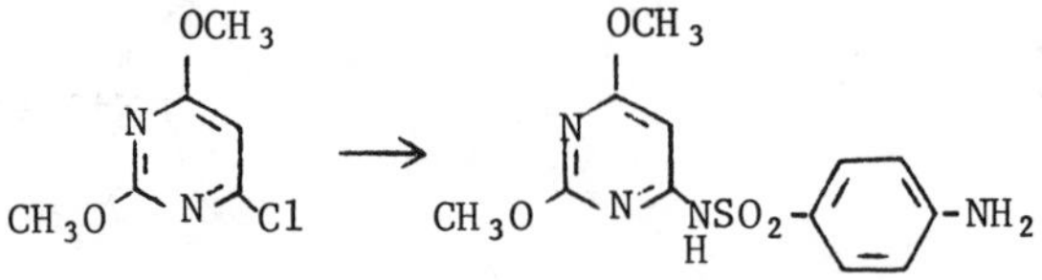

146   112

A somewhat more circuitous route is required to prepare sul-
fonamide-containing pyrimidines unsubstituted at 2. Thus, acylation of the 2-thiomethyl pyrimidine, *147*, with the sulfonyl
chloride, *88*, affords *148*. Removal of sulfur by means of Raney
nickel *(149)* followed by deacetylation gives *sulformethoxine*
(113).

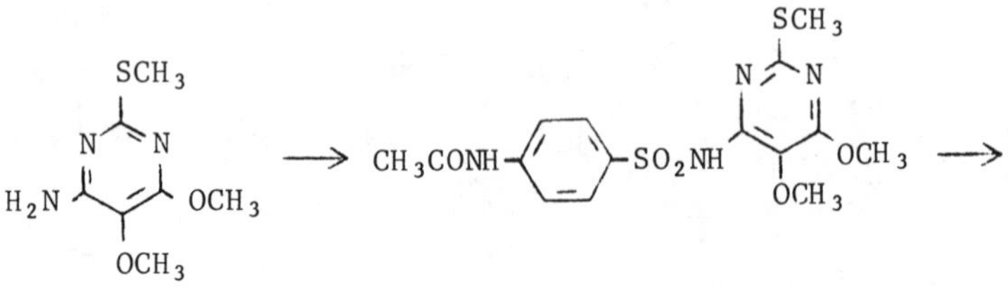

147   148

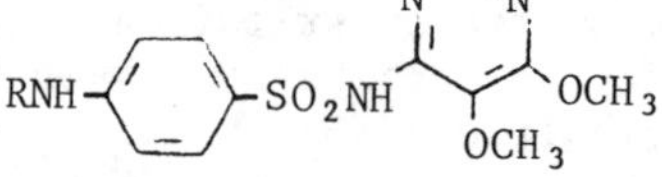

149, R=COCH$_3$
113, R=H

Preparation of the substituted piperazine required for *sulfalene (114)* starts with bromination of 2-aminopiperazine to give the dihalide *(150)*. Displacement of halogen by sodium methoxide proceeds regioselectively at the more reactive 3 position to give *151*. Hydrogenolysis over palladium on charcoal gives the desired intermediate *(152)*.

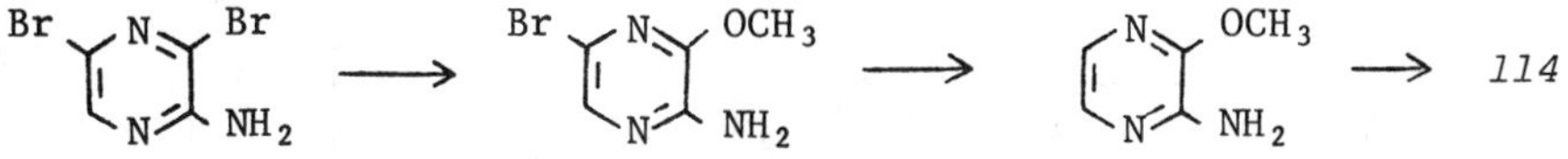

150   151   152

Similar selectivity in displacement reactions is shown by 3,6-dichloropyridazine *(153)* (available by halogenation of the product from maleic anhydride and hydrazine). Thus, reaction of the dihalide with the sodium salt from sulfanilamide *(93)* affords *sulfachloropyridazine (104)*. Reaction of this last with sodium methoxide under somewhat more drastic conditions results in displacement of the remaining chlorine to give *sulfamethoxypyridazine (105)*.

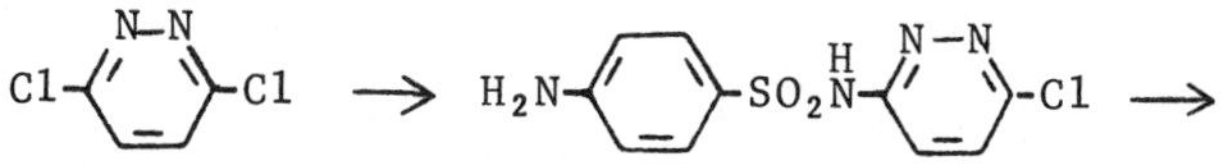

153   104

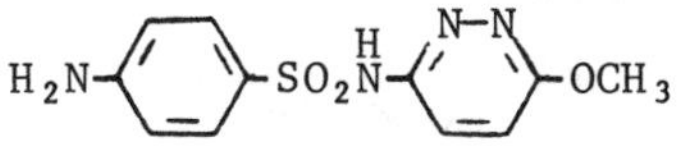

105

Acylation of a sulfonamide on the amide nitrogen serves to remove the sometimes objectionable taste of these drugs. Reaction of intermediate, *154*, with acetic anhydride followed by reduction of the nitro group affords *acetyl methoxyprazine (156)*.[51] The last, which has much the same biologic action as the parent compound, is used for oral administration in syrups.

Sterilization of the G.I. tract either in preparation for surgery or treatment of intestinal infection requires administration of an antibiotic in a form such that it will not be absorbed

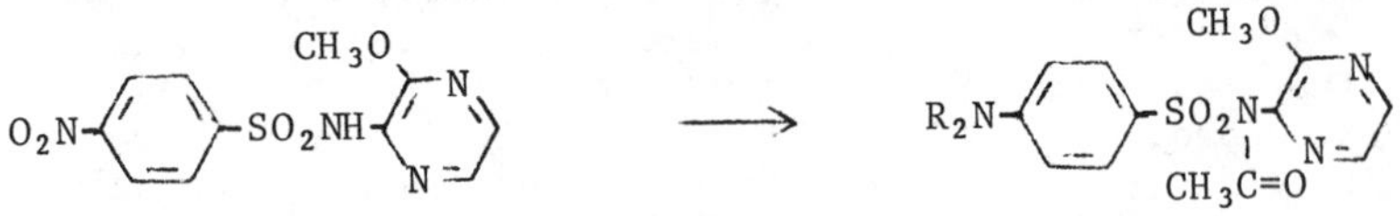

154

155, R=O
156, R=H

prior to the desired site of action. Acylation of the amine nitrogen of a sulfa antibiotic with a dibasic acid affords compounds that are not absorbed systemically following oral administration. Reaction of sulfathiazole with succinic anhydride under
rigorously controlled conditions affords directly *succinyl sulfathiazole (157)*[52]; a similar reaction with phthalic anhydride gives
phthaloyl sulfathiazole (158).[53]

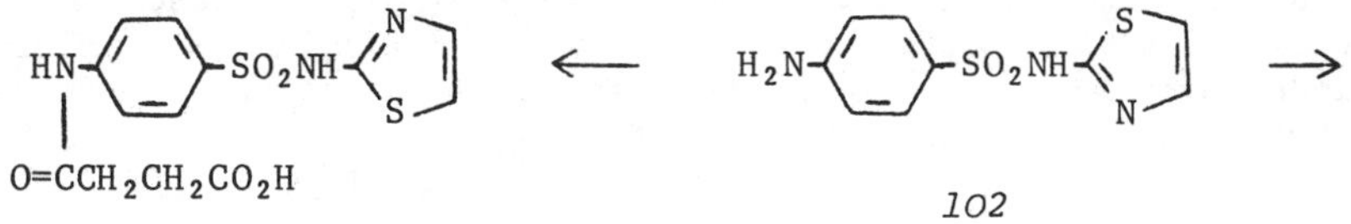

157

102

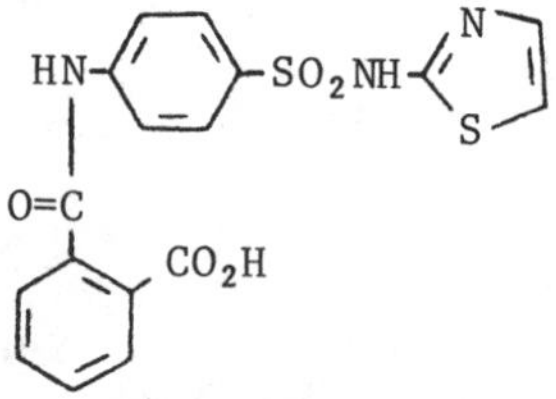

158

b. Bissulfonamidobenzenes

Among one of the more unusual side effects noticed as the use of
the sulfonamides became widespread was the increased urine output
of many patients treated with these drugs. The fact that the
urine was unusually alkaline led to the suspicion, later confirmed by independent means, that these agents were responsible
for partial inhibition of the enzyme carbonic anhydrase. Inhibition of this enzyme causes increased excretion of sodium and bi-
carbonate ions as well as water, in effect bringing about diure-

sis.

  While the use of diuretics had long been recognized as a
valuable tool for the treatment of many diseases involving water
retention, relatively few effective agents were available prior
to the development of the compounds based on the sulfonamides.
These serendipitous observations led to an intensive effort to
maximize the effect of these agents on carbonic anhydrase. It
was soon found that among the simpler compounds, the best activity is obtained by inclusion of two sulfonamide groups disposed
meta to each other on the aromatic ring. Treatment of chlorobenzene with chlorosulfonic acid under forcing conditions affords
the bis sulfonyl chloride, 159. Ammonolysis of this intermediate
gives *chlorphenamide (160)*. A similar sequence on metachloroaniline leads to *chloraminophenamide (162)*.[54] Dihalogenated aroma-
tics are apparently sufficiently inert towards the bischlorosul-
fonation reaction; thus a more elaborate sequence is required for
preparation of such analogs. Reaction of orthochlorophenol with
chlorosulfonic acid affords intermediate *(163)*; ammonolysis gives
the sulfonamide *(164)*. In an unusual reaction, treatment of the
phenol with phosphorus trichloride then replaces the hydroxyl
group by chlorine to afford *dichlorophenamide (165)*.[55]

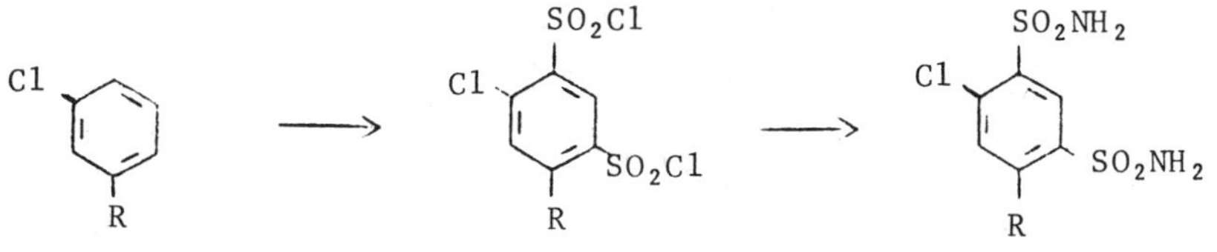

R=H, NH$_2$

159, R=H
161, R=NH$_2$

160, R=H
162, R=NH$_2$

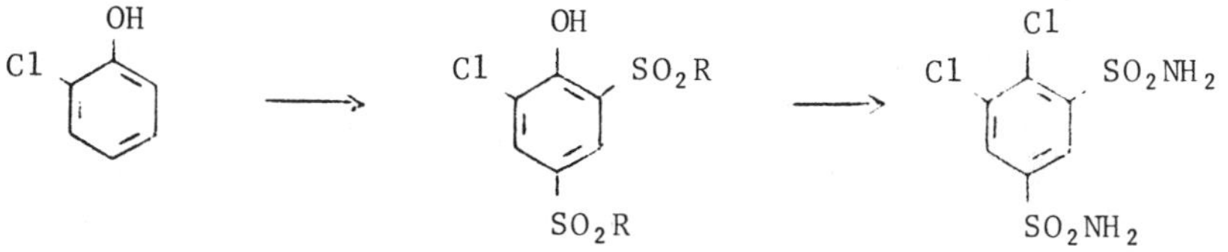

163, R=Cl
164, R=NH$_2$

165

  Chlorosulfonation of chlorobenzene under milder conditions
affords the product of monosubstitution *(166)*; reaction with

ammonia then gives the sulfonamide (167). Chlorosulfonation of
that sulfonamide then affords an intermediate (168) suitable for
preparation of diuretics containing differing substituents on
nitrogen. Thus, reduction of the cyclic cyanohydrin, 169, affords
the amine, 170; formylation by ester interchange with methyl formate (171) followed by reduction with lithium aluminum hydride
gives the N-methylated derivative (172). Acylation of the last
by the sulfonyl chloride, 168, gives the diuretic mefruside
(173).[56]

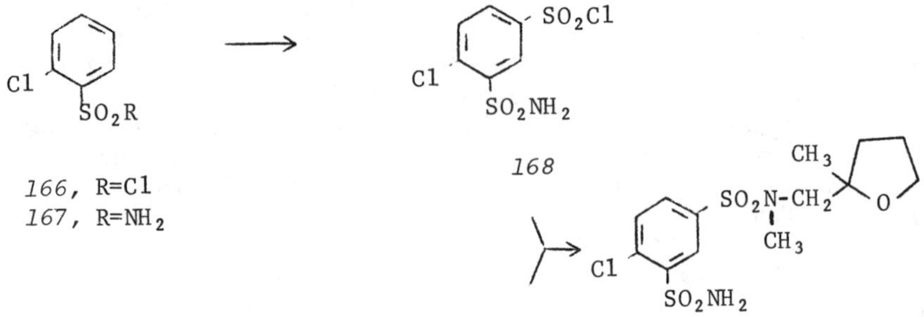

166, R=Cl
167, R=NH$_2$

168

173

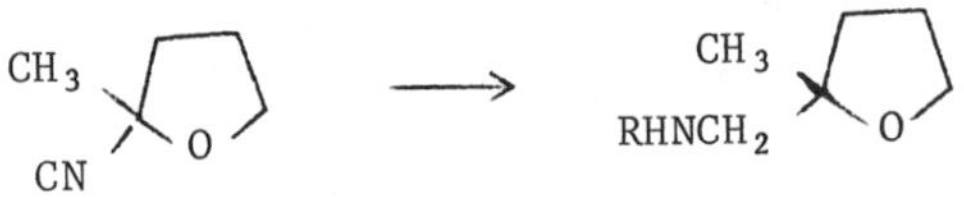

169

170, R=H
171, R=CHO
172, R=CH$_3$

c. Sulfonamidobenzoic Acids

Diuretic activity can be retained in the face of replacement of
one of the sulfonamide groups by a carboxylic acid or amide.
Reaction of the dichlorobenzoic acid, 174, with chlorsulfonic
acid gives the sulfonyl chloride, 175; this is then converted to
the amide (176). Reaction of that compound with furfurylamine
leads to nucleophilic aromatic displacement of the highly activated chlorine at the 2 position. There is thus obtained the
very potent diuretic furosemide (177).[57]
  Nitrosation of 2,6-dimethylpiperidine gives the correspond-

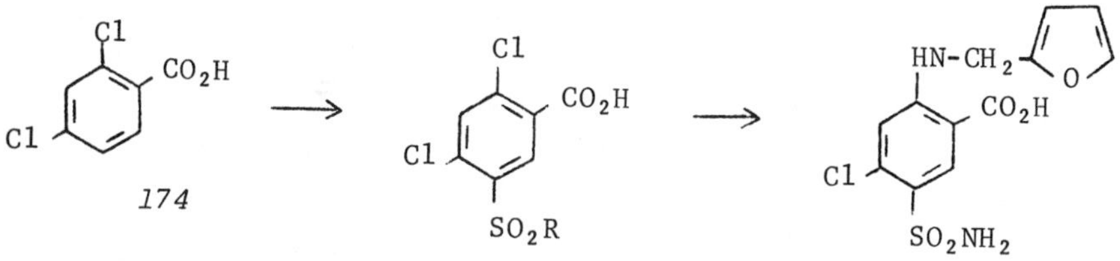

175, R=Cl
176, R=NH$_2$

177

ing N-nitroso compound (178); reduction leads to the hydrazine derivative, 179. Reaction of that intermediate with the acid chloride, 180 (available from the chlorosulfonation product of p-chlorobenzoic acid), gives the diuretic clopamide (181).[58]

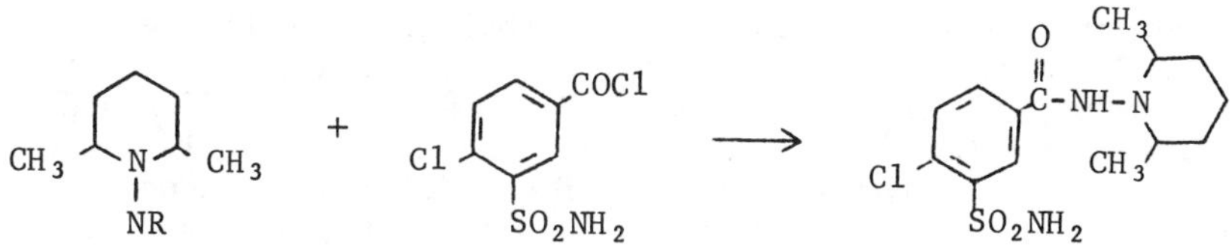

178, R=NO
179, R=NH$_2$

180

181

When penicillin was first introduced, clinicians were plagued by the extremely rapid excretion in the urine of this then extremely scarce drug. It was hoped that some other acidic compound administered along with the antibiotic might be excreted by the kidneys competitively with the drug and thus slow its loss via urine. A search for such an agent turned to a sulfonamide acid of known low toxicity, probenecid (183). In fact, administration of this compound, which has no significant antibacterial activity in its own right, along with penicillin significantly prolonged blood levels of the antibiotic. In the course of these studies it was also noted, however, that probenecid promoted excretion of uric acid. The ready availability of long-acting penicillin derivatives has long since obviated the need for probenecid as an adjunct. The drug has since found a place in the treatment of gout.

The drug can be prepared in a straightforward manner by reaction of sulfonyl chloride, 182, with di-n-propylamine followed by hydrolysis of the nitrile to a carboxylic acid.[59]

$$NC-\langle\bigcirc\rangle-SO_2Cl \quad\longrightarrow\quad HO_2C-\langle\bigcirc\rangle-SO_2N\begin{array}{l}CH_2CH_2CH_3\\CH_2CH_2CH_3\end{array}$$

182   183

d. Sulfonylureas

Diabetes is a disorder of carbohydrate metabolism traceable to
deficiencies in the production of insulin by the pancreas. Prior
to the discovery of insulin by Banting and Best in the 1930s, the
lifespan of a young diabetic was limited indeed. The finding
that those diabetics whose disease began early in life could be
maintained on insulin from animal sources was dramatic. A goodly
number of diabetics do not manifest the disease until well into
their forties. Such patients may be controlled for some time by
diet or by insulin. The finding that some of the sulfonamide
antibiotics could lower blood sugar in some individuals (hypo-
glycemia) led to the development of an additional method for
treatment of the hyperglycemia of adult-onset diabetes. (It
should be noted that the drug is without effect on individuals
lacking capacity to produce insulin—the youthful diabetics).

Systematic modification of the sulfanilamide molecule in
order to maximize the hypoglycemic activity led to the observation that the sulfonamide is best replaced by a sulfonylurea
function. Modification on both the aromatic ring and the substituent on the terminal nitrogen modulates the activity of the products.

Sulfonylureas are accessible by the many methods that have
been developed for the preparation of simpler ureas. For example,
treatment of p-toluenesulfonamide (184) with butyl isocyanate
(185) affords tolbutamide (186).[60]

Reaction of the sodium salt of p-chlorosulfonamide with

$$CH_3-\langle\bigcirc\rangle-SO_2NH_2 \quad + \quad OCNCH_2CH_2CH_2CH_3 \quad\longrightarrow$$

184   185

$$CH_3-\underset{}{\underset{}{\bigcirc}}-SO_2NH\overset{\overset{O}{\|}}{C}NHCH_2CH_2CH_2CH_3$$

186

ethyl chlorocarbonate gives the carbamate, *188*. Reaction of that intermediate with *n*-propylamine gives *chlorpropamide (189)*.[61]

$$Cl-\underset{}{\underset{}{\bigcirc}}-SO_2NH_2 \longrightarrow Cl-\underset{}{\underset{}{\bigcirc}}-SO_2NHCO_2C_2H_5 \longrightarrow$$

187   *188*

$$Cl-\underset{}{\underset{}{\bigcirc}}-SO_2NH\overset{\overset{O}{\|}}{C}NHCH_2CH_2CH_3$$

189

Treatment of piperidine with nitrous acid affords the N-nitroso derivative *(190)*; reduction gives the corresponding hydrazine *(191)*. Condensation of this intermediate with the carbamate *(192)* obtained from *p*-toluenesulfonamide leads to the oral hypoglycemic agent *tolazemide (193)*.[62] In a similar vein, reaction of the hydrazine obtained by the same sequence from azepine *(194)* with the carbamate, *188*, gives *azepinamide (195)*.[62]

$$RN\bigcirc \quad + \quad CH_3-\underset{}{\underset{}{\bigcirc}}-SO_2NHCO_2C_2H_5 \longrightarrow CH_3-\underset{}{\underset{}{\bigcirc}}-SO_2NH\overset{\overset{O}{\|}}{C}NHN\bigcirc$$

190, R=NO   *192*   *193*
191, R=NH$_2$

$$H_2N-N\bigcirc \quad + \quad 188 \quad \longrightarrow \quad Cl-\underset{}{\underset{}{\bigcirc}}-SO_2NH\overset{\overset{O}{\|}}{C}NHN\bigcirc$$

194   *195*

In another approach to the required functionality, the sodium salt of acetyl sulfanilamide *(196)* is condensed with butyl

isothiocyanate *(197)* to afford the thiourea, *198*.   Reaction with
nitrous acid serves to convert the thiourea to a urea *(199)*.
Hydrolysis of acetyl group with aqueous base affords *carbutemide*
(200).[63]   An analogous sequence starting with the meta-substituted
sulfanilamide *(200)* affords *1-butyl-3-metanylurea (202)*.[64]

$$CH_3CONH-\!\!\left\langle\bigcirc\right\rangle\!\!-SO_2NH_2 \quad + \quad SCN(CH_2)_3CH_3 \quad \longrightarrow \quad RNH-\!\!\left\langle\bigcirc\right\rangle\!\!-SO_2\overset{\overset{X}{\|}}{N}HCNHCH_2CH_2CH_2CH_3$$

196   197   *198*, R=COCH$_3$; X=S
                                                        199, R=COCH$_3$; X=O
                                                        200, R=H; X=O

$$\underset{CH_3CONH}{\left\langle\bigcirc\right\rangle}\!\!-SO_2NH_2 \qquad \longrightarrow \qquad \underset{H_2N}{\left\langle\bigcirc\right\rangle}\!\!-SO_2NH\overset{\overset{O}{\|}}{C}NHCH_2CH_2CH_2CH_3$$

201   *202*

Inclusion of a para acetyl group requires a somewhat different approach to the preparation of these compounds.   Reaction of
the diazonium salt from *p*-aminoacetophenone with sulfur dioxide
affords the sulfonyl chloride, *203*; this is then converted to the
sulfonamide, *204*.   Elaboration via the carbamate with cyclohexyl-
amine affords *acetohexamide (205)*.[65]

$$CH_3\overset{\overset{O}{\|}}{C}-\!\!\left\langle\bigcirc\right\rangle\!\!-NH_2 \quad \longrightarrow \quad CH_3\overset{\overset{O}{\|}}{C}-\!\!\left\langle\bigcirc\right\rangle\!\!-SO_2R$$

203, R=Cl
204, R=NH$_2$

$$\longrightarrow \quad CH_3\overset{\overset{O}{\|}}{C}-\!\!\left\langle\bigcirc\right\rangle\!\!-SO_2NH\overset{\overset{O}{\|}}{C}NH-\!\!\left\langle\bigcirc\right\rangle$$

205

It is of note that hypoglycemic activity is maintained even
when the aromatic ring is fused onto a carbocyclic ring.   Chlor-
sulfonation of hydrindan gives chloride, *206*.   Reaction of the
sulfonamide *(207)* obtained from that intermediate with cyclohexyl
isocyanate leads to *glyhexamide (208)*.[66]

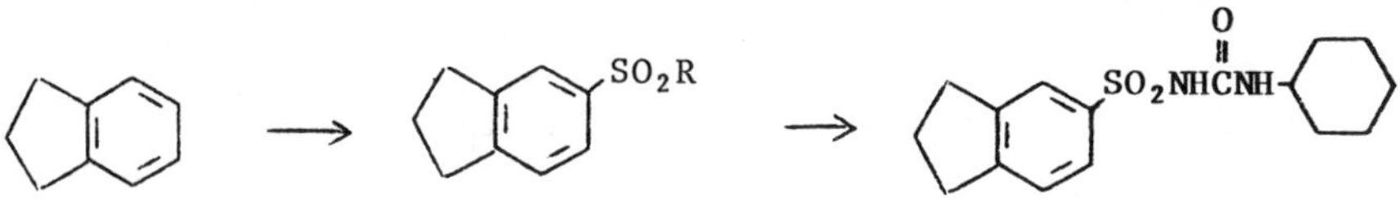

206, R=Cl
207, R=NH$_2$

208

Finally, attachment of a rather complex side chain to the para position of the benzene ring on the sulfonamide leads to the very potent, long-acting oral antidiabetic agent, *glyburide* (215).[67] Preparation of this compound starts with the chlorosulfonation of the acetamide of β-phenethylamine (209). The resulting sulfonyl chloride (210) is then converted to the sulfonamide (211) and deacylated (212). Reaction with the salicylic acid derivative, 213, in the presence of carbodiimide affords the amide, 214. Condensation of that with cyclohexylisocyanate affords *glyburide* (215).[68]

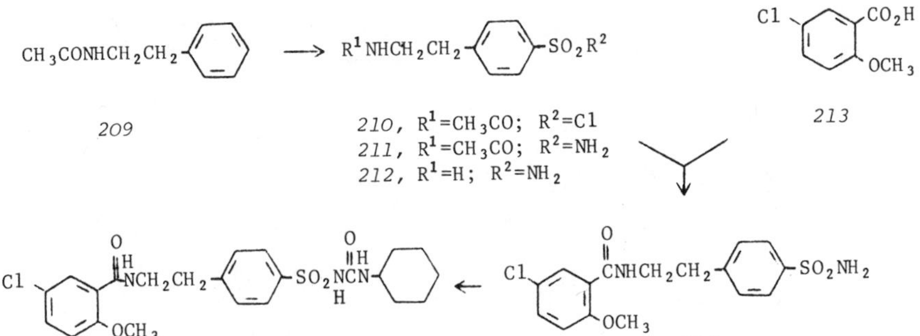

209

210, R^1=CH$_3$CO; R^2=Cl
211, R^1=CH$_3$CO; R^2=NH$_2$
212, R^1=H; R^2=NH$_2$

213

215

214

e. Diarylsulfones

Compounds closely related to the sulfonamide antibiotics proved to be the first drugs effective against *Mycobacterium leprae*, the causative agent of the disease known since antiquity, leprosy. These drugs are at least partly responsible for the decline of those horror spots, the leper colonies.

Synthesis of the first of the antileprosy drugs, *dapsone* (219), starts with aromatic nucleophilic substitution of the sodium salt of the sulfinic acid, *216*, on *p*-chloronitrobenzene to afford the sulfone *(217)*. Reduction of the nitro group *(218)* followed by deacetylation gives *dapsone (219)*. The low solubility of this drug in water makes it unsuitable for administration by injection. Reaction of *dapsone* with the sodium bisulfite adduct of formaldehyde gives the water-soluble prodrug *sulfoxone (220)*.[69] Reaction of the diamine, *219*, with the sodium bisulfite adduct from glucose gives the solubilized derivative *glucosufone (221)*.[70]

216

217, R=O
218, R=H

219

221

220

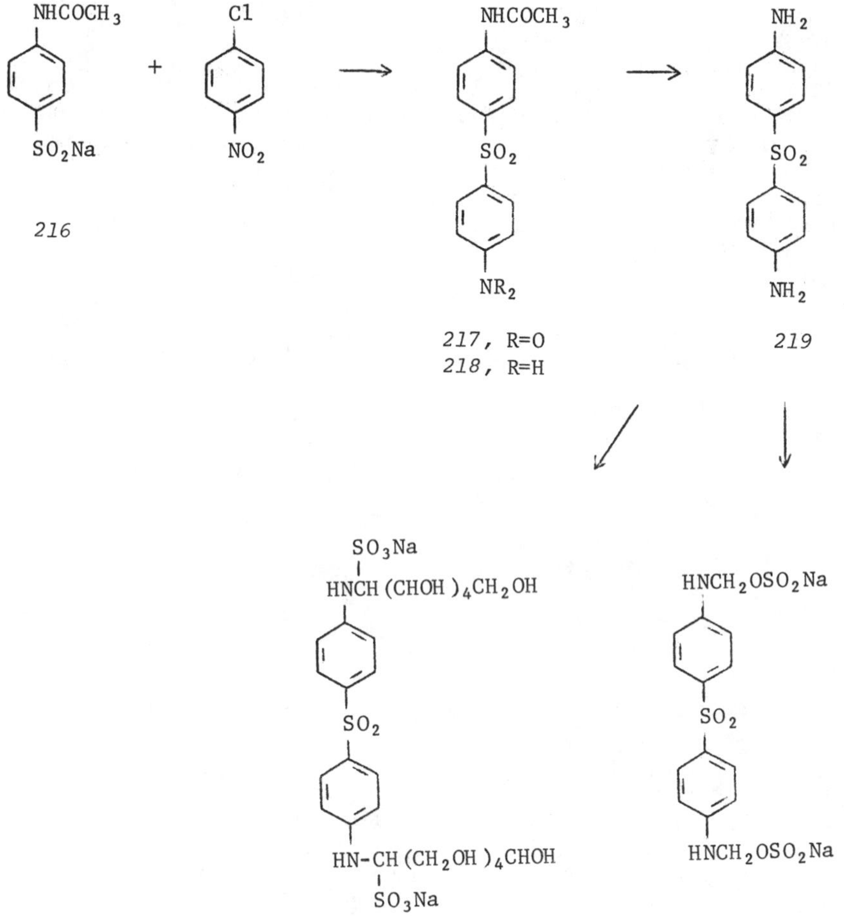

A heterocyclic ring may be used in place of one of the benzene rings without loss of biologic activity. The first step in the synthesis of such an agent starts by Friedel-Crafts-like acylation rather than displacement. Thus, reaction of sulfenyl chloride, *222*, with 2-aminothiazole *(223)* in the presence of acetic anhydride affords the sulfide, *224*. The amine is then protected as the amide *(225)*. Oxidation with hydrogen peroxide leads to the corresponding sulfone *(226)*; hydrolysis followed by reduction of the nitro group then affords *thiazosulfone (227)*.[71]

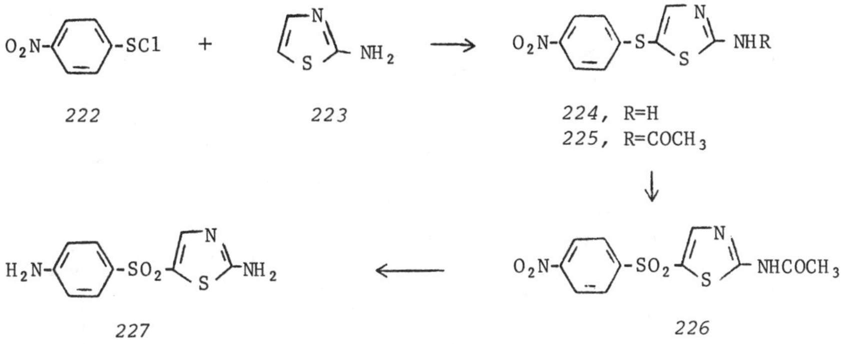

O_2N
SCl
+
N
S
NH_2
N
S
S
NHR
222
223
224, R=H
225, R=$COCH_3$
H_2N
SO_2
N
S
NH_2
N
S
SO_2
$NHCOCH_3$
227
226

REFERENCES

1. J. T. Sheehan, *J. Amer. Chem. Soc., 70*, 1665 (1943).
2. M. W. Goldberg, U. S. Patent 2,879,293 (1959).
3. J. H. Wilkinson and I. L. Finar, *J. Chem. Soc.*, 32 (1948).
4. C. V. Winder, J. Wax, L. Scotti, R. A. Scherrer, E. M. Jones, and F. W. Short, *J. Pharmacol. Exp. Ther., 138*, 405 (1962).
5. D. E. Pearson, K. N. Carter, and C. M. Greer, *J. Amer. Chem. Soc., 75*, 5905 (1953).
6. C. M. Baker and J. R. Campbell, U. S. Patent 2,887,513 (1959).
7. J. Harley-Mason and A. H. Jackson, *J. Chem. Soc.*, 3651 (1954).
8. K. Kawara, Japanese Patent 3,071 (1951).
9. F. H. S. Curd and F. L. Rose, *J. Chem. Soc.*, 729 (1946).
10. A. D. Ainsley, F. H. S. Curd, and F. L. Rose, *J. Chem. Soc.*, 98 (1949).
11. A. F. Crowther, F. H. S. Hurd, and F. L. Rose, *J. Chem. Soc.*,

1780 (1951).

12. L. C. Cheney, R. R. Smith, and S. B. Binkley, *J. Amer. Chem. Soc.*, *71*, 60 (1949).

13. Anon., British Patent 914,008 (1962); *Chem. Abst.*, *58*, 523c (1963).

14. A. Buzas, J. Teste, and J. Frossard, *Bull. Soc. Chim. Fr.*, 839 (1959).

15. Anon., Belgian Patent 629,613 (1963); *Chem. Abst.*, *60*, 14,437d (1963).

16. R. Howe and R. G. Shanks, *Nature*, *210*, 1336 (1966).

17. A. F. Crowther and L. H. Smith, *J. Med. Chem.*, *11*, 1009 (1968).

18. A. Brandstrom, N. Carrodi, U. Junggren, and T. E. Jonsson, *Acta Pharm. Suecica*, *3*, 303 (1966).

19. H. L. Yale, E. J. Pribyl, W. Braker, F. H. Bergeim, and W. A. Lott, *J. Amer. Chem. Soc.*, *72*, 3710 (1950).

20. R. S. Murphy, U. S. Patent 2,770,649 (1956).

21. H. E. Parker, U. S. Patent 3,214,336 (1965).

22. C. D. Lunsford, R. P. Mays, J. A. Ridiman, Jr., and R. S. Murphey, *J. Amer. Chem. Soc.*, *82*, 1166 (1900).

23. H. Gilman and G. R. Wilder, *J. Amer. Chem. Soc.*, *77*, 6644 (1955).

24. E. M. Schultz, E. S. Cragoe, Jr., J. B. Bricking, W. A. Bolhofer, and J. M. Sprague, *J. Med. Chem.*, *5*, 660 (1962).

25. G. Domagk, *Deut. Med. Wochenschr.*, *61*, 250 (1935).

26. J. Trefouel, J. Fourneau, F. Nitti, and D. Bovet, *Compt. Rend. Soc. Biol.*, *120*, 756 (1935).

27. M. L. Crossley, E. H. Northey, and M. E. Hultquist, *J. Amer. Chem. Soc.*, *61*, 2950 (1939).

28. H. Gysin, U. S. Patent 2,503,820 (1950).

29. P. S. Winnek, G. W. Anderson, H. W. Marson, H. E. Faith, and R. O. Roblin, Jr., *J. Amer. Chem. Soc.*, *64*, 1682 (1942).

30. L. C. Leitch, B. E. Baker, and L. Brickman, *Can. J. Res.*, *23B*, 139 (1945).

31. R. O. Roblin, Jr., J. H. Williams, P. S. Winnek, and J. P. English, *J. Amer. Chem. Soc.*, *62*, 2002 (1940).

32. H. M. Wuest and M. Hoffer, U. S. Patent 2,430,094 (1947).

33. W. Loop, E. Luhrs, and P. Hauschildt, U. S. Patent 2,809,966 (1957).

34. P. Schmidt and J. Druey, *Helv. Chim. Acta*, *41*, 306 (1958).

35. A. Adams and R. Slack, *J. Chem. Soc.*, 3070 (1959).

36. R. J. Fossbinder and L. A. Walter, *J. Amer. Chem. Soc.*, *61*, 2032 (1939).

37. R. Winterbottom, *J. Amer. Chem. Soc.*, *62*, 160 (1940).

38. M. M. Lester and J. P. English, U. S. Patent 2,790,798 (1957).

39. J. H. Clark, U. S. Patent 2,712,012 (1955).
40. H. J. Backer and A. B. Grevenstuk, *Rec. Trav. Chim. Pays Bas, 61*, 291 (1942).
41. W. T. Caldwell, E. C. Kornfeld, and C. K. Donnell, *J. Amer. Chem. Soc., 63*, 2188 (1941).
42. W. Loop and E. Luhrs, *Ann., 580*, 225 (1953).
43. K. Gutsche, A. Harwart, H. Horstmann, H. Priewe, G. Raspe, E. Schraufstatter, S. Wirtz, and U. Worffel, *Arzneimittel Forsch., 14*, 373 (1964).
44. H. Horstmann, T. Knott, W. Scholtan, E. Schraufstatter, A. Walter, and U. Worffel, *Arzneimittel Forsch., 11*, 682 (1961).
45. R. G. Shepherd, W. E. Taft, and H. M. Krazinski, *J. Org. Chem., 26*, 2764 (1961).
46. Anon., Belg. Patent 618,639 (1962); *Chem. Abs., 59*, 7,540c (1963).
47. B. Camerino and G. Palamidessi, U. S. Patent 3,098,069 (1963).
48. O. Hubner, U. S. Patent 2,447,702 (1948).
49. H. Wojahn and H. Wuckel, *Arch. Pharm., 284*, 53 (1951).
50. Anon., Brit. Patent 828,963 (1960); *Chem. Abs., 54*, 12,500i (1960).
51. B. Camarino and G. Palamidessi, *Gazz. Chim. Ital., 90*, 1815 (1960).
52. M. L. Moore and C. S. Miller, *J. Amer. Chem. Soc., 64*, 1572 (1942).
53. M. L. Moore, U. S. Patent 2,324,013 (1943).
54. F. C. Novella and J. M. Sprague, *J. Amer. Chem. Soc., 79*, 2028 (1957).
55. E. M. Schultz, U. S. Patent 2,835,702 (1958).
56. H. Horstmann, H. Wollweber, and K. Meng, *Arzneimittel Forsch., 17*, 653 (1967).
57. K. Sturm, W. Siedel, and R. Weyer, German Patent 1,122,541 (1962).
58. E. Jucker and A. Lindenmann, *Helv. Chim. Acta, 45*, 2316 (1962).
59. C. S. Miller, U. S. Patent 2,608,507 (1952).
60. H. Ruschig, W. Avmuller, G. Korger, H. Wagner, and J. Scholtz, U. S. Patent 2,968,158 (1961).
61. F. J. Marshall and M. V. Sigal, *J. Org. Chem., 23*, 927 (1958).
62. J. B. Wright and R. E. Willette, *J. Med. Chem., 5*, 815 (1962).
63. E. Haack, U. S. Patent 2,907,692 (1959).
64. E. Haack, *Arzneimittel Forsch., 8*, 444 (1958).
65. F. J. Marshall, M. V. Sigal, H. R. Sullivan, C. Cesnik, and

M. A. Root, *J. Med. Chem.*, *6*, 60 (1963).

66. H. Hoehn and H. Breur, U. S. Patent 3,097,242 (1963).
67. W. Avmuller, A. Bander, R. Heerdt, K. Muth, P. Pfaff, F. H. Schmidt, H. Weber, and R. Weyer, *Arzneimittel Forsch.*, *16*, 640 (1966).
68. R. S. P. Hsi, *J. Labeled Comp.*, *9*, 91 (1973).
69. H. Bauer, *J. Amer. Chem. Soc.*, *61*, 617 (1939).
70. Anon., Swiss Patent 234,108 (1944); *Chem. Abstr.*, *43*, 4297a (1949).
71. L. L. Bambas, *J. Amer. Chem. Soc.*, *67*, 671 (1945).

CHAPTER 9

Polycyclic Aromatic Compounds

1. INDENES

a. Indenes with Basic Substituents

The low order of structural specificity required for classical antihistaminic activity was noted earlier. It has been found possible to substitute an indene nucleus for one of the two aromatic rings that most of these agents possess. The basic side chain may be present as either dimethylaminoethyl or itself cyclized to provide an additional fused ring.

Alkylation of 1-indanone with 2-dimethylaminoethyl chloride affords the substituted ketone (1). Condensation with the lithium reagent obtained from 2-ethylpyridine affords the alcohol (2). Dehydration under acidic conditions gives *dimethylpyrindene (3)*.[1]

Mannich reaction of methylamine and formaldehyde with two equivalents of acetophenone leads to the unusual double condensation product, 4. Treatment of this diketone with base leads to the intramolecular aldol product (5). The symmetrical nature of 4 allows but one product. Strong acid serves to both cyclize the carbonyl group into the aromatic ring and to dehydrate the tertiary alcohol (although not necessarily in that order); there is thus obtained the diene, 6. Conditions for the catalytic hydrogenation of this product can be so arranged as to give the product of 1,4 addition of hydrogen, the indene, *pyrindamine (7)*.[2]

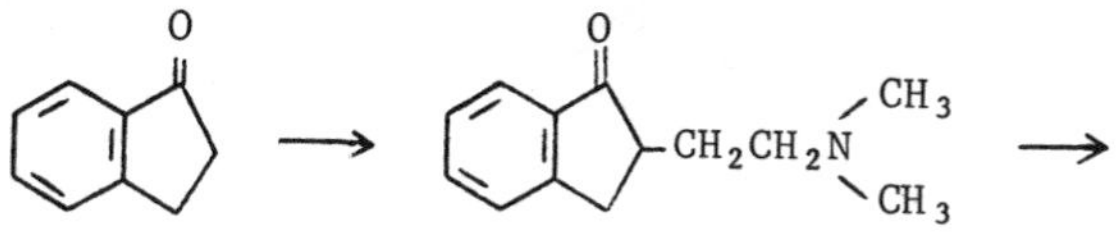

1

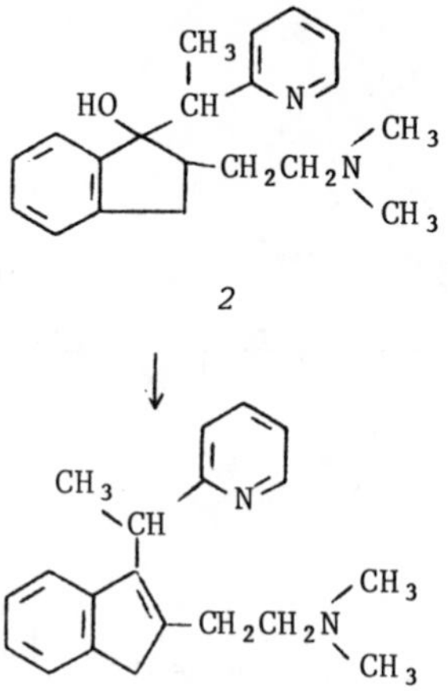

CH3
HO
CH
N
CH2CH2N
CH3
CH3
CH3
CH
N
CH2CH2N
CH3
CH3

2 → *3*

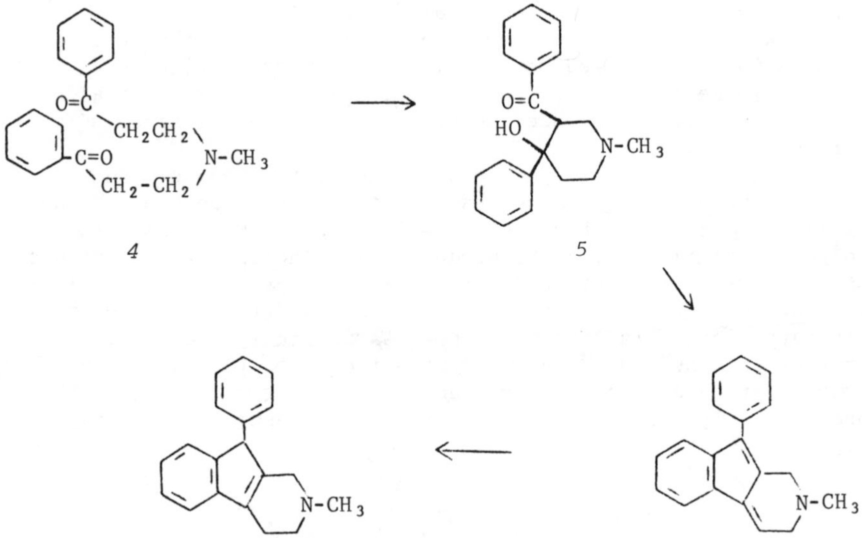

O=C
CH2CH2
C=O
N-CH3
CH2-CH2
O=C
HO
N-CH3
N-CH3
N-CH3

4 → *5* → *6* → *7*

b.   Indandiones

Anticoagulant therapy was developed with the adventitious discovery of *dicoumarol (8)*. A fuller discussion of the rationale for
the use of such compounds is found in the chapter on Five-Membered Heterocycles Fused to One Benzene Ring. The reader's attention is directed, however, at the fact that *dicoumarol* is a poly-
carbonyl compound containing a very acidic hydrogen. A series of
similarly acidic 1,3-indandiones have been found to constitute an
additional class of anticoagulant agents.

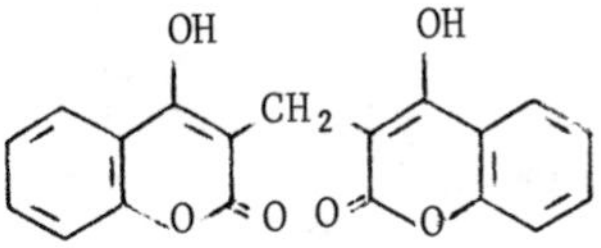

8

Condensation of an appropriately substituted phenylacetic
acid with phthalic anhydride in the presence of sodium acetate
leads to aldol-like reaction of the methylene group on the acid
with the carbonyl on the anhydride. Dehydration followed by
decarboxylation of the intermediate affords the methylenephthal-
ides *(12)*. Treatment of the phthalides with base affords directly
the indandiones, probably via an intermediate formally derived
from the keto-acid anion *(13)*. The first agent of this class to
be introduced was *phenindandione (14)*[3]; this was followed by
anisindandione (15)[4] and *chlorindandione (16)*.[5]

Replacement of the phenyl group at the 2 position by diphenylacetyl affords an anticoagulant with long duration of action
and improved therapeutic ratio. Condensation of dimethyl phthal-
ate with 1,1-diphenylacetone *(17)* in the presence of base affords
phenindandione (18).[6]

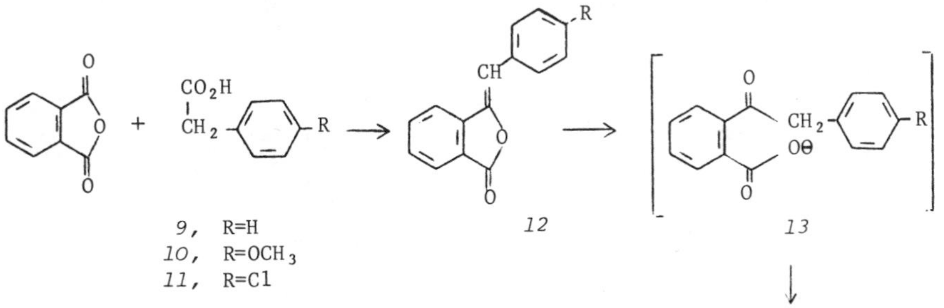

9,   R=H
10,   R=OCH$_3$
11,   R=Cl

12

13

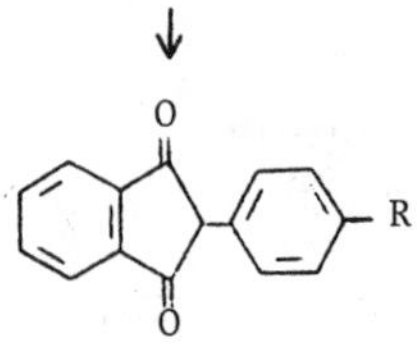

14, R=H
15, R=OCH$_3$
16, R=Cl

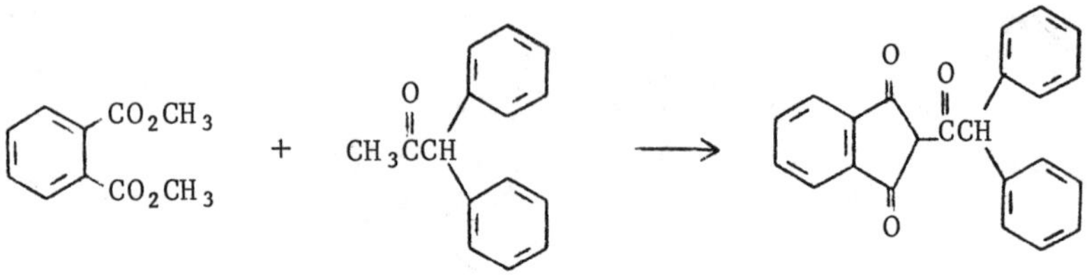

17   18

2. DIHYDRONAPHTHALENES

As noted previously, triarylethylenes substituted by a basic
group, such as *clomiphene*, exhibit estrogen antagonist activity.
Formal cyclization of that molecule to a more steroid-like, rigid
conformation enhances potency in this series.

Wittig condensation of the ylide from the phosphonium salt,
19, with the hydroxymethylene ketone, *20*, affords the product,
21, as a mixture of isomers. Catalytic hydrogenation leads to
22. Treatment of that intermediate with aluminum chloride leads
to selective demethylation of that ether para to the carbonyl
group *(23)*. Cyclization by means of tosic acid gives the dihydro-
naphthalene nucleus *(24)*. Alkylation of the phenol with N-(2-
chloroethyl)pyrrolidine affords *nafoxidine (25)*.[7]

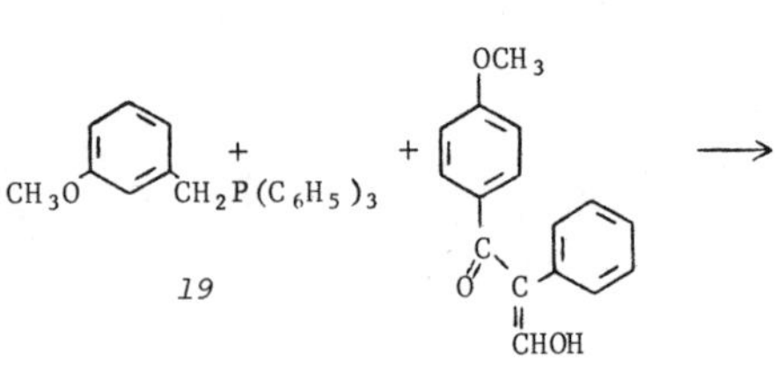

19   20

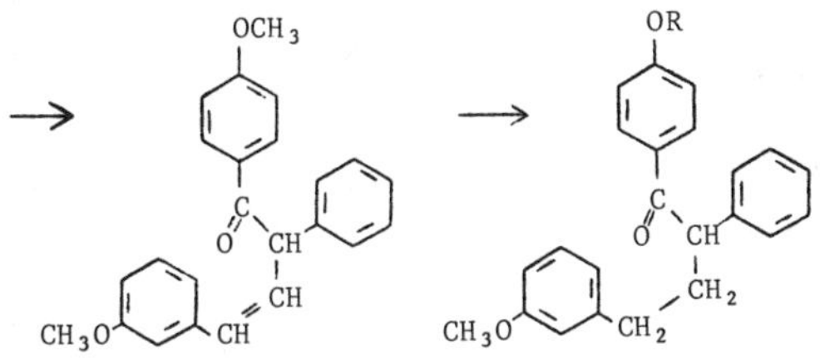

21

22, R=CH$_3$
23, R=H

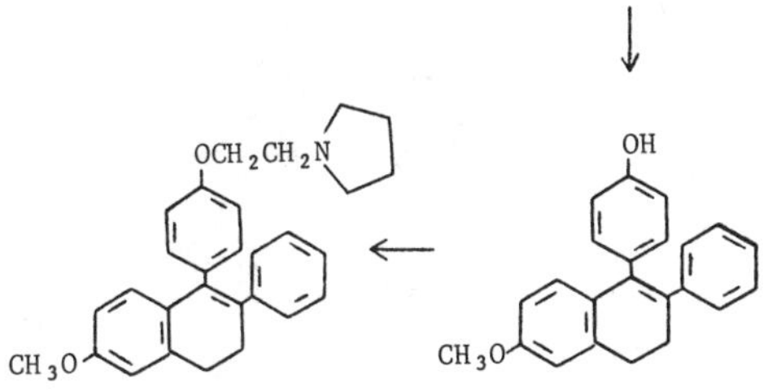

25   24

3. DIBENZOCYCLOHEPTENES AND DIBENZOCYCLOHEPTADIENES

Almost anyone who has at some time in his life met some reverses
is familiar with depression. In the normal course of events,
changing circumstances will soon lead to the replacement of this
state of mind by a more pleasant one. There exist, however, a
set of pathologic states in which depression feeds on itself in
a destructive cycle. Individuals affected with this syndrome—
whether precipitated by outside events or not—eventually find it
most difficult to function. The advent of antidepressant drugs,
first the MAO inhibitors and more recently the tricyclic antidepressants, have made this syndrome amenable to treatment.

The intent in the preparation of the first of these drugs
was possibly the synthesis of analogs of the phenothiazine tranquilizer drugs (A). It is a well-known rule of thumb in medicinal chemistry that biologic activity can often be maintained
when sulfur is replaced by an ethylene group—saturated or unsaturated—and weakly basic nitrogen by carbon (B). Careful pharmacologic evaluation of the compounds produced by this rationale
revealed them to have utility as antidepressants rather than
tranquilizers.

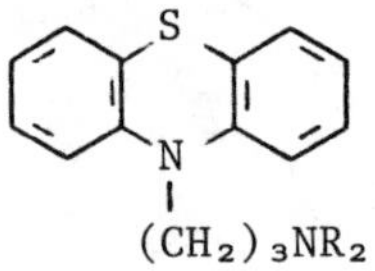

A

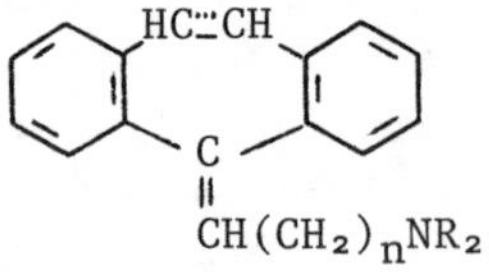

B

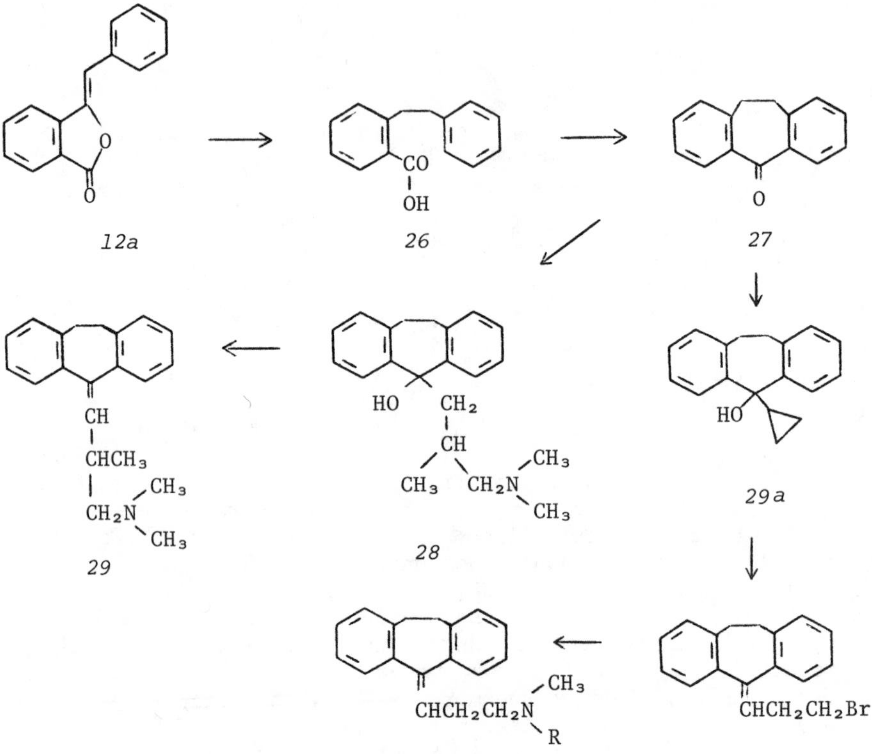

12a

$\longrightarrow$

26

$\longrightarrow$

27

29

28

29a

31, R=H
32, R=CH$_3$

30

Preparation of the key intermediate to this series begins by reduction of the methylene phthalide, *12a*, with hydriodic acid and red phosphorus. Cyclization of the acid *(26)* thus obtained affords the tricyclic ketone, *27*. Reaction with the Grignard reagent from 3-dimethylamino-2-methylpropyl chloride affords the alcohol, *28*. Dehydration of the carbinol gives *butriptyline* *(29)*.[8]

The scheme used above for attaching the side chain is not applicable to secondary amines since such compounds would not form organometallics. In an ingenious synthesis, the ketone, *27*, is first condensed with cyclopropyl-magnesium bromide *(29a)*. Solvolysis in hydrogen bromide goes to the allylic halide, *30*, via the cyclopropylcarbinyl cation (see Prostaglandins for a fuller exposition of this reaction). Displacement of the allylic halogen by means of methylamine gives *nortriptylene (31)*[9]; reaction with dimethylamine, on the other hand, gives *amytriptylene (32)*.

An alternate scheme for preparation of the last drug involves first bromination of the methylene group on *33* (obtainable by several methods from *27*). A displacement reaction of the Grignard reagent prepared from *34* on 2-dimethylaminoethyl chloride affords again *amytriptylene (32)*.[10]

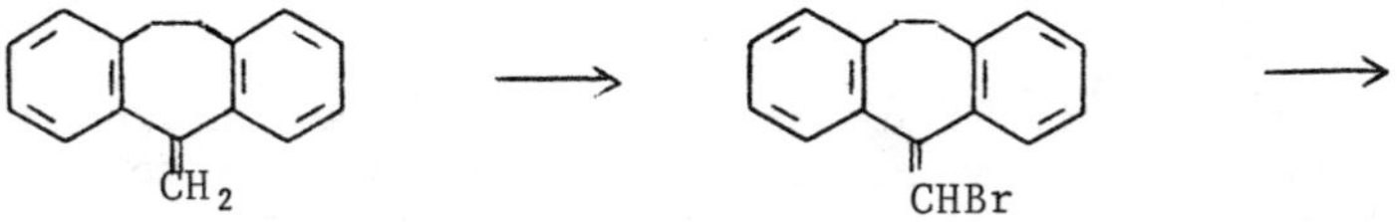

33	*34*	

To anticipate briefly, shortening the length of the side chain in the phenothiazines from three to two carbon atoms changes the activity of the products from neuroleptics to antihistaminic agents. A rather similar effect is seen in the tricyclic antidepressants. Reaction of ketone, *27*, with the Grignard reagent from 4-chloro-1-methylpipyridine *(35)* affords the tertiary alcohol, *36*. Dehydration gives the antihistamine, *cyproheptadine (37)*.[11]

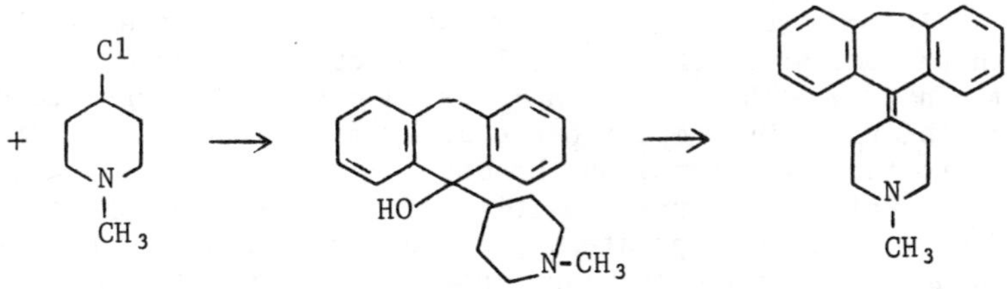

35	*36*	*37*

Introduction of an additional double bond into the tricyclic nucleus, on the other hand, is consistent with antidepressant activity. Alkylation of the potassium salt, obtained on treatment of hydrocarbon, *38*, with ammonia, with the chlorocarbamate, *39*, affords the intermediate, *40*. Basic hydrolysis leads to *protriptylene (41)*.[12]

40, R=$CO_2C_2H_5$
41, R=H

4. COLCHICINE

The active principle of the autumn crocus *(Colchicum autumnale)*, *colchicine (48)*, is one of the very few drugs that have remained in reputable medical use since ancient times. This drug was the only useful treatment available for the excruciating pain associated with crystallization of uric acid in the joints characteristic of gout until the advent of *allopurinol*. Although the precise mechanism by which *colchicine* gives this dramatic relief remains undefined, the antimitotic activity of this agent is thought to play a role in its effect. Due to the difficulty of preparation, few analogs of *colchicine* exist; it is structurally a one-drug class.

Preparation of the molecule by total synthesis is rendered unusually difficult by the presence of the two fused seven-membered rings, one of which is a tropolone. The most recent of several total syntheses of this molecule is noteworthy for building this very system in a single step.[13] The synthesis starts with the oxidative phenol coupling reaction on the diphenolic compound, *42*. This reaction, carried out in the presence of an iron chloride:DMF complex proceeds by first forming a radical para to the free phenol on the more highly oxygenated ring; addition of this to the para position of the remaining phenolic ring affords, after appropriate adjustment of electrons, the spirodienone, *43*. Treatment with diazomethane converts the phenol to the ether; reduction by means of sodium borohydride affords the alcohol, *44*, as a mixture of epimers. Methyleneation by means of the Simmons-Smith reaction (methylene iodide:zinc-copper couple) converts the olefinic bond to a cyclopropane *(45)*. Oxidation by means of Jones reagent gives the ketone, *46*.

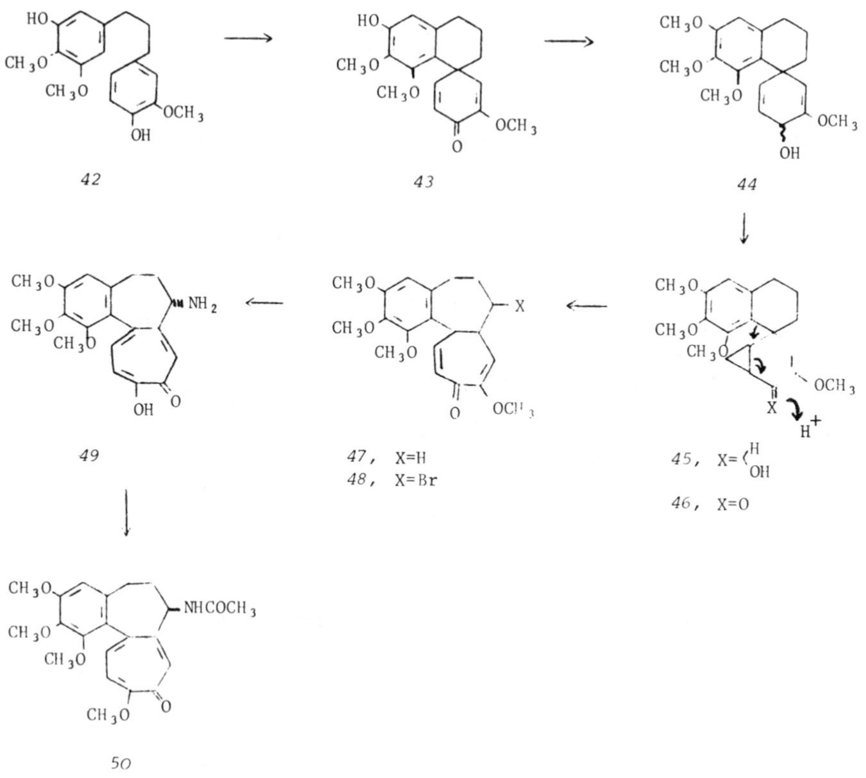

The key step in this sequence, achieved by exposure of *46* to a mixture of sulfuric acid and acetic anhydride, involves opening of the cyclopropane ring by migration of a sigma bond from the quaternary center to one terminus of the former cyclo-propane. This complex rearrangement, rather reminiscent of the dienone-phenol reaction, serves to both build the proper carbon skeleton and to provide ring C in the proper oxidation state. The synthesis concludes by the route pioneered by Eschenmoser.[14] Bromination of *47* proceeds at the position α to the tropolone ring to give *48*. Displacement of halogen by ammonia followed by base hydrolysis of the tropolone methyl ether gives trimethyl-colchicinic acid. Acetylation of the amine followed by reesterification of the tropolone yields *colchicine (50)*.

REFERENCES

1. C. F. Huebner, E. Donoghue, P. Wenk, E. Sury, and J. A. Nelson, *J. Amer. Chem. Soc., 82*, 2077 (1960).
2. J. T. Plati and W. Wenner, U. S. Patent 2,470,108 (1947).
3. C. S. Jacques, E. Gordona, and E. Lipp, *Can. Med. Assoc. J., 62*, 465 (1950).
4. A. Horeau and J. Jacques, *Bull. Soc. Chim. France*, 53 (1948).
5. H. G. Kreg, *Pharmazie, 13*, 619 (1958).
6. D. G. Thomas, U. S. Patent 2,672,483 (1954).
7. D. Lednicer, D. E. Emmert, S. C. Lyster, and G. W. Duncan, *J. Med. Chem., 12*, 881 (1969).
8. S. O. Winthrop, M. A. Davis, G. S. Myers, J. G. Gavin, R. Thomas, and R. Barber, *J. Org. Chem., 27*, 230 (1962).
9. R. D. Hoffsommer, D. Taub, and N. L. Wendler, *J. Org. Chem., 27*, 4134 (1962).
10. R. D. Hoffsommer, D. Taub, and N. L. Wendler, *J. Med. Chem., 8*, 555 (1965).
11. E. L. Engelhardt, U. S. Patent 3,014,911 (1961).
12. M. Tischler, J. M. Chemerda, and J. Kollonowitsch, Belgian Patent 634,448 (1964); *Chem. Abst., 61*, 4295a (1964).
13. E. Kotani, F. Miyazaki, and S. Tobinaga, *Chem. Commun.*, 300 (1974).
14. J. Schreiber, W. Leimgruber, M. Pesaro, P. Schudel, T. Threfall, and A. Eschenmoser, *Helv. Chim. Acta, 44*, 540 (1961).

CHAPTER 10

Steroids

The development of this class of tetracyclic alicyclic compounds into several classes of therapeutically useful drugs represents one of the most vivid illustrations of the serendipitous nature of medicinal chemistry. Each series of steroid drugs, the estrogens, the androgens, the progestins, and finally the corticoids, were first discovered during investigations of mammalian endocrine systems. The infinitesimal amounts of these agents present in mammalian tissues hampered the initial endocrinologic work; it was obvious that material would have to be obtained from some source other than isolation from animal glands in order to define the mode of action of the compounds. The potent biologic effects of these compounds, as well as the structural complexity of those for which a structure had been assigned, acted as a spur to synthetic chemists. The initial work consisted largely of partial syntheses from steroids from some other, more abundant natural source. With time, each of the natural steroids has been prepared by total synthesis. With the few exceptions noted below, the total syntheses, although often elegant, have not proved commercially competitive with partial synthesis.

Once the steroid hormones became available to endocrinologists in sizeable quantities, the pharmacology of the agents was investigated in greater detail. It was found that these drugs had unanticipated uses far beyond mere replacement therapy. Thus the corticoids, the steroids of the adrenal cortex, were to be of great value in the relief of inflammation; the androgens elaborated by the male testes were found to have anabolic effects. Finally, an appropriate combination of progestin and estrogen was found to inhibit ovulation in the female, leading eventually to the development of the oral contraceptive, the Pill.

The steroids, as found in mammalian systems, are seldom useful as drugs due to a fairly general lack of oral activity. Most of the agents exert other actions in addition to the desired one.

155

one. An androgen, for example, continues to have masculinizing
properties even though it is in use as an anabolic agent. These
reasons, as well as the search for patentable entities, led to
intensive efforts on both the synthesis and pharmacology of modified steroids. The goal of oral activity has been handily met;
the split between the desired pharmacologic activity and the
intrinsic endocrine activity has at best been only partly achieved.

1. COMMERCIAL PREPARATION OF ESTROGENS, ANDROGENS, AND
    PROGESTINS

The steroids as a class represent a structurally complex problem
for the synthetic chemist. Even a relatively simple compound
such as estrone possesses three ring fusions, two of which can
lead to isomers and four chiral centers (identified below by *).
Only one of the sixteen possible isomers possesses the desired
activity in satisfactory potency.

estrone

    Although all the main classes of steroids have now been
attained by total synthesis, most drugs are in fact, as noted
above, prepared by partial synthesis from natural products that
contain the steroid nucleus. The bulk of the world's supply of
steroid starting material is derived by differing chemical routes
from only two species of plants: the Mexican yam, a species of
Dioscorea, and the humble soybean. The advantage of using plants
rather than valuable domestic animals as raw material is fairly
obvious.
    In a process developed by the chemists at Syntex,[1] the yam
is first processed to afford the sapogenin diosgenin *(1)*. This
material, which contains the requisite tetracyclic nucleus in the
correct stereochemical array, contains six superfluous carbon
atoms in the side chain. Treatment of diosgenin with hot acetic
anhydride in the presence of a catalyst such as p-toluenesulfonic
acid leads to a reaction reminiscent of the formation of enol

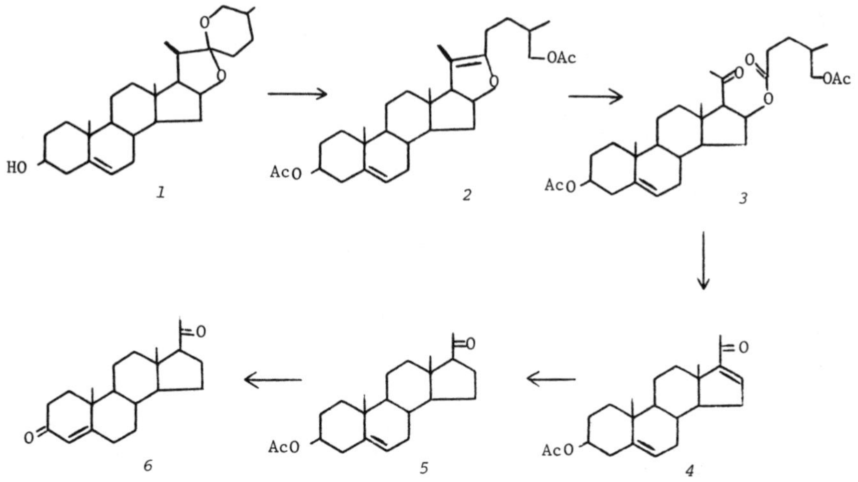

ethers from ketals. In this case the net result of the transfor-   ⑨
mation is the opening of the spiran ring to a dihydrofuran (2);
the hydroxyl at 3 is acetylated under these reaction conditions.[2]
Oxidation of (2) with chromium trioxide effects the desired scis-
sion of the side chain with formation of the desired 20 ketone.
Treatment of this ester of a β-ketoalcohol with acetic anhydride
leads to elimination of that ester grouping; there is obtained an
intermediate with functionality suitable for subsequent modification, 16-dehydropregnenolone (4). Catalytic reduction goes as
expected, preferentially at the conjugated double bond, to afford
pregnenolone acetate (5). When progesterone (6) is the target
molecule, the acetate is first removed by saponification; oxidation with an aluminum alcoholate (Oppenauer reaction), leads
initially to the unconjugated 3-keto-5-ene compound. The basic
reaction conditions serve to shift the double bond into conjugation. Progesterone is a key intermediate in the manufacture of
cortical steroids. The various intermediates listed above are
currently turned out in tonnage quantity.

    A progesterone precursor, 16-dehydropregenolone acetate,
serves as a starting material to the androgens as well. In an
ingenious scheme 4 is first converted to its oxime; treatment of
(8) under the conditions of the Beckmann rearrangement leads to
migration of the unsaturated center to nitrogen, with consequent
formation of the acylated eneamine (9). Hydrolysis affords presumably first the eneamine (10); this unstable entity further

suffers hydrolysis to give, finally, dehydroepiandrosterone acetate (11). Removal of the acetate by saponification followed by
Openauer oxidation leads to the conjugated 3-enone (12). There
is thus obtained androstenedione (12).[3],[4]

The nonsapponifiable fraction from the very abundant oil
from soybeans is known to be rich in a mixture of steroids bearing a ten carbon atom side chain at the 17 position. The chemists
at Upjohn developed an efficient and economical route for exploitation of this natural product as a source of progesterone.[5],[6]
Only stigmasterol (13), of the many steroids present in the crude
extract, bears unsaturation in the side chain; it is therefore
the only component of the mixture suitable for further processing.
Following its separation by an ingenious leaching process, this
compound is subjected to the conditions of the Openauer oxidation
to afford stigmastadienone (14). Ozonization of this compound
affects only the most electron-rich double bond, that in the
side chain; workup affords the ketoaldehyde (15) which is but one
carbon atom removed from the goal. This aldehyde is then converted selectively to the 22-eneamine (16). Oxidation of this last
under a variety of conditions (ozonization, photo-oxygenation)
affords progesterone (17).
    The structurally simplest steroids, the aromatic A ring
estrogens, have ironically proven most difficultly accessible
because this aromatic ring is not found in any of the plant
sterols available in commercial quantities. The main task of
partial synthesis from naturally occurring material thus becomes

the excision of the angular methyl group at the A-B ring junction.
In one of the earlier routes, androstenedione was first reduced
to androsterone *(18)*. (Introduction of hydrogen on the alpha
side, the side below the plane of the molecule, is determined by
attachment of the catalyst to the least-hindered side of the
molecule.) Treatment of the ketone with bromine in acetic acid
leads to formation of the 2,4-dibromide.[19] (There is good evidence that bromination affords first the 2-bromosteroids; this
then brominates again to give the 2,2-dibromo compound; the final
product is obtained after a series of rearrangements.) Treatment
of the dibromide with hot collidine leads to dehydrobromination
and formation of the 1,4-dienone *(21)*. Estrone *(25)* is obtained
in modest yield when that last compound is passed through a column at 600°C in the presence of mineral oil.[7] In an alternate
approach, the dienone is subjected to allylic bromination with
N-bromosuccinimide. The bromo compound *(22)* thus produced gives
triene *23* on treatment with collidine. Pyrolysis in mineral oil
leads to loss of the methyl group; catalytic hydrogenation reduces
the 6 double bond to afford estrone.[8] The better yield obtained
on pyrolysis of the triene apparently compensates for the additional steps in this sequence. In the most interesting and recent
modification, the dienone is first converted to its propylene
ketal *(20)*. Aromatization is accomplished by treatment of this
intermediate with the radical anion obtained from lithium and
diphenyl in refluxing tetrahydrofuran. Since the methyl group in
this case leaves as methyl lithium, diphenylmethane is included

in the reaction mixture to quench this by-product in order to prevent its reaction with starting material.[9] Workup of the reaction
mixture under acidic conditions results in hydrolysis of the ketal
at 17; estrone is then obtained directly in a quite respectable
yield.

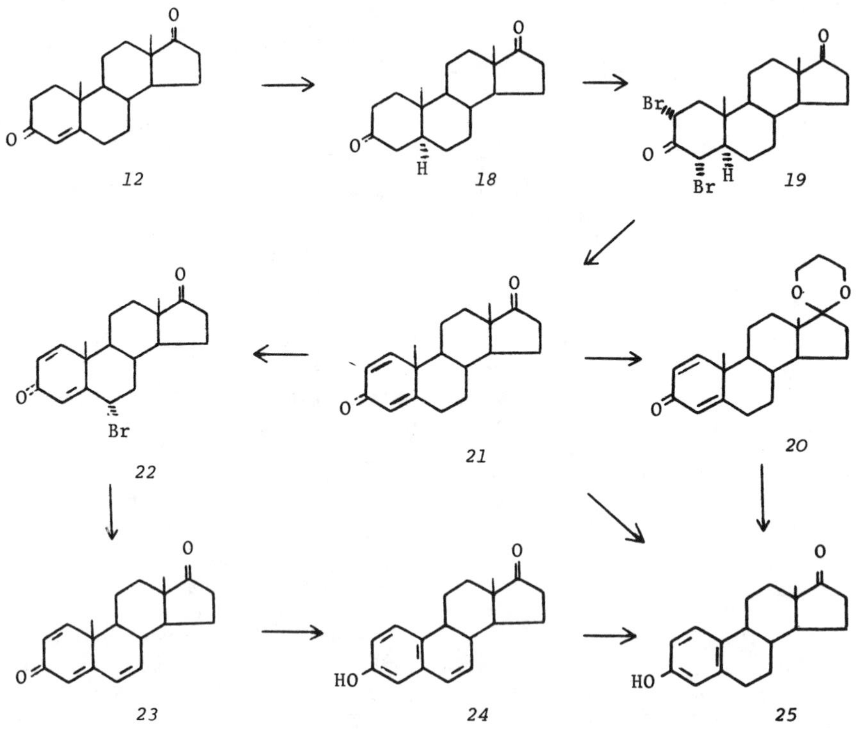

2. AROMATIC A-RING STEROIDS

The female of mammalian species secretes a series of steroid hormones characterized by an aromatic A ring and the lack of a side
chain at the 17 position. These compounds serve as regulators
in the reproductive processes of the species. The name (estrogens) comes from the fact that in some lower animals the elaboration of this type of compound is directly involved with the phe-

nomenon of heat estrus. In humans, these hormones are involved
not only in the menstrual cycle, but also in such diverse processes as implantation in the uterus of fertilized ova and calcium
metabolism. Estrogen deficiency has an adverse effect on general
health; the psychic manifestations of menopause, for example, are
at least partly traceable to the rapidly changing estrogen titers
characteristic of that time of life.

Although estrone and estradiol (26) have both been isolated
from human urine, it has recently been shown that it is the latter
that is the active compound that binds to the so-called estrogen
receptor protein.[10] Reduction of estrone with any of a large
number of reducing agents (for example, any of the complex metal
hydrides) leads cleanly to estradiol. This high degree of stereoselectivity to afford the product of attack at the alpha side of
the molecule is characteristic of many reactions of steroids.
This tendency is particularly marked at the 17 position; attack
at the alpha side meets only hydrogen interactions but approach
from the opposite side is hindered by the adjacent 18 methyl
group.

Although both *estrone* and estradiol are available for replacement therapy, they suffer the disadvantage of poor activity on
oral administration and short duration of action even when administered parenterally, because of ready metabolic disposition. In
order to overcome these deficiencies, there was developed a series
of esters of estradiol with long-chain fatty acids. These esters
are oil-soluble and correspondingly water-insoluble compounds.
They are usually administered intramuscularly by injection. Since
they are not soluble in water they form a so-called depot that
remains at or near the site of injection. As the esters slowly
hydrolyze by exposure to body fluids, the relatively water-soluble
estrone is released and finds its way into the bloodstream. In
this way the patient is provided with a reasonably constant low-
level dose of the hormone.

The esters are prepared by first treating estradiol with the
appropriate acid chloride. The resulting diester, 27, is then
subjected to mild acid or basic hydrolysis; in this way, the
phenolic ester group is removed selectively.

It has been established that both the 17 hydroxy androgens
and estrogens, when administered orally, are quickly converted
to water-soluble inactive metabolites by intestinal bacteria,
usually by reactions at the 17 position. It is this inactivation
process that is largely responsible for the low-order oral potency
observed with these agents. Incorporation of an additional carbon atom at the 17 position should serve to make the now tertiary
alcohol less susceptible to metabolic attack and thus potentially
confer oral activity to these derivatives.

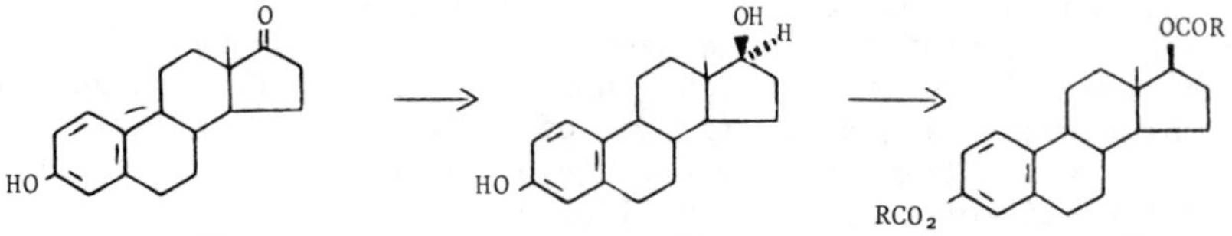

compound	R	generic name
27a	CH₂CH₃	*estradiol dipropionate*
28a	CH₂CH₂CH₂CH₃	*estradiol valerate*
28b	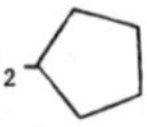 CH₂CH₂⟨cyclopentyl⟩	*estradiol cypionate*
28c	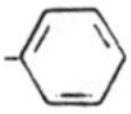 ⟨phenyl⟩	*estradiol benzoate*
28d	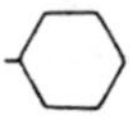 ⟨cyclohexyl⟩	*estradiol hexahydrobenzoate*

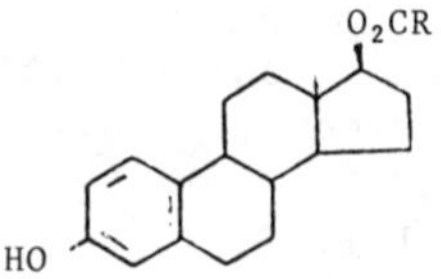

Reaction of estrone with a metal acetylide affords 17α-ethynyl-17β-hydroxy-estradiol (*ethynylestradiol, 30a*; EE).[12] This compound is equipotent with estradiol by subcutaneous administration, but it is 15 to 20 times as active when administered orally. Ethynylation of the methyl ether of estradiol analogously affords *mestranol (30b)*.[13] It should be noted that the same factors apply in these reactions as in previously discussed reductions at 17; almost the sole products of these reactions are those which result from attack of reagent from the least hindered α side of the steroid. *Ethynylestradiol* and *mestranol* are of special commercial significance since the majority of the oral contraceptives now on sale incorporate one or the other of the compounds as the estrogenic component.

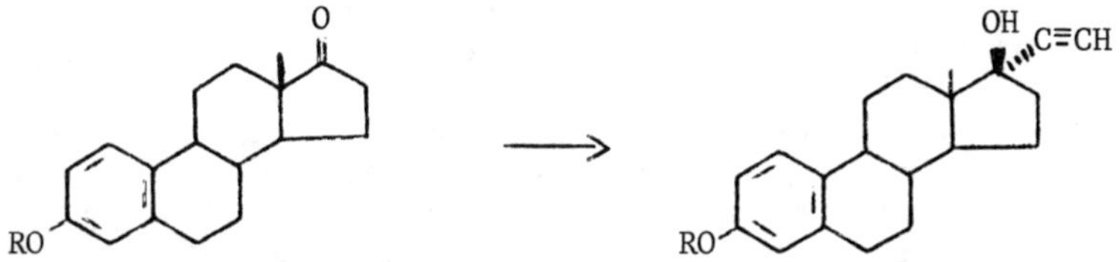

29a, R=H
29b, R=CH$_3$

30a, R=H, *ethynylestradiol*
30b, R=CH$_3$, *mestranol*

3. 19-NORSTEROIDS

a. 19-Norprogestins

Progesterone *(17)* possesses poor activity when administered by
mouth. This fact was particularly frustrating since it was known
as early as the late 1930s that this compound effectively inhib-
ited ovulation in rabbits when administered subcutaneously. The
development of an orally effective progestin thus seemed to hold
out the promise of the long looked for oral contraceptive. In
the following decade two compounds were indeed reported to show
oral progestational activity. The first of these, *ethisterone*
(31), was not suitable for use since it elicited androgenic
responses as well; the second compound, product of a long
and involved degradation of the difficultly attainable natural
product strophanthidin, was formulated at the time as 19-nor-
progesterone *(32)*.[16] (This product has since been shown to be
isomeric with progesterone at both C-14 and C-17). Both these
leads served to spur further synthetic efforts in this area.

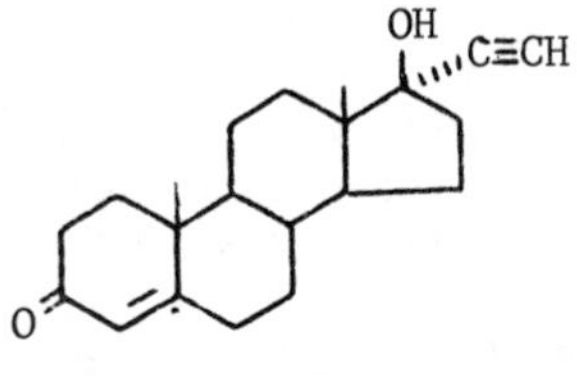

31

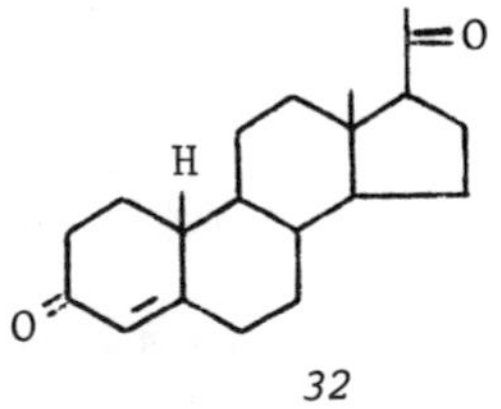

32

The elaboration of a method for the reduction of aromatic
rings to the corresponding dihydrobenzenes under controlled conditions by A. J. Birch opened a convenient route to compounds
related to the putative norprogesterone. This reaction, now
known as the Birch reduction,[17] is typified by the treatment of

the monomethyl ether of estradiol with a solution of lithium
metal in liquid ammonia in the presence of an alcohol as a proton
source. Initial reaction consists in 1,4 metalation of the most
electron-deficient positions of the aromatic ring—in the case of
an estrogen, the 1 and 4-positions. Reaction of the intermediate
with the proton source leads to the dihydrobenzene; a special
virtue of this sequence in steroids is the fact that the double
bond at 2 in effect becomes an enol ether moiety. Treatment of
that product (34) with weak acid, for example, oxalic acid, leads
to hydrolysis of the enol ether, producing β,γ-unconjugated
ketone 35. Hydrolysis under more strenuous conditions (mineral
acids) results in migration of the double bond as well to yield
19-nortestosterone (36, nandrolone).[18]

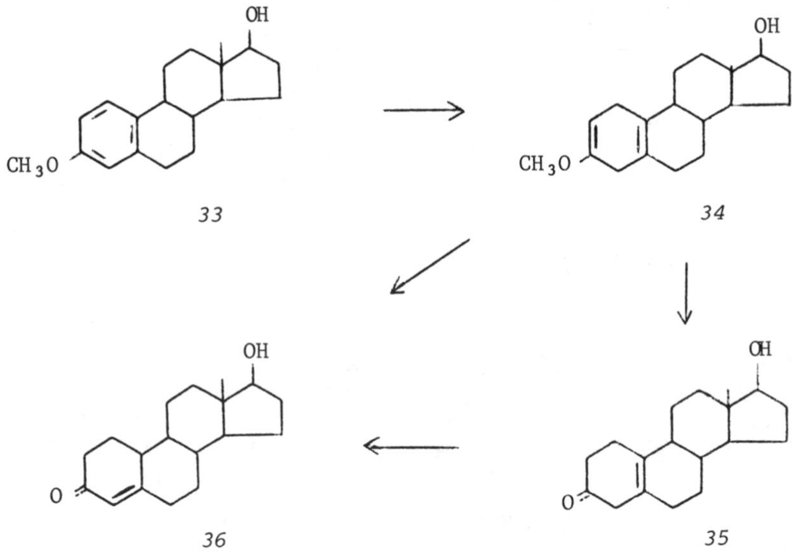

Oppenauer oxidation of the enol ether (34) affords the
corresponding 17 ketone (37) (the enol ether is stable to the
basic oxidation conditions). This ketone affords the corresponding 17α-ethynyl compound on reaction with metal acetylides.
Hydrolysis of the enol ether under mild conditions leads directly
to ethynodrel (39),[19] an orally active progestin. This is the
progestational component of the first oral contraceptive to be
offered for sale. Treatment of the ethynyl enol ether with strong
acid leads to yet another oral progestin employed as a contraceptive, norethindrone (40).[20] In practice these and all other so-
called combination contraceptives are mixtures of 1-2% mestranol

or ethynylestradiol and an oral progestin (see Table 1 in Section
f). It has been speculated that the discovery of the necessity
of estrogen in addition to progestin for contraceptive efficacy
is due to the presence of a small amount of unreduced estradiol
methyl ether in early batches of 37. This, when subjected to
oxidation and ethynylation, would of course lead to mestranol.
In any event, the need for the presence of estrogen in the mixture is now well established experimentally.

In further modifications of these norprogestins, reaction of
norethindrone with acetic anhydride in the presence of p-toluenesulfonic acid, followed by hydrolysis of the first-formed enol
acetate, affords norethindrone acetate (41).[21] This in turn
affords, on reaction with excess cyclopentanol in the presence
of phosphorus pentoxide, the 3-cyclopentyl enol ether (42),[22] the
progestational component of Riglovic®. Reduction of norethindrone affords the 3,17-diol. The 3β-hydroxy compound is the
desired product; since reactions at 3 do not show nearly the
stereoselectivity of those at 17 by virtue of the relative lack
of stereo-directing proximate substituents, the formation of the
desired isomer is engendered by use of a bulky reducing agent,
lithium aluminum-tri-t-butoxide. Acetylation of the 3β,17β-diol
affords ethynodiol diacetate, one of the most potent oral progestins (44).[23]
        In another approach to analogs, nortestosterone is first
converted to the thioketal by treatment with ethylene dithiol in
the presence of boron trifluoride. (The mild conditions of this
reaction compared to those usually employed in preparing the
oxygen ketals probably accounts for the double bond remaining at
4,5.) Treatment of this derivative with sodium in liquid ammonia

affords the 3-desoxy analog *(46)*. Oxidation by means of Jones reagent followed by ethynylation of the 17 ketone leads to the orally active progestin, *lynestrol (48)*.[24]

40 *41* *42* *43* *44* *36* *45* *46* *47* *48*

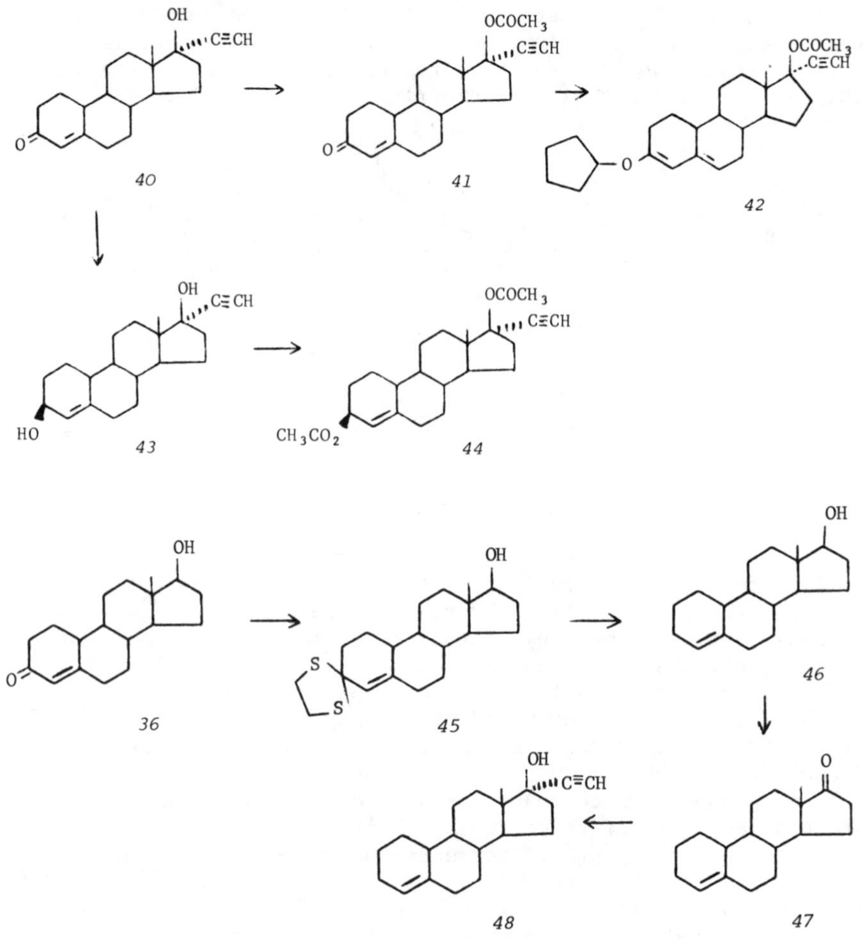

b. 19-Norsteroids by Total Synthesis

Steroids not readily accessible by modification of plant starting materials, for example, those possessing unusual substituents at the angular positions, are made available by total synthesis.

It is probable, too, that intensive-process research development on the reactions involved in these syntheses may have made these routes commercially competitive with partial syntheses based on plant sterols.

In the first of these sequences, often called the Torgov-Smith synthesis, the initial step consists in condensation of a 2-alkyl-cyclopentane-1,3-dione with the allyl alcohol obtained from 6-methoxy-1-tetralone and vinylmagnesium chloride. Although this reaction at first sight resembles a classic SN_i displacement, the reaction is actually carried out with only a trace of base. It is not at all unlikely that the extremely acidic dione causes the allyl alcohol to lose hydroxide and form the allyl cation; this then reacts with the anion of the dione. Cyclization of the condensation product under acid conditions affords, where the starting material was 2-methylcyclopentanedione, the complete carbon skeleton of the 19-norsteroids; when 2-ethylcyclopentane-1,3-dione is used instead, an intermediate to a commercial progestin is obtained. Catalytic reduction of the 14 double bond proceeds at the α side due to the presence of the bulky angular group at 13. This step has the additional important consequence of establishing the important trans C/D ring juncture. There is evidence to suggest that this is the thermodynamically unfavored configuration. Reduction of the ketone proceeds as expected for such steroids to give the β-alcohol. Birch reduction of the remaining superfluous double bond at 8 proceeds to establish the trans B/C ring juncture. Although this happens to be the thermodynamically favored product, an argument based on kinetics will predict the same product. There has thus been produced the 18 methyl homolog of estrone methyl ether as a racemate. This compound, when subjected to the same series of transformations used to prepare norethindrone, affords racemic *norgestrel (54)*.[25] It is of note that although the synthesis has involved the formation of no fewer than 6 chiral centers, only two of the 64 possible isomers are formed.

Extension of the conjugation of the 3 ketone in the 19 norprogestins has been found to increase significantly the potency of these agents. A total synthesis has been evolved for preparing one of these agents that was first obtained by partial synthesis.[26] This consists in adding each of the steroid rings sequentially starting at D. Reaction of the unsaturated ketone, 55, with 2-methylcyclopentane-1,2-dione in a Robinson annelation (conjugate addition followed by aldol cyclization) affords the C/D fragment, 56. This is then saponified and resolved into its optical isomers. Reduction of the S isomer proceeds at the α face opposite the angular methyl group, as in the steroids, to establish in one step the stereochemistry at 8 and 13. The 17

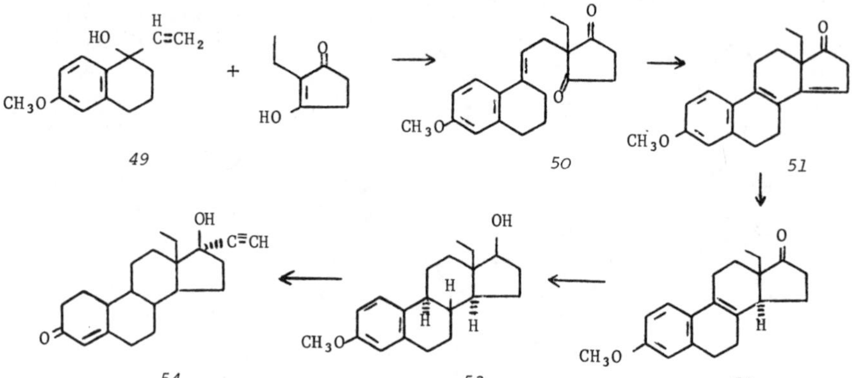

ketone is then converted to the 17β benzoate in several steps and
the keto acid cyclized to the enol lactone, *58*. Reaction of *58*
with the Grignard reagent from halide, *59*, affords after deketalization the diketone, *60*. (This last presumably proceeds by addition of the Grignard to the lactone carbonyl, followed by opening
to a 1,5-diketone and then cyclization.) Treatment of the tricyclic diketone, *60*, with pyrrolidine affords the tetracyclic steroid skeleton as the enamine, *61*. Exposure of this last to weak
acid results in hydrolysis of the enamine to the ketone *(62)* without subsequent migration of the double bonds. This is then converted to triene, *63*, with dichlorodicyanoquinone. (An alternate
procedure consists in forming the 11 hydroxy-4,9-diene by oxidation of the diene with molecular oxygen in the presence of triethylamine followed by reduction of the intermediate hydroper-
oxide; dehydration of the alcohol affords the triene.) The triene is then oxidized to the 3,17-diketone. This compound regioselectively forms a cyanohydrin at 17; the 3 ketone is then protected as its oxime. The cyanohydrin is removed with mild base
and the resulting ketone ethynylated at 17. Removal of the oxime
affords chiral *norgestatriene (66)*.[27]

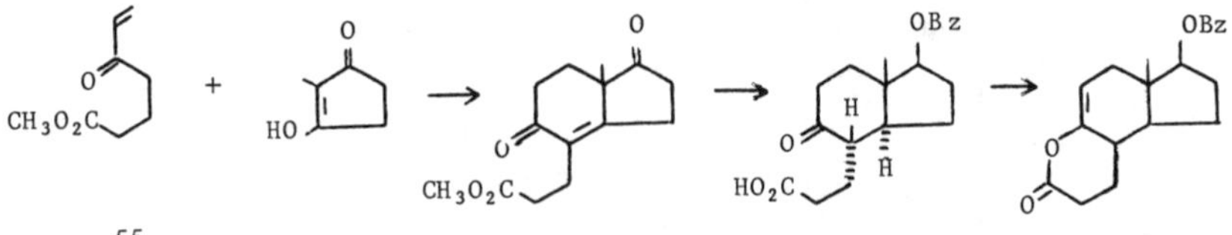

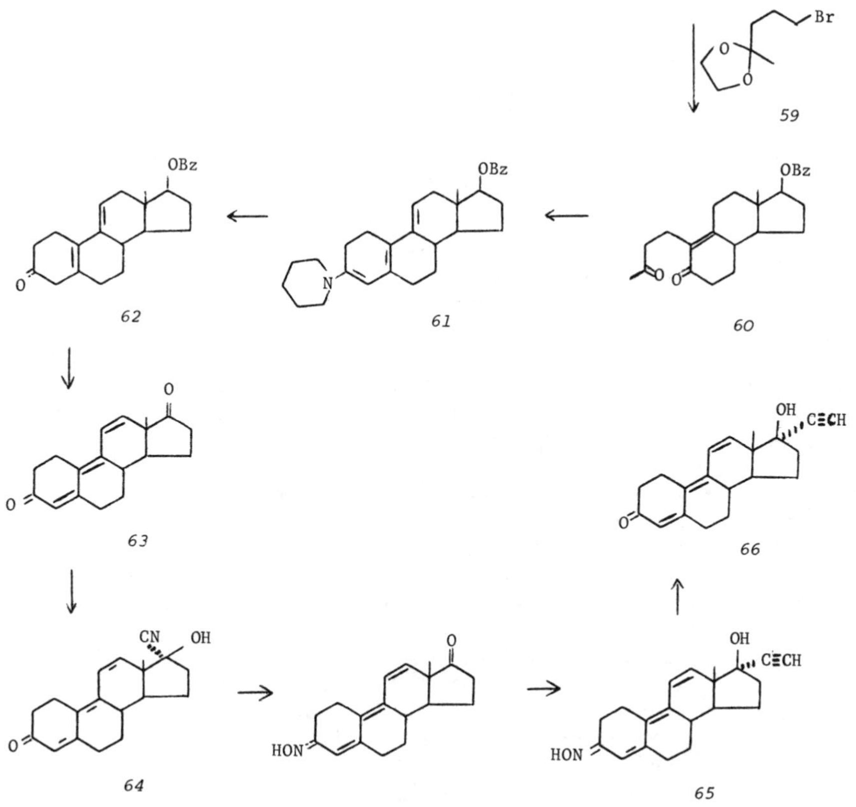

c.   19-Norandrogens

The integrity of the reproductive system as well as that of the
male accessory sex organs of mammalian species is supported by a
series of steroid hormones secreted largely in the testes, known
collectively as the androgens.   These compounds are C-19 steroids,
and, like the estrogens, lack a side chain at C17; the series is
typified by testosterone *(67)*.

     As with the other sex hormones, the first clinical use of
androgens was for support therapy in individuals deficient in the
endogenous hormone.   The discovery that androgens exert an anabolic effect greatly extended the indications for their use.

67

These agents promised utility by prompting a decreased excretion
of nitrogenous metabolites by causing an increase in protein
synthesis in various pathologic conditions marked by wastage of
muscle tissue. Before such use could be undertaken, the problems
of the low order of oral activity and ready metabolism and excretion of the natural androgens had to be overcome. Additionally,
since use as anabolic agents would not necessarily be restricted
to males, means had to be found to overcome the androgenic or
masculinizing effect of these agents. Oral activity and metabolism were first tackled by the preparation of oil-soluble esters
as detailed in Section b.

      The goal of oral activity was first met not in the 19-nor
series but in the compounds possessing the 10 methyl group of
natural products. Androgens containing the 17α-alkyl grouping
are active on oral administration for much the same reason the
corresponding estrogens show activity by that route—inhibition of
transformation at 17 in the gut. It was found early that the
same sort of argument applied to the 19-nor compounds.

      Reaction of estrone methyl ether with methyl Grignard reagent
followed by Birch reduction and hydrolysis of the intermediate
enol ether affords the prototype orally active androgen in the
19-nor series, *normethandrolone (69)*.[20] (Note that here again
the addition of the methyl group proceeded stereoselectively by
approach from the least hindered side.) The preparation of the
ethyl homolog starts by catalytic reduction of *mestranol*; treatment of the intermediate, *70*, under the conditions of the Birch
reduction and subsequent hydrolysis of the intermediate enol
ether yields *norethandrolone (71)*.[13]

      Condensation of the lynestrol intermediate *(47)* with ethyl-
magnesium bromide affords the oral androgen *ethylestrenol (72)*.[24]
Animal experiments on the various drugs above have all shown
increased anabolic effects relative to androgenicity.

      In the case of androgens as with estrogens there is occasion-
ally need for treatment of patients with chronic sustained doses
of these drugs. Resort is made to esters of the androgen with
long-chain fatty acids in order to provide oil-soluble agents;

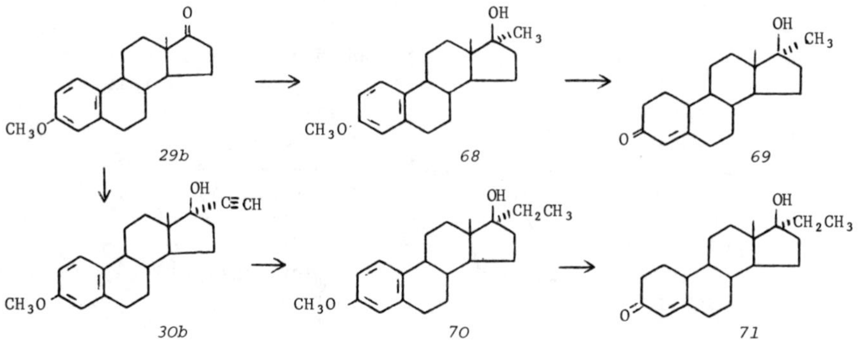

these are then used as solutions in oil to provide a depot of drug. For example, treatment of 19-nortestosterone with decanoic anhydride and pyridine affords *nandrolone decanoate (74a)*.[28] Acylation of *73* with phenylpropionyl chloride yields *nandrolone phenpropionate (74b)*.[29]

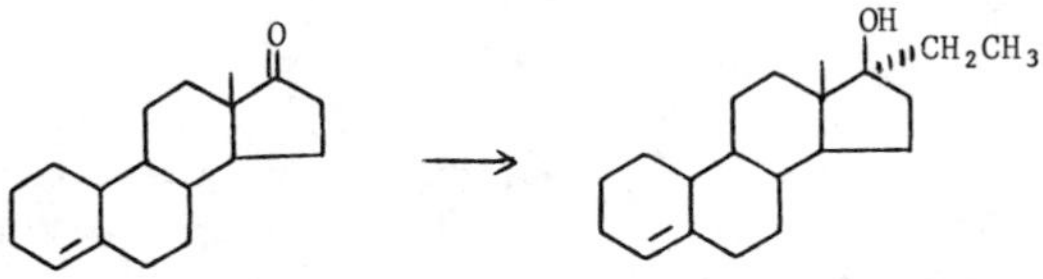

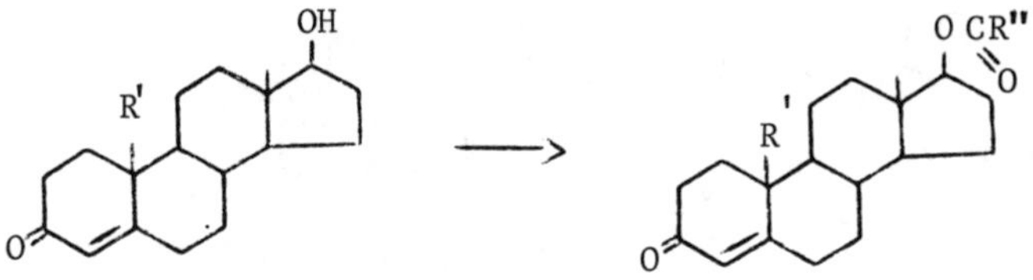

73, R'=H
75, R'=CH$_3$

74a, R'=H, R''=(CH$_2$)$_8$CH$_3$
74b, R'=H, R''=CH$_2$CH$_2$C$_6$H$_5$
76a, R'=CH$_3$, R''=CH$_2$CH$_3$
76b, R'=CH$_3$, R''='CH$_2$)$_8$CH$_3$

76c, R'=CH$_3$, R''=CH$_2$CH$_2$-⬠

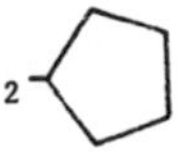

4.   STEROIDS RELATED TO TESTOSTERONE

Oil-soluble derivatives of testosterone itself predate those of
its 19-nor congener; these agents too are used to administer
depot injections so as to provide in effect long-term blood
levels of drug. Thus, acylation of testosterone with propionyl
chloride in the presence of pyridine yields *testosterone propionate (76a)*[30]; acylation by means of decanoic anhydride yields
testosterone decanoate (76b).[31] Finally, reaction of *75* with 3-
cyclopentylpropionyl chloride affords *testosterone cypionate
(76c)*.[32] This last undergoes hydrolysis unusually slowly because
of the presence of two substituents at the δ position (see
Newman's Rule of 6).[33]
      Reaction of dehydroepiandrosterone with an excess of methyl-
magnesium bromide affords the 17α-methyl compound; again the
aforementioned steric effects lead to high stereoselectivity.
Oppenauer oxidation of the resultant intermediate *(77a)* proceeds
with a shift of the double bond into conjugation to yield *methyl-
testosterone (78a)*.[34] When the initial condensation is carried
out with the Grignard reagent from allyl bromide instead, this
sequence yields *allylestrenol (78b)*.[36] Perhaps most startling
is the fact that the product obtained from the use of a metal
acetylide in this synthesis, *ethisterone (78c)*, shows little, if
any androgenic potency. Instead, the compound is an orally effective progestin.

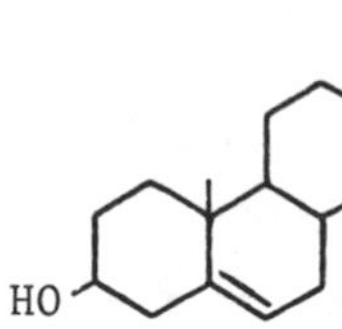

11

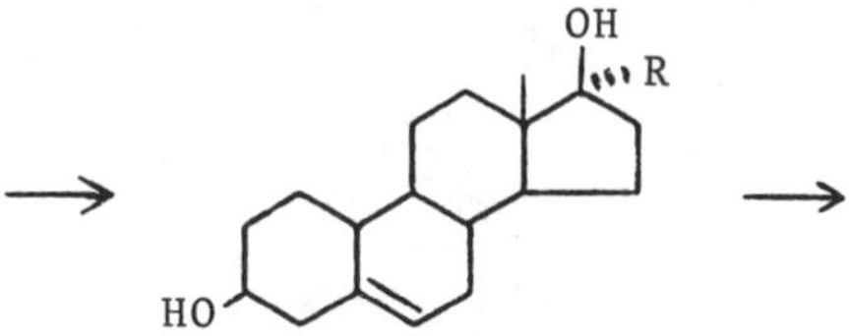

77a, R=CH$_3$
77b, R=C≡CH

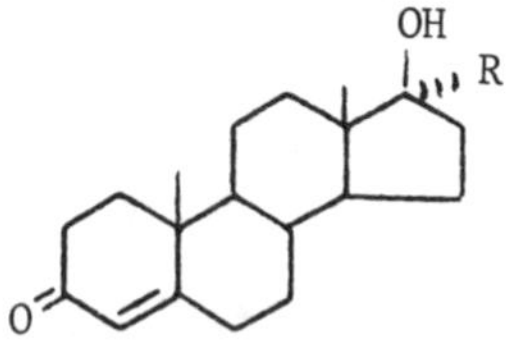

78a, R=CH$_3$
78b, R=CH$_2$CH=CH$_2$
78c, R=C≡CH

These agents, as well as those discussed below, have all
been used at one time as orally active anabolic-androgenic agents.
Dehydrogenation of methyl-testosterone by means of chloranil
extends the conjugation to afford the 4,6-diene-3-one system of
79. This compound in turn undergoes 1,6 conjugate addition of
methylmagnesium bromide in the presence of cuprous chloride to
afford largely the 6α-methyl product (80), known as *bolasterone*.[37]
Dehydrogenation with selenium dioxide, on the other hand, affords
the cross-conjugated diene, *methandrostenolone (81)*.[38]

Hydroxylation of the double bond of methyltestosterone by
means of osmium tetroxide and hydrogen peroxide affords the 4,5
diol. This undergoes beta elimination on treatment with base to
yield *oxymestrone (83)*.[39]

Catalytic reduction of dehydroepiandrosterone goes as
expected largely from the unhindered side of the molecule to
afford a trans A/B ring fusion, 84. Reaction with methyl Grignard
reagent followed by oxidation of the intermediate yields *androstanolone (86)*.[40] (There is some evidence that the corresponding
dihydrotestosterone lacking the 17 methyl group may in fact be
the physiologic androgen.) Formylation of 86 with ethyl formate
and base gives *oxymetholone (87)*.[41] Catalytic reduction of the
analogous hydroxmethylene compound from dihydrotestosterone propionate gives first the 2β-methyl product. Treatment with base
leads this to isomerize to the thermodynamically favored equatorial 2α-methyl compound, *dromostanolone propionate (88)*.[41] The
formyl ketone (87) undergoes a reaction typical of this functional
array on treatment with hydrazine, leading to formation of the

anabolic steroidal pyrazole (89), stanazole.[42] Bromination of 86
with a single equivalent of bromine under carefully buffered conditions permits the isolation of the monobromide (90). Dehydrohalogenation with lithium chloride in DMF affords the enone
(91),[43] an important intermediate to compounds discussed below.

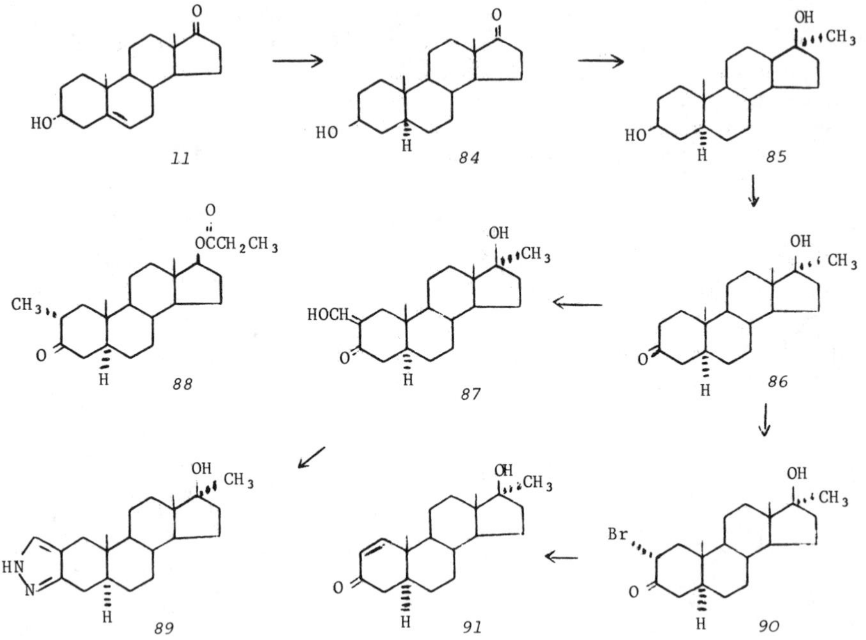

Conjugate addition of methyl magnesium iodide in the presence of cuprous chloride to the enone (91) leads to the 1α-methyl
product mesterolone (92).[44] Although this is the thermodynamically unfavored axially disposed product, no possibility for
isomerization exists in this case, since the ketone is once removed from this center. In an interesting synthesis of an oxa
steroid, the enone (91) is first oxidized with lead tetraacetate;
the carbon at the 2 position is lost, affording the acid aldehyde.
Reduction of this intermediate, also shown in the lactol form,
with sodium borohydride affords the steroid lactone oxandrolone
(94),[45] a potent anabolic agent. The 17-desmethyl analog of 91—
obtainable by the same route as 91—like many other conjugated
ketones, reacts with diazomethane, possibly by a 1,3-dipolar
addition reaction, to form the pyrazole (96). This, on treatment
with silica gel, followed by acetylation of the product, affords

methenolone acetate (97).[46] It should be noted that the product in this case is the vinyl methyl group rather than the cyclopropane often observed on decomposition of pyrazoles not adjacent to a ketone.

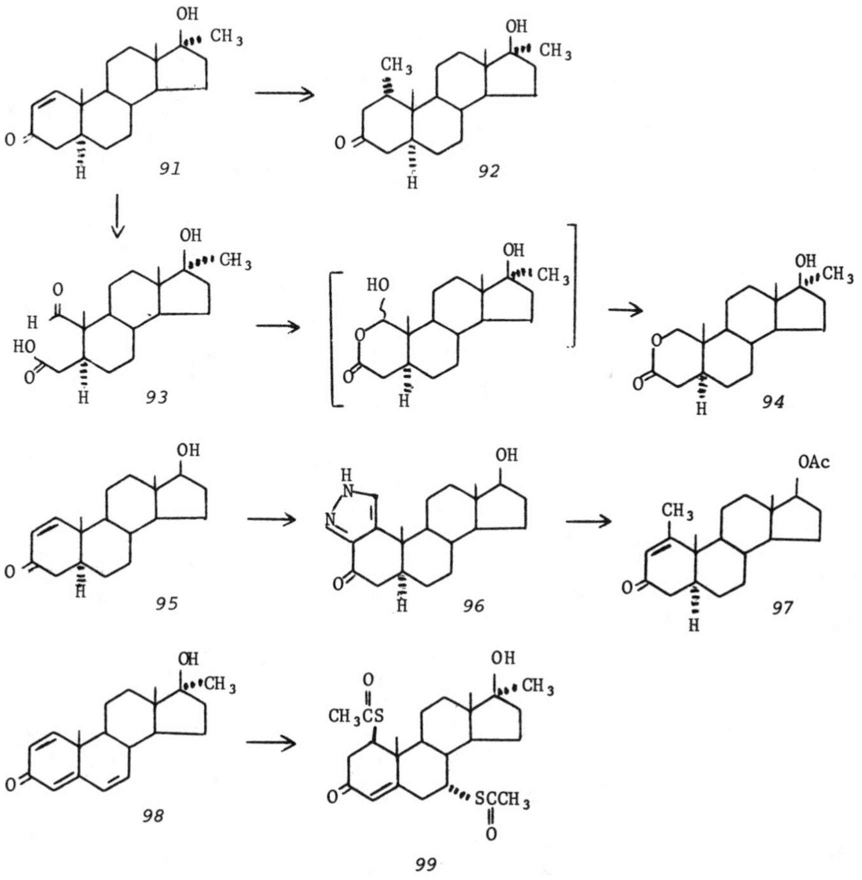

Another example of resort to heteroatoms to obtain both oral potency and a split between androgenic and anabolic activities is *tiomestrone (99)*. Trienone, *98*, prepared in much the same way as *23*, undergoes sequential 1,6 and 1,4 conjugate addition of thioacetic acid under either irradiation or free radical catalysis to afford the compound containing two sulfur atoms.[47]

The chemistry of *fluoxymestrone* is more typical of that of

the corticoids we meet below than it is of the androgens. This
potent androgenic anabolic agent was in fact developed in parallel with the corticoids. The present discussion, however, allows
an examination of some of this chemistry unencumbered by the
excess functionality of the corticoids. Although several routes
to this agent have been published, we only consider the most
direct.

One of the stumbling blocks in the early work on the synthesis of corticoids was the introduction of the 11-β-hydroxy group
necessary for activity. Because of its remoteness from existing
functionality, there were few ways in which this could be introduced chemically. The signal discovery of the microbiologic
conversion of progesterone to 11-α-hydroxy progesterone by
Peterson and Murray at Upjohn[48] made such compounds readily
accessible. Analogous microbiologic oxidation of androstenedione
(12) affords the 11-α-hydroxy derivative, 100. Oxidation with
chromium trioxide yields adrenosterone (101). (This compound can
also be obtained directly from cortisone by scision of the dihydroxyacetone side chain with sodium bismuthate.) Treatment with
a limited amount of pyrrolidine under carefully controlled conditions leads to selective eneamine formation at the least hindered
ketone—at 3 (102). (The 11 ketone is highly hindered and will
not form an eneamine using any of the common methods.) Reaction
with methylmagnesium bromide followed by removal of the eneamine
yields the familiar 17α-methyl 17β-hydroxy derivative (103)—note
again the resistance of the extremely hindered 11 ketone to addition reactions. The ketone at 3 is then again converted to
its eneamine. Treatment of this intermediate with lithium aluminum hydride, followed by hydrolysis of the eneamine, gives the
dihydroxyketone (104). The secondary alcohol at 11 is next
selectively converted to the toluenesulfonate ester; this last
affords the 9(11) olefin (105) on treatment with base. When 105
is subjected to N-bromoacetamide in water—in effect, hypobromous
acid—the 9α-bromo, 11β-hydroxy compound (106) is obtained. It is
presumed that the initial bromonium ion is formed on the less-
hindered side; diaxial opening with hydroxide at 11 will lead to
the observed product. Treatment with base leads to displacement
of bromine by the alkoxide ion and consequent formation of the
9,11 epoxide (109). This scheme then is a strategem allowing
specific synthesis of the alternate epoxide than would be obtained
on direct treatment of 105 with a peracid. Ring opening of the
oxirane with hydrogen fluoride affords the key 9α-fluro-11β-
hydroxy function in 108 and completes the synthesis of fluoxymestrone,[49] an anabolic-androgenic agent.

The inclusion of a 6α-methyl group is known to potentiate
the effect of progestins. Dimethisterone represents an applica-

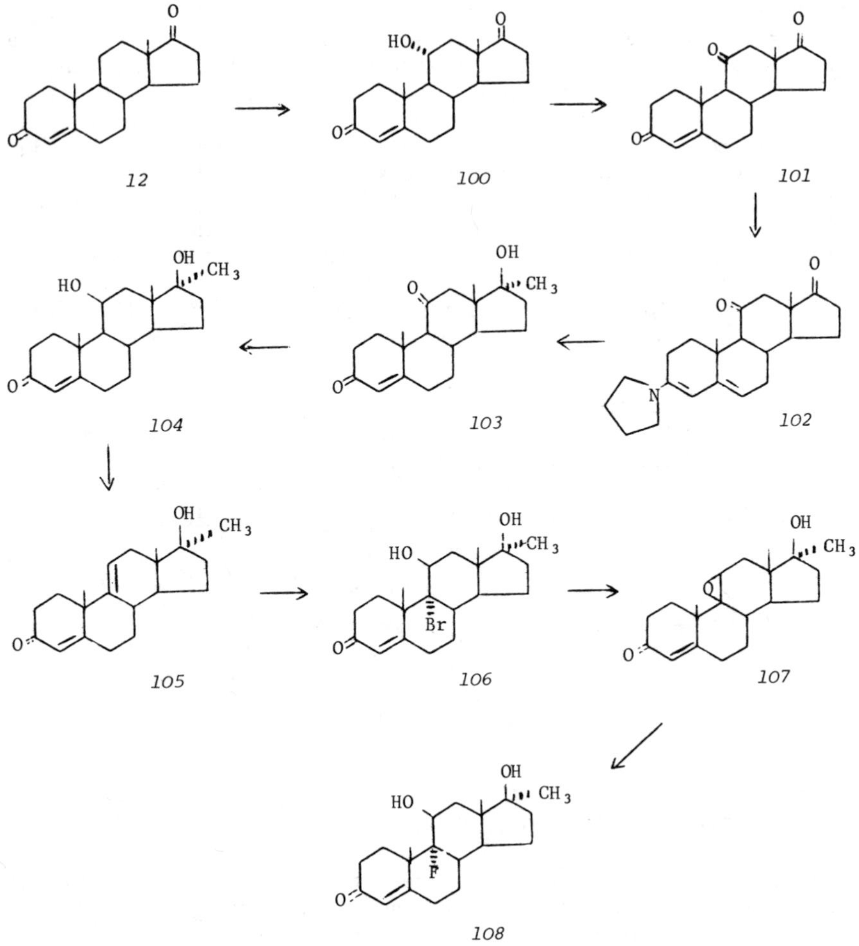

tion of this modification to the *ethisterone* molecule. Oxidation
of *109*—obtained by acetylation of *77b*—with perphthalic acid
affords largely the α-epoxide *110*, by reason of the approach of
the bulky reagent from the unhindered side of the molecule. Reaction of this oxide with methyl Grignard reagent proceeds by the
well-known diaxial opening of oxiranes with nucleophiles to
afford the 6β-methyl 5α-hydroxy compound (*111*); the acetate is
lost during this transformation by reaction with excess Grignard
reagent. The resulting triol is then allowed to react with an

excess of dihydropyran in order to mask the hydroxyls as their
tetrahydropyranyl ether. The acetylene is converted to its anion
with sodium amide and alkylated with methyl iodide to afford the
propyne side chain. Treatment with dilute acid to remove the
tetrahydropyranyl ether groups followed by oxidation with chromium trioxide:pyridine complex converts the secondary alcohol at
3 to the corresponding ketone *(113)*. This β-hydroxyketone undergoes dehydration to the conjugated ketone when subjected to
strong acid. The previously isolated methyl group at 6 now occupies an epimerizable position by virtue of its vinylogous relation to the ketone. The methyl group in fact isomerizes to the
more stable equatorial 6α position, to afford *dimethisterone*
(114).[50],[51] This agent, like its prototype, is an orally effective progestin.

5.   STEROIDS RELATED TO PROGESTERONE

The lack of oral activity of progesterone proper has already been
mentioned. Even after the orally active 19-nor agents, which
showed progestational activity, had been elaborated, the search
continued for an orally active compound that contained the full
pregnane nucleus *(115)*. At the time such a compound would have
had the economic advantage of sidestepping the then burdensome
ring A aromatization reactions.
    The first indication that such a goal was attainable came
from the observation that 17α-methylprogesterone *(116)* was more
potent than progesterone itself as a progestin.[52] A systematic
investigation of substituents at 17 revealed that although the
17α-hydroxyl analog is only weakly active, the corresponding 17α-
acetoxy compound is in fact a relatively active progestin.

115   116

Epoxidation of one of the early intermediates from the diosgenin route, pregnenolone (4), with alkaline hydrogen peroxide
selectively affords, as this reagent usually does, the product of
attack at the conjugated ketone (117).[53] Diaxial opening of the
oxirane with hydrogen bromide proceeds both regio- and stereospecifically to the bromohydrin (118). Catalytic reduction of
this last in the presence of ammonium acetate removes the halogen
while leaving the unsaturation at 5,6 unaffected. The 17α-hy-
droxypregnenolone (119) thus obtained is formylated at 3 under
relatively mild conditions; this formate is then treated with
acetic anhydride in the presence of p-TSA to afford the 3-for-
mate- 17 -acetate (120). Oppenauer oxidation of the formate-
acetate leads directly to hydroxyprogesterone acetate (121).[54]
In a modification of this scheme, hydroxypregnenolone is first
acetylated under mild conditions to the 3-acetate and then under
forcing conditions with caproic anhydride to give the acetate-
caproate (122). Ester interchange with methanol removes the
acetate at 3; Oppenauer oxidation affords hydroxyprogesterone
caproate (124).[55]

Introduction of a substituent at the 6 position serves, as
we have seen in the case of dimethisterone, to increase markedly
the potency of progestins. In the first of these efforts,
acetoxyprogesterone, an agent known to have oral activity, was
the molecule so modified. Treatment of hydroxyprogesterone
(125)—obtained by Oppenauer oxidation of 17α-hydroxypregnenolone
(119)—with an excess of ethylene glycol leads to the bis ketal,
126. The shift of the double bond to 5,6 is characteristic of the
3-keto-4-ene chromophore. The olefin gives a mixture of the α-
and β-epoxides when subjected to peracid, with the former predominating. Treatment of the α-oxide with methyl Grignard
reagent leads to the familiar diaxial opening and thus the product 128. Deketalization reveals the β-ketoalcohol grouping at
positions 3 and 5 in 129. This readily dehydrates to 130 on
treatment with base. The methyl group equilibrates to the
thermodynamically more stable equatorial 6α position on exposure
to acid. Acetylation under forcing conditions affords 132,

medroxyprogesterone acetate.[55] Dehydrogenation of this compound with chloranil affords *133, megesterol acetate.*[56] Both these agents are potent orally active progestins.

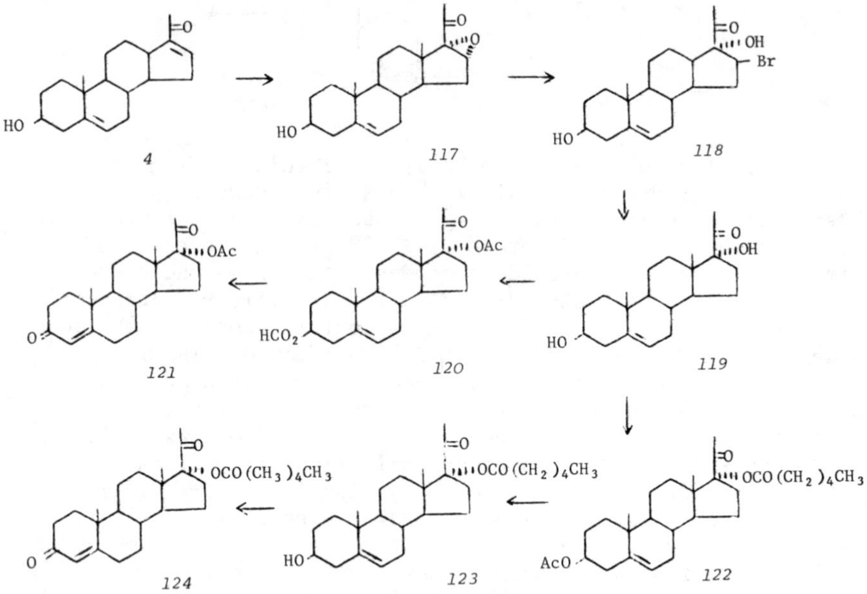

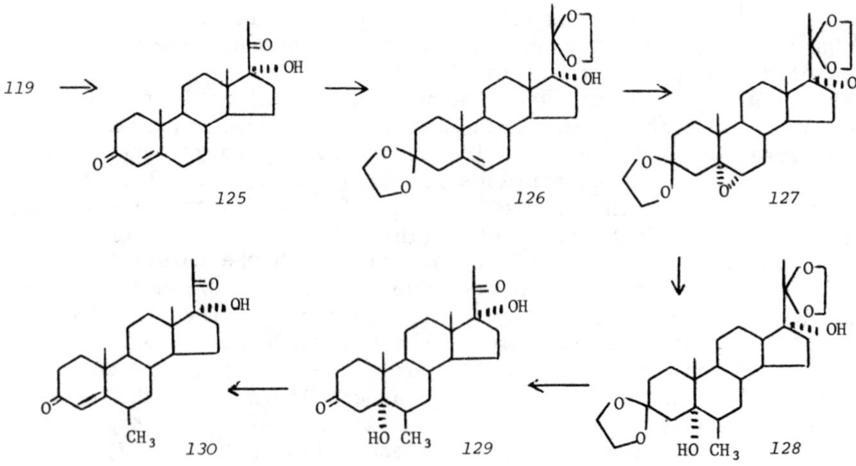

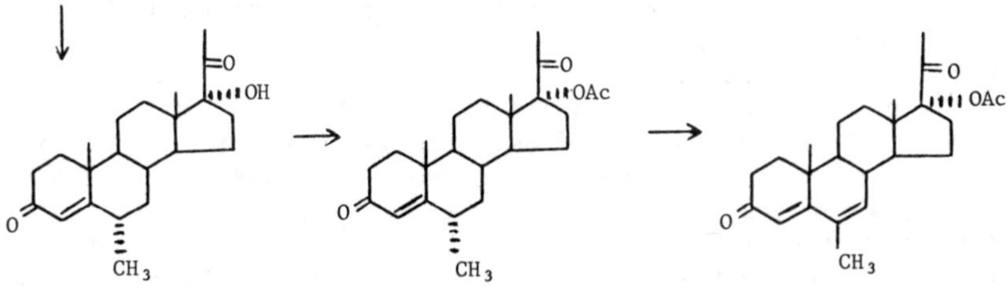

131   132   133

Replacement of the 6 methyl of *133* by a chlorine atom proves
to be compatible with biologic activity. Epoxidation of
diene, *134*–obtained from hydroxyprogesterone acetate by chloranil
dehydrogenation–with a bulky peracid gives the 6,7α-oxide, *135*.
Ring opening with hydrochloric acid in aqueous dioxane affords
the intermediate chlorohydrin *136*; this is not isolated, since it
dehydrates to *chlormadinone acetate (137)* under the reaction conditions.[57] This last agent, incidentally, has undergone extensive clinical trial as a contraceptive in its own right without
added progestin. Reports from these trials were said to be
encouraging. The high potency of the compound permitted the use
of low doses, hence the sobriquet, "minipill."

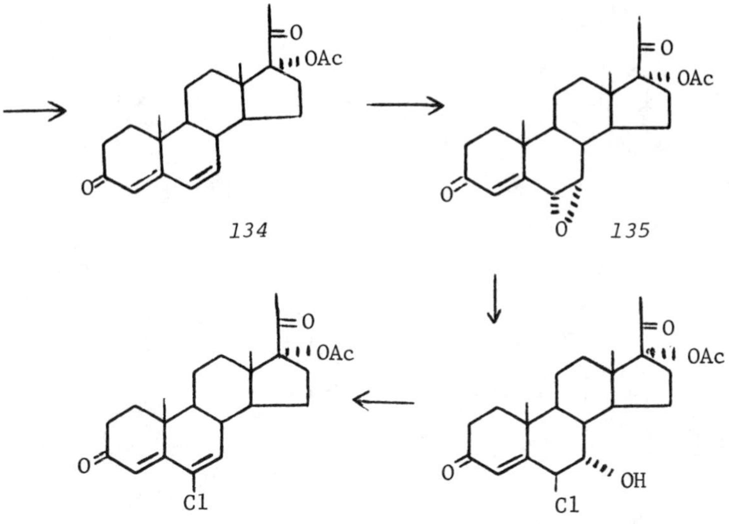

134   135

137   136

6-Methyl-16-dehydropregnenolone, the key intermediate to the preparation of both *melengesterol acetate* and *medrogestone,* is not readily prepared from any of the intermediates described thus far. Petrov and his collaborators have devised several interesting schemes that go back to diosgenin *(1)* as the starting point. These schemes perform the necessary modifications in rings A and B with the sapogenin side chain still in place. In essence this approach employs this side chain as a protecting group for the future 16-dehydro-20-ketone function. In one of these routes, diosgenin *(1)* is first converted to the 3-toluenesulfonate. Solvolysis of this homoallylic alcohol derivative *(138)* affords the 3,5-cyclosteroid, *140,* via the cyclopropyl carbinyl ion, *139.* (This general reaction was probably first found in the steroids and bore the name of "*i*-steroid rearrangement.") Oxidation of the product by means of the chromium trioxide-pyridine complex affords ketone, *141.* Reaction of this with methyl magnesium iodide affords two isomeric carbinols with the α-isomer predominating. Solvolysis in the presence of a nucleophile such as acetic acid reverses the cyclopropylcarbinyl transformation to afford homoalylic acetate, *143.* Removal of the sapogenin side chain much as in the case of *1* leads to the desired product, *144.*[58]

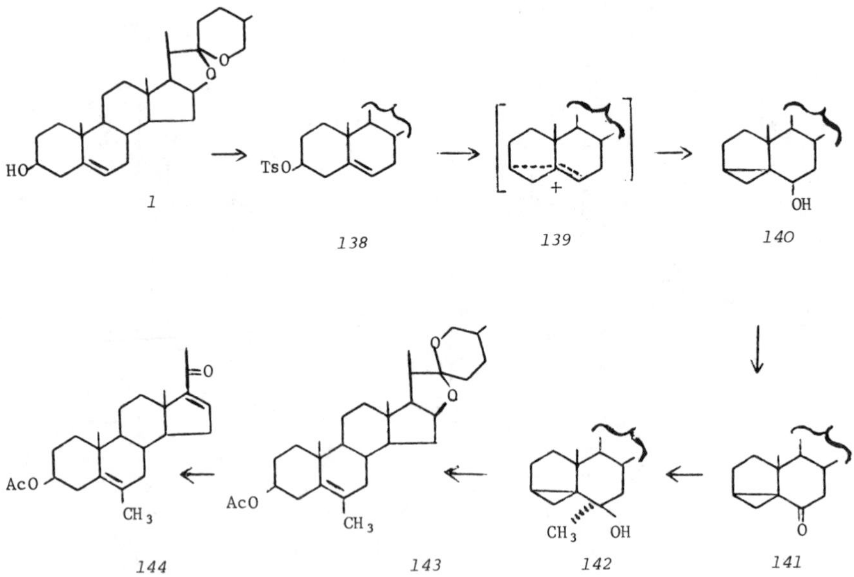

Substitution at the 16 position was found to lead to further potentiation of progestational activity. Reaction of *144* with diazomethane at the conjugated double bond at 16 gives first the pyrazole, *145*. This heterocycle affords the 16 methyl enone on pyrolysis [analogous to the reaction observed at the 1 position cited earlier (95-97)]. Selective epoxidation of the conjugated double bond to the 16,17α-epoxide over that at 5,6 is achieved by oxidation with basic hydrogen peroxide. Opening of this tetra-substituted oxirane ring in acid proceeds with loss of a proton from the β position (16 methyl) to afford the desired 16-methyl-ene-17α-hydroxy-20-ketone functionality in the D ring. Oppenhauer oxidation of the saponified product gives *149*; this is then dehy-drogenated to the 4,6-diene with chloranil. Acetylation under forcing conditions completes the synthesis of *melengesterol acetate (151).*[59]

The oral activity of 17α-methyl progesterone *(116)* has al-ready been alluded to. This agent, which may well owe this property to the inhibition of metabolism in a manner analogous to the gonadal steroids, is not sufficiently potent in its own right to constitute a useful drug. Incorporation of known poten-tiating modifications yields the commercially available oral progestin *medrogestone (154).* Reduction of the conjugated 16, 17 double bond of 6-methyl-16-dehydropregnenolone acetate by means of lithium in liquid ammonia leads initially to the 17 enolate ion, *152*; this is alkylated in situ with methyl iodide. The now-familiar steric control asserts itself to afford the 17α-methyl compound, *153*. The acetate group is lost as a side reaction. In an interesting modification on the usual scheme, *153* is treated with aluminum isopropoxide and a ketone (Oppenauer conditions) as well as chloranil in a single reaction; the 4,6 diene, *154 (medrogesterone)*, is obtained directly from this step.[60]

144 →

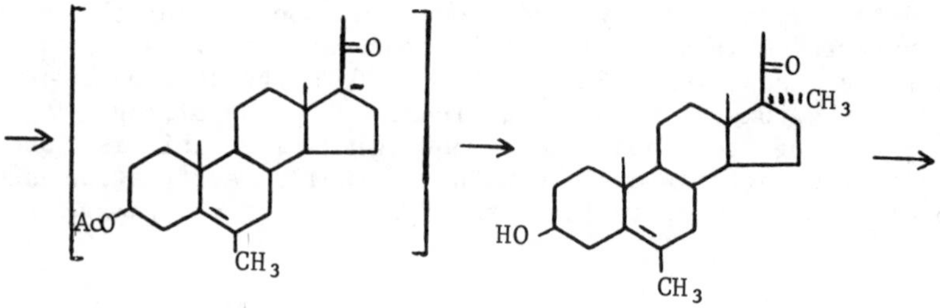

152

153

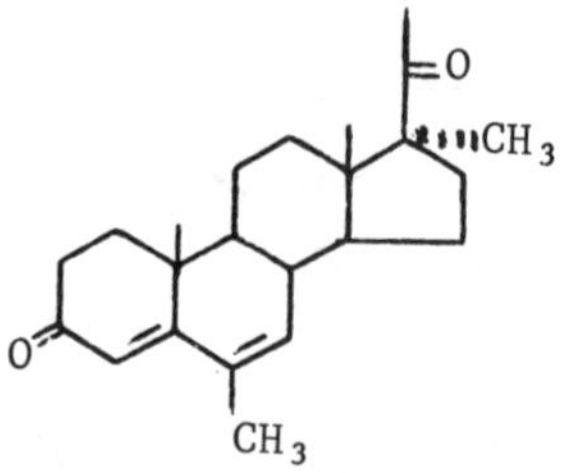

154

It should be noted that the stereochemistry of the B/C and C/D junctions has remained inviolate in all the modifications discussed to date. It was in fact assumed that changing either of these was a quick path to loss of activity. Just such a modification, however, led to a progestin with a unique pharmacologic profile.

Allylic bromination of pregnenolone acetate with dibromodimethylhydantoin affords the 7-bromo compound *(155)* of undefined stereochemistry. Dehydrobromination by means of collidine followed by saponification affords the 5,7 endocyclic cis,cis-diene, *156*. This compound contains the same chromophore as ergosterol, a steroid used as a vitamin D precursor. The latter displays a complex series of photochemical reactions; among the known products is lumisterol, in which the stereochemistry at both C_9 and C_{10} is inverted. Indeed, irradiation of *156* proceeds to give just such a product *(158)*. This reaction can be rationalized by

assuming first a light-induced ring opening to an intermediate
such as the triene, *157*; such a species would be predicted to
ring close in conrotatory fashion with the formation of the
observed stereochemistry. Oppenauer oxidation of the product
goes in the usual fashion, although one double bond remains out
of conjugation *(159)*. Treatment with acid gives the fully conjugated diene of *dydrogesterone (160)*.[61]

It is a common property of progestins that they will inhibit
ovulation when combined with estrogens. *Dydrogesterone* has no
effect on ovulation either by itself or in combination with estrogens. Some progestins, particularly those which possess the full
progesterone skeleton, will induce masculinizing changes in the
female offspring of treated female animals. *Dydrogesterone* differs in this respect, too, since no such effects are observed
after its administration.

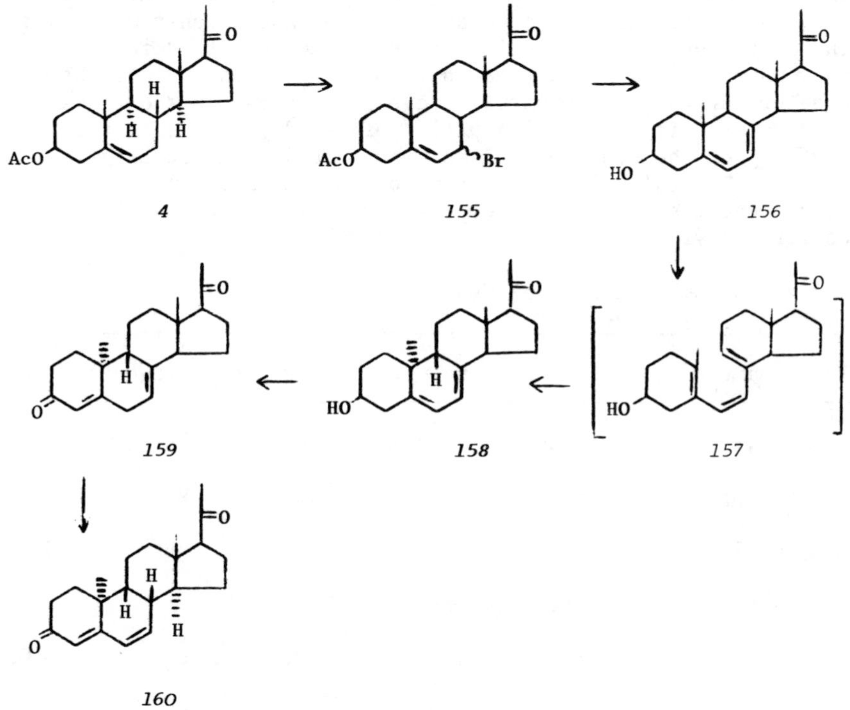

6. THE ORAL CONTRACEPTIVES

The original rationale for the use of progestins as oral contraceptives—besides the animal experiments previously alluded to—
resided in the fact that females do not ovulate during pregnancy—
a time in which there are known to exist high levels of circulat-
ing blood progesterone. It was therefore intended to mimic the
hormonal state of pregnancy by administration of exogenous progestational agents; as we have already seen, it was found empirically that an estrogen was needed to combine with the progestin
in order to achieve full efficacy. In a normal menstrual cycle,
the lining of the uterus undergoes a series of morphologic
changes, whether ovulation occurs or not, characterized by pro-
liferation of the blood vessels and tissues of the walls. The
phenomenon of menstruation represents the periodic sluffing of
this buildup in the absence of conception. It was thus thought
inadvisable to maintain a woman in a continued amenstrual state.
The almost universal practice has been adopted of administering
the contraceptive for a time that roughly corresponds to the
greater part of the menstrual cycle—20-21 days. Discontinuance
of drug at this point for a period of 4-5 days leads to the
sluffing of the uterine wall and the bleeding characteristic of
menses. Table 1 below lists some of the combination (estrogen
plus progestin) oral contraceptives that have been available
commercially.

Table 1. Combination Oral Contraceptives

Trade Name[d]	Progestin	mg[a]	Estrogen	mg[a]
Anovlar	norethindrone acetate	4.0	EE[b]	.05
Enovid-E	norethinodrel	2.5	ME[c]	0.1
Lyndiol	lynestrol	5.0	ME	0.15
Norinyl	norethindrone	1.0	EE	0.05
Ovral	norgestrel	0.5	EE	0.05
Ovulen	ethynodiol diacetate	1.0	ME	0.1
Planor	norgestrienone	2.0	ME	0.1
Provest	medroxyprogesterone acetate	10.0	EE	0.05

Table 1, continued

| Riglovis | Riglovis | 0.5 | EE | 0.05 |
| Volidan | *melengesterol acetate* | 4.0 | EE | 0.05 |

[a]Mg in daily dose. [b]EE, ethinyl estradiol. [c]ME, mestranol.
[d]Registered trademarks.

Advances in reproductive physiology as well as empirical observations suggested that the progestational component of the Pill need not be administered for the full 21 days. In analogy to the normal menstrual cycle it was considered that the progestin need be included for only the last few days. Such a regimen would have the advantage of reducing exposure to the progestational component of these drugs. This expectation was borne out in practice. The so-called sequential contraceptives consist of a series of 15 doses of estrogen alone; these are followed by five dosages of the estrogen-progestin combination. In practice this regime has been well tolerated, although it may be fractionally less efficacious than the more traditional contraceptives. Some of the commercially available sequential contraceptives are listed below in Table 2.

Table 2. Sequential Oral Contraceptives

Trade Name[a]	Progestin	mg	Estrogen	mg
C-Quens	*chlormadinone acetate*	2.0	ME	0.08
Norquens	*norethindrone*	2.0	ME	0.08
Oracon	*dimethisterone*	25.0	EE	0.10
Ortho-Novum	*norethindrone*	2.0	ME	0.08

[a]Registered trademark.

In addition, several progestins have been used in the absence of estrogens for purposes of contraception. It is clear that they owe their efficacy, which is not as high as that of the combination or sequential treatments, to some mechanism other than inhibition of ovulation. These are not yet represented by marketed entities for that indication.

Several progestins have been formulated for administration

as depot injections; the low water solubility of these compounds
allows the agent to be deposited intramuscularly in a microcrys-
talline form.   Slow dissolution provides a chronic blood level of
the compound.   At least one of these agents, *medroxyprogesterone
acetate* (Depo Provera®), has shown promise in the clinic as an
injectable contraceptive of relatively long duration.   Its mechanism of action is probably a combination of inhibition of ovulation and some other effect on the reproductive process.

7.   CORTISONE AND RELATED ANTIINFLAMMATORY STEROIDS

It was known as early as 1927 that the adrenal glands of mammalian species secrete a series of substances essential to the survival of the individual.   The hormonal nature of these secretions
was suggested by the observation that extracts of the adrenal
gland and more specifically of the outer portion of that organ
(cortex) would ensure survival of animals whose adrenals had been
excised.   By 1943 no fewer than 28 steroids had been isolated
from adrenal cortical extracts.   These compounds were found to be
involved in the regulation of such diverse and basic processes as
electrolyte balance, carbohydrate metabolism, and resistance to
trauma, to name only a few.
     Again, as in the case of the other steroid hormones, the
quantities of these compounds isolable from animal sources was
barely sufficient for structural characterization.   Complete
biologic characterization therefore depended on material made
available by synthesis.   Approaches to these compounds by classical steroid chemistry were greatly hampered by the finding that
one of the principal cortical steroids, *cortisone (161)*, possessed
oxygen substitution at the 11 position.   There was at the time no
obvious way for functionalizing C_{11} by chemical means; at this
writing, in fact, this is still not readily accomplished.[94]   As
we saw earlier, plant materials provided an efficient starting
point for the steroids discussed previously; unfortunately, the
corresponding C-ring oxygenated plant sterols are not available
in comparable supply.   Instead, early syntheses fell back on a
starting material from animal sources; cholic acid *(162)*, one of
the bile acids, possessing oxygenation at C_{12}.   This material
available in tonnage quantities from ox bile from slaughterhouses,
was used as starting material for the synthesis of the initial
quantities of cortisone.[62]   Briefly, this partial synthesis
devolves conceptually on three basic operations: degradation of
the bile acid side chain to the required dihydroxyacetone moiety,
transposition of oxygen from C_{12} to C_{11}, and finally generation
of the 3-keto-4-ene system from the 3,7 diol.   Once cortisone was

found to have important therapeutic uses, this process (which
will not be detailed here; see reference 63 for a detailed discussion) was considerably modified and the process developed to a
point of quite high efficiency. There is reason to believe, however, that the bile acid route was finally supplanted by the
route that included microbiologic oxidation.

161   162

The availability of cortisone in sizeable quantities made it
possible for Kendall and Hench at the Mayo Clinic to follow up on
their clinical observation that patients suffering from rheumatoid arthritis showed symptomatic relief in the presence of high
endogenous cortisone levels. Indeed, they were soon able to
describe the dramatic relief afforded arthritics by treatment
with pharmacologic doses of cortisone. As this drug came into
use for this, as well as for treatment of other inflammation,
side effects were found that were perhaps a manifestation of the
important physiologic role of this class of steroids. There were
seen, for example, disturbances in electrolyte balance and glucose metabolism as well as more bizarre effects, such as the
development at high chronic doses of the so-called moon face and
dowagers hump. An intense effort was mounted on the part of most
large pharmaceutical companies to prepare analogs that would
emphasize the antiinflammatory activity without increasing the
side effects due to hormonal potency. It cannot be disputed that
dramatic increases in potency over cortisone were finally achieved;
it is equally clear that the purely antiinflammatory corticoid
has yet to be found.

It had been known for some time from studies of biosynthesis
that corticoids rise physiologically from progesterone by hydroxylation at both C_{11} and in the side chain. In fact, perfusion of
steroids with the preformed side chain through isolated beef
adrenal glands effects just that reaction. Reasoning that microorganisms might well possess some enzyme system analogous to that
which carries out that hydroxylation, a group at Upjohn undertook
a systematic search to screen for such activity. They were

rewarded by the observation that the soil organisms, *Rhizopus arrhizus* or *nigricans*, effected conversion of progesterone to 11α-hydroxyprogesterone in 50% yield. This conversion became the keystone in a synthesis of cortisone from progesterone—and thus from stigmasterol and eventually soybean sterols.

Large-scale commercial production of modified corticoids starts with just that microbiologic oxidation of progesterone to yield 11α-hydroxyprogesterone *(163)*. Oxidation of the alcohol leads to the trione, *164*. In the first step for conversion of the progesterone side chain to that of cortisone, the compound is condensed with ethyl oxalate. Selectivity is achieved due to the great steric hindrance about C_{12} and the increased reactivity of the methyl ketone at C_{21} over the corresponding 2 position. (Formation of an enolate at the latter would decrease the nucleophilicity of that position by distributing the charge over the conjugated system.) Formation of enolate *165* serves to activate the 21 position selectively towards halogenation. In an essentially one-pot reaction, the sodium salt of the enolate is first treated with two equivalents of bromine. The crude bromo compound obtained from this reaction *(166)* is then treated with a metal alkoxide. The dibromoketone undergoes the characteristic Favorsky reaction as well as dehydrohalogenation to yield the unsaturated ester, *167*. The ketone at 3 is then protected as either its ketal or enamine. Reduction with lithium aluminum hydride simultaneously reduces the ester to the alcohol and the ketone at 11 to the 11β-alcohol; acetylation followed by removal of the protecting group affords compound *169*, two oxygens removed from the goal. Osmium tetroxide is well known to oxidize olefins to the corresponding diols. This reagent in the presence of hydrogen peroxide carries this oxidation one step further in the case of allylic acetates such as those present in *169* and oxidizes the secondary alcohol to a ketone.[64] Thus, reaction of *169* with either the above reagent or phenyliodosoacetate in the presence of osmium tetroxide affords directly *hydrocortisone acetate (170a)*,[85] an important drug in its own right and starting material for other antiinflammatory agents. Several products of relatively lower importance are derived from *170a*. Saponification of the acetate at 21 gives *hydrocortisone (170b)*. Oxidation of the 11 alcohol yields *cortisone acetate (171a)*; *cortisone (171b)* is obtained when this last is saponified.

As is apparent at a glance, cortisone is an intricate molecule with a wealth of functionality. Steroid transformations in the corticoid series require serious strategic planning in order to provide the appropriate protecting groups and to introduce substituents in the proper order. It is therefore easy in a discussion of this chemistry to get lost in a welter of detail.

17 → 163 → 164 → 165 → 166 → 167 → 168 → 169 → 170a, R=Ac; 170b, R=H → 171a, R=Ac; 171b, R=H

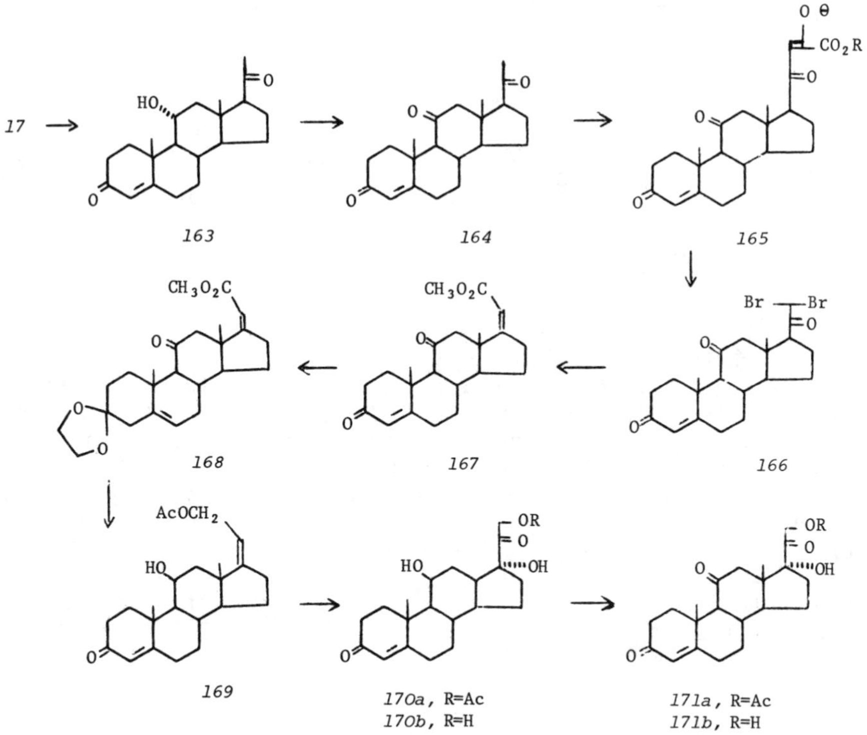

For this reason in this section we depart from our practice of discussing each synthesis in detail. Certain standard operations, for example, introduction of 9-fluoro substituents, are referred to as though they were a single reaction; only the salient points of the syntheses are dwelt on. Examination of some of these syntheses strongly suggests that these were aimed at preparing compounds for biologic assay. It is more than likely that the commercial preparations have only the final product in common with the published route.

One of the first indications that the antiinflammatory potency of the corticoids could be increased was the observation that incorporation of a 9α-fluoro group in hydrocortisone resulted in a tenfold increase in activity. Treatment of hydrocortisone acetate *(170a)* with phosphorus oxychloride in pyridine yields the corresponding olefin, *172*. This, on being subjected to the reaction sequence depicted in the transformation of *104* to *108* (addition of HOBr, closure to the epoxide and ring opening with HF), affords *fludrocortisone acetate (173)*.[66]

170a $\longrightarrow$ $\longrightarrow$

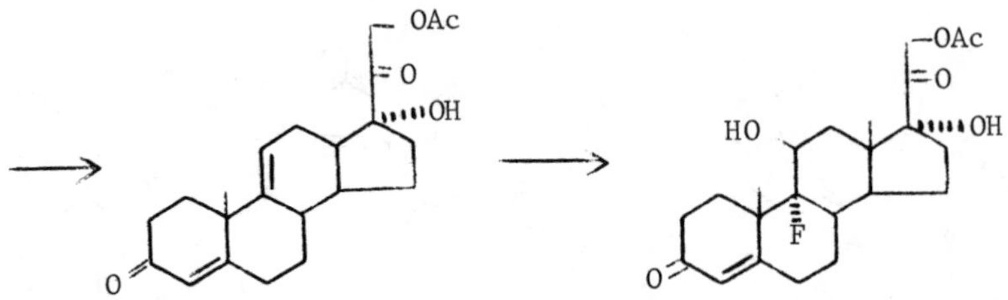

172   173

    Incubation of cortisone with *Corynebacterium simplex* results
in dehydrogenation of the bond at 1,2 and the isolation of the
corresponding 1,4-diene, *prednisone (174)*; hydrocortisone affords
prednisolone (175a) when subjected to this microbiologic transformation.[67] Both these agents as well as the ester, *prednisolone acetate (175b)*, were found to show increased potency over
the parent compounds; there is also a suggestion that other hormonal activities may be decreased. The subsequent finding that
modifications in corticoids that lead to increased potency are
often additive in effect led to inclusion of this feature in most
later clinical agents.

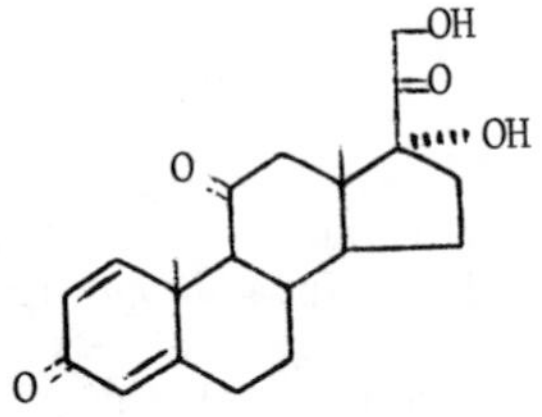

174

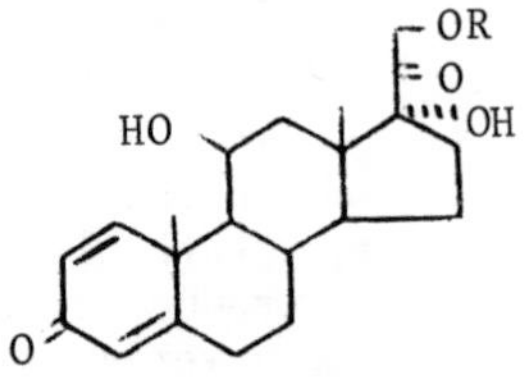

175a, R=H
175b, R=COCH$_3$

    Both the above potentiating modifications were next included
in a single molecule. Catalytic reduction of *173* affords the
corresponding 5α-derivative. This is then taken on to the 2,4-
dibromo compound (see the transformation of 12 to 21 for discussion); dehydrohalogenation gives the 1,4 diene, *9α-fluoropred-
nisolone acetate (176)*,[69,70] a potent antiinflammatory agent.
    We have already seen that incorporation of a 6 methyl group
into progestins increases the biologic activity of these mole-

cules (see *112*, *132*, and *133*); the analogous modification of corticoids has a similar effect on potency. Condensation of cortisone *(171b)* with formaldehyde converts the dihydroxyacetone moiety of the steroids to a double internal acetal, referred to as
the bismethylenedioxy group, a common protecting group for the
corticoid side chain (see inset). Ketalization of the steroid
thus protected shifts the double bond to the 5 position. Treatment of *178* with peracid affords a mixture of the two epoxides.
This mixture is then rearranged to ketone, *180*, by treatment with
formic acid. This last gives the methyl carbinol, *181*, with
methyl Grignard reagent (the 11 ketone is too hindered to undergo
Grignard addition under all but the most forcing conditions).
Dehydration of the tertiary alcohol followed by reduction with
lithium aluminum hydride leads to the ketal, *182*; it should be
noted that the double bond of *178* has in effect been restored.
Indeed, deketalization of *182* leads to the conjugated ketone containing now an additional methyl group at the 6α position. The
additional double bond at the 1 position is introduced in this
case by treatment with selenium dioxide. Removal of the protecting group with acetic acid affords *methylprednisolone (185)*,[71,72]
a widely used corticoid.

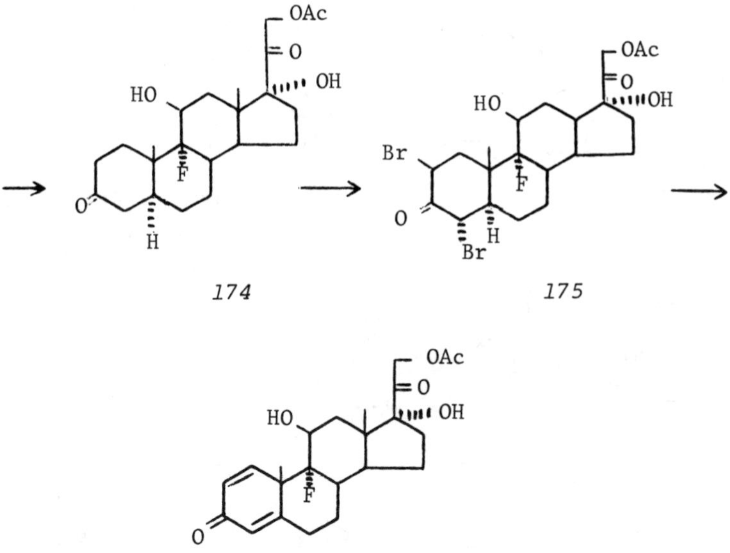

The corresponding 6β-fluoro steroid also exhibits potent

171b   →   177   →   178

181   ←   180   ←   179

182   →   183   →   184

185

antiinflammatory activity. Rather than carrying the dihydroxyacetone side chain through the synthesis in a protected form, the
route to the fluoro compound intercepts an intermediate towards
formation of that side chain; the cortical side chain in this
case is carried along in latent form. Epoxidation of the isolated
double bond of *168a* (obtained by reduction of the ketone of *168*)
affords in this case largely the α-epoxide. Opening of the oxirane with hydrogen fluoride gives fluorohydrin, *187*, stereospeci-
ficity and regiospecificity depending on diaxial opening of the
ring. The acrylic acid side chain is next elaborated to the dihydroxyacetone in the same manner as the transformation of *168* to
170a. Deketalization of *188* leads to the β-hydroxyketone, *189*;
this readily dehydrates to *190* with base. Dehydrogenation to the
1,4-diene by means of selenium dioxide followed by equilibration
of the fluorine to the more stable 6α position completes the
synthesis of *fluprednisolone acetate (191)*.[73]

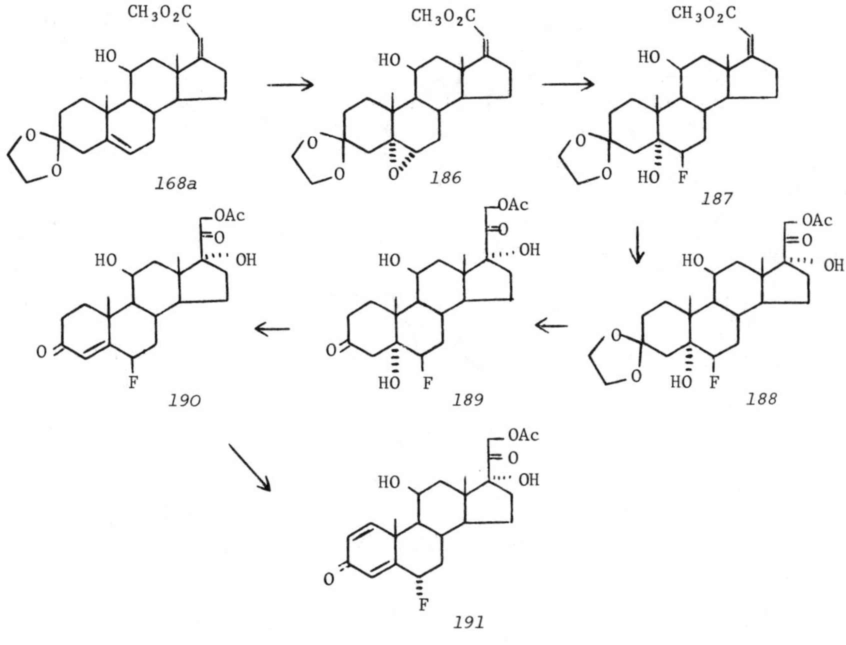

Important pathways for biologic deactivation of cortical
steroids in humans involve reduction of the ketone at 21 and
scision of the entire side chain at C_{17}. Substitution at C_{16}, it

was hoped, would interfere with this degradation by providing
steric hindrance to the degradative enzymes. One of the early
applications of this strategem involved the preparation of *16β-
methylprednisone (199)*. Condensation of the enone, *192*, an intermediate from the synthesis of cortisone by the bile acid route,
with diazomethane followed by pyrolysis of the intermediate pyrazole gives the 16-methyl enone *(193)* (see transformation of *95*
to *97* and *144* to *146* for discussion of this reaction). Catalytic
reduction results in addition of hydrogen from the less-hindered
side and formation of the 16β-methyl intermediate *(194)*. The
progesterone side chain in this case is elaborated to the dihydroxyacetone by the so-called Gallagher chemistry. In this, the
ketone at 20 is first converted to the enol acetate *(195)*; epoxidation affords an oxirane that is essentially a masked derivative
of a ketal at C_{20}. Hydrolytic opening of the epoxide can be
viewed, at least formally, as leading first to the alcohol at 17
and a hemiketal at 20; final product is the hydroxyketone, *196*.
Bromination, because of the great hindrance about the ketone at
C_{11}, proceeds exclusively at the methyl ketone. Displacement of
the halogen with acetate completes the side chain *(198)*. Saponification followed by oxidation with *N*-bromosuccinide surprisingly
goes exclusively at C_3 to give the ketone. Introduction of the
double bonds at 1 and 4 (in this case by the bromination debro-
mination sequence) leads to the potent corticoid, *16β-methyl prednisone (199)*.[74,75]

192   193   194

197   196   195

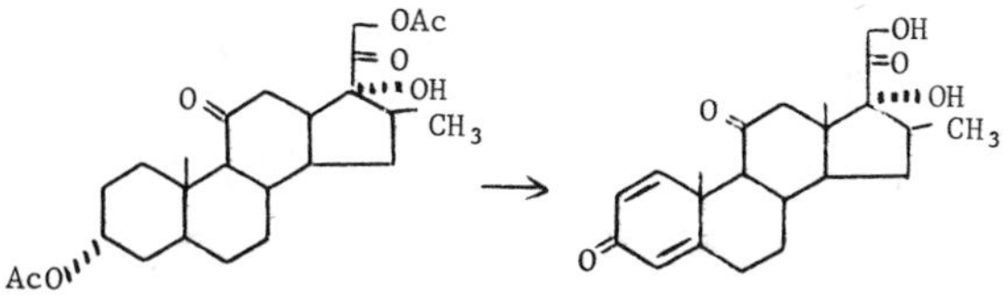

198   199

In another scheme to block metabolism of the cortical side
chain, the steroid is equipped with a methylene substituent at
16.   Thus, 16-dehydropregnenolone acetate *(4)* is first converted
to the corresponding 16 methyl derivative by the diazomethane
addition-pyrolysis scheme alluded to above.   This is then taken
on to 16-methylene-17α-hydroxy progesterone *(201)* by a route
analogous to that outlined earlier (transformation of *144* to *148)*
for the corresponding 6 methyl analog.   Bromination of the methyl
group at 21 followed by displacement of the halogen with acetate
completes the preparation of the side chain *(202)*.   This scheme
differs from others we have seen in the late introduction of the
oxygen at 11.   Thus, incubation of *202* with a *Curvularia* affords
in this case the 11β-hydroxy compound *(203)*.   Oxidation of that
alcohol followed by saponification and finally introduction of
the 1,2 double bond—by a second microbiologic step—yields *predny-
lene (204)*.[76]

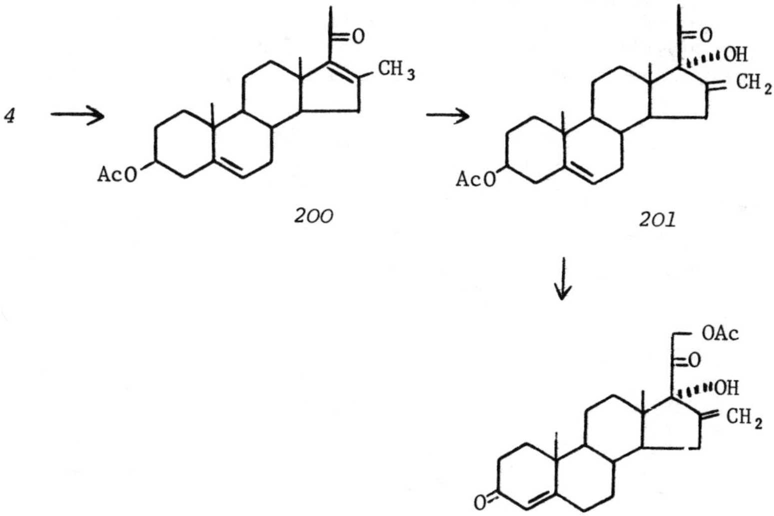

200   201

202

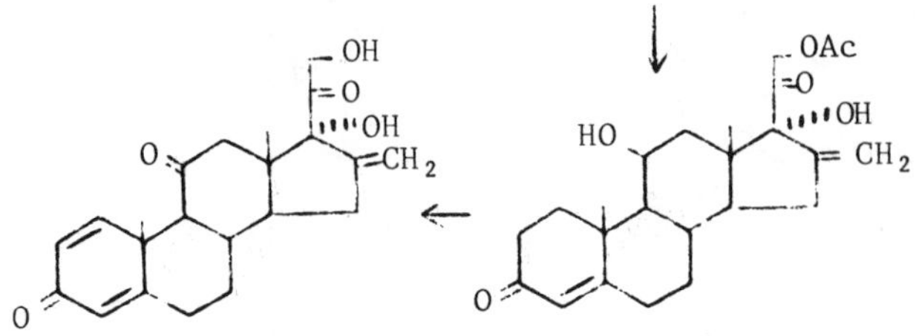

204   203

Incorporation of some of the traditional potentiating groups into the 16-methyl corticoids leads to a series of exceedingly active compounds. Ketalization of the 16β-methylprednisone intermediate, *196*, followed by reduction with sodium in alcohol affords the product of thermodynamic control at 11, the equatorial 11α-hydroxy derivative (metal hydride reduction usually gives 11β alcohols). This compound is then deketalized; the methyl ketone at 21 is brominated and the halogen displaced with acetate ion to afford the compound containing the requisite side chain *(206)*. Oxidation with *N*-bromoacetamide selectively leads to the 3-ketone; this is then converted to the 1,4-diene by the bromination-dehydrobromination scheme *(208)*. The 11-hydroxyl group is then converted to the tosylate; treatment with base affords the 9,11 olefin *(209)*. This last is converted to the 9α-fluoro-11β-hydroxy grouping by the now-familiar scheme *(105 to 108)* to afford, after saponification, *betamethasone (210)*.[77]

The substituents we have seen thus far have all shown stereoselective demands—only one isomer of a given set is compatible

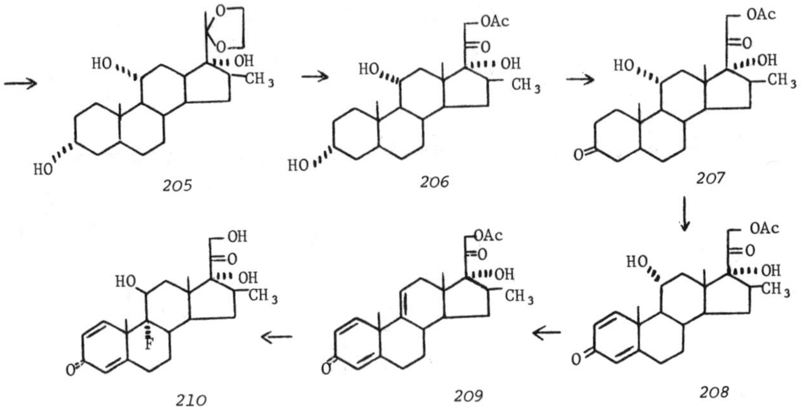

205   206   207

210   209   208

with biologic activity. The 16 position represents an exception
to this rule. The agents isomeric at 16 to the above are fully
as active as the 16β compounds. Condensation of the intermediate
192 with methyl Grignard reagent leads (by conjugate addition
from the least-hindered side) to the free alcohol analog of *194*,
epimeric at 16, that is, the 16α-isomer. This compound is then
converted to cortisone analog *212*, lacking the double bond in the
A ring, by a sequence identical to that described above for the
16β compound (*194* to *199*). That double bond is introduced by a
modification of the bromination dehydrohalogenation procedure
using a single equivalent of bromine (*213*).[78] Protection of the
ketone at 3 followed by reduction gives the 11-hydroxy intermediate. This last is dehydrated to the 9,11 olefin and transformed to the 9,11 fluorohydrin in the usual way. The second
double bond in ring A in this case is introduced by means of
selenium dioxide; saponification completes the synthesis of *dexamethasone (216)*.[79,80]

The potentiation of activity due to the 16α-methyl group
also proved additive with that which had been observed earlier
on incorporation of the 6α-fluoro substituent. Reaction of 16-
dehydropregnenolone with methyl Grignard reagent proceeds as with
the more complex substrate to give, in this case, 16α-methylpreg-
nenolone, *217*. Reacetylation followed by epoxidation gives the
5α,6α-epoxide. Opening of the oxirane ring with hydrogen fluoride followed by acetylation gives intermediate, *218*. This is
then subjected to the side-chain elaboration reaction discussed
earlier (transformation of *194* to *198*) to give triacetate, *219*.
Selective saponification at 3 followed by oxidation gives an

intermediate β-hydroxyketone; this, on treatment with base, goes
to the conjugated ketone *220* with simultaneous epimerization of
fluorine to 6α. In the original work, the 11β-hydroxy function
of *221* was introduced by perfusion of *220* through isolated beef
adrenals; this is presumably not the commercial route. Selenium
dioxide oxidation serves to introduce the 1,2 double bond; *paramethasone (222)*[81] is thus obtained.

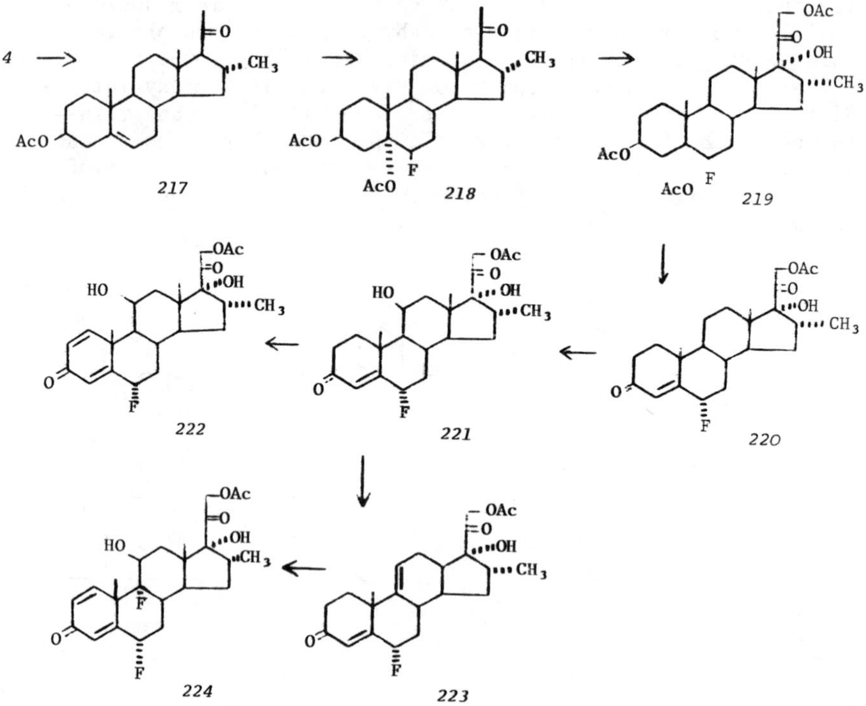

Dehydration of *221* affords the corresponding 9,11 olefin,
223. When this compound is subjected to the series of reactions
for introduction of the 9,11 fluorohydrin, there is obtained the
antiinflammatory steroid *flumethasone (224)*.[82] As might be
expected from the incorporation of a group in almost every position known to increase potency *224* is an extremely active agent.

Incorporation of a hydroxyl group at the 16 position has
been fully as fruitful of active corticoids as the corresponding
methyl derivatives. In this case, however, only the 16α-isomers
seem to have reached the stage of the clinic. The key to entry

into this series is a clever dehydration reaction that eliminates
water in the same reaction from both 11 and 17.[83] Ketalization
of hydrocortisone acetate *(170a)* affords the ketal, *225*. Treatment of this compound with thionyl chloride in pyridine at -5°C
affords intermediate, *226*. Deketalization leads to the true
starting material of this series *(227)*. Oxidation of this compound with either osmium tetroxide or potassium premanganate in
acetone selectively attacks only the 16,17 double bond and that
from the α side, presumably for steric reasons. Thus, in one
step, the substituent at 17 is restored and the new one at 16
introduced. Acetylation under mild conditions leads to *228*. The
9α-fluoro-11β-alcohol is then introduced by the customary scheme.
The 1,2 double bond is introduced by means of selenium dioxide;
saponification completes the synthesis of *triamcinolone (230)*.
Reaction of this 16,17 diol with acetone forms the ketal, *231*;
this last is the widely used antiinflammatory steroid *triamcinolone acetonide (231).*[84]

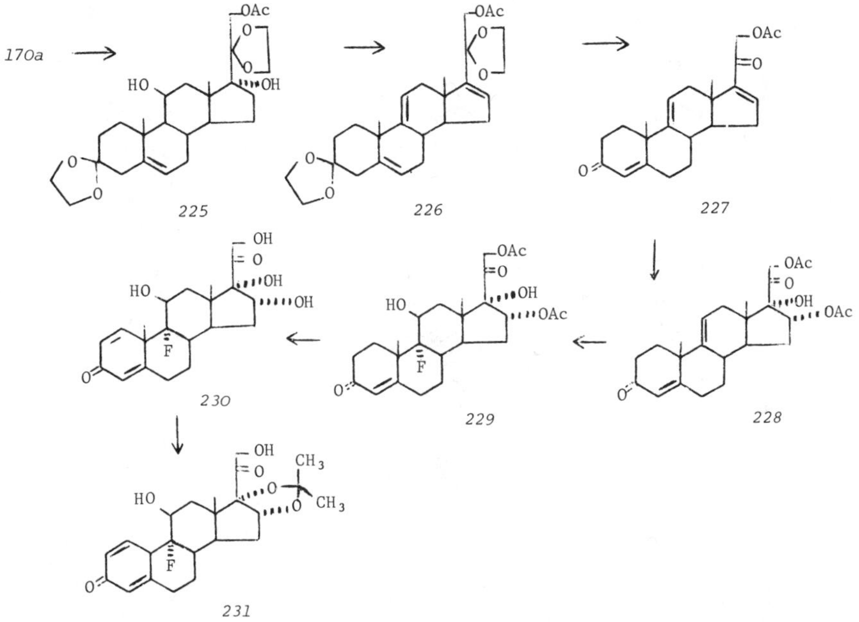

The potentiation obtained with 6α-fluoro group was found to
be additive to that of the 16 hydroxy group, just as in the case
of the corresponding methyl compounds. The synthesis of these
agents relies on introduction of the corresponding hydroxyl group

at a relatively late stage. As in the case of some of the other
6α-fluoro compounds, one must wonder whether the method used for
introducing this function (perfusion through beef adrenals) is in
fact that used for commercial production. Hydroxylation of the
21 acetoxy derivative of 16-dehydropregnenolone (232)—obtainable
from the parent compound in a few steps[85]—affords the 16α,17α-
glycol; this is protected for subsequent reactions as its acetonide (223). Epoxidation gives mainly the 5α,6α-oxide. This is
then transformed to the 6β-fluoro enone by the customary reaction
sequence (see transformation of 186 to 190). The acetonide is
removed during the course of this sequence to afford 235. The
above-mentioned biotransformation serves to introduce the 11 oxygen of 236. Fludroxycortide (237) is obtained from the latter by
dehydrogenation at 1,2 and then conversion to its acetonide.[86]
Alternately, 236 is subjected first to the procedures leading to
introduction of the 9α-fluoro grouping (238). Introduction of
the 1,2-double bond followed by acetonide formation yields flucinolone acetonide (239).[87]

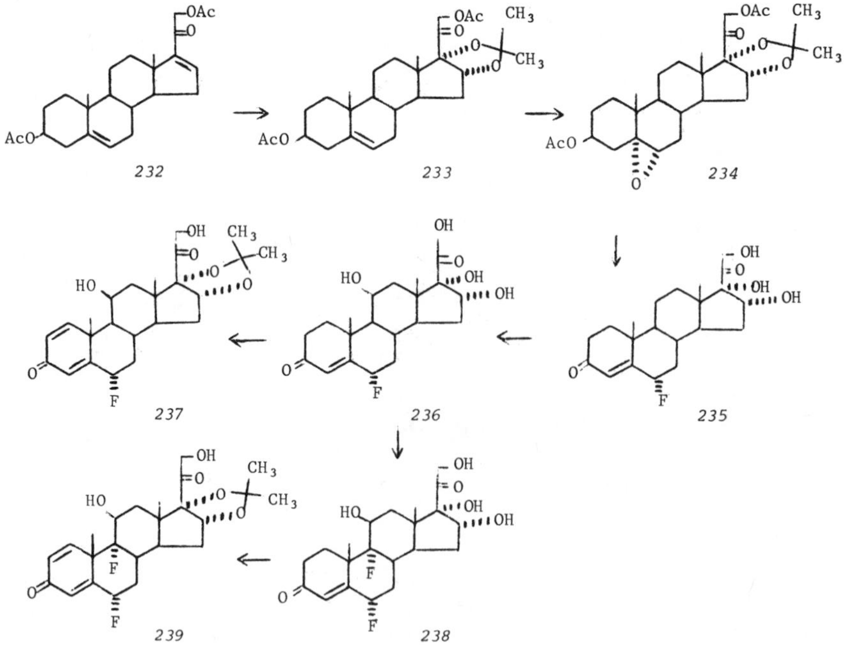

The early structure-activity correlations in the corticoids
suggested that the functionality present in cortisone or dihydro-
cortisone was a minimum for biologic activity; that is, analogs
in which any of the keto or hydroxyl groups were deleted tended
to be inactive. We saw earlier that, in the case of both the
progestins and the androgens, a similar rule apparently fell down
for the 3-desoxy compounds, at least one example in each class
showing sufficient activity to be marketed as a drug. There are
similar exceptions to the rule in the corticoid series: steroids
that lack some apparently crucial structural feature, yet sufficiently active to be used as drugs. It is of note that the
examples shown below are used mainly as topical antiinflammatory
agents.

Dehydration of prednisolone acetate *(175b)* yields the corresponding 9,11 olefin. As a variation on the chemistry we have
seen previously, this olefin is allowed to react with chlorine
in the presence of lithium chloride. If this addition is assumed
to proceed by the customary mechanism, the first intermediate
should be the 9α,11α-chloronium ion. Axial attack by chloride
anion from the 11β position will lead to the observed stereochemistry of the product *dichlorisone (240)*.[88]

175b →

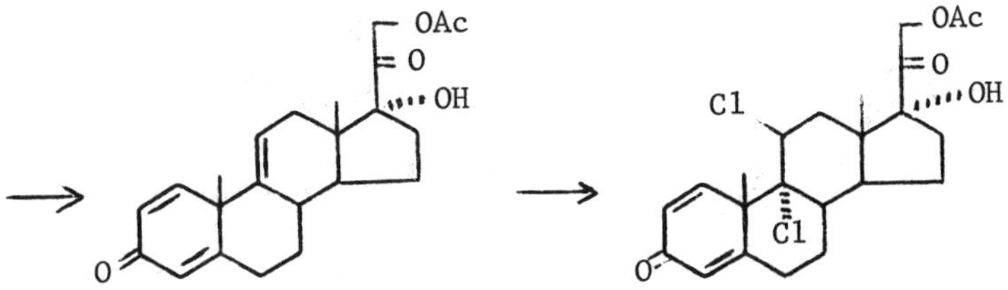

239   *240*

The oxygen atom at 21 is similarly an expendable group.
Reaction of *241* (obtained from *185* by the usual procedure for
introduction of the 9α-fluoro group) with methanesulfonyl chloride affords the 21 mesylate *(242a)*. Replacement of the leaving
group at 21 with iodine by means of potassium iodide in acetone
followed by reduction of the halogen with zinc in acetic acid
leads to *fluorometholone (243)*.[89]

Deletion of the 17α-hydroxy group similarly leads to an
effective topical antiinflammatory agent. Treatment of 16α-
methylpregnenolone *(244)* (obtained by conjugate addition of an
organometallic to pregnenolone) sequentially with bromine and
acetate ion affords the 21 acetate, 245 (see, for example, the
transformation of *196* to *198*). In an interesting variation on
the method for the introduction of a fluorine atom at 6, the

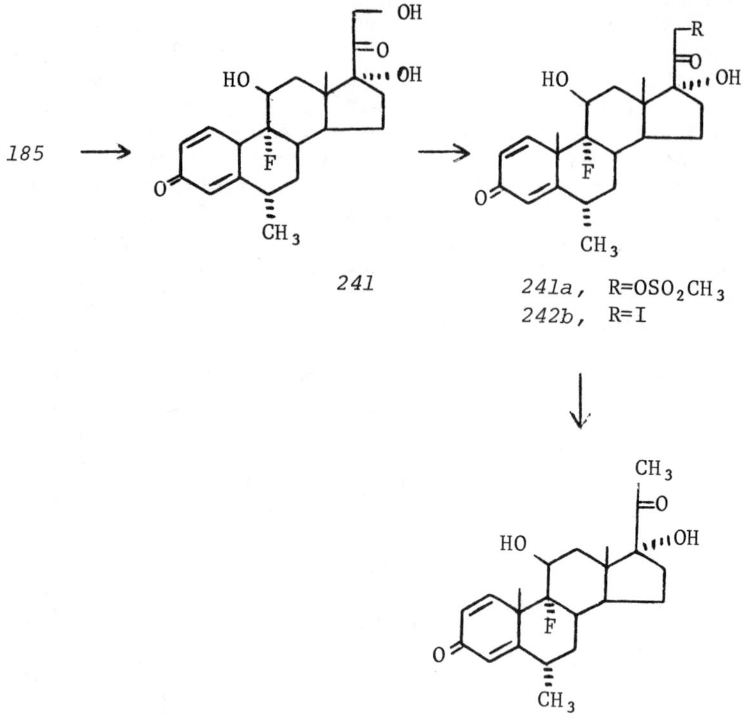

185 → *241* → *241a,* R=OSO$_2$CH$_3$
                     242b, R=I

243

intermediate is first treated with HF in the presence of *N*-bromo-
acetamide; this in effect results in the addition of BrF, presumably, as judged by the stereochemistry of the product, initiated
by formation of the α-bromonium ion. Oxidation of the hydroxyl
at 3, followed by elimination of the halogen β to the ketone,
isomerization of fluorine to the equatorial 6α configuration, and
finally saponification lead to *247*. Incubation of this with a
Curvularia introduces the 11β-hydroxy group. Fermentation of *248*
with *C simplex* serves to dehydrogenate the 1,2 bond. There is
thus obtained *fluocortolone (249)*.[90]
        Examination of the dates on the references to this chapter
will quickly reveal that publications on the corticoids, as indeed all other steroids, reached a steep maximum in the late
1950s to about 1960. After that, publication dropped off to a
comparative trickle. It should be kept in mind when examining

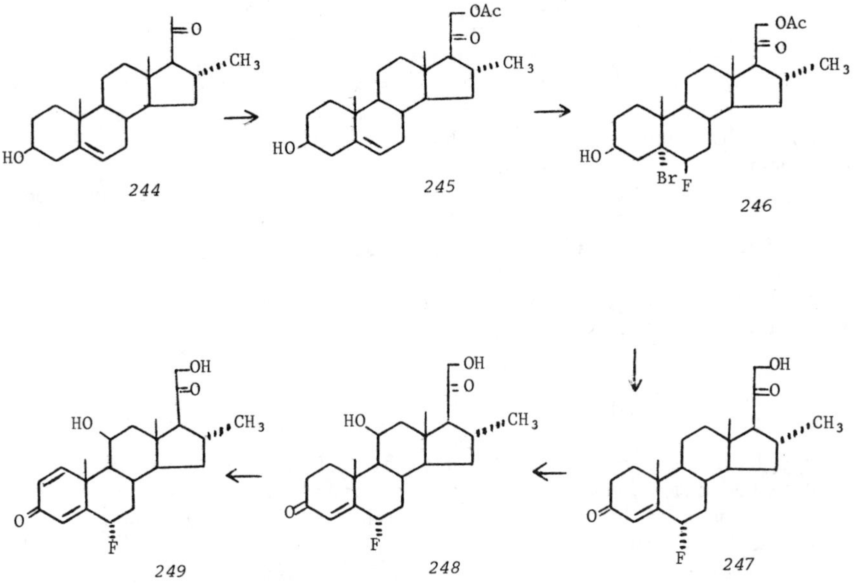

these dates that they represent a skewed sample in that the only
publications cited are those which led finally to either drugs or
agents that almost made the market. Work on steroids did not
cease quite as abruptly as the bibliography suggests.

The apparent peaking of research in this area is an interesting phenomenon that deserves some comment. To begin with, it is
true that within each of the classes of steroids discussed drugs
had been found that met most of the demands of the practicing
clinician. However, none of these entities was free from some
troublesome side effects in some fraction of the patients. Under
normal circumstances this might well have led to continuing work
at some lower level of activity. Two reasons can be invoked for
the decreased effort in this field. In the first place the very
large number of analogs tested—this chapter of course barely
skims the surface of these—served to convince a number of influ-
ential pharmacologists that the splits between the various activities that were being so strenuously sought were probably not
achievable. Thus, no pure anabolic androgen, for example, was
ever uncovered. Excellent splits achieved in experimental animals
had a way of diminishing during clinical trials.

A factor at least as important as those above is the passage

of the Drug Amendments of 1962. The increasing difficulty and
expense of placing a drug on the market made manufacturers chary
of developing drug that did not have promise of impressive sales
figures. Entering a market such as the corticoids with an agent
that might not be readily distinguishable pharmacologically from
existing entries was clearly too expensive to contemplate seri-
ously. This state of affairs has its silver lining in the fact
that much "me-too" research went by the boards. On the other
hand, the true utility of many pharmacologic agents has only been
discovered during the course of clinical trials, often for the
wrong indication. The high cost of developing a drug for the
submission of an NDA and the current trend on the part of the FDA
in the United States greatly decreases the chances of such serendipitous discoveries.

8. MISCELLANEOUS STEROIDS

Although the era of intensive steroid research saw many efforts
to develop compounds with activities other than those catalogued,
this work met with scant success. One such line of research did,
however, bear fruit.

It was known for some time that even after the corticoids
had been separated from crude extracts of the adrenal cortex, the
remaining material, the so-called "amorphous fraction" still possessed considerable mineralocorticoid activity. Aldosterone
(250), one of the last steroids to be isolated from this fraction,
proved to be the active principle. This compound proved to be an
extremely potent agent for the retention of salt, and thus water,
in body fluids. An antagonist would be expected to act as a
diuretic in those edematous states caused by excess sodium retention. Although aldosterone has been prepared by both total[91]
and partial[92] synthesis, the complexity of the molecule discour-
aged attempts to prepare antagonists based directly on the parent
compound.

The much simpler steroid, 253, was fortuitously found to fulfill this role when injected into animals. Its lack of oral
activity was overcome by incorporation of the 7α-thioacetate
group. Reaction of the ethisterone intermediate, 77b, with a
large excess of an organomagnesium halide leads to the corresponding acetylide salt; carbonation with CO_2 affords the carboxyllic
acid, 251. This is then hydrogenated and the hydroxy acid cyclized to the spirolactone. Oppenauer oxidation followed by
treatment with chloranil affords the 4,6-dehydro-3-ketone (254).
Conjugate addition of thiolacetic acid completes the synthesis of
spironolactone (255), an orally active aldosterone antagonist.[93]

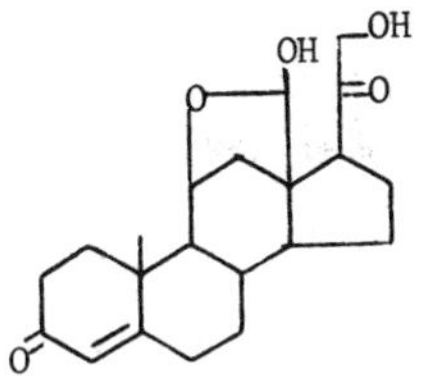

250

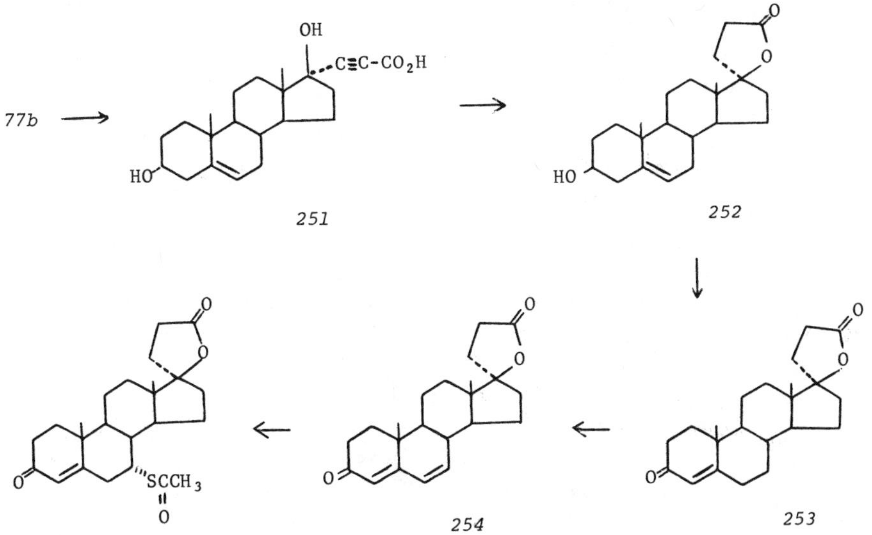

77b $\longrightarrow$

251

$\longrightarrow$

252

255

$\longleftarrow$

254

$\longleftarrow$

253

REFERENCES

1. R. E. Marker, R. B. Wagner, P. R. Ulshafer, E. L. Wittbecker, D. P. J. Goldsmith, and C. H. Ruof, *J. Amer. Chem. Soc.*, *69*, 2167 (1947).
2. For a modification of this step, see A. F. B. Cameron, R. M. Evans, J. C. Hamlet, J. S. Hunt, P. G. Jones, and A. G. Long, *J. Chem. Soc.*, 2807 (1955).
3. F. H. Tendick and E. J. Lawson, U. S. Patent 2,335,616 (1943).
4. G. Rosenkranz, O. Mancera, F. Sondheimer, and C. Djerassi, *J. Org. Chem.*, *21*, 520 (1956).

5. F. W. Heyl and M. E. Herr, *J. Amer. Chem. Soc.*, *72*, 2617 (1950).

6. G. Slomp, Jr., and J. L. Johnson, *J. Amer. Chem. Soc.*, *80*, 915 (1953).

7. E. B. Hershberg, M. Rubin, and E. Schwenk, *J. Org. Chem.*, *15*, 292 (1950).

8. S. Kaufmann, J. Pataki, G. Rosenkranz, J. Romo, and C. Djerassi, *J. Amer. Chem. Soc.*, *72*, 4531 (1950).

9. H. L. Dryden, Jr., G. M. Webber, and J. Weiczovek, *J. Amer. Chem. Soc.*, *86*, 742 (1964).

10. E. V. Jensen and H. I. Jacobson, *Rec. Progr. Hormone Res.*, *18*, 387 (1962).

11. See, for example, A. C. Ott, U. S. Patent 2,611,773 (1952).

12. H. H. Inhofen, W. Logeman, W. Hohlweb, and A. Serini, *Chem. Ber.*, *71*, 1024 (1938).

13. F. B. Colton, L. N. Nysted, B. Riegel, and A. L. Raymond, *J. Amer. Chem. Soc.*, *79*, 1123 (1957).

14. A. W. Makepeace, G. L. Weinstein, and M. H. Friedman, *Amer. J. Physiol.*, *119*, 512 (1937).

15. H. H. Inhoffen, W. Logemann, W. Holway, and A. Serini, *Chem. Ber.*, *71*, 1024 (1938).

16. W. M. Allen and M. Ehrenstein, *Science,* *100*, 251 (1944).

17. A. J. Birch, *Quart. Rev.*, *4*, 69 (1950).

18. A. L. Wilds and N. A. Nelson, *J. Amer. Chem. Soc.*, *75*, 5366 (1953).

19. F. B. Colton, U. S. Patent 2,655,518 (1952).

20. C. Djerassi, L. Miramontes, G. Rosenkranz, and F. Sondheimer, *J. Amer. Chem. Soc.*, *76*, 4092 (1954).

21. J. Iriarte, C. Djerassi, and H. J. Ringold, *J. Amer. Chem. Soc.*, *81*, 436 (1959).

22. A. Ercoli and R. Gardi, *J. Amer. Chem. Soc.*, *82*, 746 (1960).

23. P. D. Klimstra and F. B. Colton, *Steroids,* *10*, 411 (1967).

24. M. S. DeWinter, C. M. Siegmann, and C. A. Szpilfogel, *Chem. Ind.*, 905 (1959).

25. G. H. Douglas, J. M. H. Graves, D. Hartley, G. A. Hughes, B. J. McLaghlin, J. B. Siddall, and H. Smith, *J. Chem. Soc.*, 5072 (1963).

26. R. Joly, J. Warnant, J. Jolly, and J. Mathieu, *Comp. Rend.*, *258*, 5669 (1964).

27. L. Velluz, G. Nomine, R. Bucourt, and J. Mahieu, *Comp. Rend.*, *257*, 569 (1963).

28. E. D. DeWyt, O. Overbeek, and G. A. Overbeek, U. S. Patent 2,998,423 (1961).

29. R. A. Donia and A. C. Ott, U. S. Patent 2,868,809 (1960).

30. Anon., Swiss Patent 206,119 (1939).

31. K. Junkmann, J. Kahol, and H. Richter, U. S. Patent 2,840,508

(1958).

32. A. C. Ott, M. H. Kuizinga, S. C. Lyster, and J. L. Johnson, *N. Y. IUPAC Congress, Abstracts of Papers*, p. 294 (1951).
33. M. S. Newman, *J. Amer. Chem. Soc.*, *72*, 4783 (1950).
34. L. Ruzicka, M. W. Goldberg, and H. R. Rosenberg, *Helv. Chim. Acta*, *18*, 1487 (1935).
35. H. H. Inhoffen, W. Logemann, W. Holweg, and A. Serini, *Chem. Ber.*, *71*, 1024 (1938).
36. H. H. Inhoffen and W. Logemann, German Patent 882,398 (1953).
37. J. A. Campbell and J. C. Babcock, *J. Amer. Chem. Soc.*, *81*, 4069 (1959).
38. C. Megstre, H. Frey, W. Vosser, and A. Wottstein, *Helv. Chim. Acta*, *39*, 734 (1956).
39. B. Camerino, M. B. Patelli, and G. Sala, U. A. Patent 3,060,201 (1962).
40. L. Ruzicka, M. W. Goldberg, H. R. Rosenberg, *Helv. Chim. Acta*, *18*, 1487 (1935).
41. H. J. Ringold, E. Batres, O. Halpern, and E. Necoechea, *J. Amer. Chem. Soc.*, *81*, 427 (1959).
42. R. O. Clinton, A. J. Manson, F. W. Stonner, A. L. Beyler, G. O. Potts, and A. Arnold, *J. Amer. Chem. Soc.*, *81*, 1513 (1959).
43. R. E. Counsell, P. D. Klimstra, and F. B. Colton, *J. Org. Chem.*, *27*, 248 (1962).
44. R. Wiechert, German Patent 1,152,100 (1963).
45. R. Pappo and C. J. Jung, *Tetrahedron Lett.*, 365 (1962).
46. R. Wiechert and E. Kaspar, *Chem. Ber.*, *93*, 1710 (1960).
47. J. M. Kramer, K. Bruckner, K. Irmscher, and K. H. Bork, *Chem. Ber.*, *96*, 2803 (1963).
48. D. H. Peterson, H. C. Murray, S. H. Eppstein, L. M. Reinecke, A. Weintraub, P. D. Meister, and H. M. Leigh, *J. Amer. Chem. Soc.*, *74*, 5933 (1952).
49. M. E. Herr, J. A. Hogg, and R. H. Levin, *J. Amer. Chem. Soc.*, *78*, 501 (1956).
50. M. Ackroyd, W. J. Adams, B. Ellis, V. Petrow, and I. A. Stuart Webb, *J. Chem. Soc.*, 4049 (1957).
51. S. P. Barton, D. Burn, G. Cooley, B. Ellis, and V. Petrow, *J. Chem. Soc.*, 1957 (1959).
52. H. Heusser, C. R. Engel, P. T. Herzig, and P. A. Plattner, *Helv. Chim. Acta*, *33*, 2229 (1950).
53. P. L. Julian, E. W. Meyer, W. J. Karpel, and I. R. Waller, *J. Amer. Chem. Soc.*, *72*, 5145 (1950).
54. H. J. Ringold, B. Löken, G. Rosenkranz, and F. Sondheimer, *J. Amer. Chem. Soc.*, *78*, 816 (1956).
55. J. C. Babcock, E. S. Gutsell, M. E. Herr, J. A. Hogg, J. C. Stucki, L. E. Barnes, and W. E. Dulin, *J. Amer. Chem. Soc.*,

80, 2904 (1958).

56. H. J. Ringold, J. P. Ruelas, E. Batres, and C. Djerassi, *J. Amer. Chem. Soc., 81,* 3712 (1959).

57. K. Bruckner, B. Hampel, and V. Johnson, *Chem. Ber., 94,* 1225 (1961).

58. D. Burn, B. Ellis, V. Petrow, I. A. Stuart Webb, and D. M. Williamson, *J. Chem. Soc.,* 4092 (1957).

59. D. N. Kirk, V. Petrow, and D. M. Williamson, *J. Chem. Soc.,* 2821 (1961).

60. R. Deghenghi, C. Revesz, and R. Gaudry, *J. Med. Chem., 6,* 301 (1963).

61. M. P. Rappoldt and P. Westerhoff, *Rec. Trav. Chim. Pays Bas, 80,* 43 (1961).

62. L. H. Sarett, *J. Biol. Chem., 162,* 601 (1946).

63. L. F. Fieser and M. Fieser, "Steroids," p. 651, Reinhold, N. Y. (1959).

64. K. Miescher and J. Schmidlin, *Helv. Chim. Acta, 33,* 1840 (1950).

65. J. A. Hogg, P. F. Beal, A. H. Nathan, F. H. Lincoln, W. P. Schneider, B. J. Magerlein, A. R. Hanze, and R. W. Jackson, *J. Amer. Chem. Soc., 77,* 4436 (1955).

66. J. Fried and E. F. Sabo, *J. Amer. Chem. Soc., 76,* 1455 (1954).

67. A. Nobile, W. Charney, P. L. Perlman, H. L. Herzog, C. C. Payne, M. E. Tully, M. A. Jernik, and E. B. Hershberg, *J. Amer. Chem. Soc., 77,* 4184 (1955).

68. H. L. Herzog, C. C. Payne, M. A. Jernik, D. Gould, E. L. Shapiro, E. P. Oliveto, and E. B. Hershberg, *J. Amer. Chem. Soc., 77,* 4781 (1955).

69. R. F. Hirschmann, R. Miller, R. E. Beyler, L. H. Sarrett, and M. Tischler, *J. Amer. Chem. Soc., 77,* 3166 (1955).

70. J. Fried, K. Florey, E. F. Sabo, J. E. Herz, A. R. Restivo, A. Borman, and F. M. Singer, *J. Amer. Chem. Soc., 77,* 4181 (1955).

71. J. H. Fried, G. E. Arth, and L. H. Sarett, *J. Amer. Chem. Soc., 81,* 1235 (1959).

72. For an alternate synthesis, see G. B. Spero, J. L. Thompson, B. J. Magerlein, A. R. Hanze, H. C. Murray, O. K. Sebek, and J. A. Hogg, *J. Amer. Chem. Soc., 78,* 6213 (1956).

73. J. A. Hogg and G. B. Spero, U. S. Patent 2,841,600 (1958).

74. E. P. Olivetto, P. Rausser, A. L. Nussbaum, W. Gerbert, E. B. Hershberg, S. Tolksdorf, M. Eisler, P. L. Perlman, and M. M. Pechet, *J. Amer. Chem. Soc., 80,* 4428 (1958).

75. D. Taub, R. D. Hoffsomer, H. L. Slates, and N. L. Wendler, *J. Amer. Chem. Soc., 80,* 4435 (1958).

76. H. J. Mannhardt, F. V. vWerder, K. H. Bork, H. Metz, and

K. Bruckner, *Tetrahedron Lett.*, *16*, 21 (1960).

77. E. P. Olivetto, P. Rausser, H. L. Herzog, E. B. Hershberg, S. Tolksdorf, M. Eisler, P. L. Perlman, and M. M. Pechet, *J. Amer. Chem. Soc.*, *80*, 6687 (1958).

78. G. E. Arth, D. B. R. Johnston, J. Fried, W. Spooner, D. Hoff, and L. H. Sarett, *J. Amer. Chem. Soc.*, *80*, 3160 (1958).

79. G. E. Arth, D. B. R. Johnston, D. R. Hoff, L. H. Sarrett, R. H. Silber, H. C. Stoerk, and C. A. Winter, *J. Amer. Chem. Soc.*, *80*, 3161 (1958).

80. For an alternate route, see E. P. Olivetto, P. Rausser, A. L. Nussbaum, W. Gerbert, E. B. Hershberg, S. Tolksdorf, M. Eisler, P. L. Perlman, and M. M. Pechet, *J. Amer. Chem. Soc.*, *80*, 4430 (1958).

81. J. A. Edwards, H. J. Ringold, and C. Djerassi, *J. Amer. Chem. Soc.*, *82*, 2318 (1960).

82. J. A. Edwards, H. J. Ringold, and C. Djerassi, *J. Amer. Chem. Soc.*, *81*, 3156 (1959).

83. W. S. Allen and S. Bernstein, *J. Amer. Chem. Soc.*, *77*, 1028 (1955).

84. S. Bernstein, R. H. Lenhard, W. S. Allen, M. Heller, R. Littel, S. M. Stollar, L. I. Feldman, and R. H. Blank, *J. Amer. Chem. Soc.*, *81*, 1689 (1959).

85. P. L. Julian, E. W. Meyer, W. J. Karpel, and I. R. Waller, *J. Amer. Chem. Soc.*, *72*, 5145 (1956).

86. J. S. Mills, A. Bowers, C. Casas-Campillo, C. Djerassi, and H. J. Ringold, *J. Amer. Chem. Soc.*, *81*, 1264 (1959).

87. J. S. Mills, A. Bowers, C. Djerassi, and H. J. Ringold, *J. Amer. Chem. Soc.*, *82*, 3399 (1960).

88. C. H. Robinson, L. Finckenor, E. P. Olivetto, and D. Gould, *J. Amer. Chem. Soc.*, *81*, 2191 (1959).

89. F. H. Lincoln, Jr., W. P. Schneider, and G. B. Spero, U. S. Patent 2,867,638 (1959).

90. A. Domenico, H. Gibbian, U. Kerb, K. Kieslich, M. Kramer, F. Newman, and G. Raspe, *Arzneimittel Forsch.*, *15*, 46 (1965).

91. W. S. Johnson, J. C. Collins, R. Pappo, and M. B. Rubin, *J. Amer. Chem. Soc.*, *80*, 2585 (1958).

92. D. H. R. Barton and J. M. Beaton, *J. Amer. Chem. Soc.*, *83*, 4083 (1961).

93. J. A. Cella and R. C. Tweit, *J. Org. Chem.*, *24*, 1109 (1959).

94. For a very recent method for introduction of this functionality by chemical methods, see R. Breslow, *J. Amer. Chem. Soc.*, *96*, 6792 (1974).

CHAPTER 11

Tetracyclines

The tetracyclines are valuable orally active broad-spectrum antibiotics prepared by isolation from the fermentation liquors of
various strains of *Streptomyces* or by chemical transformation of
fermentation-derived substances. The basic ring system and num-
bering pattern is as follows:

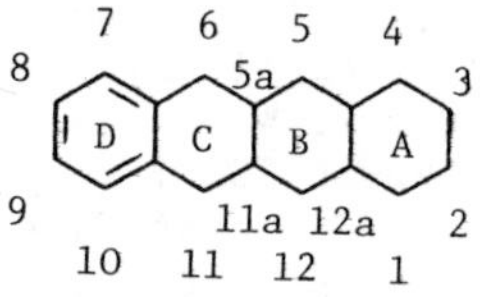

The first three of these agents to be discovered, *tetra-*
cycline (1),[1] *chlortetracycline (2)*,[2] and *oxytetracycline (3)*,[3]
are subject to two major modes of degradation under conditions
occurring during their isolation, purification, formulation, and
administration. These are dehydration and epimerization. Each
of these reactions leads to inactivation of the antibiotic; thus,
considerable effort has been expended in attempts to prevent or
minimize these reactions.

The dehydration reaction leads by an E_2 process to *8* and is
promoted by the tertiary, benzylic nature of the OH group at C_6
and its antiperiplanar trans relationship to the H atom at C_{5a}.
Furthermore, one of the cannonical forms of the enolizable β-
dicarbonyl system present at C_{11} and C_{12} has a double bond in the
C ring. Thus, dehydration leads to aromatization of the C ring,
and this factor must provide some of the driving force for the
reaction.

Work on mutant cultures provided the first practical,
although partial, solution to the dehydration phenomenon. A
mutant strain whose parent produced *chlortetracycline (2)* was

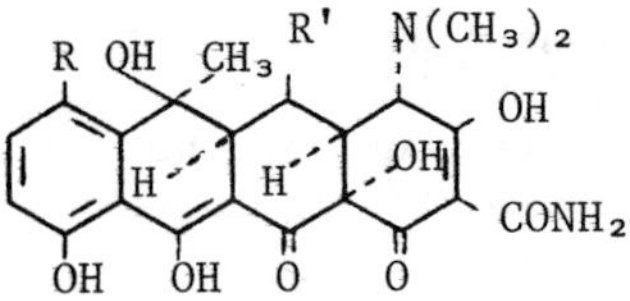

1, R=R'=H
2, R=Cl, R'=H
3, R=H, R'=OH

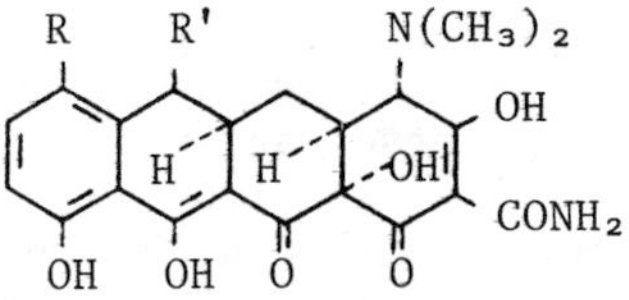

4, R=Cl, R'=OH
5, R=R'=H
6, R=NO₂, R'=H
7, R=NMe₂, R'=H

found to produce a new antibiotic, *6-demethylchlortetracycline (4)*.[4] This strain was ultimately shown to lack a necessary enzyme for the incorporation of methionine-derived carbon into the antibiotic at the C_6 position. Having a secondary rather than a tertiary OH at C_6, this agent is much more stable to dehydration in aqueous acidic solutions than its progenitor. It also has some pharmacodynamic advantages because of its enhanced lipophilicity and was soon introduced into clinical use. This led to a considerable exploration of the chemistry of the tetracyclines with the object of improving still further their pharmacodynamic and therapeutic properties.

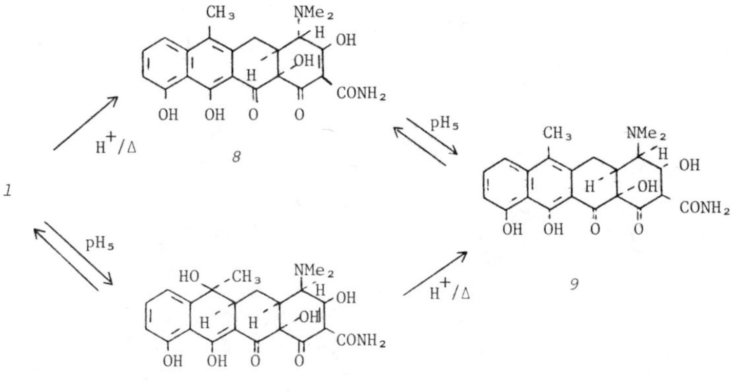

A practical process had earlier been developed for the transformation of *chlortetracycline (2)* into *tetracycline (1)* by catalytic hydrogenolysis of the aromatic chloro group.[5] Application of the reaction under suitable conditions to *demethylchlortetra-*

cycline (4) was found to hydrogenolyze both the chlorine and the benzylic hydroxyl group.[6] The product, 6-demethyl-6-deoxytetracycline *(5)*, is the simplest reported tetracycline with essentially intact antibiotic properties. Its structure defines the minimum known structural requirements for bioactivity in this series. Although the agent has not seen clinical use in the United States, it is an exceptionally valuable chemical intermediate. In contrast to antibiotics *1-4*, it is sufficiently acid stable to be recovered unchanged from solutions in concentrated sulfuric acid. This allows for a wider range of electrophilic reactions than was previously possible. The most successful application of such reactions led to the preparation of *7-dimethylamino-6-demethyl-6-deoxytetracycline (minocycline) (7)*.

Nitration of *5* by a mixture of KNO_3 and concentrated H_2SO_4 produces a mixture of the 7- *(6)* and 9-nitro-6-demethyl-6-deoxytetracyclines *(11)*. The former *(6)* is reductively methylated by catalytic hydrogenation in the presence of formaldehyde to give *minocycline (7)*.[7] This substance has broadened antibacterial activity compared to *demethylchlortetracycline (4)*, especially against Gram-negative organisms resistant to the other tetracyclines by R-factor-mediated mechanisms. In addition, lower daily doses are required because of its relatively low excretion rate.

Similar transformations have not as yet been successfully applied to the tetracyclines bearing a hydroxy group at C_5, and no mutant culture has been reported that biosynthesizes a 6-deoxy-5-oxytetracycline. However, other means have been found to avoid 5a,6-dehydration in this subfamily. Treatment of *3* with *N-*

chlorosuccinimide, or other sources of positive halogen, in anhydrous acidic media results in good yields of the 11a-chloro derivative *(12)*, in which enolization of the carbonyl group at C_{11} is
not possible, and part of the driving force for the aromatization
reaction is removed. When dehydrating agents such as anhydrous
HF are used, *12* dehydrates exocyclically to give *13*. Careful
reduction removes the blocking halo group while leaving the exocyclic double bond intact to give *6-methylene-5-oxytetracycline
(14)*, an antibiotic in clinical use.[8]

Treatment of *14* with hydrogen and a catalyst converts it to
a mixture of epimeric 6-deoxy-5-oxytetracyclines (*15* and *16*),
each of which is active as an antibiotic. The more active isomer
has the natural tetracycline configuration of the methyl group at
C_6 and is in clinical use as *α-6-deoxyoxytetracycline (15)*.[9]
This highly lipophilic tetracycline is the first "one-a-day"
tetracycline (when used to treat mild infections).

$$3 \longrightarrow$$

12

13

14

15, R=H, R'=CH_3
16, R=CH_3, R'=H

The second major mode of degradation of this class of antibiotics is epimerization. The dimethylamino function at C_4 is
axial and subject to a 1,3-diaxial nonbonded interaction with the
C_{12a}-OH group (which is also axial). Being α to the resonance-
stabilized β-tricarbonyl system in ring A, the dimethylamino
function can relieve this strain by epimerization. This reaction,
which occurs most rapidly in aqueous solutions of pH 3-5, results
in an equilibrium mixture consisting of nearly equal amounts of
the two epimers. All clinically significant tetracyclines have
this property to a greater or lesser extent. Unfortunately, the
4-epitetracyclines are essentially inactive as antibiotics and,
in addition, 4-epianhydrotetracycline *(9)*, formed by dehydration

of 4-epitetracycline *(10)*, or by the epimerization of anhydro-
tetracycline *(8)*, has been shown to be toxic. Those tetracyclines
which cannot dehydrate (such as *7* and *15*) should be free from
this kind of toxicity. No chemical technique has yet emerged
that prevents epimerization at C_4 while preserving bioactivity.
This is clearly a worthwhile objective for further work.

Since the tetracyclines are not soluble enough for convenient administration in parenteral solutions, derivatives have been
sought that have enhanced water solubility. A variety of "prodrugs," of which the pyrrolidinomethyl analog of *tetracycline*
(17) is representative, have been prepared by a Mannich-type reaction to fill this need.[10] This derivative is much more water
soluble than the other tetracyclines and is used clinically. It
is quite unstable at physiologic pH values and reverts rapidly to
tetracycline after administration. Amides are not usually nucleo-
phillic enough to participate in a Mannich reaction; however, the
A-ring β-tricarbonyl system of tetracyclines is unusual in several
respects. For example, this group has a pKa of about 3, making it
as acidic as many carboxyllic acids. Thus, at the pH of the
Mannich reaction, this part of the molecule supports a negative
charge and can react with the intermediate methylene imine of
pyrrolidine. Attachment of the new group to the nitrogen atom
rather than to C_2 or to one of the oxygens allows the system to
retain its resonance stabilization *(rolitetracycline)*.

17

REFERENCES

1.   J. H. Boothe, J. Morton, J. P. Petisi, G. R. Wilkinson, and
     J. H. Williams, *J. Amer. Chem. Soc.*, 75, 4621 (1953); L. H.
     Conover, W. T. Moreland, A. R. English, C. R. Stephens, and
     F. J. Pilgrim, *J. Amer. Chem. Soc.*, 75, 4622 (1953); P. P.
     Minieri, M. C. Firman, A. G. Mistretta, A. Abbey, C. E.
     Bricker, N. E. Rigler, and H. Sokol, *Antibiot. Ann.*, 81
     (1953-4).

2. R. W. Broschard, A. C. Dornbush, S. Gordon, B. L. Hutchings, A. R. Kohler, G. Krupka, S. Kushner, D. V. Lefemine, and C. Pidacks, *Science, 109*, 199 (1949); B. M. Duggar, *Ann. N. Y. Acad. Sci., 51*, 177 (1948).

3. A. C. Finlay, G. L. Hobby, S. Y. P'an, P. P. Regna, J. B. Routien, D. B. Seeley, G. M. Shull, B. A. Sobin, I. A. Solomons, J. W. Vinson, and J. H. Kane, *Science, 111*, 85 (1950); P. P. Regna, I. A. Solomons, K. Murai, A. E. Timreck, K. J. Brunings, and W. A. Lazier, *J. Amer. Chem. Soc., 73*, 4211 (1951).

4. J. R. D. McCormick, N. O. Sjolander, U. Hirsch, E. R. Jensen, and A. P. Doerschuk, *J. Amer. Chem. Soc., 79*, 4561 (1957).

5. L. H. Conover, W. T. Moreland, A. R. English, C. R. Stephens, and F. J. Pilgrim, *J. Amer. Chem. Soc., 75*, 4622 (1953).

6. J. R. D. McCormick, E. R. Jensen, P. A. Miller, and A. P. Doerschuk, *J. Amer. Chem. Soc., 82*, 3381 (1960).

7. M. J. Martel, Jr. and J. H. Boothe, *J. Med. Chem., 10*, 44 (1967); R. F. Church, R. E. Schaub, and M. J. Weiss, *J. Org. Chem., 36*, 723 (1971).

8. R. K. Blackwood, J. J. Beereboom, H. H. Rennhard, M. Schach von Wittenau, and C. R. Stephens, *J. Amer. Chem. Soc., 85*, 3943 (1963).

9. C. R. Stephens, J. J. Beereboom, H. H. Rennhard, P. N. Gordon, K. Murai, R. K. Blackwood, and M. Schach von Wittenau, *J. Amer. Chem. Soc., 85*, 2643 (1963).

10. W. Seidel, A. Soder, and F. Linder, *Munchen Med. Wochenschrift, 17*, 661 (1958); W. J. Gottstein, W. F. Minor, and L. C. Cheney, *J. Amer. Chem. Soc., 81*, 1198 (1959).

CHAPTER 12

Acyclic Compounds

It has become almost an article of faith among both pharmacologists and medicinal chemists that drugs (and for that matter, hormones) owe their action to interaction with some receptors. Much evidence has accumulated to indicate that such receptors consist of specific sites on polypeptide molecules. As such, the receptor site is in all probability a highly organized location with specifically located complexation sites and stereochemistry. It would therefore follow that the best fit to such a receptor could be accomplished by a molecule with correspondingly high organization. Deliberate arrangement of the spacing of functionality is most simply accomplished efficiently by the use of some cyclic nucleus as the foundation for potential medicinal agents. Empirically at least, the vast majority of drugs used in clinical practice incorporate at least one ring. However, there are several exceptions to this rule. We have noted drugs that seem to owe their action to some specific functionality rather than to the carbon skeleton to which they are attached. Many of these agents have counterparts in the acyclic series. A very few agents occur only as acyclic molecules.

Derivatives of 1,2 and 1,3 glycols have found extensive use as drugs to relieve mild anxiety. Many of these, in addition, have some activity as muscle-relaxing agents and are used for relief of muscle spasms. The prototype in this series, *meprobamate (4)*, gained some renown in the folklore of the 1950s under the trade name of Miltown®. Reduction of malonic ester, *1*, by means of lithium aluminum hydride affords the corresponding glycol *(2)*. (An alternate route to this intermediate goes through formylation of aldehyde, *5*, with formaldehyde.) Reaction of the glycol with phosgene affords the intermediate, *3*; this gives *meprobamate (4)*[1] on treatment with ammonia. A similar sequence using the malonic ester, *6*, as starting material affords the tranquilizer, *mebutamate (7)*.[2] It has proven possible to prepare

218

derivatives bearing different substitution on the two hydroxyl groups in this series. Thus, reaction of the glycol, 2, with dimethyl carbonate affords the cyclic carbonate, 8, in an exchange reaction. Ring opening of this compound by means of isopropylamine proceeds regiospecifically to give the monocarbamate, 9. An exchange reaction of 9 at the remaining hydroxyl group with the carbamate of ethanol affords *carisoprodol (10)*.[3]

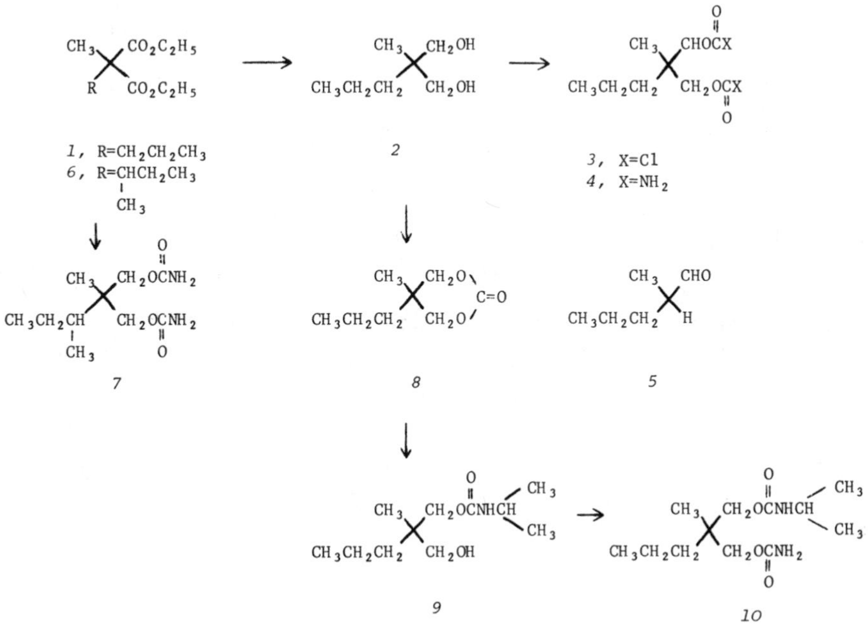

Although the following derivatives of 1,2-glycols do in fact contain an aromatic ring, they are presented here because they are so closely related in structure and activity to their acyclic counterparts. Hydrolysis of the cyanohydrin *(12)* of p-chloroacetophenone with concentrated sulfuric acid affords the hydroxy amide *(13)*. This amide is first hydrolyzed to the acid *(14)* and then esterified. Reaction of the ester *(15)* with methylmagnesium iodide gives *phenaglycodol (16)*,[4] a minor tranquilizer with some activity as an anticonvulsant agent for petit mal epileptic seizures.

Reaction of the glycol *(17)* from hydroxylation of styrene with ethyl chloroformate affords the carbonate ester, *18*. Treatment of this last with ammonia at elevated temperature gives the sedative, *styramate (19)*.[5] A similar sequence on the ethyl ana-

$$\text{Cl}\!-\!\!\bigcirc\!\!-\!\text{COCH}_3 \longrightarrow \text{Cl}\!-\!\!\bigcirc\!\!-\!\underset{\text{CH}_3}{\overset{\text{OH}}{\text{CCN}}} \longrightarrow \text{Cl}\!-\!\!\bigcirc\!\!-\!\underset{\text{CH}_3}{\overset{\text{OH}\ \text{O}}{\text{C-CR}}}$$

11   12   13, R=NH$_2$
                                                          14, R=OH
                                                          15, R=OC$_2$H$_5$

$$\text{Cl}\!-\!\!\bigcirc\!\!-\!\underset{\text{CH}_3\ \text{CH}_3}{\overset{\text{OH}\quad\text{OH}}{\text{C-C-CH}_3}}$$

16

log, *20* (obtainable by metal hydride reduction of the homolog of
14), gives *hydroxyphenamate (21)*.[5]

$$\bigcirc\!\!-\!\underset{}{\overset{\text{OH}}{\text{CHCH}_2\text{OH}}} \longrightarrow \bigcirc\!\!-\!\underset{}{\overset{\text{OH}\quad\text{O}}{\text{CHCH}_2\text{OCOC}_2\text{H}_5}} \longrightarrow \bigcirc\!\!-\!\underset{}{\overset{\text{OH}\quad\text{O}}{\text{CHCH}_2\text{OCNH}_2}}$$

17   18   19

$$\bigcirc\!\!-\!\underset{\text{CH}_2\text{CH}_3}{\overset{\text{OH}}{\text{C-CH}_2\text{OH}}} \longrightarrow \bigcirc\!\!-\!\underset{\text{CH}_2\text{CH}_3}{\overset{\text{OH}\quad\text{O}}{\text{C-CH}_2\text{OCNH}_2}}$$

20   21

Replacement of the carbamate function by an amide seems to
be compatible with meprobamate-like activity in a compound formally derived from a 1,2-glycol. Oxidation of the commercially
available aldehyde, *22*, under controlled conditions affords the
corresponding acid *(23)*. This is then converted to its amide
(24) via the acid chloride. Epoxidation by means of perphthalic
acid affords *oxanamide (25)*.[6]
Acylureas (A) are among the oldest known sedative-hypnotic

$$CH_3CH_2CH_2CH=C \begin{smallmatrix} \diagup CH_2CH_3 \\ \diagdown CHO \end{smallmatrix} \longrightarrow CH_3CH_2CH_2CH=C \begin{smallmatrix} \diagup CH_2CH_3 \\ \diagdown \underset{O}{\overset{}{C}}-R \end{smallmatrix}$$

22

23, R=OH
24, R=NH$_2$

$$\downarrow$$

$$CH_3CH_2CH_2CH-\overset{\overset{\displaystyle O}{\diagup\diagdown}}{C} \begin{smallmatrix} \diagup CH_2CH_3 \\ \diagdown \underset{\overset{\parallel}{O}}{CNH_2} \end{smallmatrix}$$

25

drugs. Similar in action to the better-known barbiturates (B), these agents may owe their action to the fact that they incorporate in open form a good portion of the functionality of the barbituric acids:

$$R^1-\underset{\underset{Br}{|}}{\overset{\overset{\displaystyle R^2}{\diagdown}}{C}} \begin{smallmatrix} \overset{\displaystyle O}{\parallel} \\ NH \end{smallmatrix} \underset{\underset{H_2}{N}}{\diagdown} O$$

$$R^2-\overset{\overset{\displaystyle R^1}{\diagdown}\overset{\displaystyle O}{\parallel}}{} \begin{smallmatrix} NH \\ O \end{smallmatrix} \underset{\underset{H}{N}}{\diagdown} O$$

A   B

Bromination of the substituted butyric acid, 26, by the Hell-Volhardt-Zelinsky procedure affords the α-halo acid bromide (27). Reaction of this with urea affords directly bromisovalum (28). An analogous sequence on acid, 29 (obtained by decarboxylative hydrolysis of the malonic ester), leads to carbromal (30). Dehydrohalogenation of 30 by means of silver oxide affords the corresponding olefin, ectylurea (31),[7] itself a sedative-hypnotic.

The activity of compounds incorporating the biguanide function as oral antidiabetic agents has been alluded to previously. A very simple alkyl side chain in fact can serve as the carbon moiety of such drugs. Buformin (32),[8] obtained by reaction of

$$CH_3CHCH_2CO_2H \longrightarrow CH_3CHCHCOBr \longrightarrow CH_3CH-CHCNHCNH_2$$

CH₃ column under first: CH_3 Br over second with CH_3 Br, O with CH_3, O

26   27   28

$$CH_3CH_2 \diagdown CHCO_2H \longrightarrow CH_3CH_2 \diagup CCNHCNH_2 \longrightarrow CH_3CH_2 \diagdown C-CNHCNH_2$$

with Br, O, O groups

29   30   31

butylamine and dicyanamide, has found use as an agent for the
treatment of adult-onset diabetes.

$$CH_3CH_2CH_2CH_2NH_2 \;+\; NCNC-NH_2 \longrightarrow CH_3CH_2CH_2CH_2NHCNHCNH_2$$

with NH and NH NH groups

32

    Control of tuberculosis, long one of the scourges of mankind,
began with the introduction of effective antibacterial agents.
Thus, this disease was treated initially with some small measure
of success with various sulfa drugs; the advent of the antibiotic,
streptomycin, provided a major advance in antitubercular therapy,
as did the subsequent discovery of *isoniazid* and its analogs.
One of the most recent drugs effective against tuberculosis,
ethambutol (35), stands out not only for its lack of structural
features common to other antituberculars but also by the fact that
it is one of the few acyclic medicinal agents with no cyclic
counterpart. (By a stretch of the imagination the amino alcohols
in this agent may be said to bear some relation to the corresponding functions in the aminoglycoside antibiotics.) Reduction of
the ethyl ester of racemic alanine homolog, *33*, by means of
lithium aluminum hydride affords the amino alcohol *(34)*. The (+)
isomer is then separated by means of optical resolution. This
resolved base is used to effect a double alkylation reaction on

ethylene dichloride. It is of note that the product, *ethambutol*
(36),[9] contains both chiral centers in the (+) form. The meso
isomer (+,-) is some 16 times less active, while the levo isomer
(-,-) is all but inactive.

$$CH_3CH_2CHNH_2 \xrightarrow{} CH_3CH_2 \text{—} C \text{—} NH_2 \xrightarrow{} (CH_3CH_2 \text{—} C \text{—} NHCH_2\text{—})_2$$

with groups:

$CO_2C_2H_5$ above $CHNH_2$ for compound **33**

CH_2OH / H for compound **34**

CH_2OH / H for compound **35**

Disulfiram, an agent whose structure is more inorganic than
organic, constitutes yet another medicinal agent with no cyclic
counterpart. This compound, which was actually first patented as
an accelerating agent for the vulanization of rubber, has at various times been used to combat chronic alcoholism. The mode of
action depends on the simple fact that ingestion of alcohol causes
violent sickness in patients treated chronically with *disulfiram*.
Treatment of diethylamine with carbon disulfide and sodium hydroxide affords the salt, *36*. Oxidation of this with sodium hypochlorite gives the corresponding disulfide, *disulfiram (37)*.[10]

$$\begin{array}{c} C_2H_5 \\ \diagdown \\ C_2H_5 \diagup \end{array} N\overset{\overset{S}{\parallel}}{C}\text{-SNa} \xrightarrow{} \begin{array}{c} C_2H_5 \\ \diagdown \\ C_2H_5 \diagup \end{array} N\overset{\overset{S}{\parallel}}{C}\text{-S-S-}\overset{\overset{S}{\parallel}}{C}N\begin{array}{c} \diagup C_2H_5 \\ \\ \diagdown C_2H_5 \end{array}$$

36   **37**

Organometallic compounds occupy a venerable place in medicinal chemistry. Paul Ehrlich devoted the better part of his
efforts to the search for "the magic bullet" in the late nineteenth century. That is, he was seeking an agent that would des-
troy microbes without harming the host. He scored success in this
quest by the discovery of the antisyphilitic agent, *salvarsan*
(38). As the field of medicinal chemistry advanced, and more
specific and potent drugs became available, organometallic agents
have tended to diminish in importance. *Salvarsan*, for example,
has long since been supplanted by antibiotics. In the area of
diuretics, too, the initial drugs were organometallics, in this
case organomercurial compounds. Most of these have long since
been replaced by sulfonamides and thiazides. As a general rule,
however, the newer diuretic agents tend to cause excretion of not

only water and sodium ion, which is desirable, but other ions
such as potassium and sometimes urea. Loss of these sometimes
causes metabolic disturbances. The fact that the mercurial diuretics lead to an almost ideal diuresis in which ions are excreted
in concentration mirroring their presence in serum has led to
small-scale continued use of these drugs.

Condensation of allyl isocyanate with succinimide affords
the cyclic diacylurea *39*. Acid hydrolysis leads to ring opening
of the succinimide *(40)*. Oxymercuration of the terminal olefin
bond with mercuric acetate in methanol solution affords the diuretic *meralluride (41)*.[11]

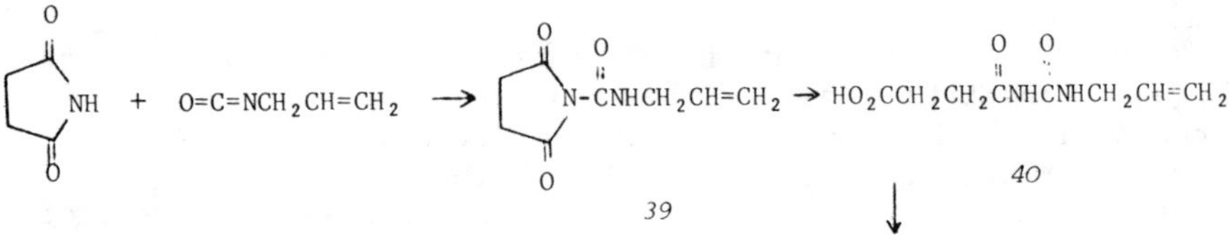

38

39

40

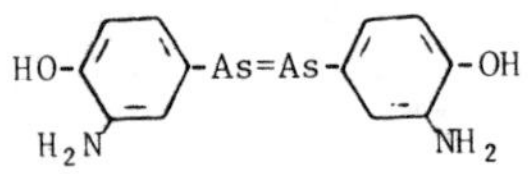

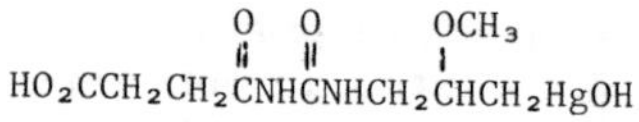

The cyclized analog of *meralluride* is prepared by a similar
synthesis. Thus, condensation of camphoric acid *(42)* (obtained
by oxidation of camphor) with ammonia gives the bicyclic succinimide *(44)*. Reaction with allyl isocyanate followed by ring
opening and then reaction with mercuric acetate affords the mercury derivative *(45)* as the acetate rather than the hydroxide as
above. Reaction with sodium chloride converts that acetate to
the halide *(46)*. Displacement on mercury with the disodium salt
of thioglycollic acid affords the diuretic *mercaptomerine (47)*.[12]

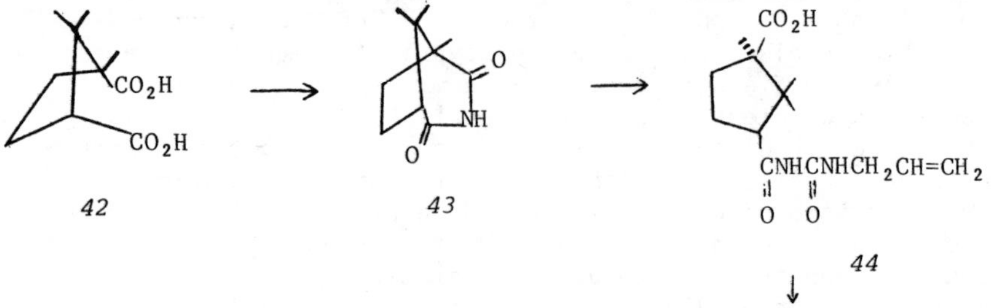

42   43   44

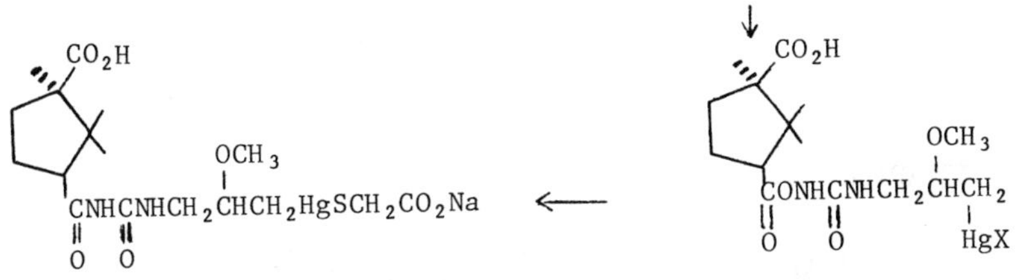

$$\text{CNHCNHCH}_2\text{CHCH}_2\text{HgSCH}_2\text{CO}_2\text{Na}$$

47

45, X=OCOCH$_3$
46, X=Cl

REFERENCES

1. B. J. Ludwig and E. C. Piech, *J. Amer. Chem. Soc.*, *73*, 5779 (1951).
2. F. M. Berger and B. J. Ludwig, U. S. Patent 2,878,280 (1959).
3. F. M. Berger and B. J. Ludwig, U. S. Patent 2,937,119 (1960).
4. J. Mills, U. S. Patent 3,812,363 (1957).
5. R. H. Sifferd and L. D. Braitberg, U. S. Patent 3,066,164 (1962).
6. K. W. Wheeler, J. G. VanCampen, and R. S. Shelton, *J. Org. Chem.*, *25*, 1021 (1960).
7. D. E. Fancher, U. S. Patent 2,931,832 (1960).
8. S. L. Shapiro, V. A. Parino, and L. Freedman, *J. Amer. Chem. Soc.*, *81*, 3728 (1959).
9. R. G. Wilkinson, M. B. Cantrall, and R. G. Shepherd, *J. Med. Chem.*, *5*, 835 (1962).
10. G. C. Bailey, U. S. Patent 1,796,977 (1931).
11. D. E. Pearson and M. V. Sigal, *J. Org. Chem.*, *15*, 1055 (1955).
12. G. Wendt and W. F. Bruce, *J. Org. Chem.*, *23*, 1448 (1958).

CHAPTER 13

Five-Membered Heterocycles

---

1. DERIVATIVES OF PYRROLIDINE

Derivatives of pyrrolidine containing the ring in its fully
reduced form are discussed in earlier sections of this book. To
recapitulate, compounds containing this moiety seldom show activities that differ greatly in kind from the corresponding open-
chain tertiary amine.

Oxidation of the ring to a pyrrolidone or succinimide endows
the derivatives with CNS activity. Double alkylation on ethylamine by 1,4-dibromo-2-hydroxybutane affords the hydroxypyrroli-
dine, 1. Treatment with thionyl chloride gives the corresponding
chloro compound (2). Alkylation of the carbanion of diphenylacetonitrile with 2 gives the aminonitrile, 3. Acid hydrolysis
of the nitrile yields the acid (4). This last undergoes rearrangement to the pyrrolidone (7) on treatment with thionyl chloride. This reaction may be rationalized by assuming that the
acid chloride (5) first forms in the normal fashion; internal
acylation would then lead to the strained bicyclic quaternary
salt, 6. Attack by the chloride ion on the ethylene bridge carbon adjacent to the positive nitrogen affords the observed product (7). Displacement of the halogen with morpholine affords
doxapram (8),[1] an agent used as a respiratory stimulant, particularly in patients with postanesthetic respiratory depression.

Formal oxidation of pyrrolidine to the succinimide stage
affords a series of compounds used as anticonvulsant agents for
treatment of seizures in petit mal epilepsy. Knoevnagel condensation of benzaldehyde with ethyl cyanoacetate affords the unsaturated ester, 9. Conjugate addition of cyanide ion leads to the
di-nitrile ester (10). Hydrolysis in mineral acid affords the
succinic acid (11), presumably by decarboxylation of the intermediate tricarboxyllic acid. Lactamization with methylamine gives
phensuximide (12).[2]

226

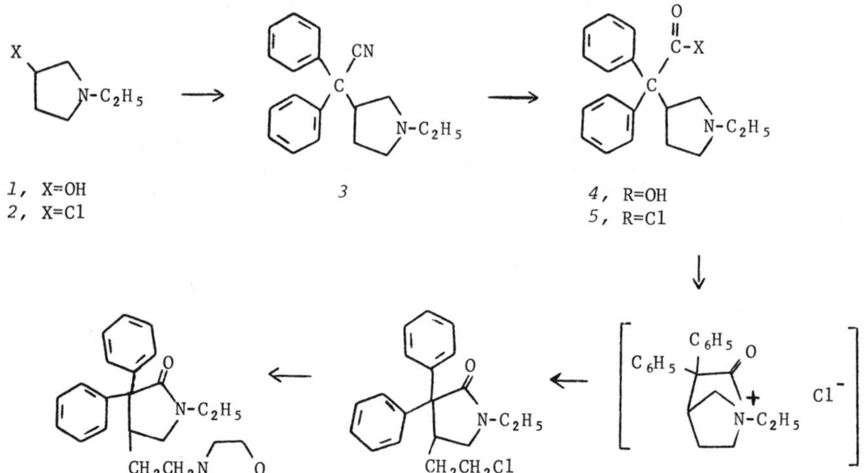

1, X=OH
2, X=Cl

3

4, R=OH
5, R=Cl

6

7

8

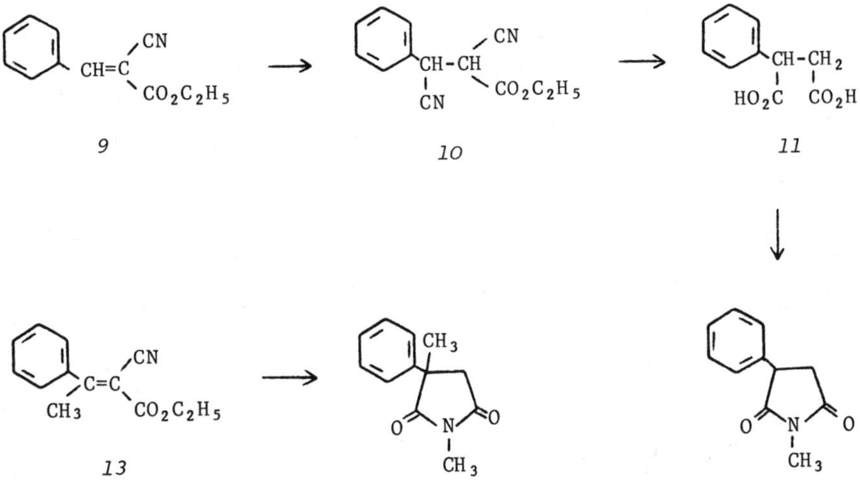

9

10

11

13

14

12

Use of acetophenone rather than benzaldehyde in the Knoevnagel condensation reaction affords the unsaturated ester, *13*. Elaboration of this to the succinimide by a scheme analogous to that above leads to the anticonvulsant agent *methsuximide (14)*.[2] Although actually a compound known for quite some time, the aliphatic analog, *ethosuximide*, was in fact introduced after the above agents. This compound can be attained by first subjecting the condensation product, *15*, to the succinic acid synthesis used above. Cyclization by means of ammonia gives *ethosuximide (17)*.[3]

15

16

17

2. NITROFURANS

Derivatives of 2-nitrofurans are known to possess both bacteriostatic and bacteriocidal properties. That is, the agents will halt and to some degree reverse multiplication of bacteria responsible for infections. In contrast to the antibiotic agents, derivatives of nitrofuran are used largely for topical infections. It should be noted, however, that the word topical is used here in the embriologic sense. Suitable derivatives have found use for treatment of both urinary and digestive tract infections. Considerable ingenuity has been used to design derivatives of nitrofuran so that they will reach some specific site such as the urinary tract following oral administration.

The first drugs in this class to be introduced into clinical practice are simple derivatives of 5-nitrofurfural *(18)*. Thus, the oxime is known as *nitrofuroxime (19)*, while the semicarbazone is called *nitrofurazone (20)*. In order to maintain better control over the distribution and metabolism of these antibacterial agents, increasingly complex side chains and rings have been grafted onto the hydrazone.

Thus, in one such example, hydroxyethylhydrazine *(21)* is first converted to the carbamate *(22)*. Condensation with *18* yields *nidroxyzone (23)*.[4]

Cyclization of *21* by means of diethyl carbonate gives the corresponding aminooxazolidone *(24)*. This compound is then condensed with benzaldehyde to Shiff base *(25)*. An exchange reac-

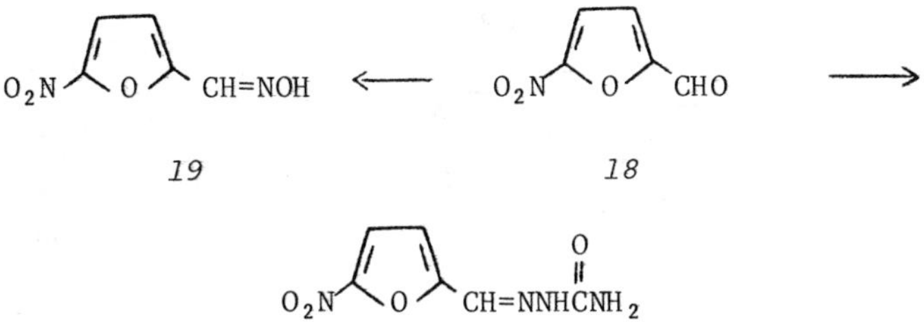

19   18

20

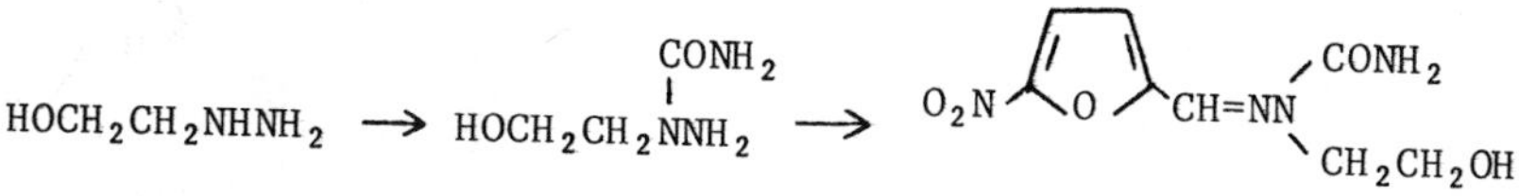

21   22   23

tion of this last with the oxime, *19*, affords *furazolidone (26)*.[5]

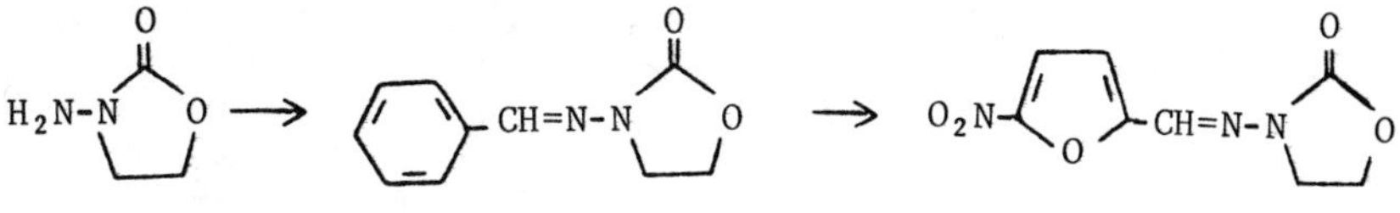

24   25   26

In a scheme intended to produce a more highly substituted oxazolidone, epichlorohydrin is condensed with morpholine in the presence of strong base to give the aminoepoxide, *27*.[6] Ring opening of the oxirane by means of hydrazine gives the hydroxy-hydrazine *(28)*. Ring closure with diethyl carbonate leads to the substituted oxazolidone *(29)*. Condensation with *18* affords *furaltadone (30)*.[7]

In much the same vein, treatment of the hydroxyhydrazine, *31* (obtained by ring opening of the thiomethyl epoxide with hydrazine), with diethyl carbonate gives the oxazolidone, *32*. Condensation with the ubiquitous *18* leads to *nitrofuratel (33)*.[8]

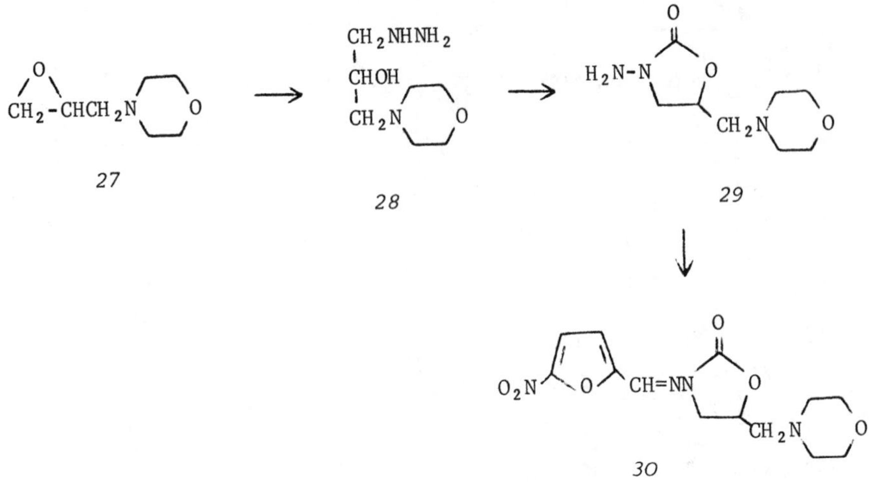

$$CH_2\text{-}CHCH_2N \quad O \quad \rightarrow \quad \begin{array}{c} CH_2NHNH_2 \\ | \\ CHOH \\ | \\ CH_2N \quad O \end{array} \quad \rightarrow \quad H_2N\text{-}N \quad O \quad CH_2N \quad O$$

27   28   29

30

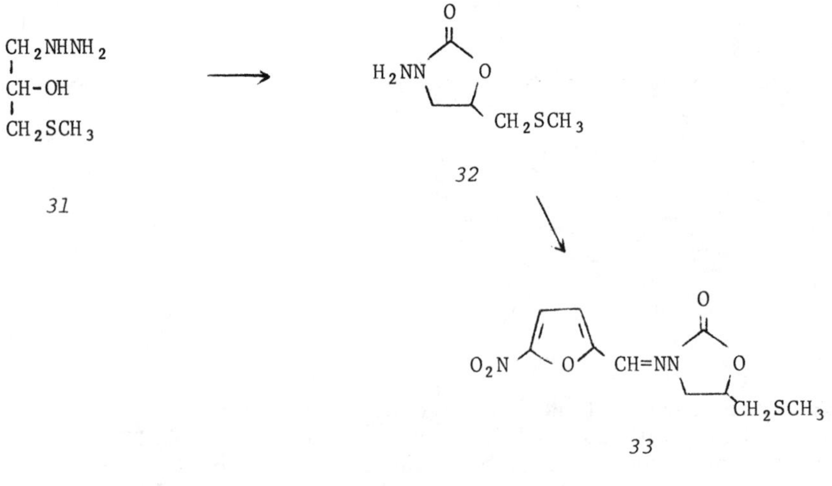

$$\begin{array}{c} CH_2NHNH_2 \\ | \\ CH\text{-}OH \\ | \\ CH_2SCH_3 \end{array} \quad \longrightarrow \quad H_2NN \quad O \quad CH_2SCH_3$$

31   32

$$O_2N \quad O \quad CH=NN \quad O \quad CH_2SCH_3$$

33

Reaction of hydrogen cyanide with the α-hydrazinoester, *34*, leads to the carbamate *(35)*. Cyclization by means of strong acid affords the corresponding aminohydantoin *(36)*.[9] Condensation with *18* affords *nitrofurantoin (37)*.[10]

Treatment of the heterocycle, *38* (obtained from ethylene-diamine and carbon disulfide), with nitrous acid affords the *N*-nitroso compound, *39*. Reduction with zinc leads to the corre-

34, 35, 36, 37

sponding amine *(40)*. This affords, on condensation with *18*, the antibacterial agent *thiofuradene (41)*.[11]

38   *39*, R=NO; *40*, R=NH_2 *41*

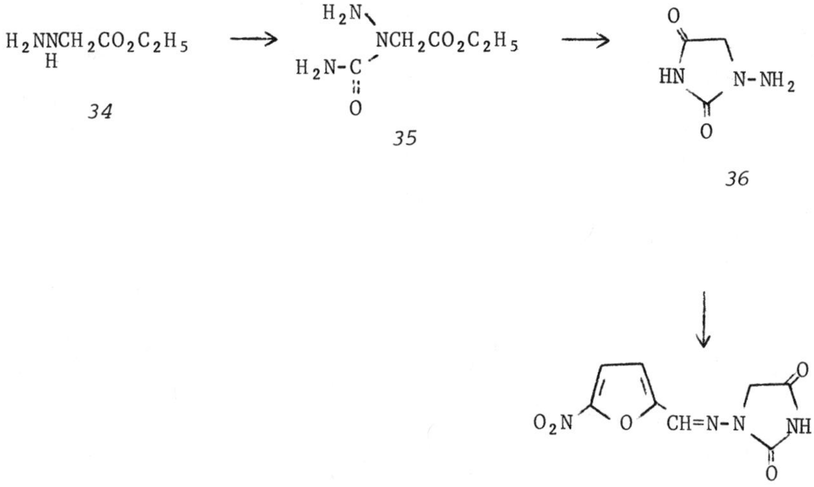

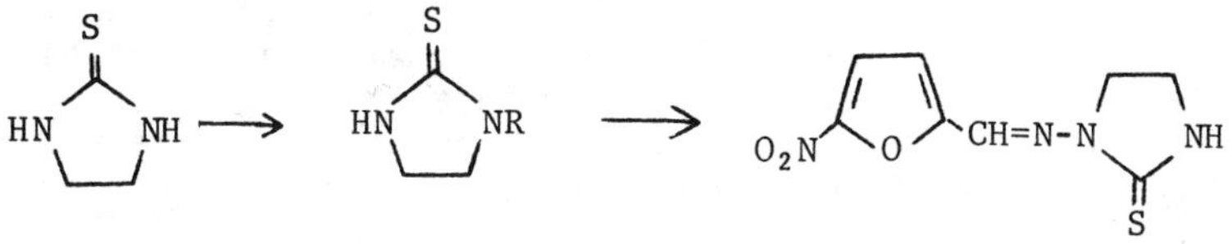

It will of course have been noted that all the above nitrofurans that contain a second heterocyclic ring are linked to that moiety by what is essentially a hydrazone function. Attachment of the second heterocycle by means of a carbon-carbon bond is apparently consistent with biologic activity. Treatment of the thiosemicarbazone of acetaldehyde *(42)* with acetyl chloride leads that compound to cyclize to the thiadiazole (perhaps by way of the enol form, *43*). Condensation of the active methyl group on that heterocycle *(44)* with the aldehyde in *18* by means of strong base gives the olefin, *44*. Removal of the acetyl group by saponification gives *nifurprazine (46)*.[13]

$$CH_3CH=NNHC(=S)NH_2 \longrightarrow \left[CH_3CH \overset{N-N}{\underset{HS}{\diagup}} C-NH_2 \right] \longrightarrow CH_3 \overset{N-N}{\underset{S}{\diagup}} NHCOCH_3$$

42   43   44

$$O_2N \overset{}{\diagup} O \overset{}{\diagup} CH=CH \overset{N-N}{\underset{S}{\diagup}} NHR$$

45, R=COCH$_3$
46, R=H

3. OXAZOLIDINEDIONES AND AN ISOXAZOLE

As we have seen previously, succinimides containing a quaternary
carbon form the basis for a series of anticonvulsant drugs.   In
the course of research in this series, it was found that the
inclusion of additional hetero atoms in the ring was quite compatible with anticonvulsive activity.   We consider here the oxa-
zolidinediones; a discussion of the hydantoins is found later in
this section.

One of the standard methods for construction of the basic
heterocyclic ring was elaborated not long after the turn of the
century.   Thus, condensation of ethyl lactate with guanidine
leads to the imine of the desired ring system (47), possibly by
a reaction scheme such as that outlined below.   Hydrolysis affords
the oxazolidinedione (48).[14] Methylation in the presence of base
gives 49.

Treatment of 49 with a strong base such as sodium ethoxide
serves to remove the last proton on the heterocyclic ring.   Alkylation of the resulting carbanion with allyl bromide affords
aloxidone (50)[15]; methyl sulfate on the carbanion gives trimethadione (51),[16] while ethyl sulfate yields paramethadione (52).[17]

Hydrazides of isonicotinic acid have been used as antidepressant agents by virtue of their monoamine oxidase-inhibiting activity; the pyridine ring has been shown to be replaceable by an

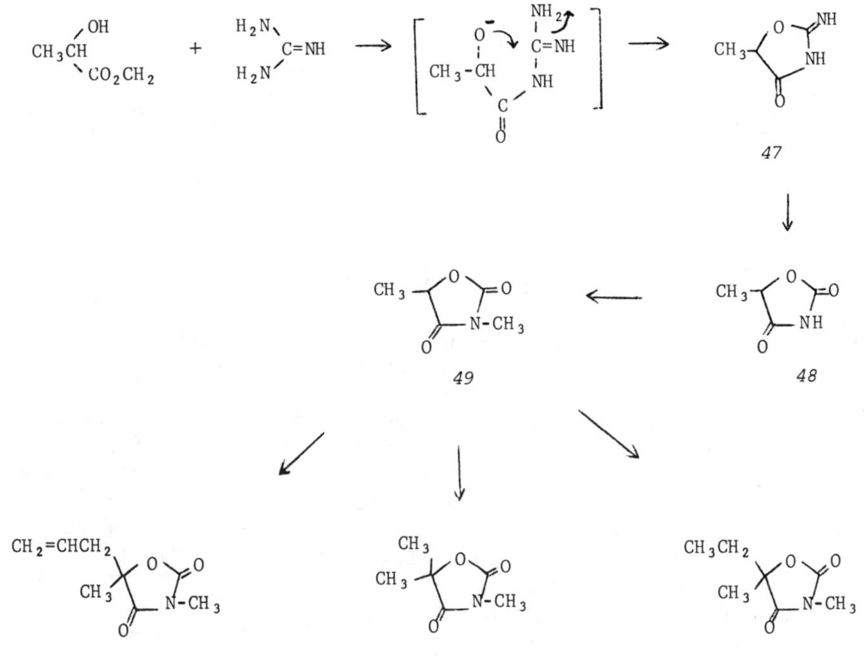

isoxazole nucleus. The properly functionalized ring system (54) is obtained by condensation of the diketone ester, 53 (itself a product of condensation of acetone and diethyl oxalate in the presence of base) with hydroxylamine. This ester is then converted to the hydrazide (55) via the acid and acid chloride. Condensation with benzaldehyde affords the corresponding Shiff base (56). Catalytic reduction of that intermediate affords the MAO inhibitor *isocarboxazine* (57).[18]

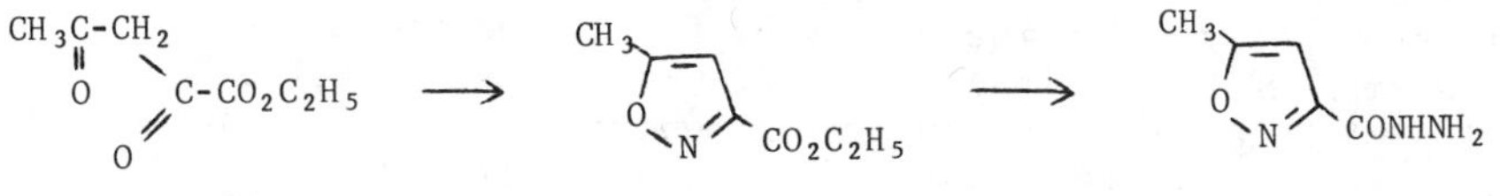

57

56

4. PYRAZOLONONES AND PYRAZOLODIONES

One of the first synthetic organic compounds to find use as an important drug was, in fact, a heterocycle. First prepared in 1887, *antipyrine*, as its name implies, was first used as an agent to reduce fever. One may conjecture that its analgesic and anti-inflammatory properties were uncovered in the course of subsequent clinical application. The pharmacologic spectrum of both classes of heterocyclic compounds is very similar to that of *aspirin* and some other nonsteroidal antiinflammatory agents. Some of the later agents do show better activity against arthritis than does *aspirin*, although it should be added that side effects still present a problem in these structural classes.

Condensation of ethyl acetoacetate with phenyl hydrazine gives the pyrazolone, 58. Methylation by means of methyl iodide affords the prototype of this series, *antipyrine (59)*. Reaction of that compound with nitrous acid gives the product of substitution at the only available position, the nitroso derivative (60); reduction affords another antiinflammatory agent, *aminopyrine (61)*. Reductive alkylation of 61 with acetone in the presence of hydrogen and platinum gives *isopyrine (62)*.[19] Acylation of 61 with the acid chloride from nicotinic acid affords *nifenazone (63)*.[20] Acylation of 61 with 2-chloropropionyl chloride gives the amide, 64; displacement of the halogen with dimethylamine leads to *aminopropylon (65)*.[21]

Antipyretics that carry an alkyl substituent on the remaining carbon atom rather than nitrogen are accessible by condensation of phenylhydrazine with substituted acetoacetates. Thus, reaction of the acetoacetate, 66, with phenylhydrazine followed by N-methylation leads to *propylphenazone (67)*.[22] An analogous reaction on the β-ketoester, 68, affords *mofebutazone (69)*.[23]

Substitution of a second benzene ring onto the nitrogen atoms of the pyrazoles and incorporation of a second carbonyl group leads to a small series of drugs that have proven quite

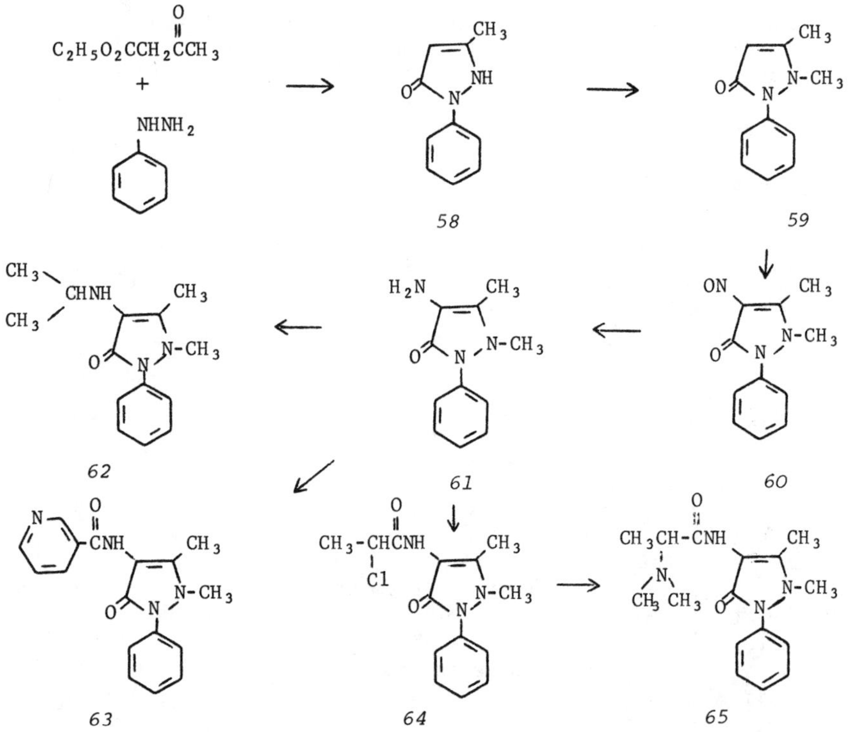

58 59 60 61 62 63 64 65

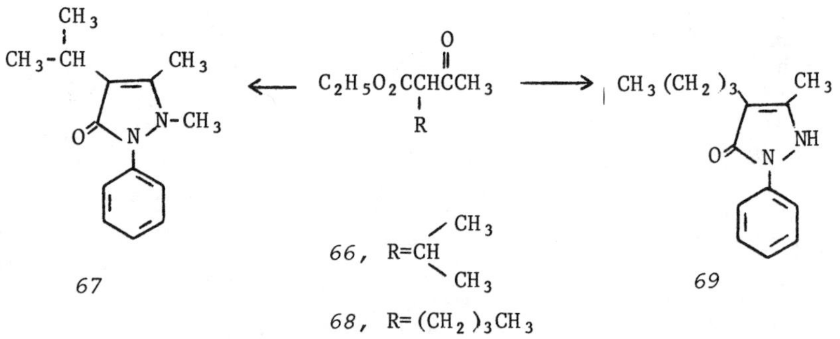

67

66, R=CH(CH$_3$)$_2$

68, R=(CH$_2$)$_3$CH$_3$

69

effective in the treatment of the pain associated with rheumatoid
arthritis. The side effects of these agents, particularly their
propensity to cause gastric irritation, has limited their use to
some extent. The prototype for this class, *phenylbutazone (70)*,[24]
is obtained in straightforward manner by condensation of diethyl
n-butylmalonate with hydrazobenzene in the presence of base; in
effect, this represents the formation of the heterocyclic system
by simple lactamization.

$$CH_3(CH_2)_3CH \begin{array}{c} \diagup CO_2C_2H_5 \\ \diagdown CO_2C_2H_5 \end{array} \quad + \quad \begin{array}{c} HN \\ | \\ HN \end{array} \quad \longrightarrow \quad CH_3(CH_2)_3-$$

                                                                                        70

     Drugs are seldom excreted in the same form as they are admin-
istered. Since such compounds are essentially chemicals foreign
to the body, they are processed chemically by the body's detoxi-
fication system so as to render them more easily excretable. One
of the more common chemical changes observed on aromatic rings
consists in hydroxylation to a phenol. Since metabolism is by no
means synonymous with inactivation, it sometimes happens that
metabolism affords a derivative more active than the drug that was
in fact administered. (It might be added that cases have actually
been recorded in which the administered agent is intrinsically
inactive before some metabolically induced chemical reaction.)
Careful study of the metabolic fate of *phenylbutazone* revealed
that in this case there was an agent produced that was more active
than the original drug. This agent is now available as a drug in
its own right. Condensation of the protected aminophenol, *71*,
with nitrobenzene affords the corresponding azo compound *(72)*;
reduction gives the hydrazobenzene *(73)*. Condensation of this
with diethyl butylmalonate gives the heterocycle *(74)*. Removal
of the benzyl group by hydrogenolysis gives *oxyphenbutazone (75)*.[25]

$$H_2N-\!\!\!\!\bigcirc\!\!\!\!-OCH_2C_6H_5 \longrightarrow \bigcirc\!\!-N=N-\!\!\!\!\bigcirc\!\!\!\!-OCH_2C_6H_5 \longrightarrow \bigcirc\!\!-NHNH-\!\!\!\!\bigcirc\!\!\!\!-OCH_2C_6H_5$$

      71   72   73

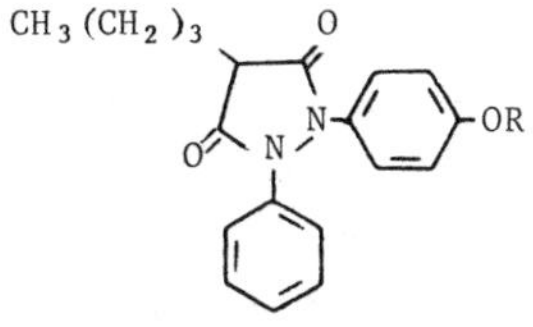

74, R=CH$_2$C$_6$H$_5$
75, R=H

Incorporation of a carbonyl group into the alkyl side chain also proved compatible with biologic activity. The key intermediate (76) is obtainable by Michael addition of the anion from diethyl malonate to methylvinyl ketone followed by ketalization with ethylene glycol. Condensation of 76 with hydrazobenzene leads to the pyrazolodione; hydrolysis of the ketal group affords *ketasone (78)*.[26]

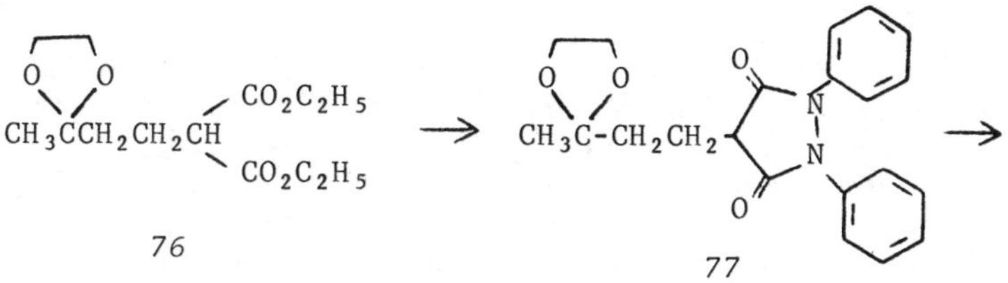

76   77

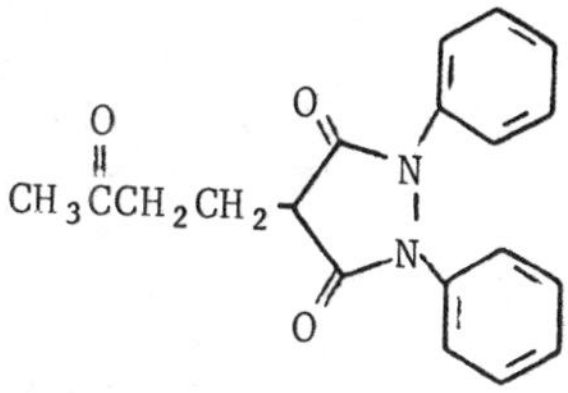

78

Replacement of the methyl ketone moiety in 78 by a phenyl sulfoxide, interestingly, leads to a relatively potent uricosuric agent with diminished antiinflammatory action. This effect in lowering serum levels or uric acid leads to the use of this drug in the treatment of gout. Alkylation of diethyl malonate with the chlorosulfide, 79, gives the intermediate, 80. The pyrazolodione (81) is prepared in the usual way by condensation with hydrazobenzene. Careful oxidation of the sulfide with one equivalent of hydrogen peroxide affords *sulfinpyrazone (82)*.[27]

5. IMIDAZOLES

The use of nitrofurans and their derivatives as antibacterial agents has been touched upon above. Nitro derivatives of another relatively simple five-membered heterocycle (imidazole) have an important place in the clinic as antitrichomonal agents. While infections due to trichomonas, a protozoan, are seldom life threatening, they can cause serious physical discomfort. Agents to combat such infections are therefore in some demand. One of the simpler agents, *azomycin (87)*, interestingly, was first iso- lated from the culture broth from a *Streptomyces* strain. Struc- ture determination established this compound to be one of the rare, naturally occurring nitro compounds. Total synthesis of this agent begins with the condensation of cyanamide with the aminoacetal, *83*. Treatment of the intermediate *(84)* with acid unmasks the aldehyde group; condensation of that function with the primary amino groups affords 2-aminoimidazole *(85)*.[28] Diazo- tization of the amino group in *85* followed by displacement of the diazonium salt *(86)* by means of sodium nitrite in the presence of copper affords *azomycin (87)*.[29]

Synthetic work in the imidazole series is complicated by the ready tautomeric equilibrium that can be set up among the double bond isomers (A, B). Thus, even if a reaction designed to afford the 5 isomer (A) is accomplished regiospecifically, tautomeriza- tion of the product affords either the 4 isomer (B) or a mixture of the two. (This tautomerism is, of course, no problem in azo- mycin because of the symmetry of that molecule.)

Thus, nitration of 2-methylimidazole *(88)* affords a mixture of the 4- and 5-nitro isomers *(89,90)*. It is possible, however, to take advantage of the above mobile equilibrium in such a way as to lead the mixture to predominantly a single alkylation product (a process reminiscent of the C versus O alkylation problem in carbocyclic chemistry). It has been found empirically that

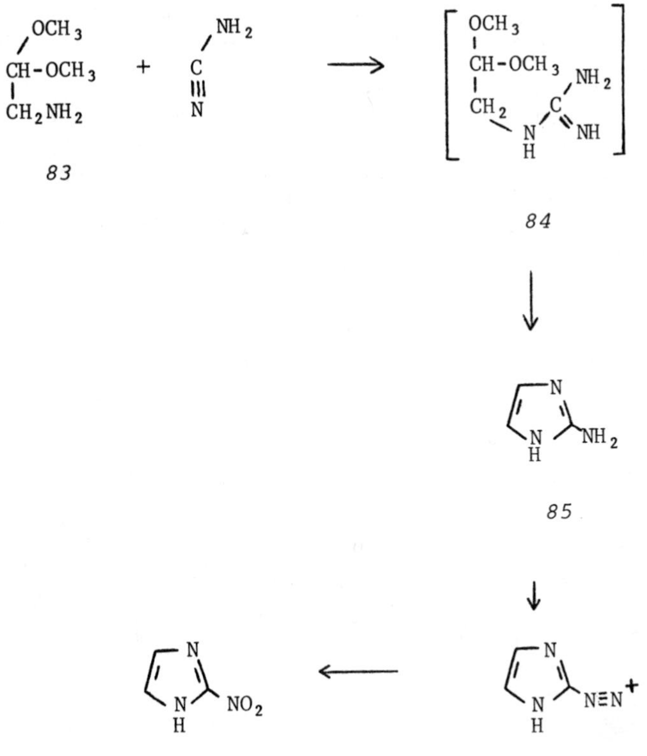

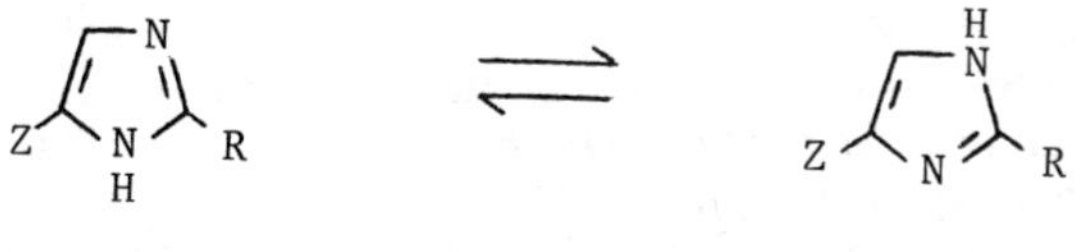

alkylation of the mixture *(89,90)* in nonpolar solvents favors formation of the product from the 5-nitro isomer. Conversely, alkylation of the preformed anion in solvents such as DMF favor the
4-nitro product.

Alkylation of the 5(4)-nitro compound with methyl sulfate in
nonpolar solvents affords *dimetridazole (91)*,[30] an antitrichomonal
agent used in veterinary practice. Alkylation with chlorohydrin
leads to *metronidazole (92)*,[31] a drug that has found widespread
use in the treatment of vaginal trichomoniasis. Finally, alkylation by means of *N*-(2-chloroethyl)morpholine affords *nitrimidazine (93)*.

Hyperthyroidism, that is, the overproduction of thyroid hormones, is usually treated by surgical removal of the thyroid
gland. Before such a procedure is undertaken, the hyperthyroidism is usually first brought under control by treatment with so-
called antithyroid agents.

Condensation of the aminoacetal, *83*, with methylisocyanate
affords the substituted thiourea, *94*. Treatment with acid leads
to cyclization of the masked aldehyde with the amino group to
afford the antithyroid agent *methimazole (95)*. An alternate
route consists in reaction of the methylated acetal *(96)* with
thiocyanic acid.[32] Reaction of the product with ethyl chloroformate leads to the S-acylated product *(97)*. This undergoes S to
N migration with concomitant tautomerization in the presence of
a slight excess of ethyl chloroformate. There is thus obtained
carbimazole (98).[33] The presence of an enolizable thioamide
linkage in all other known antithyroid agents led to the specula-
tion that *98* may have to undergo metabolic deacylation in order

to express its activity.

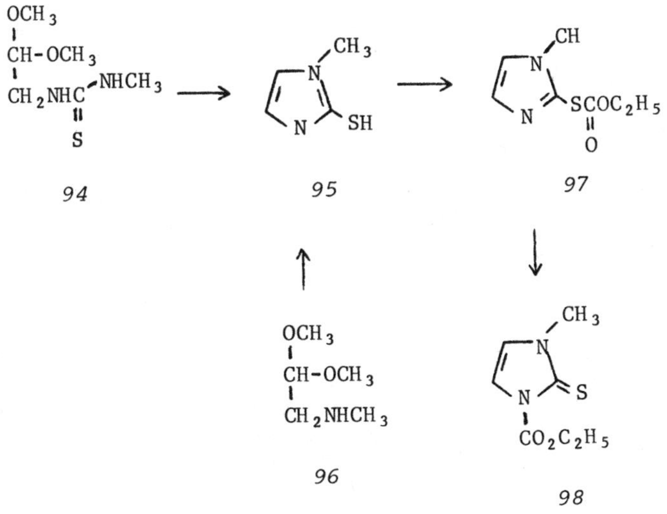

OCH$_3$
|
CH-OCH$_3$
|
CH$_2$NHC$^{\diagup}$NHCH$_3$
‖
S

94

95

97

96

98

6. IMIDAZOLINES

The biologic effects of the imidazolines are reminiscent of those
of the biogenic amines such as epinephrine and norepinephrine.
Although these heterocyclic agents bear almost no structural
similarity to the endogenous substances, they show marked effects
on the vessels of the circulatory system. The exact effect is
highly sensitive to the structure of the side chain. Several of
these agents are effective as local vasoconstrictors; these are
used extensively as nasal decongestants. Those agents which act
as adrenergic blocking agents have been used experimentally in
the treatment of hypertension. One such compound, *clonidine*, is
an effective hypertensive agent in man.

Condensation of the iminoether *(99)*, obtained by methanolysis
of phenylacetonitrile, with ethylendiamine affords *tolazoline*
(100).[33] This drug shows the behavior of an adrenergic blocking
agent and has been used in the treatment of peripheral vascular
disease due to its vasodilating effect. An analogous reaction on
iminoether, *101*, yields *naphazoline (102).*[33] This drug paradoxically acts as a topical vasoconstricting agent; it is therefore
used extensively as a nasal decongestant.

Preparation of the analog of *102* containing a saturated ring

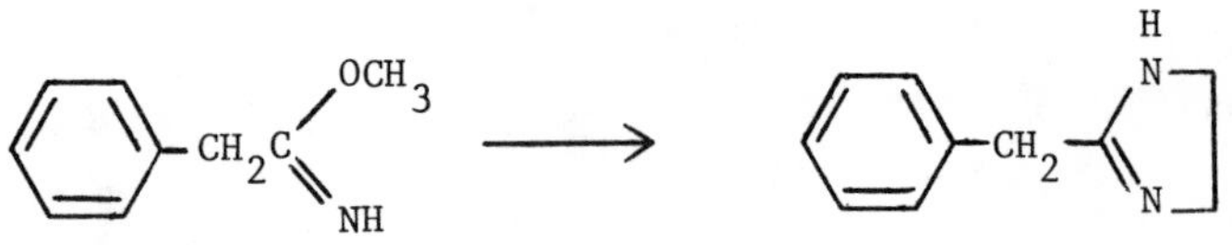

99   *100*

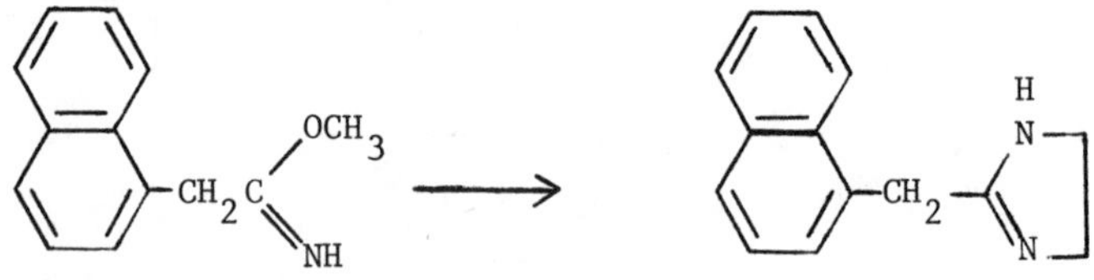

101   *102*

starts with conversion of the carboxylic acid, *103*, to the corresponding amide *(104)*; this is then dehydrated to the nitrile *(105)*. Reaction of the nitrile with ethylenediamine affords *tetrahydrozoline (106)*,[34] a drug used as a nasal decongestant.

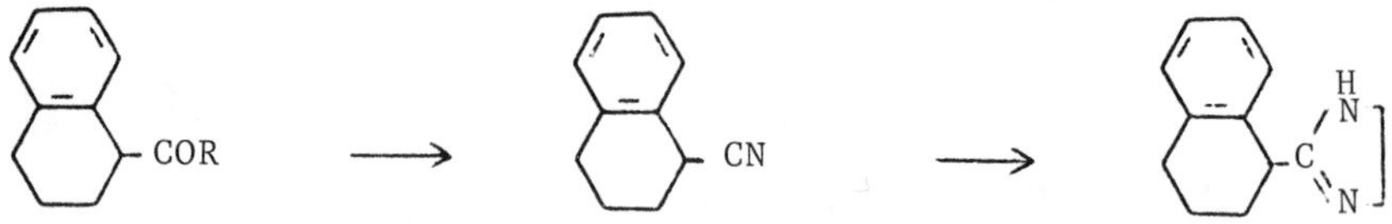

103, R=OH   *105*   *106*
104, R=NH$_2$

Inclusion of additional alkyl groups on the aromatic ring leads to decongestants with longer duration of action. Thus, reaction of the arylacetonitrile, *109*, obtainable from hydrocarbon, *107*, by chloromethylation *(108)*, followed by displacement of the halogen by means of cyanide ion with ethylenediamine, leads to *xylometazoline (111)*.[35] The analogous reaction of the oxygenated derivative, *110*, affords *oxymetazoline (112)*.[36]

Employment of the imidazoline fragment as one of the basic nitrogen atoms in the ethylenediamine antihistamine structure leads to a molecule in which the cardiovascular effects have been supplanted by antihistaminic activity. Alkylation of benzylaniline *(113)* with the halogenated imidazoline, *114*, affords *antazoline (115)*,[37] a drug used as an antihistamine. Shortening one of the side chains on the aromatic nitrogen and inclusion of a phenol function markedly changes the biologic activity; this product, *phentolamine (118)*, shows α-adrenergic blocking action superior

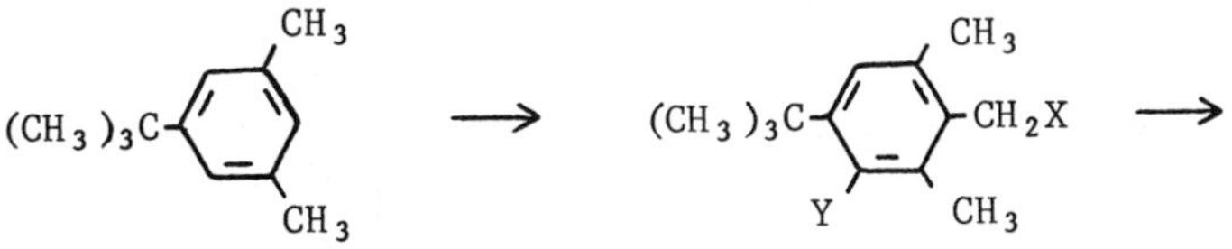

107

108, X=Cl;Y=H
109, X=CN;Y=H
110, X=CN;Y=OH

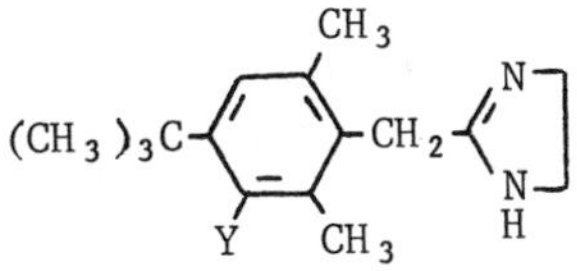

111, Y=H
112, Y=OH

to *tolazoline*. The agent can be prepared by alkylation of the aminophenol, *116*, by the halide, *114*. An interesting alternate synthesis consists in first using *116* as the amine component in the condensation with hydrogen cyanide and formaldehyde to give the α-aminonitrile derivative of formaldehyde *(117)*. Condensation of *117* with ethylene diamine gives *phentolamine (118)*.[38]

Replacement of the methylene group at the 2 position of the imidazoline ring by nitrogen results in compounds whose main action is that of a hypotensive agent. Although these act to some degree as suppressors of the sympathetic nervous system, the mechanism by which they reduce high blood pressure is thought to lie elsewhere. It is of note that the additional nitrogen in effect builds a guanidine-like function into the molecule. Reaction of ethylenediamine with carbon disulfide gives the heterocycle, *119*; methylation proceeds on the nucleophilic sulfur to afford the imidazoline, *120*. Condensation of that intermediate with the aromatic amine, *121* (obtained by reduction of one of the two nitration products of tetralin) leads to apparent displacement of methylmercaptan *(122)*. There is evidence to indicate that reactions of this type in fact involve an addition-elimination sequence. There is thus obtained *tramazoline (122)*.[39] An analogous sequence on 2,6-dichloroaniline *(123)* affords *clonidine (124)*.

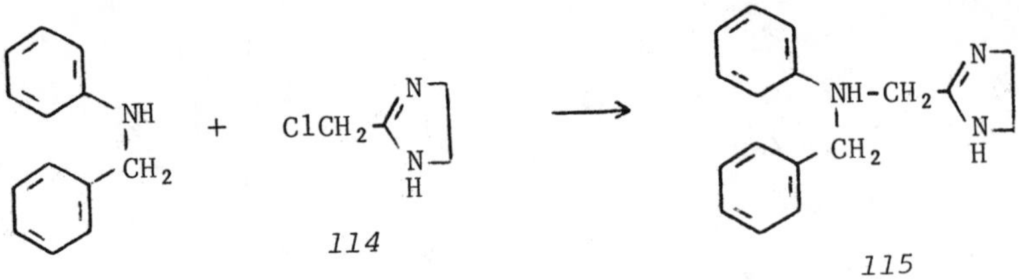

113 + 114 → 115

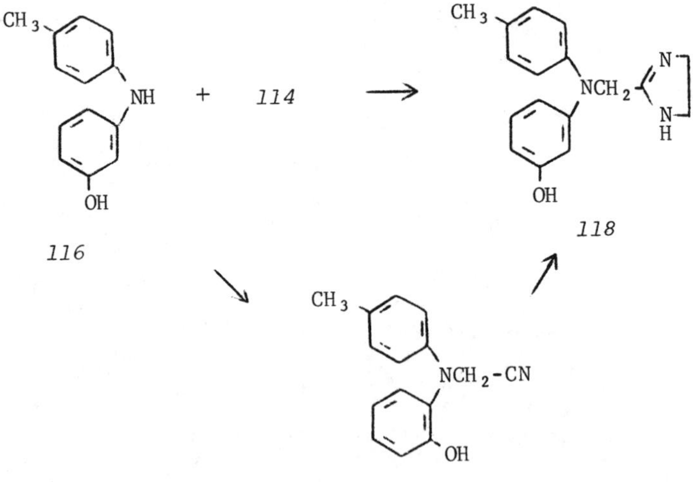

116 + 114 → 118

117

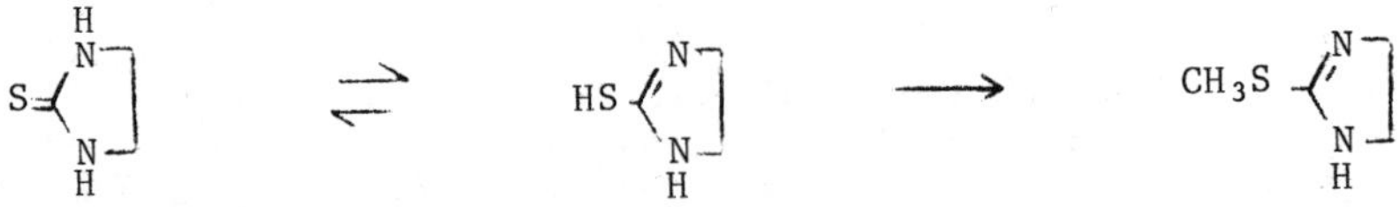

119a ⇌ 119b → 120

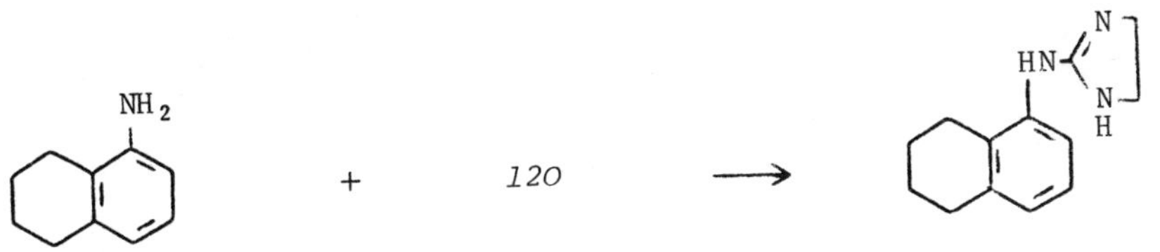

121 + 120 → 122

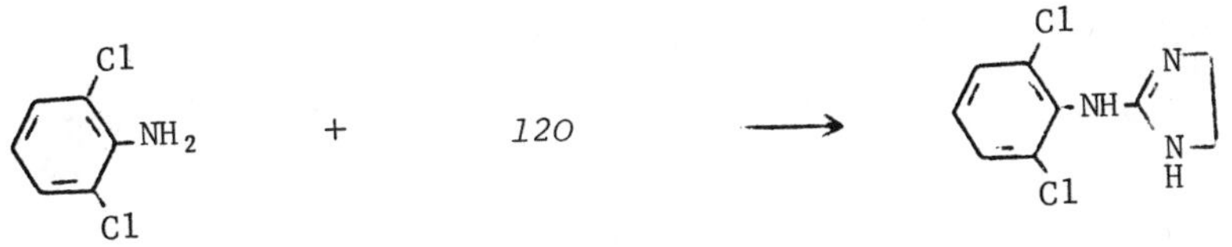

123 + 120 → 124

7. HYDANTOINS

The discovery of the hypnotic activity of the barbiturates led to
an intensive examination of related heterocyclic systems in the
search for agents with a better pharmacologic ratio. Although
the hydantoin ring is smaller by one atom than that of the barbiturates, these two heterocycles do share the cyclic acylurea
functionality. As shown previously, this functional array leads
to hypnotic activity even when present in acyclic form. Although
barbiturates had found some use in resolving the convulsions
resulting from grand mal epileptic seizures, their hypnotic activity severely restricted their general use. The hydantoins, interestingly, show increased anticonvulsant activity at the expense
of the hypnotic effect.

      One of the earliest preparations of this ring system starts
with displacement of the hydroxyl of benzaldehyde cyanohydrin
(125) by urea. Treatment of the product (126) with hydrochloric
acid leads to addition of the remaining urea nitrogen to the
nitrile. There is thus obtained, after hydrolysis of the imine
(127), the hydantoin (128). Alkylation by means of ethyl iodide
affords ethotoin (129).[40]

      A more direct route to this ring system consists in the
treatment of a ketone with an aqueous solution of potassium cya-

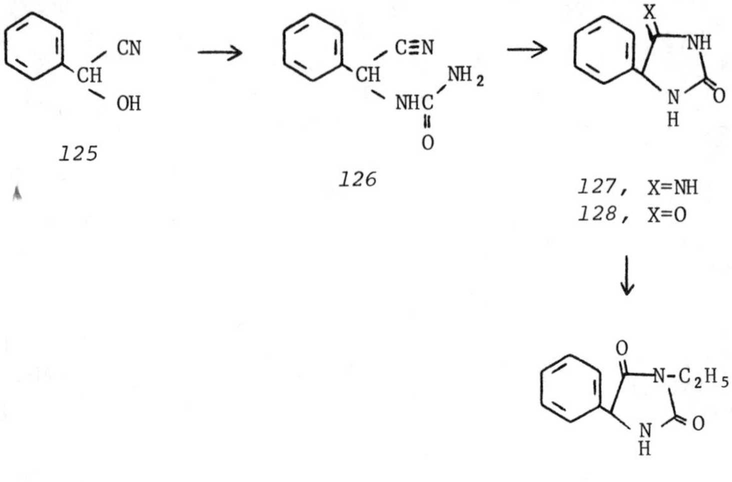

125

126

127, X=NH
128, X=O

129

nide and ammonium carbonate to afford the hydantoin directly.
Thus, acetophenone affords the hydantoin, *132*. The reaction can
be rationalized by assuming that the first step consists in formation of the α-aminonitrile *(132)*; addition of ammonia to the
nitrile will then give the amino-amidine, *131*. The remaining
carbonyl group is then provided by either the carbonate ion or
the carbon dioxide, with which it is in equilibrium. Methylation
of the product affords *mephenytoin (133)*. In a similar fashion,
benzophenone leads to *diphenylhydantoin (134)*,[41] while β-tetra-
lone gives the spirocyclic hydantoin *tetratoin (135)*.[42]

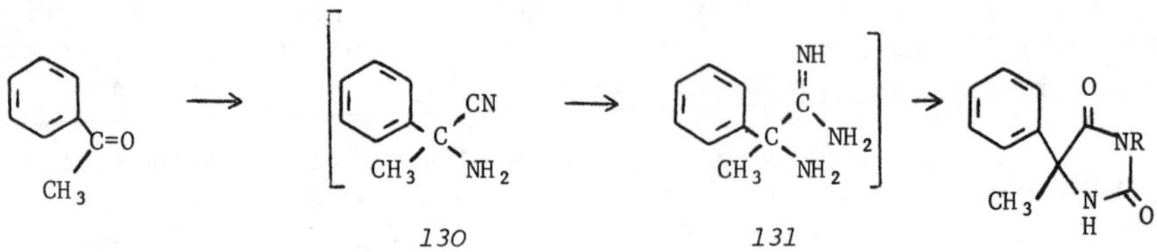

130

131

132, R=H
133, R=CH$_3$

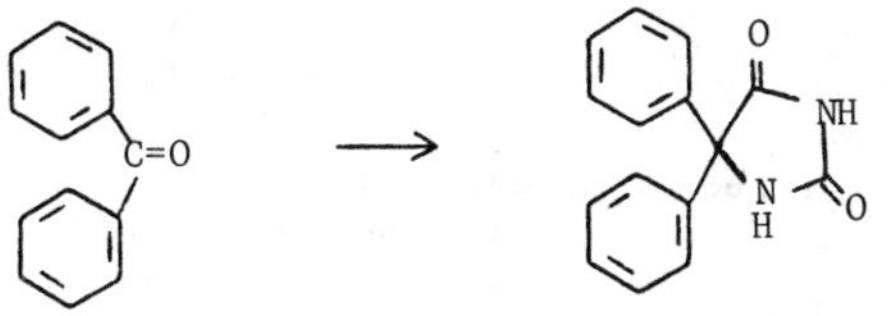

134

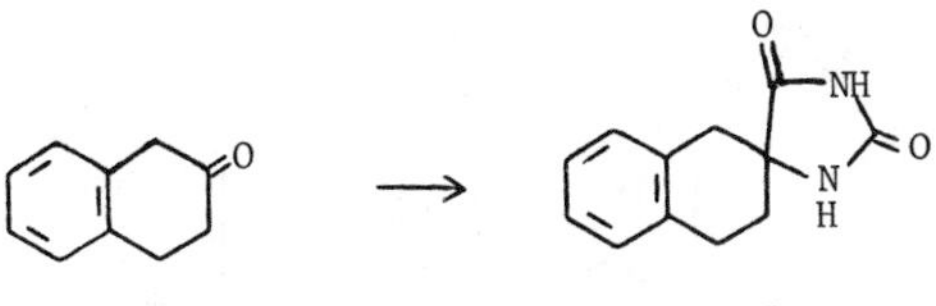

135

8. MISCELLANEOUS FIVE-MEMBERED HETEROCYCLES

As demonstrated above, nitro derivatives of five-membered heterocycles have found extensive use as antiinfective agents. It is
therefore of interest that the nitro derivative of a substituted
thiazole was at one time used as an antitrichomonal agent. Bromination of 2-aminothiazole *(136)* (obtained from condensation of
thiourea with chloroacetaldehyde) gives the 4-bromo derivative
(138); this is then acetylated to *139*. Treatment of *139* with
nitric acid leads to an interesting displacement of bromine by a
nitro group to afford *aminitrazole (140)*.[43]

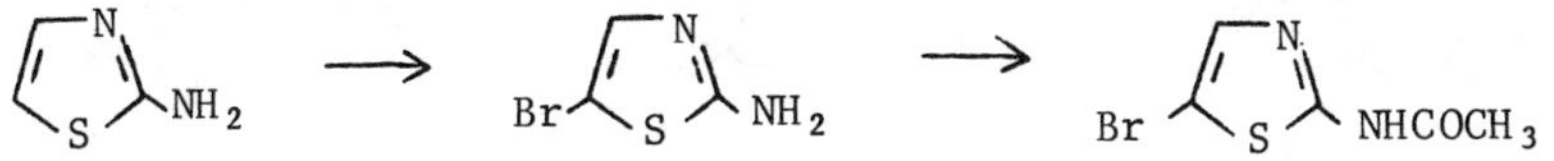

136   *138*   *139*

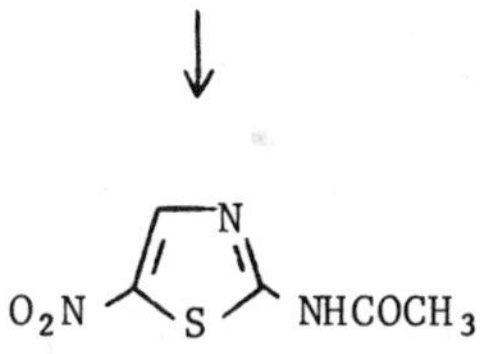

140

A thiazole derivative that incorporates a fragment of the amphetamine molecule shows some CNS stimulant activity; more specifically, the compound antagonizes the depression caused by overdoses of barbiturates and narcotics. Reaction of benzaldehyde with sodium cyanide and benzenesulfonyl chloride gives the toluenesulfonyl ester of the cyanohydrin (141). Reaction of this with thiourea leads directly to *aminophenazole (143)*.[44] It is probable the reaction proceeds by displacement of the tosylate by the thiourea sulfur to give *142*; addition of the amino group to the nitrile followed by tautomerization affords the observed product.

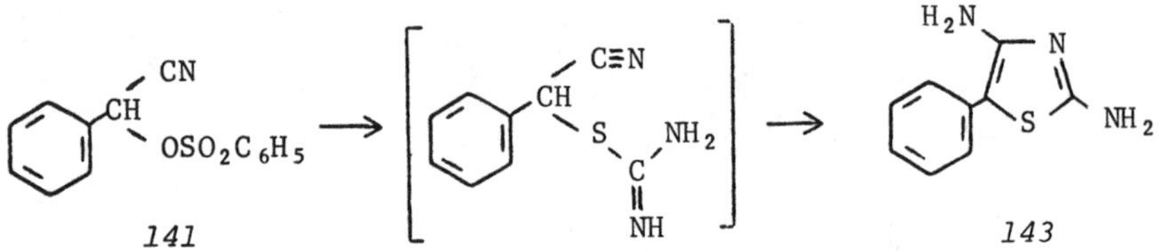

Acylation of benzamidoxime (144) with chloropropionyl chloride gives the O-acylated derivative (145). Reaction of that intermediate with diethylamine serves first to cyclize the molecule to the 1,2,4-oxadiazole heterocycle; subsequent displacement of the halogen on the side chain gives *oxolamine (146)*,[45] a drug with antitussive and spasmolytic activity.

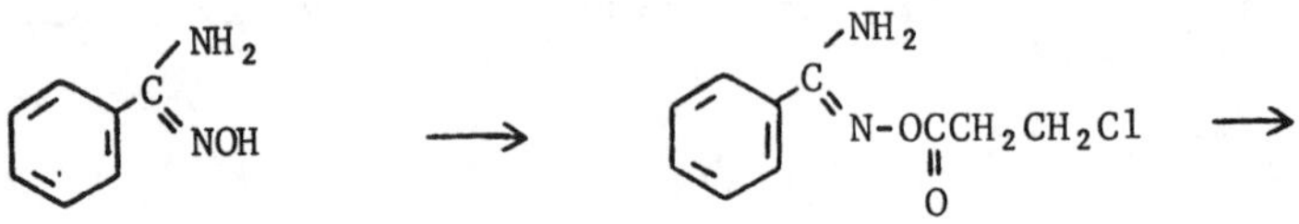

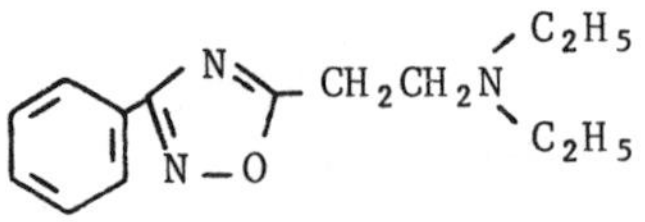

Shifting the side chain to the 4 position (with the necessary tautomeric change) affords an agent with local anesthetic and coronary vasodilator activity. Cyclization of compound *147* by means of phosphorus oxychloride gives the amino-1,2,4-oxodiazole *(148)*.[45] Alkylation of that compound with 2-chlorotriethylamine in the presence of sodium hydroxide proceeds via the tautomer, *149*, rather than the fully conjugated isomer. There is thus obtained *imolamine (150)*.[46]

One of the side effects noted in the clinical use of the sulfonamide antibacterial agents was a diuretic effect caused by inhibition of the enzyme carbonic anhydrase. Attempts to capitalize on this side effect so as to obtain agents with greatly enhanced diuretic activity first met success when a heterocyclic ring was substituted for the benzene ring of the sulfonamide. Treatment of the hydrazine derivative, *151*, with phosgene leads to the 1,3,4-thiadizole, *152*.[47] (Phosgene possibly acylates one of the amino groups and thus converts this to a leaving group subsequent to attack by the sulfur on the remaining thioamide.) Acylation of the amine gives the amide, *153*. Oxidation of the thiol by means of aqueous chlorine goes directly to the sulfonyl chloride *(154)*. Finally, amonolysis of the halide with ammonia affords *acetazolamide (155)*.[48] The same scheme starting with the butyramide *(156)* yields *butazolamide (157)*.[49]

In a further development on this theme, the thiol, *153*, is first alkylated to the corresponding benzyl ether *(158)*. Treatment with sodium methoxide removes the proton on the amide nitrogen to afford the ambient anion *(159)*. This undergoes alkylation with methyl bromide on the ring nitrogen; thus it locks amide into the imine form *(160)*. Chlorolysis serves both to oxidize the sulfur to the sulfone stage and to cleave the benzyl ether linkage; there is thus obtained the sulfonyl chloride, *161*.

Amonolysis affords the diuretic agent *methazolamide (162)*.[50]

151

152

153, $R=CH_3$
156, $R=CH_2CH_2CH_3$

159

158

154

160

161, X=Cl
162, $X=NH_2$

155, $R=CH_3$
157, $R=CH_2CH_2CH_3$

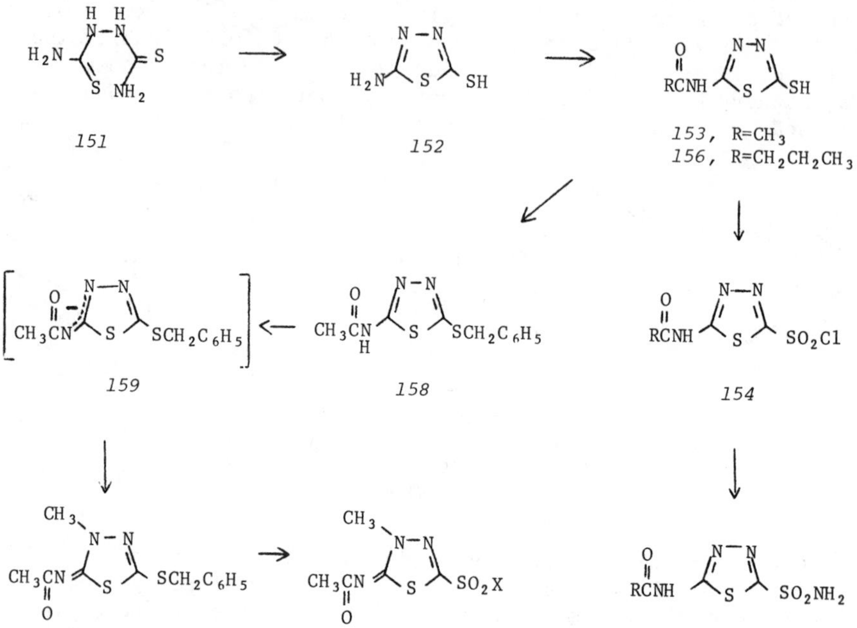

REFERENCES

1. C. D. Luns, A. D. Cale, J. W. Ward, B. V. Franko, and H. Jenkins, *J. Med. Chem.*, *7*, 302 (1964).
2. C. A. Miller and L. M. Long, *J. Amer. Chem. Soc.*, *73*, 4895 (1951).
3. S. S. G. Sircar, *J. Chem. Soc.*, 600 (1927).
4. W. B. Stillman and A. B. Scott, U. S. Patent 2,416,634 (1947).
5. G. Gever and C. J. O'Keefe, U. S. Patent 2,927,110 (1960).
6. O. Eisleb, U. S. Patent 1,790,042 (1931).
7. G. Gever, U. S. Patent 2,802,002 (1957).
8. Anon., Belgian Patent 635,608 (1963).
9. W. Treibe and E. Hoffa, *Chem. Ber.*, *31*, 162 (1898).
10. K. J. Hayes, U. S. Patent 2,610,181 (1952).

11. J. G. Michels, U. S. Patent 2,290,074 (1960).
12. J. Goerdler, J. Ohm, and O. Tegtmeyer, *Chem. Ber.*, *89*, 1534 (1956).
13. Anon., Belgian Patent 630,163 (1963).
14. W. Trabe and R. Aschar, *Chem. Ber.*, *46*, 2077 (1913).
15. J. S. H. Davies and W. Hook, British Patent 632,423 (1949).
16. M. A. Spielman, *J. Amer. Chem. Soc.*, *66*, 1244 (1944).
17. M. A. Spielman, U. S. Patent 2,575,693 (1951).
18. T. S. Gardner, E. Wenis, and J. Lee, *J. Med. Chem.*, *2*, 133 (1960).
19. E. Skita and W. Stummer, German Patent 930,328 (1955).
20. A. Pongrantz and K. L. Zirm, *Monatsh.*, *88*, 330 (1957).
21. Anon., Japanese Patent 8770 (1958).
22. Y. Sawa, *J. Pharm. Soc. Japan,* *57*, 953 (1937).
23. J. Buchi, J. Amman, R. Lieberherr, and E. Eichenberger, *Helv. Chim. Acta,* *36*, 75 (1953).
24. H. Stenzl, U. S. Patent 2,562,830 (1951).
25. R. Pfister and F. Hafliger, *Helv. Chim. Acta,* *40*, 395 (1957).
26. R. Deuss, R. Pfister, and F. Hafliger, U. S. Patent 2,910,481 (1959).
27. R. Pfister and F. Hafliger, *Helv. Chim. Acta,* *44*, 232 (1961).
28. G. C. Lancini, E. Lazari, and R. Pallanza, *Farm. Ed. Sci.,* *21*, 278 (1966).
29. G. C. Lancini and E. Lazari, *Experientia,* *21*, 83 (1965).
30. V. K. Bhagwat and F. L. Pyman, *J. Chem. Soc.,* *127*, 1832 (1928).
31. R. M. Jacob, G. L. Regnies, and C. Crisan, U. S. Patent 2,994,061 (1960).
32. R. G. Jones, E. C. Kornfeld, K. C. McLaughlin, and R. C. Anderson, *J. Amer. Chem. Soc.,* *71*, 4000 (1949).
33. A. Sohn, U. S. Patent 2,161,938 (1939).
34. M. E. Synerholm, L. H. Jules, and M. Sayhun, U. S. Patent 2,731,471 (1956).
35. A. Hueni, U. S. Patent 2,868,802 (1959).
36. W. Frushtorfer and H. Mueler-Calgan, German Patent 1,117,588 (1961).
37. K. Miescher and W. Klaver, U. S. Patent 2,449,241 (1943).
38. K. Miescher, A. Marxer, and E. Urech, U. S. Patent 2,503,509 (1950).
39. A. Berg, German Patent 1,191,381 (1963).
40. A. Pinner, *Chem. Ber.,* *21*, 2320 (1888).
41. H. R. Henze, U. S. Patent 2,409,754 (1946).
42. L. H. Jules, J. A. Faust, and M. Sayhun, U. S. Patent 2,716,648 (1955).
43. C. D. Hurd and H. L. Wehrmeister, *J. Amer. Chem. Soc.,* *71*, 4007 (1949).

44. R. M. Dodson and H. W. Turner, *J. Amer. Chem. Soc.*, *73*, 4517 (1951).
45. G. Ponzio, *Gazz. Chim. Ital.*, *62*, 859 (1932).
46. M. D. Aron-Samuel and J. J. Sterne, French Patent M2033 (1963).
47. P. C. Guha, *J. Amer. Chem. Soc.*, *44*, 1502 (1922).
48. R. O. Roblin and J. W. Clapp, *J. Amer. Chem. Soc.*, *72*, 4890 (1950).
49. J. R. Vaughan, J. A. Eichler, and G. W. Anderson, *J. Org. Chem.*, *21*, 700 (1956).
50. R. W. Young, K. H. Wood, J. A. Eichler, J. R. Vaughan, and G. W. Robinson, *J. Amer. Chem. Soc.*, *78*, 4649 (1956).

CHAPTER 14

Six-Membered Heterocycles

1. PYRIDINES

Nicotinic acid (2), the oxidation product of the coal tar chemical, β-picoline, has shown activity in man in lowering elevated cholesterol levels. This property has led to some use of this drug for the treatment of the hyperlipidemias associated with atherosclerosis. It is of interest that the drug, in addition, has a remarkable effect in alleviating the symptoms of pellagra, a vitamin B-deficiency disease. Administration of nicotinic acid is sometimes limited by the facial flushing observed on ingestion of the drug, a phenomenon associated with vasodilation. *Nicotinyl alcohol (3)*, obtained by reduction of 2 with lithium aluminum hydride, capitalizes on this effect; this drug is used as a peripheral vasodilator.

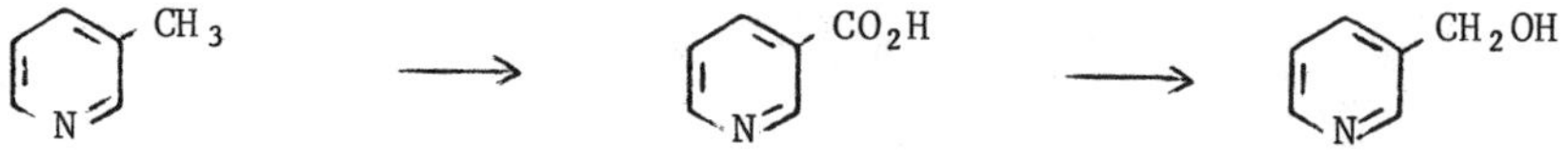

Conversion of the carboxylic acid to the diethyl amide interestingly leads to an agent that exhibits the properties of a respiratory stimulant. One synthesis of this agent starts with the preparation of the mixed anhydride of nicotinic and benzenesulfonic acid *(4)*. An exchange reaction between the anhydride and diethyl benzenesulfonamide affords *nikethemide (5)*.[1]

Although the advent of the antibiotics revolutionized the treatment of bacterial infections, tuberculosis has proven unusually resistant to chemotherapeutic attack. Although many antibiotics are effective to some extent in arresting the progress of

253

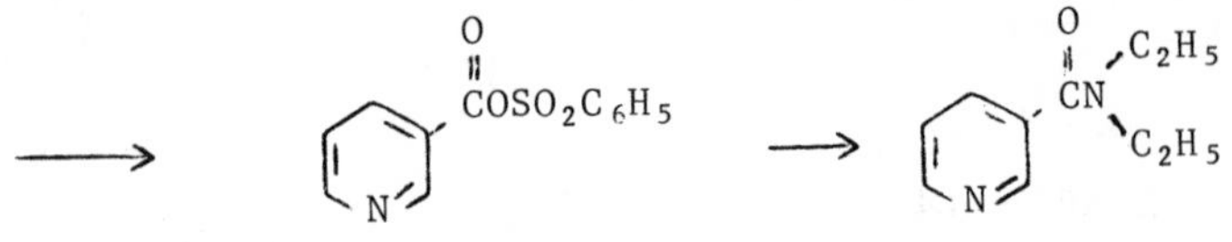

this disease, none is uniformly successful. It had been observed
that nicotinamide showed some effect on the tubercule bacillus
in vitro. A systematic investigation of related pyridine derivatives led to the discovery of one of the most successful antitubercular agents, *isoniazide (7)*. This hydrazide can be obtained
in a straightforward manner by treatment of methyl isonicotinate
(6) with hydrazine. Extensive clinical use of this agent showed
the drug to possess a wholly unanticipated antidepressant effect
in addition to its antibacterial action. This action, later
attributed to inhibition of the enzyme monoamine oxidase, led to
intensive efforts on the preparation of hydrazides in many heterocyclic series in order to obtain antidepressant agents.

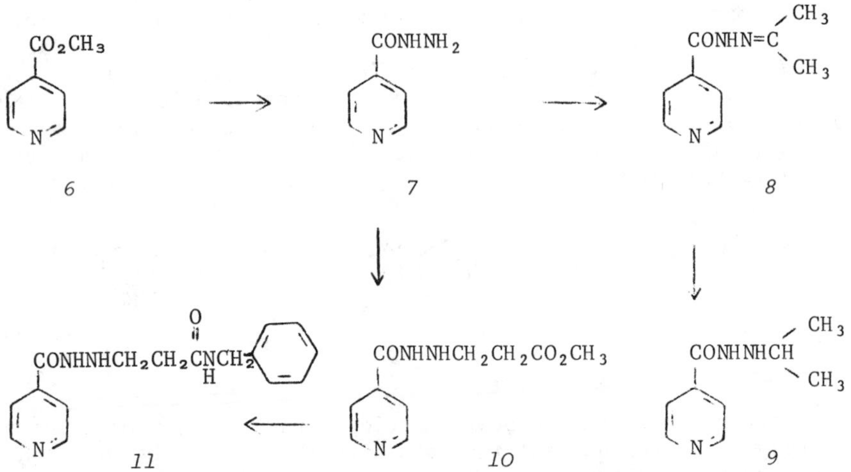

Thus, condensation of *isoniazide* with acetone at the basic
nitrogen gives the corresponding Shiff base *(8)*. Catalytic reduction affords the antidepressant, *iproniazid (9)*.[2] Addition of
the same basic nitrogen to methyl acrylate by Michael condensation leads to the β-amino ester *(10)*. This is converted to the
amide, *nialamide (11)*,[3] on heating with benzylamine.

A thioamide of isonicotinic acid has also shown tuberculo-
static activity in the clinic. The additional substitution on
the pyridine ring precludes its preparation from simple starting
materials. Reaction of ethyl methyl ketone with ethyl oxalate
leads to the ester-diketone, 12 (shown as its enol). Condensation of this with cyanoacetamide gives the substituted pyridone,
13, which contains both the ethyl and carboxyl groups in the
desired position. The nitrile group is then excised by means of
decarboxylative hydrolysis. Treatment of the pyridone (14) with
phosphorus oxychloride converts that compound (after exposure to
ethanol to take the acid chloride to the ester) to the chloro-
pyridine, 15. The halogen is then removed by catalytic reduction
(16). The ester at the 4 position is converted to the desired
functionality by successive conversion to the amide (17), dehydration to the nitrile (18), and finally addition of hydrogen sulfide. There is thus obtained *ethionamide (19)*.[4]

In an unusual variant on the Chichibabin reaction, treatment
of 3-hydroxypyridine with sodium amide at 200° affords 2,6-di-
aminopyridine (21). Coupling of the product with benzenediazo-
nium chloride gives *phenazopyridine (22)*.[5] This drug is used as
an analgesic for the urinary tract in conjunction with antibacterial agents for treatment of urinary infections.

Replacement of one of the benzene rings by pyridine in the
fenamic acid-type analgesics leads to an agent with full pharmacologic activity. Treatment of the N-oxide of nicotinic acid
with phosphorus trichloride followed by hydrolysis of the acid

chloride gives the 2-chlorinated analog *(24)*.[6] Nucleophilic aromatic substitution on the halide by *m*-trifluoromethylaniline
affords *nifluminic acid (25)*.[7]

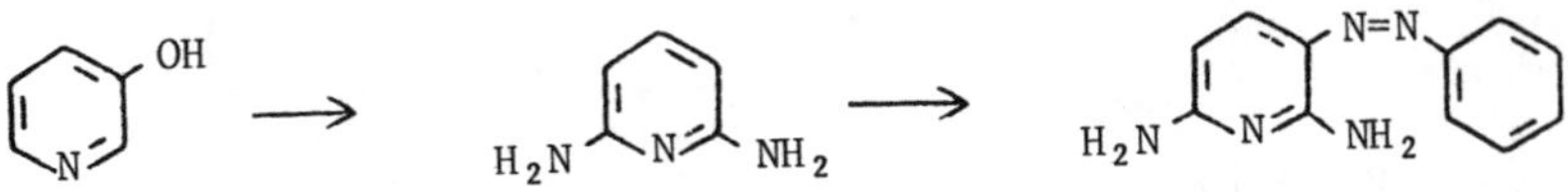

20   21   22

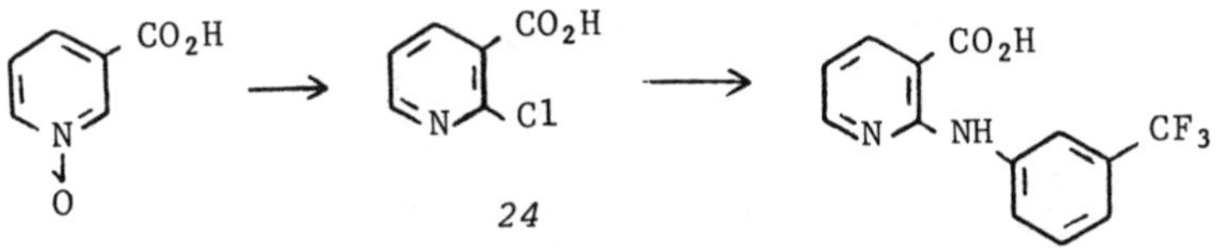

23   24

25

Vinylpyridine *(26)* exhibits many of the properties of a
Michael acceptor. Thus, this molecule will undergo conjugate
addition of methoxide ion. There is thus obtained *methyridine*
(27),[8] an antinematodal agent used in veterinary practice.

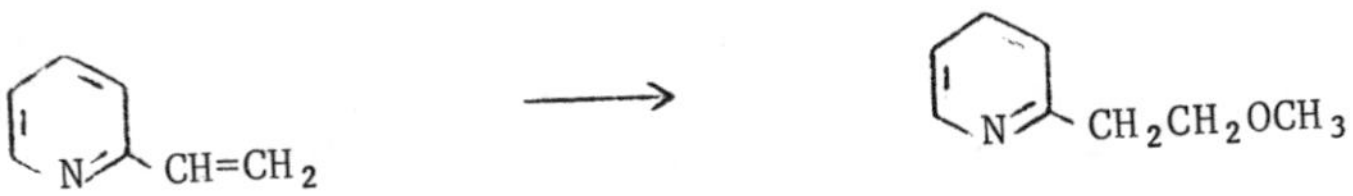

26   27

2. DERIVATIVES OF PIPERIDINE

The continuing search for molecules that possess the sedative-
hypnotic properties of the barbiturates but show a better pharmacologic ratio has, as shown above, taken many directions. To
name only two variants, the ring has been contracted and even
opened entirely; in each case some activity of the parent was
retained. Although at one time the acylurea functional array was
thought necessary for activity, the work below shows that even

this requirement is not ironclad. This lack of structural specificity is in many ways reminiscent of the wide structural latitude that has proven compatible with antihistaminic activity.
     Conjugate addition of the carbanion from 2-phenylbutyroni-
trile *(28)* to methyl acrylate gives the condensation product *29*.
Saponification affords the corresponding acid *(30)*. Further
hydrolysis of the product in acetic acid affords the glutarimide
(the formal product of cyclization of the amide with the acid),
glutethemide (31).[9] Nitration of the butyronitrile gives the *p*-
derivative *(32)*. This, when subjected to the same series of
transformation as *28*, gives the glutarimide, *33*. Catalytic reduction of the nitro group affords *aminoglutethemide (34)*.[10] Both
these agents have found use as sedative-hypnotic agents.

the glutarimide best known to the lay public, *thalidomide*

     Attachment of a basic amino group to the side chain leads to
a compound with antiparkinsonian activity. Alkylation of the
carbanion from phenylacetonitrile with 2-chlorotriethylamine
affords the product, *36*. Conjugate addition of the anion from
this to acrylonitrile gives the glutarodinitrile *(37)*. Partial
hydrolysis of this in a mixture of sulfuric and acetic acid leads
to *phenglutarimide (38)*.[11]
     The glutarimide best known to the lay public, *thalidomide*
(40), owes its reputation not to efficacy, but to the wholly
unanticipated and tragic teratogenic effects elicited by this compound. It might be noted that the very efficacy and lack of the
usual barbiturate side effects shown by this drug led to its prescription as a hypnotic for expectant mothers. Condensation of
the phthalimide of glutamic acid *(39)* with ammonia at elevated

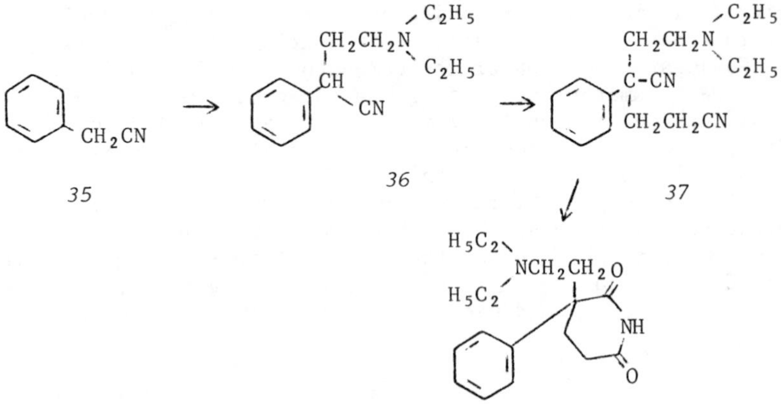

35   36   37

38

temperature leads directly to *thalidomide* (40).[12]

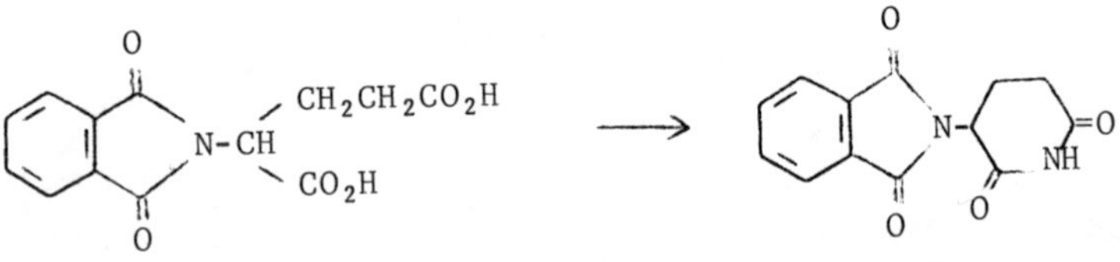

39   40

Displacement of the geminal substitution to the 4-position of the glutarimide ring interestingly leads to a drug that antagonizes the effects of the barbiturates. As such, the agent is used in the treatment of barbiturate intoxication. The original synthesis involves first the condensation of ethyl methyl ketone with two equivalents cyanoacetamide. The product can be rationalized by assuming first an aldol condensation of the ketone and active methylene compound followed by dehydration to give 41. Conjugate addition of a second molecule of cyanoacetamide would afford 42. Addition of one of the amide amines to the nitrile would then afford the iminonitrile (43). The observed product (44) can be rationalized by assuming the loss of the carboxamide group under strongly basic conditions. Decarboxylative hydrolysis of 44 leads to *bemigride* (45).[13]

The wide structural latitude permitted for hypnotic activity is made particularly clear by the observation that the two carbonyl groups in the piperidine ring need not be disposed to form a glutarimide. *Methyprylon (51)*, an effective sedative-hypnotic, actually contains isolated lactam and ketone functions. Formylation of ethyl diethylacetoacetate *(46)* by means of ethyl formate and strong base affords the derivative, *47*. Reaction of this intermediate with ammonia gives the corresponding enamine *(48)*; this cyclizes to the unsaturated lactam on heating *(49)*. Reaction of *49* with formaldehyde in the presence of sodium sulfite proceeds at the activated position α to the ketone carbonyl. Catalytic reduction of the product *(50)* results first in hydrogenolysis of the allyl alcohol; reduction of the olefinic double bond gives *methyprylon (51)*.[14]

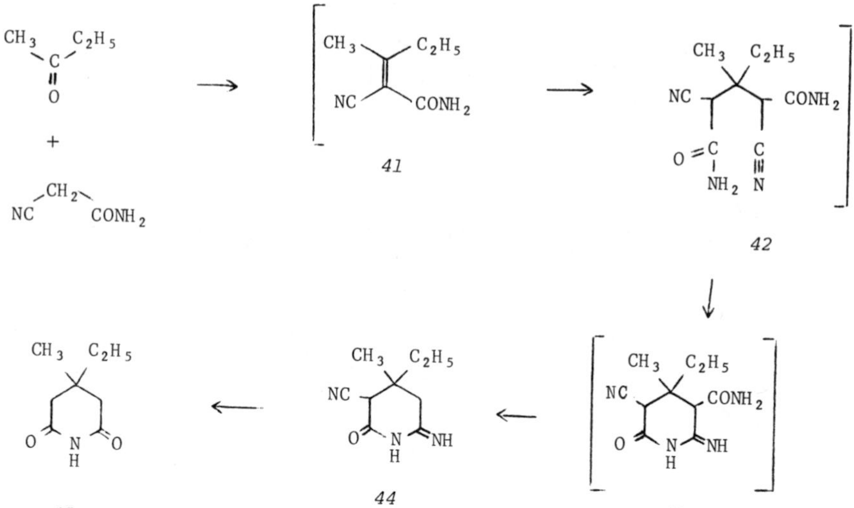

The association of a specific pharmacologic activity with certain functionality was remarked on earlier. The guanidino group, for example, often yields compounds that show hypotensive activity because of peripheral sympathetic blockade (see, for example, *bethanidine*). Attachment of a piperidine group to the side chain proves compatible with retention of this activity.

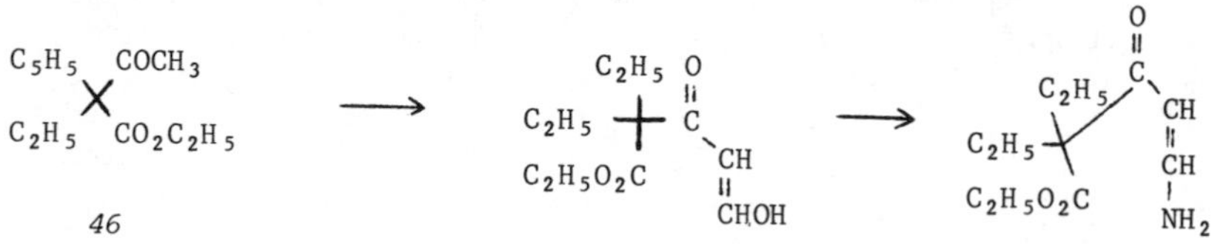

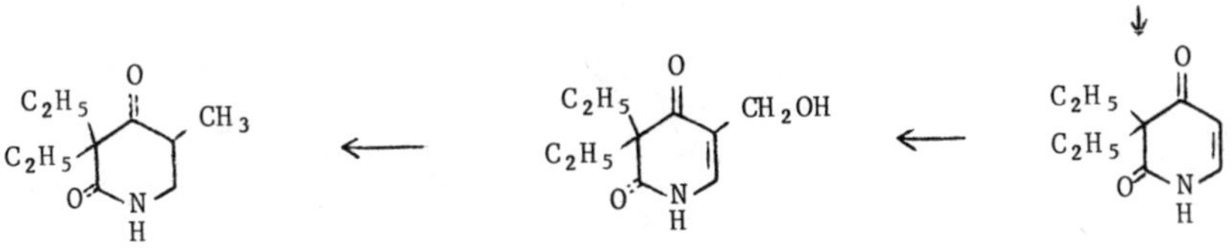

51   50   49

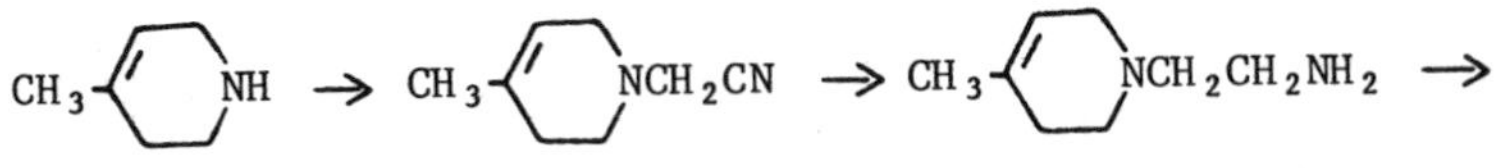

52   53   54

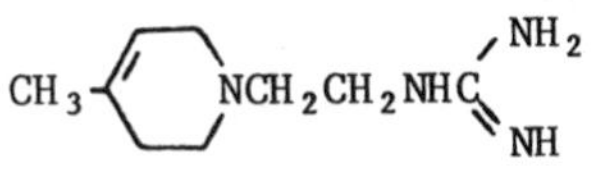

55

Alkylation of the tetrahydropyridine, 52 (obtained by reaction of
a suitable protected derivative of 4-piperidone followed by dehydration and deprotection), with chloroacetonitrile affords 53.
Reduction of the cyano group gives the diamine (54). Reaction of
this intermediate with the S-methyl ether of thiourea affords
guancycline (55).[15]

3. MORPHOLINES

Although the morpholine ring is often used as a modified version
of a tertiary nitrogen, the ring system finds only rare use as a
nucleus for medicinal agents. Both compounds below, in fact, may
be regarded as more properly related to cyclized forms of hydroxy-
phenethylamines.
    Acylation of *norephedrine (56)* with the acid chloride from
benzoylglycolic acid leads to the amide *(57)*. Reduction with
lithium aluminum hydride serves both to reduce the amide to the
amine and to remove the protecting group by reduction *(58)*.
Cyclization by means of sulfuric acid (probably via the benzylic
carbonium ion) affords *phenmetrazine (59)*.[16] In a related process, alkylation of ephedrine itself *(60)* with ethylene oxide
gives the diol, *61*. (The secondary nature of the amine in *60*
eliminates the complication of dialkylation and thus the need to
go through the amide.) Cyclization as above affords *phendimetrazine (62)*.[17] Both these agents show activity related to the
parent acyclic molecule; that is, the agents are CNS stimulants

and as such are used as appetite suppressants. It has been demonstrated, incidentally, that the phenyl and methyl ring substituents both occupy the equatorial positions, leading to the formulation of these compounds as the trans isomers.[18]

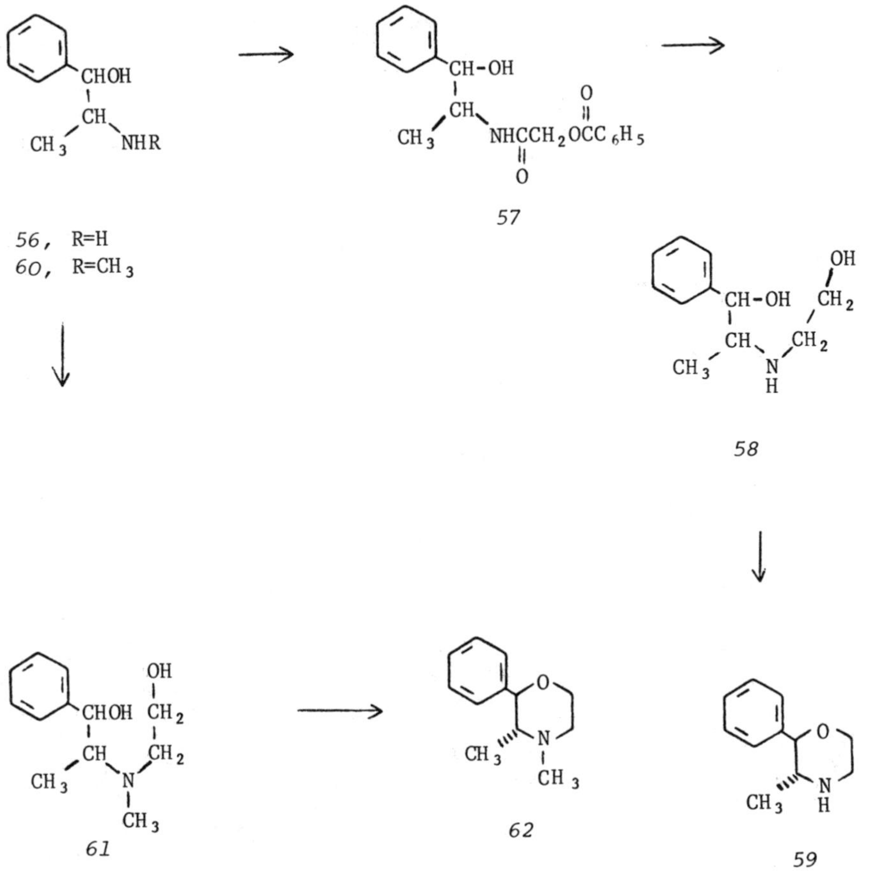

56, R=H
60, R=CH$_3$

57

58

61

62

59

4. PYRIMIDINES

The finding that 2,4-diaminopyrimidines inhibit the growth of microorganisms by interfering with their utilization of folic acid led to an intensive search for antiinfective agents in this class of heterocyclic compounds. This work led to the development of at least two successful antimalarial agents. Condensation of phenylacetonitrile with ethyl propionate in the presence of sodium ethoxide gives the cyanoketone (63). Treatment with diazomethane affords the methyl enol ether of that compound (64). Condensation with guanidine affords *pyrimethamine* (65).[19] (The reaction may well involve reaction of an amino group at the enol ether by an addition-elimination scheme followed by addition of the remaining amino group on guanidine to the nitrile.)

63   64

65

Bishomologation of benzaldehyde, 66 (for example, by reduction to the alcohol, conversion to the halide, and then malonic ester synthesis), affords the hydrocinamic acid, 67. Formylation with ethyl formate and base gives the hydroxymethylene derivative, 68. Condensation of that intermediate with guanidine gives the pyrimidine, 69, by a scheme similar to that above. The hydroxyl group is then converted to the amine by successive treatment with phosphorus oxychloride (70) and ammonia. There is thus obtained the antimalarial agent, *trimethoprim* (71). A shorter route to the same agent consists in first condensing the benzaldehyde with 3-ethoxypropionitrile to afford the cinamonitrile (72). Reaction with guanidine gives 71 directly.[20] The reaction probably involves displacement of the allylic ethoxy group in 72 by guanidine followed by addition to the nitrile; the double bond then shifts into the pyrimidine ring.

A change in the substitution pattern on the pyrimidine ring as well as conversion of one of the ring nitrogen atoms to its N-oxide affords an agent with markedly altered biologic activity. This drug, *minoxidil* (74), is an extremely effective hypotensive agent acting by means of vasodilitation. (It is of interest that

66 67 68 72 71 69, X=OH 70, X=Cl

the agent was actually discovered by way of the desoxy analog; although this compound shows some hypotensive activity in its own right, biochemical work revealed the fact that this undergoes *N*-oxide formation in vivo to afford *74*.) Condensation of ethyl cyanoacetate with guanidine in the presence of sodium ethoxide affords the starting pyrimidine *(71)*. Reaction with phosphorus oxychloride then serves to replace the hydroxyl group by chlorine *(72)*. Treatment of that intermediate with *meta*chloroperbenzoic acid results in specific oxidation of the nitrogen at the 1 position *(73)*. Displacement of the halogen with piperidine affords *minoxidil (74)*.[21]

71 72 74 73

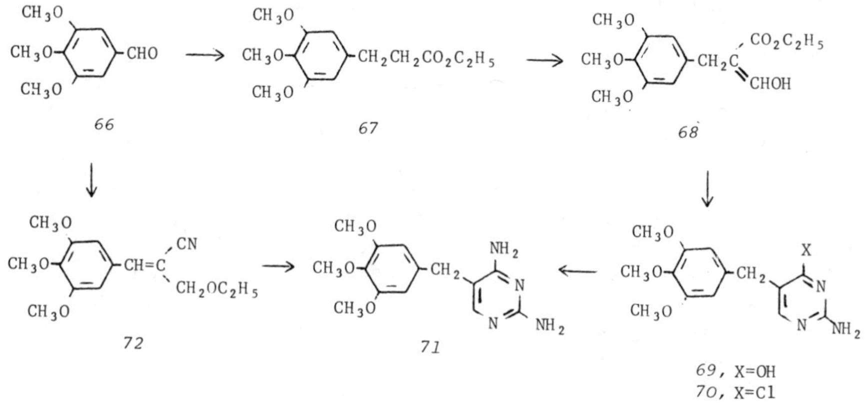

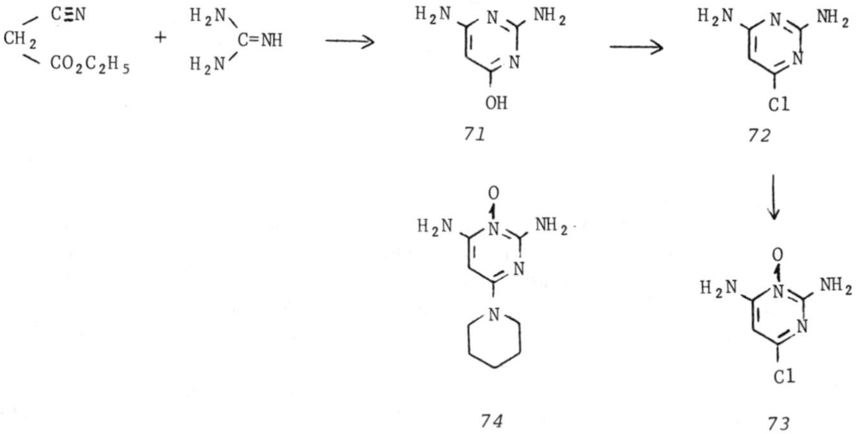

Coccidia are protozoans that can wreak havoc in a flock of poultry by the infection known as coccidiosis. Agents that control this disease—coccidiostats—are in view of the world's heavy dependence on poultry as a source of protein, of great economic significance. One of the more important drugs for treatment of this disease incorporates the pyrimidine nucleus. Condensation of ethoxymethylenemalononitrile with acetamidine affords the substituted pyrimidine, 75. This reaction may well involve conjugate addition of the amidine nitrogen to the malononitrile followed by loss of ethoxide; addition of the remaining amidine nitrogen to one of the nitriles will then lead to the pyrimidine. Reduction of the nitrile gives the corresponding aminomethyl compound (76). Exhaustive methylation of the amine (77) followed by displacement of the activated quaternary nitrogen by bromide ion affords the key intermediate (78).[22] Displacement of the halogen by α-picoline gives amprolium (79).[23]

Although the antithyroid activity of compounds incorporating an enolizable thioamide function was discussed earlier, this activity was in fact first found in the pyrimidine series. The simplest compound to show this activity, methylthiouracil (80) (shown in both enol and keto forms), is prepared quite simply by condensation of ethyl acetoacetate with thiourea.[24] Further work in this series shows that better activity was obtained by incorporation of a lipophilic side chain. Preparation of the required dicarbonyl compound starts with acylation of the magnesium enolate of the unsymmetrically esterified malonate, 81, with butyryl chlo-

ride. Treatment of the product (82) with mild acid leads to loss
of the tertiary butyl ester as isobutylene. The resulting acid
quickly decarboxylates to afford 83. Condensation of that product with thiourea affords propylthiouracil (84),[25] sometimes
known simply as PTU.

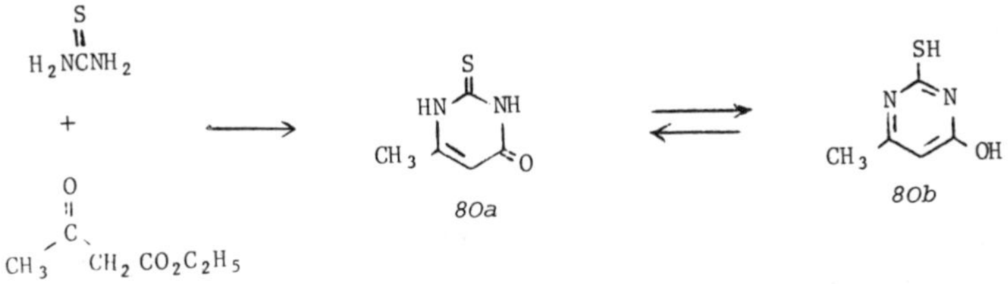

Inclusion of iodine in the thiouracyl molecule similarly
proves compatible with antithyroid activity. Alkylation of thiouracyl proper (85) with benzyl chloride affords the thioether,
86. Treatment of this with elemental iodine affords the nuclearly
substituted iodo derivative (87). Removal of the benzyl ether by
reduction leads to iodothiouracil (88).[26]

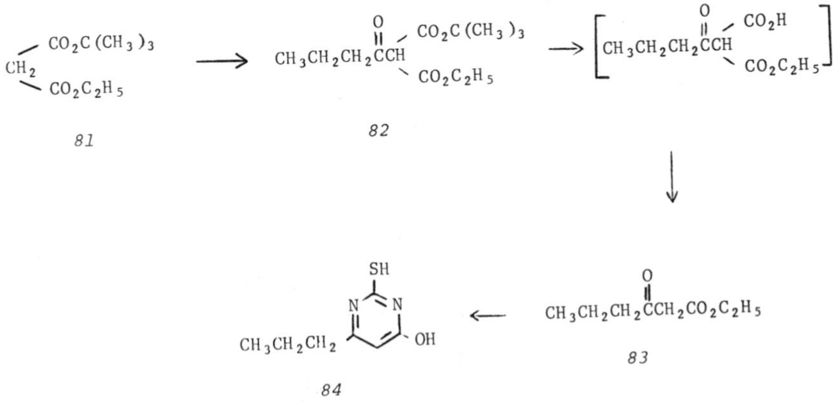

Alkyl uracyls have been known for some time to act as diuretic agents in experimental animals. The toxicity of these
agents precluded their use in the clinic. Appropriate modification of the molecule did, however, yield diuretic agents with
application in man. Reaction of allylamine with ethyl isocyanate
affords the urea, 89 (the same product can of course be obtained
from the same reagents with reversed functionality). Condensation with ethyl cyanoacetate affords aminotetradine (90).[27] In

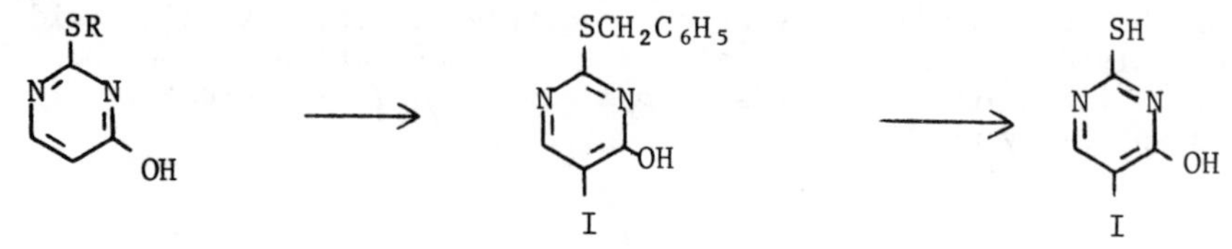

85, R=H
86, R=CH$_2$C$_6$H$_5$

87   88

much the same vein, *amisotetradine (91)*[27] is obtained by cyclization of the urea obtained from methallylamine and methylisocyanate
The latter agent has largely replaced *90* in the clinic because of
a lower incidence of side effects.

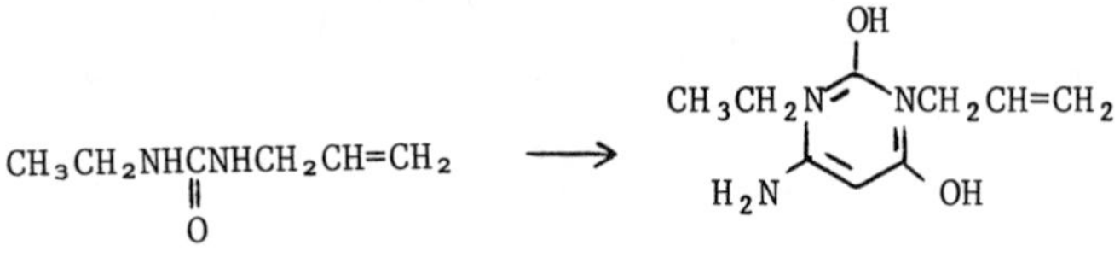

CH$_3$CH$_2$NHCNHCH$_2$CH=CH$_2$
                    ‖
                    O

89   90

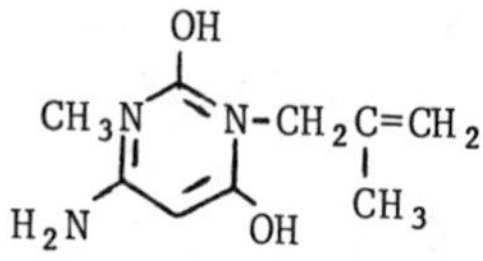

91

Although many medicinal agents incorporate the imidazoline
ring, the homologous tetrahydropyrimidine moiety has found little
use in medicinal chemistry. The exception is a pair of closely
related antihelmintic agents used in veterinary practice.
Knoevenagel-type condensation of thiophene-2-carboxaldehyde with
cyanoacetic acid gives the corresponding unsaturated nitrile *(92)*.
This is then methanolyzed in the presence of strong acid to afford
the imino-ether, *93*. Condensation with *N*-methylpropylene-1,3-
diamine proceeds probably by addition-elimination of each amino
group in turn with the imino ether. There is thus obtained *pyrantel (92)*.[28] The analog, *morantel (94)*,[29] is obtained by the same
sequence using 3-methylthiophene-2-carboxaldehyde.

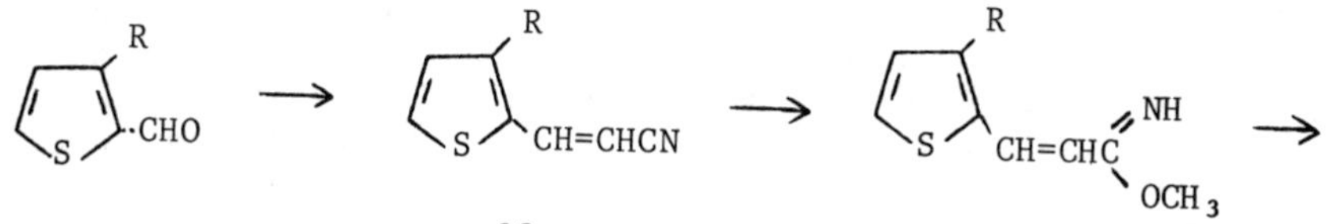

92 93

R=H, CH$_3$

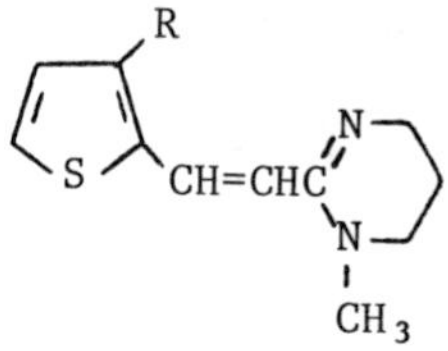

94, R=H
95, R=CH$_3$

5. BARBITURIC ACID DERIVATIVES

Derivatives of barbituric acid constitute one of the more venerable families of medicinal agents; the first member of the series,
barbital (96), has been in continuous use since 1903. This class
of sedative hypnotics is also one of the most widely used, and
it should be added, abused series of drugs. Although the
agents are generally quite effective in inducing sedation and
sleep, all barbiturates share, to a greater or lesser degree, a
similar set of disadvantages. To begin with, barbiturates tend
to have a relatively low pharmacologic ratio; news reports of
suicide by means of barbiturates are not at all uncommon. Sustained use of barbiturates is known to lead to addiction in certain individuals. Finally, use of barbiturates as sleeping
agents frequently leads to the so-called hangover on awakening.
Unlike the more traditional hangover from alcohol, this syndrome
often consists of a dulling of awareness for a considerable time.
The large number of these analogs available for purchase attests
to the great effort that has gone into attempts to circumvent the
limitations of this series of drugs.
     The final step in the synthesis of all barbiturates consists
in either condensation of a suitably substituted malonic or cyanoacetic ester with urea by means of sodium ethoxide (scheme a) or

analogous condensation of such an ester with guanidine followed
by hydrolysis of the imine thus produced (scheme b). The chemistry of this class of agents devolves on the preparation of the
required disubstituted esters. The reader will recognize that
methods for the preparation of the bulk of the intermediates are
fairly obvious. The synthesis of the majority of these drugs is
therefore not considered in detail; the products are listed in
Table 1 below. The preparations of some of the less-obvious
malonic esters are, however, found below.

Table 1. Derivatives of Barbituric Acid

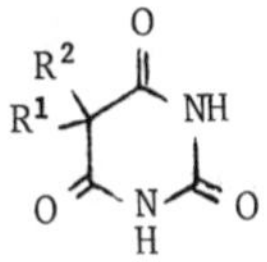

No.	Generic Name	R^1	R^2	Duration of Action
96	barbital	CH_2CH_3	CH_2CH_3	L[a]
97	butethal	CH_2CH_3	$-(CH_2)_3CH_3$	I[b]
98	hexethal	CH_2CH_3	$-(CH_2)_5CH_3$	S[c]
99	probarbital	CH_2CH_3	$CH\langle^{CH_3}_{CH_3}$	I
100	butabarbital	CH_2CH_3	$-\overset{CH_3}{\underset{}{C}}HCH_2CH_3$	I
101	pentobarbital	CH_2CH_3	$-\overset{CH_3}{\underset{}{C}}HCH_2CH_2CH_3$	S
102	amobarbital	CH_2CH_3	$CH_2CH_2CH\langle^{CH_3}_{CH_3}$	I
103	phenobarbital	$-CH_2CH_3$	C_6H_5	L
104	aprobarbital	$CH_2CH=CH_2$	$CH\langle^{CH_3}_{CH_3}$	I
105	butalbital	$CH_2CH=CH_2$	$CH_2CH\langle^{CH_3}_{CH_3}$	I

Table 1, continued

105	secobarbital	$CH_2CH=CH_2$	$\overset{CH_3}{\overset{\mid}{C}HCH_2CH_2CH_3}$	S
106	allobarbital	$CH_2CH=CH_2$	$CH_2CH=CH_2$	I
107	cyclopal	$CH_2CH=CH_2$	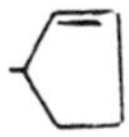	S
108	butylallonal	$-CH_2CH=CH_2$	$\underset{Br}{CH_2C=CH_2}$	I
109	methohexital	$CH_2CH=CH_2$	$\underset{CH_3}{-CHC\equiv CCH_2CH_3}$	L
110	butylvinal	$-CH=CH_2$	$\underset{CH_3}{CHCH_2CH_3}$	L
111	vinbarbital	$\underset{CH_3}{-C=CHCH_2CH_3}$	CH_2CH_3	S
112	cyclobarbital	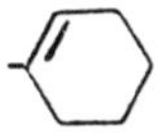	CH_2CH_3	S
113	heptabarbital	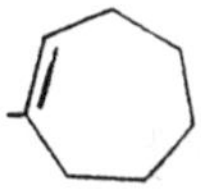	CH_2CH_3	S
114	carbubarbital	$-(CH_2)_3CH_3$	$\overset{O}{CH_2CH_2O\overset{\parallel}{C}NH_2}$	L

[a] Long acting (more than 6 hr). [b] Intermediate (3-6 hr).
[c] Short acting (less than 3 hr).

At least one of the protons on the nitrogens flanked by the two carbonyl groups is in fact quite acidic; many of the barbiturates are actually used as their sodium salts, particularly when these drugs are formulated for use by injection. The reader is referred to more specialized texts for this specific information. The duration of action of a barbiturate following administration has an important bearing on its clinical use. The long-acting compounds tend to be used as sleeping pills, while the short-acting drugs are used in surgery in conjunction with an inhalation anesthetic.

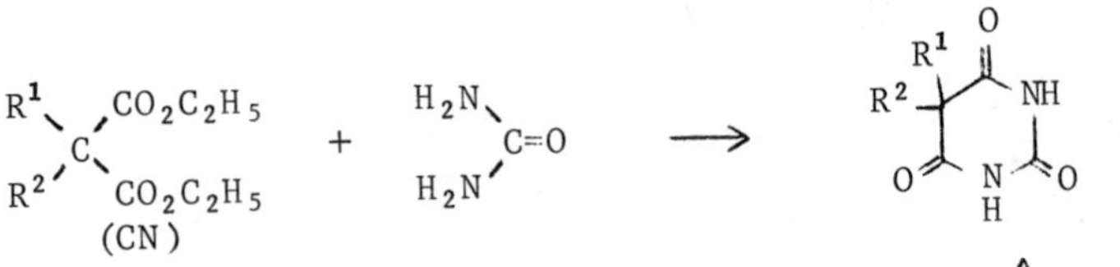

scheme a

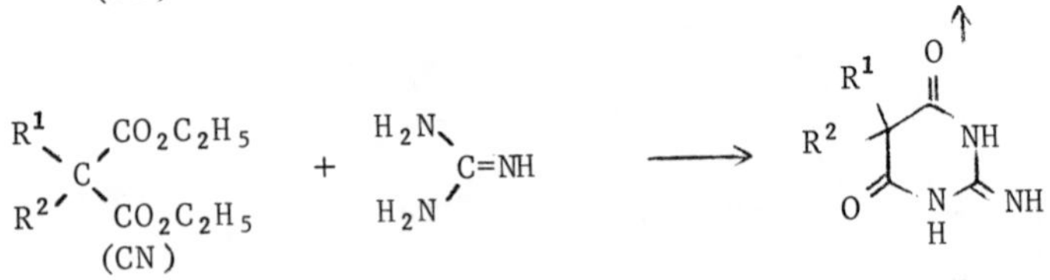

scheme b

The malonic ester required for synthesis of *cyclopal (107)*[29] can be obtained by alkylation of diethyl allylmalonate *(115)* with 1,2-dibromocyclopentane in the presence of excess base. It is probable that the reaction proceeds by elimination of hydrogen bromide from the dihalide as the first step. The resulting allilic halide *(116)* would be the most reactive electrophile in the reaction mixture and thus would quickly alkylate the anion of the malonate to afford *117*.

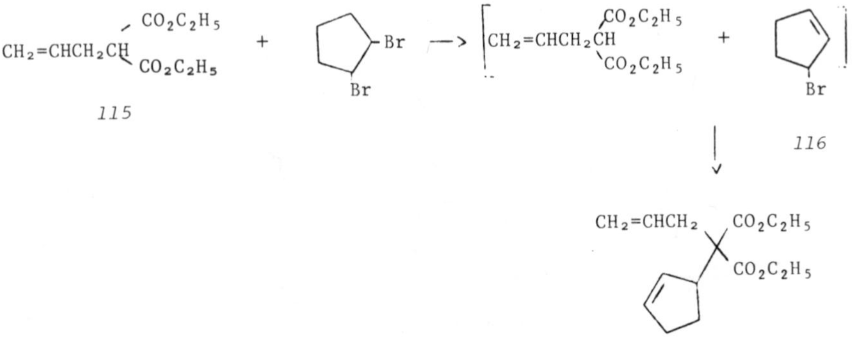

Condensation of the organometallic reagent obtained by reaction of 1-butyne and ethylmagnesium bromide with acetaldehyde affords the carbinol, *118*. Treatment with phosphorus tribromide gives the corresponding propargyl halide *(119)*. Alkylation of diethyl malonate with this reagent, followed then by alkylation with allyl bromide, gives the starting material *(120)* for *metho-*

hexital (109).[30]

$$CH_3CH_2C\equiv CMgBr \quad + \quad \underset{H}{O=CCH_3} \quad \longrightarrow \quad \underset{X}{CH_3CH_2C\equiv CCHCH_3} \quad \longrightarrow$$

118, X=OH
119, X=Br

$$\underset{CH_3-C\equiv C-CH}{\overset{CH_3CH=CH_2}{\diagdown}} \underset{\underset{CH_3}{|}}{\overset{CO_2C_2H_5}{\diagup}} CO_2C_2H_5$$

120

Treatment of an ethylidene malonic ester such as (a) with strong bases results in loss of a proton from the allylic position to produce the ambient ion (b). Alkylation of such carbanions usually occurs at the carbon bearing the carbonyl groups, resulting in the establishment of a quaternary center and deconjugation of the double bond (c).

$$\underset{a}{\overset{\diagdown}{\underset{\diagup}{CH_2}}\underset{\diagup}{\overset{\diagdown}{C=C}}\underset{CO_2R}{\overset{CO_2R}{\diagup}}} \quad \longrightarrow \quad \underset{b}{\overset{\diagdown}{C}\overset{-}{\underset{\diagup}{C}}\overset{\diagdown}{C=C}\underset{CO_2R}{\overset{CO_2R}{\diagup}}} \quad \longrightarrow \quad \underset{c}{\overset{\diagdown}{C}\overset{CO_2R}{\underset{R^1}{\overset{|}{\underset{|}{C-C-COR}}}}}$$

An early application of this reaction to the preparation of barbiturates starts by the condensation of the ketone, *121*, with ethyl cyanoacetate by Knoevenagel condensation. Alkylation of the product *(122)* with ethyl bromide by means of sodium ethoxide affords *123*. Condensation of this intermediate with guanidine in the presence of sodium ethoxide gives the diimino analog of a barbiturate *(124)*. Hydrolysis affords *vinbarbital (111).*[31,32]

Application of this scheme to condensation products of cyclo-alkanones affords the cycloalkenyl-substituted barbiturates. Thus, the condensation product of cyclohexanone and ethyl cyano-acetate *(125)* affords the intermediate *(126)* for the synthesis of *cyclobarbital (112)*[33] on alkylation with ethyl bromide. The condensation product of cycloheptanone *(127)* affords the starting

$$CH_3 \atop C_2H_5CH_2 \!\! >\!\!=\!\!O \qquad \longrightarrow \qquad CH_3 \diagdown\diagup CN \atop C_2H_5CH_2 \diagup\diagdown CO_2C_2H_5 \qquad \longrightarrow$$

121   122

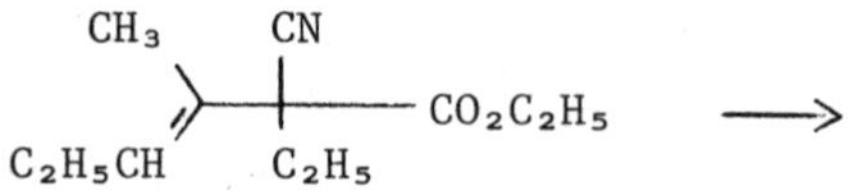

$$CH_3 \quad CN \atop C_2H_5CH \diagdown\!\!>\!\!\! = \!\!\!\mid \!\!\!\!- CO_2C_2H_5 \atop C_2H_5 \qquad \longrightarrow$$

123

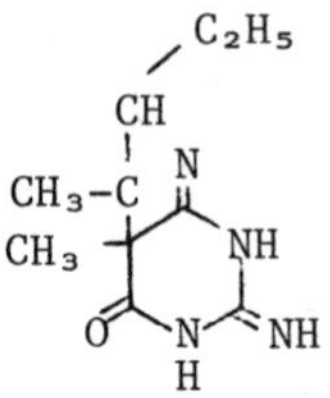

124

material (128) for *heptabarbital* (113).[34]

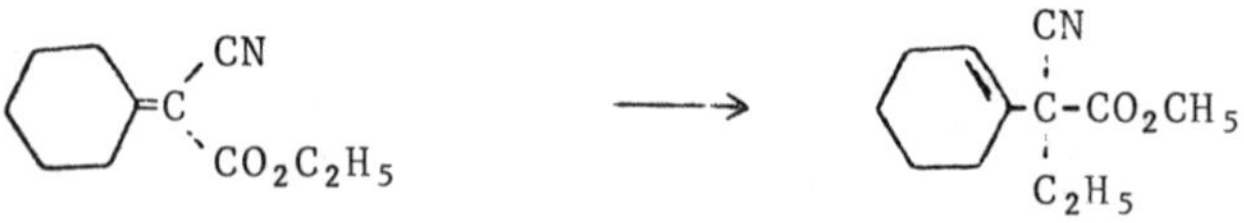

125   126

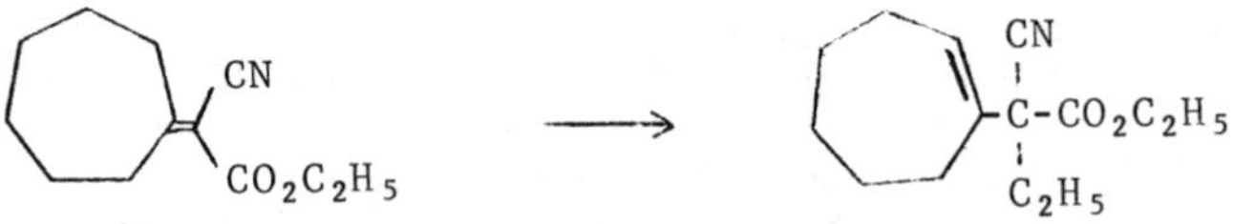

127   128

The parent compound in this series, that is, the agent substituted by a vinyl group, is obtained by direct vinylation.
Reaction of the monosubstituted barbiturate, 129, with ethylene
at elevated temperature and pressure in the presence of a zinc
catalyst affords *butylvinal* (110).[35]

Alkylation of the anion from diethyl butylmalonate with

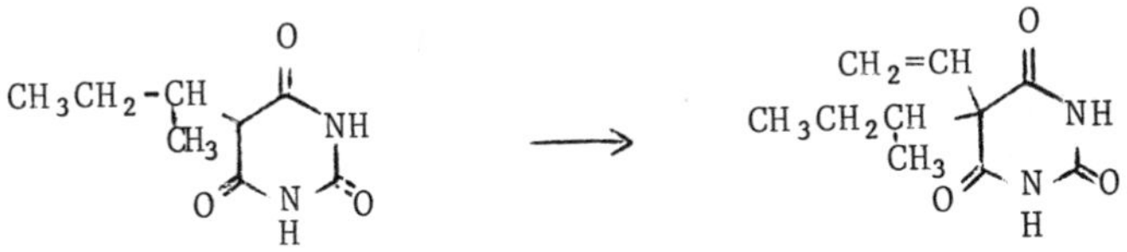

129 → 130

with ethylene oxide affords the malonate containing an hydroxyethyl side chain (131). This is then converted to the barbiturate (132) in the usual way. Treatment of the product (132)
first with phosgene and then ammonia affords the carbamate *carbubarbital* (114).[36]

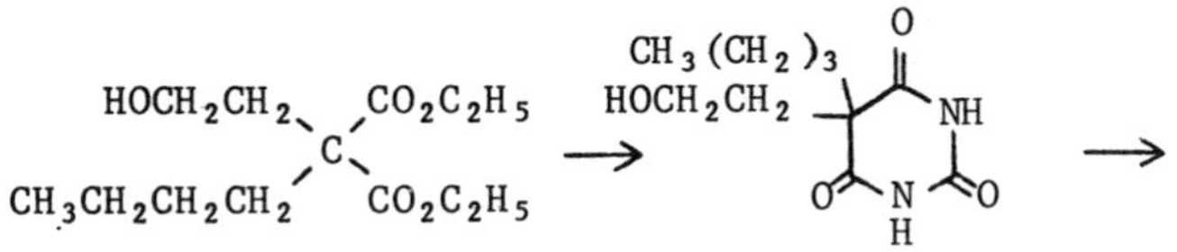

131   132

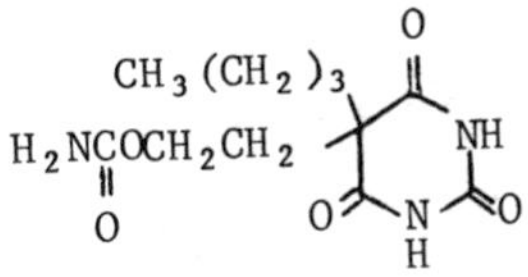

114

Condensation of disubstituted malonic ester with N-methyl
urea yields the corresponding barbituric acids bearing a methyl
group on nitrogen. (The plane of symmetry that bisects these
molecules, of course, makes both nitrogens identical.) Carbethoxylation of ethylphenylacetate (sodium hydride and ethyl chloroformate) affords diethyl phenylmalonate (133). Alkylation with
ethyl bromide gives 134. Condensation of this with N-methyl urea
in the presence of base gives *mephobarbital* (135).[37] In much the
same way, reaction of the ester, 136, with N-methyl urea affords
hexobarbital (137).[38]
    In an interesting variation on this theme, the bis acid chlo-
ride of diethylmalonate (138) is condensed with the O-methyl ether
of urea to afford the imino ether of the barbituric acid (139).
Heating this ether at 200°C results in O to N migration of the
methyl group and formation of *metharbital* (140).[39]

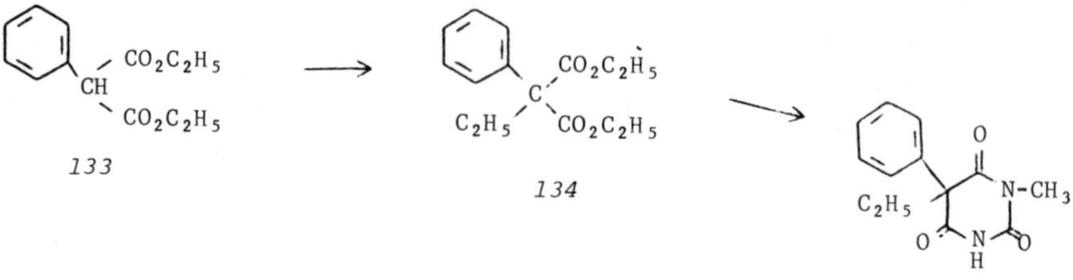

133 → 134 → 135

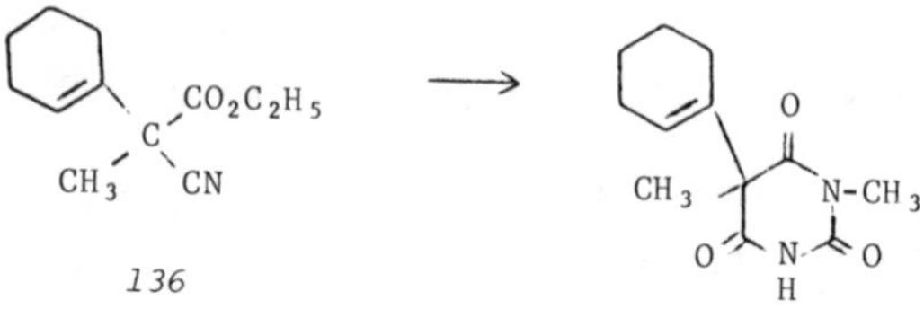

136 → 137

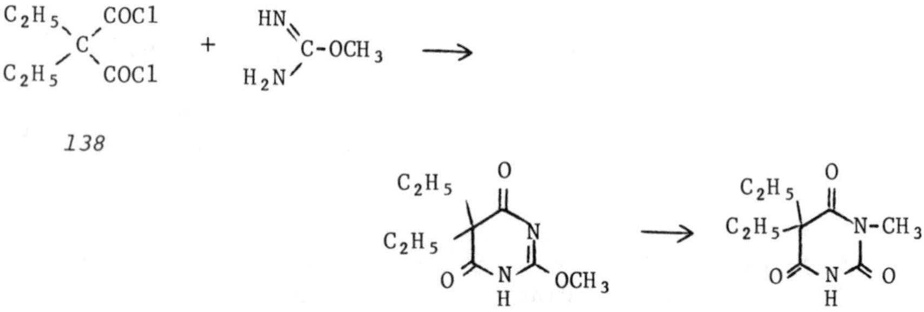

138

139 → 140

Replacement of the oxygen on the carbonyl group at the 2 position by sulfur affords a series of sedative-hypnotic agents that tend to show both faster onset and shorter duration of action than their oxygenated counterparts. These compounds are obtained in a manner quite analogous to the oxygenated analogs, that is, by condensation of the appropriate malonic ester with thiourea in the presence of a strong base. Thus, reaction of 141 with thiourea gives thiopental (142).[40] (The sodium salt of the latter is sometimes known as sodium pentothal, the "truth serum" known to all lovers of whodunits.) In a similar vein, 143 affords thiamylal *(144)*,[40] and the ester, *145*, leads to *thialbarbital (146)*.[41] It is of note that although the drug can be prepared by the above route, reaction of *barbital (96)* with phosphorus pentasulfide constitutes an alternate route to *thiobarbital (147)*.[42]

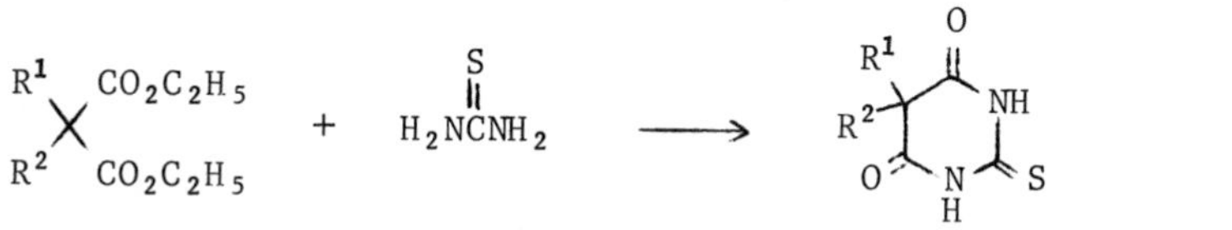

141, $R^1 = C_2H_5$
$R^2 = $ CHCH$_2$CH$_2$CH$_3$
       |
       CH$_3$

142, $R^1 = C_2H_5$
$R^2 = $ CHCH$_2$CH$_2$CH$_3$
       |
       CH$_3$

143, $R^1 = CH_2CH=CH_2$
$R^2 = $ CHCH$_2$CH$_2$CH$_3$
       |
       CH$_3$

144, $R^1 = CH_2CH=CH_2$
$R^2 = $ CHCH$_2$CH$_2$CH$_3$
       |
       CH$_3$

145, $R^1 = CH_2CH=CH_2$
$R^2 = $

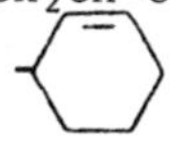

146, $R^1 = CH_2CH=CH_2$
$R^2 = $

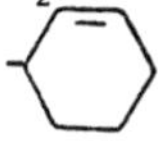

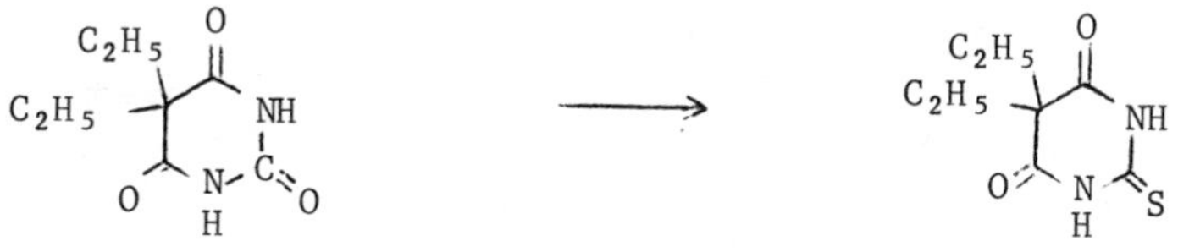

96

147

A somewhat more complex side chain is incorporated by alkylation of the carbanion of the substituted cyanoacetate, *148*, with 2-chloroethylmethyl sulfide. Condensation of the resulting cyanoester *(149)* with thiourea followed by hydrolysis of the resulting imine *(150)* affords *methitural (151)*.[42]

Cyclization of the two pendant alkyl side chains on barbiturates to form a spiran is consistent with sedative-hypnotic activity. The synthesis of this most complex barbiturate starts by alkylation of ethyl acetoacetate with 2-chloropentan-3-one to give *152*. Hydrolysis and decarboxylation under acidic conditions gives the diketone, *153*.[43] This intermediate is then reduced to the diol *(154)*, and that is converted to the dibromide *(155)* by means of hydrogen bromide. Double internal alkylation of ethyl

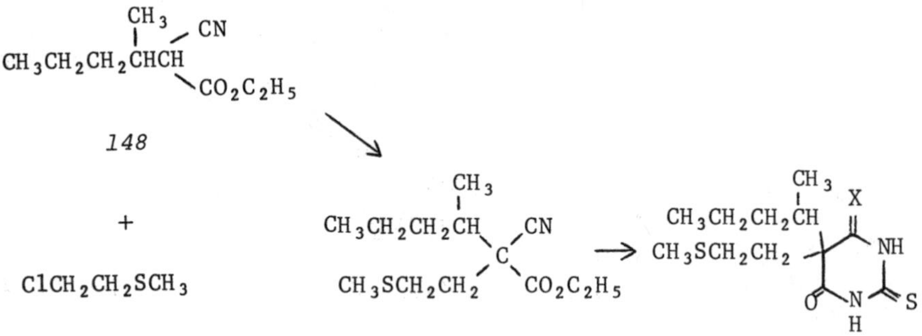

CH₃ and CN on CH₃CH₂CH₂CHCH with CO₂C₂H₅:

$$CH_3CH_2CH_2\overset{\overset{\displaystyle CH_3}{|}}{CH}CH\overset{\diagdown CN}{\diagup}_{CO_2C_2H_5}$$

148

+

$ClCH_2CH_2SCH_3$

$\longrightarrow$

$$CH_3CH_2CH_2\overset{\overset{\displaystyle CH_3}{|}}{CH}\underset{CH_3SCH_2CH_2}{\diagup}C\overset{\diagup CN}{\diagdown}_{CO_2C_2H_5}$$

149

$\longrightarrow$

$$\begin{array}{c}CH_3\\ CH_3CH_2CH_2\overset{|}{CH}\\ CH_3SCH_2CH_2\end{array}\overset{X}{\underset{O}{\diagup}}\underset{\overset{N}{H}}{\diagup}\overset{NH}{\diagdown}_S$$

150, X=NH
151, X=O

malonate with *155* affords the substituted cyclopentane, *156*, of unspecified stereochemistry. Reaction of the ester with thiourea in the presence of strong base gives *spirothiobarbital (157)*.[44]

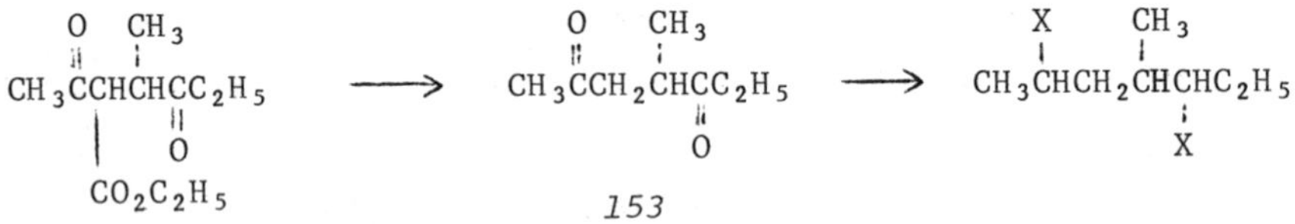

$$\begin{array}{c}O\quad CH_3\\ \overset{\|}{CH_3}\overset{\,}{C}CHCHCC_2H_5\\ \overset{\|}{\underset{|}{O}}\\ CO_2C_2H_5\end{array}$$

152

$\longrightarrow$

$$\begin{array}{c}O\quad CH_3\\ \overset{\|}{CH_3}\overset{\,}{C}CH_2CHCC_2H_5\\ \overset{\|}{O}\end{array}$$

153

$\longrightarrow$

$$\begin{array}{c}X\quad CH_3\\ CH_3\overset{|}{CH}CH_2\overset{|}{CH}CHC_2H_5\\ \overset{\,}{X}\end{array}$$

154, X=OH
155, X=Br

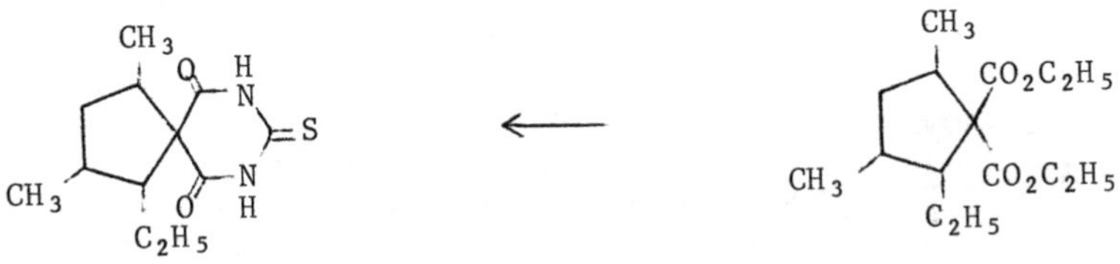

157

$\longleftarrow$

156

The close structural resemblance between the sedative-hypnotic and anticonvulsant agents was mentioned earlier. It is interesting that the two activities can be related in at least one case by a simple chemical transformation. Thus, reductive desulfurization of the thiobarbituric acid, *158*, affords *primi-*

done (159),[45] a drug used in the treatment of grand mal epilepsy.

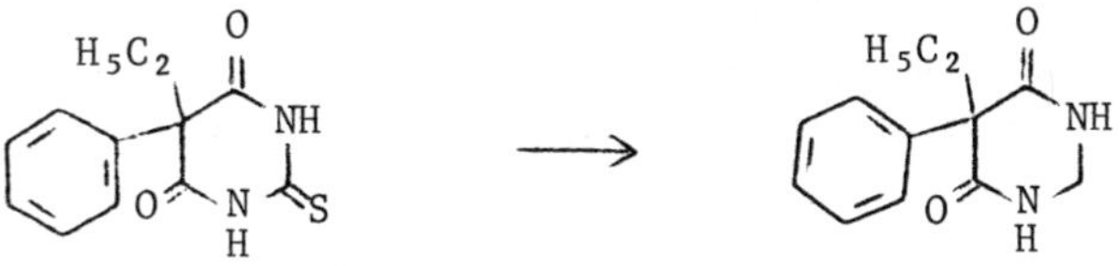

158   159

6. PYRAZINES AND PIPERAZINES

Pyridine and the ring system containing an additional nitrogen
atom at the 4 position—pyrazine—are to some extent interchange-
able as nuclei for antitubercular carboxamides. Preparation of
the requisite acid starts by condensation of phenylenediamine
with glyoxal to afford quinoxalin (160). Oxidation of this molecule interestingly proceeds at the carbocyclic aromatic ring to
afford the heterocyclic dicarboxylic acid (161). Decarboxylation
followed by esterification gives 162. Ammonolysis of the ester
affords *pyrazineamide (163)*.[46] Mannich reaction on that amide
with formaldehyde and morpholine yields *morphazineamide (164)*.[47]

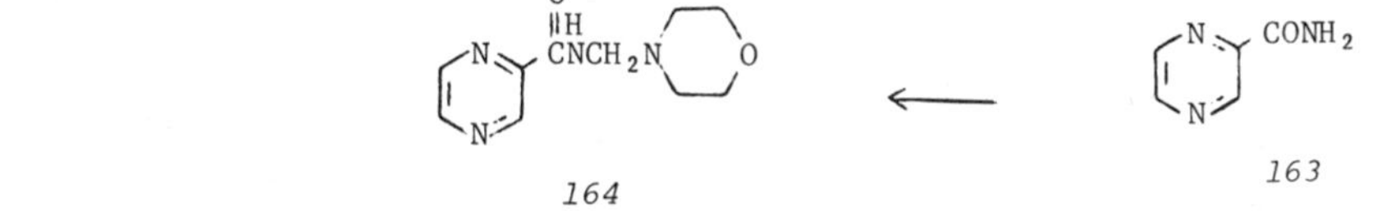

160   161   162

164   163

Carboxylic acid, 161, also serves as starting material for a
substituted pyrazine that has proven to be an important diuretic
agent. As the first step in the synthesis the acid is converted
to the corresponding amide (165). Treatment with a single equivalent of hypobromous acid effects Hoffmann rearrangement of only
one of the amide groups. Ethanolysis of the intermediate carbamate leads directly to the amino ester (166). Exposure of the

ester to sulfuryl chloride affords the dichloro derivative (167).
Ammonolysis of that dihalide proceeds to afford the product of
displacement of that halogen activated by the para carboxyl group
(168). Heating that intermediate with a salt of guanidine results
in the formation of an amide of that base. There is thus obtained
amiloride (169).[48]

161 $\longrightarrow$

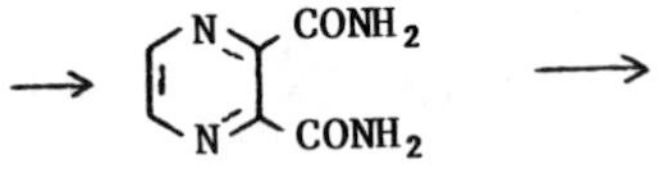

165

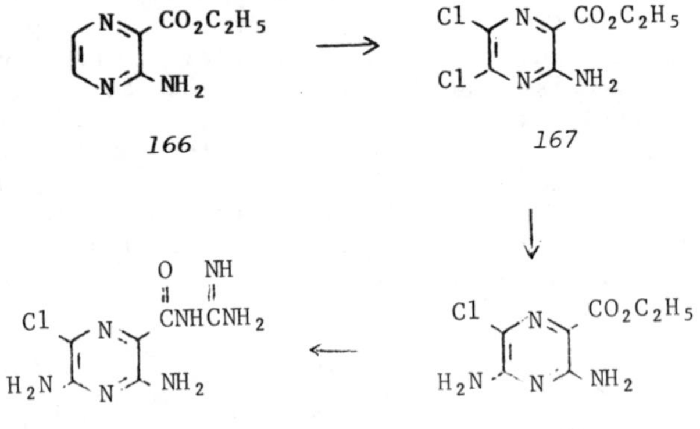

166 $\longrightarrow$ 167

169 $\longleftarrow$ 168

The piperazine ring, like both the pyrrolidine and piperidine heterocycles, is often used in drugs in place of some acyclic
tertiary amine. Since no unique properties of the piperazine ring
seem to be involved in the biologic activity of those agents, the
discussion of those compounds has been relegated to the broader
drug classes within which they occur. A small number of pipera-
zines,do, however, defy this rough classification.

Reaction of N-methylpiperazine with phosgene affords the
carbamoyl chloride (170). Treatment of this intermediate with
diethylamine affords the antiparasitic agent diethyl carbamazine
(171).[49]

Treatment of a mixture of ortho anisidine and bis(2-hydroxy-
ethyl)amine with hydrogen chloride affords the aryl-substituted
piperazine, 171. (The first step in this reaction probably consists in conversion of at least one hydroxyl group to the chloride; this then serves to alkylate the aromatic amine.) Alkyla-

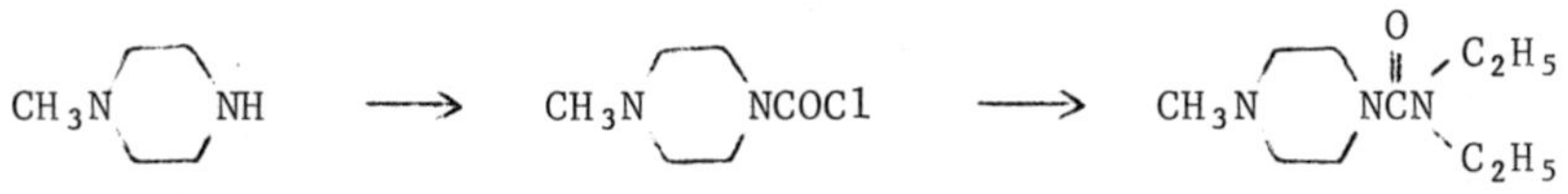

170   171

tion of the secondary nitrogen with 4-chloro-*p*-fluorobutyrophe-
none (obtained by acylation of fluorobenzene with 4-chlorobutyryl
chloride) gives the atarctic agent *fluanisone (172).*[50]

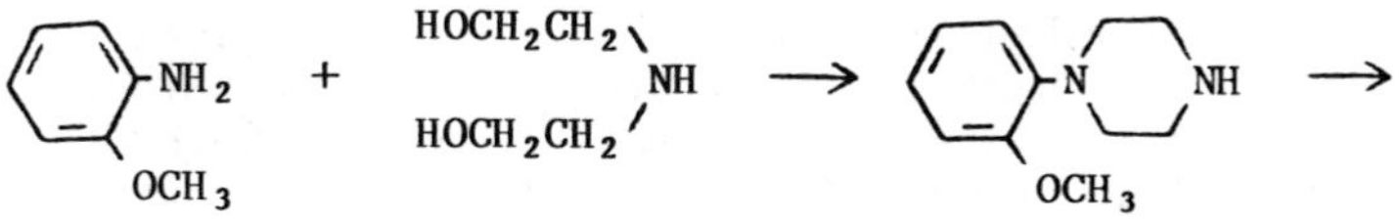

171

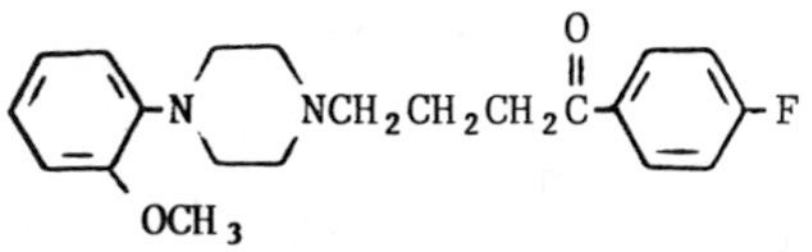

172

Alkylation of the monocarbamate of piperazine with the halide, *173*, affords *174* after removal of the protecting group by
saponification. Alkylation of the amine with the chloroamide,
175 (obtained from amine, *176*, and chloroacetyl chloride) gives
the local anesthetic *lidoflazine (177).*[51]

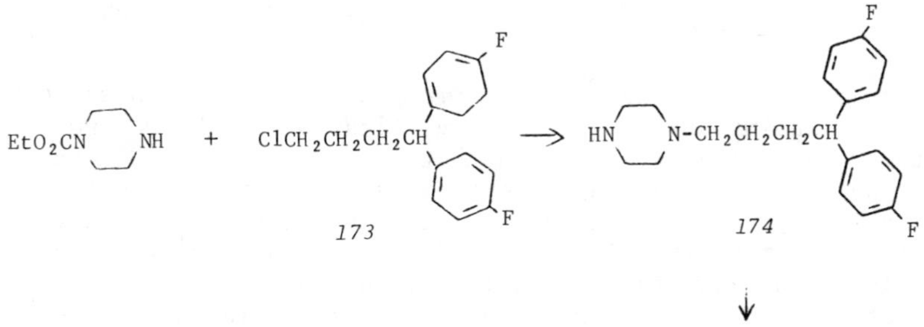

173   174

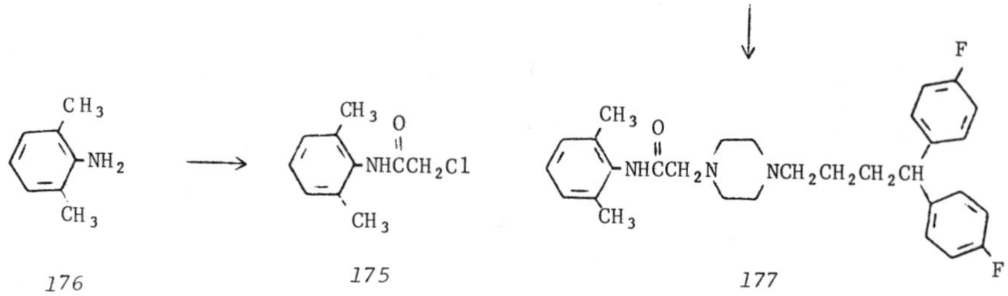

176   *175*   *177*

7. MISCELLANEOUS MONOCYCLIC HETEROCYCLES

Condensation of *p*-chlorobenzaldehyde with 3-mercaptopropionic
acid in the presence of ammonium carbonate leads to the thiazi-
none, *179*. The reaction very probably proceeds by the intermediacy of the carbonyl addition product, *178*; lactamization completes formation of the observed product. Oxidation of *179* to
the sulfone by means of potassium permanganate in acetic acid
gives *chlormezanone (180)*,[52] a minor tranquilizer with muscle-
relaxant properties.

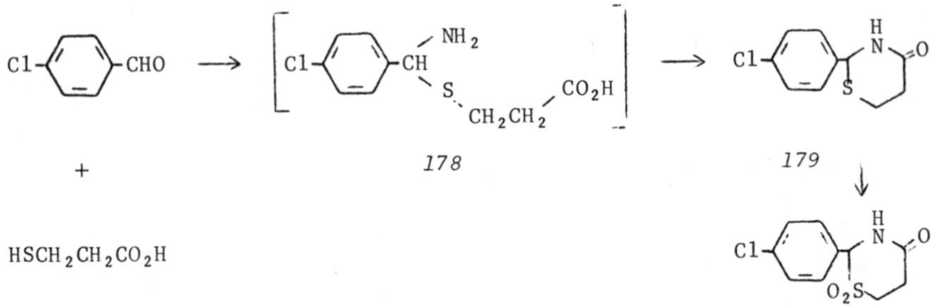

178

179

180

Aromatic biguanides such as *proguanil (181)* have been found
useful as antimalarial agents. Investigation of the metabolism
of this class of drugs revealed that the active compound was in
fact the triazine produced by oxidative cyclization onto the
terminal alkyl group. The very rapid excretion of the active
entity means that it cannot be used as such in therapy. Consequently, treatment usually consists in administration of either
the metabolic precursor or, alternately, the triazine as some
very insoluble salt to provide slow but continual release of drug.

Reaction of *p*-chloroaniline with dicyanamide affords the biguanide, *182*. This is condensed immediately with acetone to form the
aminal *cycloguanil (183)*.[53] The compound is usually used as a
salt with *pamoic acid (184)*.

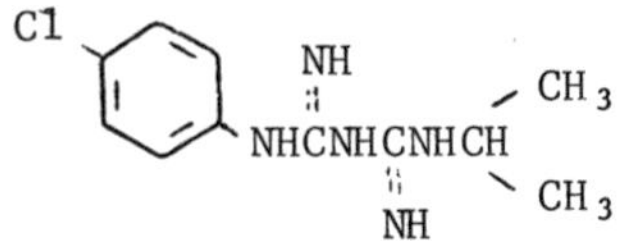

181

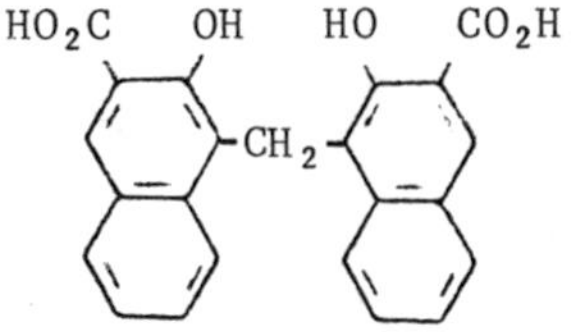

184

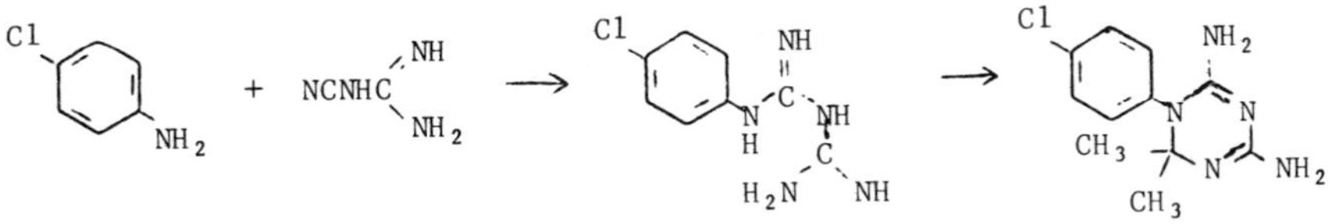

182

183

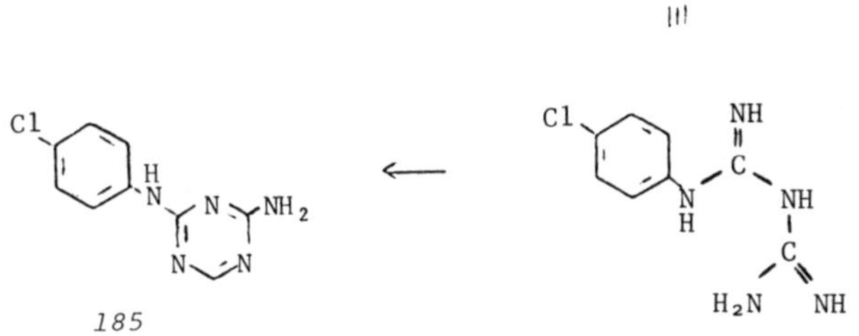

185

Cyclization of the intermediate, *182*, by means of ethyl
orthoformate takes a quite different course. The nitrogen on the
aromatic ring in this case becomes one of the exocyclic groups
to afford the *chorazanil (185)*,[54] a compound that shows diuretic
activity.

Pentylenetetrazol *(188)* is a drug with profound stimulatory
activity on the central nervous system. As such, the agent was
at one time used in shock therapy for treatment of mental disease.
Although it has since been supplanted by safer methods, the
agents still occupy an important role in various experimental
animal models in pharmacology. Addition of hydrazine to the
imino ether *(186)* obtained from caprolactam affords *187*. Treat-

ment of that hydrazine with nitrous acid affords *pentylenetetra-zol (188)*,[55] probably via the azide.

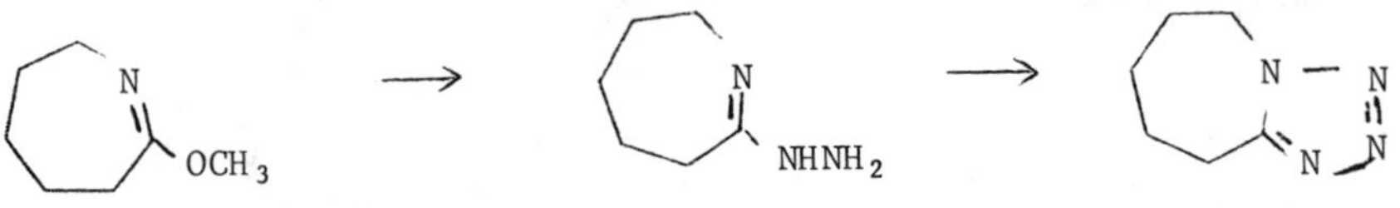

186   187   188

Guanidines with substituents of appropriate lipophilicity have proven quite useful in treatment of hypertension due to their activity as peripheral sympathetic blocking agents. One of the more important drugs in this category is *guanethidine (191)*. Alkylation of the saturated azocine with chloroacetonitrile affords the intermediate, *189*. Catalytic reduction of the nitrile gives the diamine *(190)*. Condensation of that with the S-methyl ether of thiourea affords *guanethidine (191)*.[56]

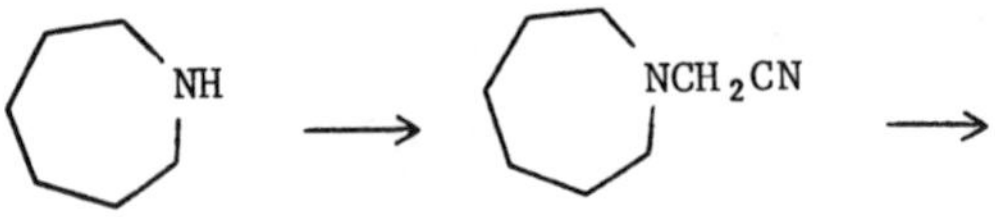

189

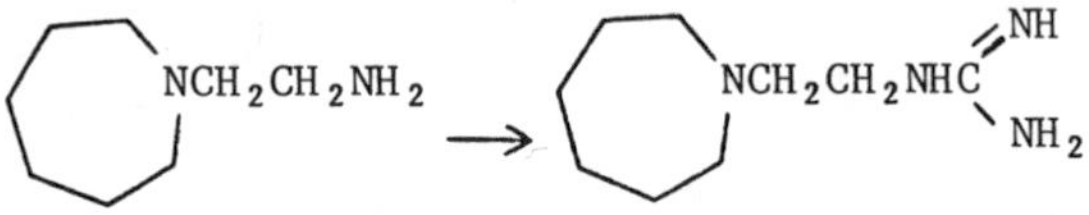

190   191

The lack of structural specificity within the sympathetic blocking agents is particularly well illustrated by a drug that is based on a heterocycle in only the loosest sense. Ketaliza-tion of cyclohexanone with 1-chloro-2,3-propanediol affords *192*. Displacement of halogen by means of the sodium salt of phthali-mide leads to the intermediate, *193*; removal of the phthaloyl protecting group by treatment with hydrazine leads to the primary amine *(194)*. This amine gives the hypotensive agent *guanadrel (195)*,[57] on reaction with the S-methyl ether of thiourea. Like all other hypotensive agents containing the guanidine function, this agent acts by blockade of the sympathetic nervous system.

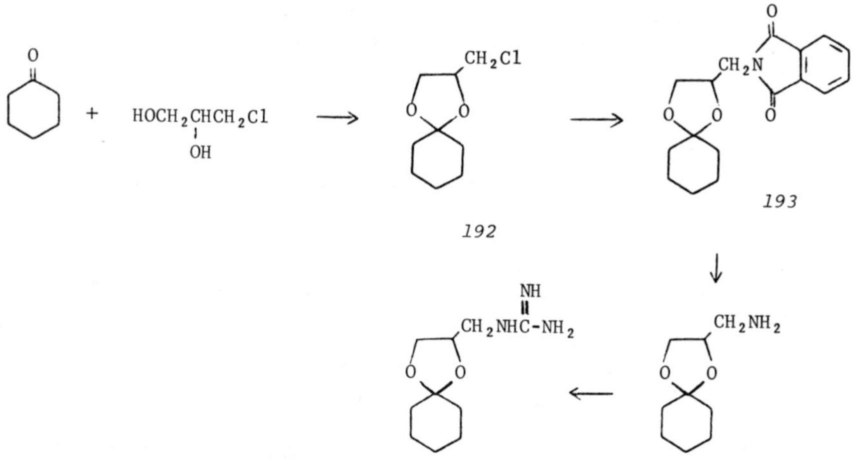

REFERENCES

1. P. Oxley, M. W. Partridge, T. D. Robinson, and W. F. Short, *J. Chem. Soc.*, 763 (1946).
2. H. H. Fox and T. Gibbas, *J. Org. Chem.*, *18*, 994 (1953).
3. B. M. Bloom and R. E. Carnham, U. S. Patent 3,040,061 (1962).
4. D. Libermann, N. Rist, F. Grumbach, S. Cals, M. Moyeux, and A. Rouaix, *Bull. Soc. Chim. Fr.*, 687 (1958).
5. R. N. Shreve, W. M. Swaney, and E. H. Riechers, *J. Amer. Chem. Soc.*, *65*, 2241 (1943).
6. E. C. Taylor and A. J. Crovetti, *J. Org. Chem.*, *19*, 1633 (1954).
7. C. Hoffmann and A. Faure, *Bull. Soc. Chim. Fr.*, 2316 (1966).
8. N. Greenlagh and P. Arnall, U. S. Patent 3,233,710 (1965).
9. E. Tagmann, E. Sury, and K. Hoffmann, *Helv. Chim. Acta,* *35*, 1541 (1952).
10. K. Hoffmann and E. Urech, U. S. Patent 2,848,455 (1958).
11. E. Tagmann, E. Sury, and K. Hoffmann, *Helv. Chim. Acta,* *35*, 1235 (1952).
12. Anon., British Patent 788,821 (1957).
13. F. B. Thole and J. F. Thorpe, *J. Chem. Soc.*, *99*, 422 (1911).
14. O. Schnider, H. Frick, and A. H. Lutz, *Experientia,* *10*, 135 (1954).
15. Anon., French Patent M3016 (1965).

16. F. H. Clarke, *J. Org. Chem.*, *27*, 3251 (1962).

17. W. G. Otto, *Angew. Chem.*, *68*, 181 (1956).

18. D. Dvornik and G. Schilling, *J. Med. Chem.*, *8*, 466 (1965).

19. P. B. Russell and G. H. Hitchings, *J. Amer. Chem. Soc.*, *73*, 3763 (1951).

20. P. Stenbuck and H. M. Hood, U. S. Patent 3,049,544 (1962).

21. W. C. Anthony and J. J. Ursprung, U. S. Patent 3,461,461 (1969).

22. R. Grewe, *Z. Physiol. Chem.*, *242*, 89 (1936).

23. L. H. Sarett, et al., *J. Amer. Chem. Soc.*, *82*, 2994 (1960).

24. H. I. Wheeler and D. F. McFarland, *Amer. Chem. J.*, *42*, 105 (1909).

25. G. W. Anderson, I. F. Halverstadt, W. H. Miller, and R. O. Roblin, *J. Amer. Chem. Soc.*, *67*, 2197 (1945).

26. H. Barrett, I. Goodman, and K. Dittmer, *J. Amer. Chem. Soc.*, *70*, 1753 (1948).

27. V. Papesh and E. F. Schroeder, U. S. Patent 2,729,669 (1956).

28. Anon., Belgian Patent 658,987 (1965).

29. R. Chaux and C. Dufraise, U. S. Patent 1,869,666 (1931).

30. W. J. Doran, U. S. Patent 2,872,448 (1959).

31. A. C. Cope and E. M. Hancock, *J. Amer. Chem. Soc.*, *60*, 2644 (1938).

32. A. C. Cope and E. M. Hancock, *J. Amer. Chem. Soc.*, *61*, 776 (1939).

33. Z. Eckstein, *Przemysl Chem.*, *9*, 390 (1953).

34. W. Taub, U. S. Patent 2,501,551 (1950).

35. M. Seefelder, *Chem. Abstr.*, *56*, 9927i (1962).

36. Anon., French Patent M1059 (1962).

37. L. Taub and W. Kropp, German Patent 537,366 (1929).

38. W. Kropp and L. Taub, U. S. Patent 1,947,944 (1934).

39. J. A. Snyder and K. P. Link, *J. Amer. Chem. Soc.*, *75*, 1831 (1953).

40. G. H. Donnison, U. S. Patent 2,876,225 (1959).

41. E. H. Vollwiller and D. L. Tabern, U. S. Patent 2,153,730 (1939).

42. O. Zima and F. VonWerder, U. S. Patent 2,561,689 (1951).

43. M. A. Youtz and P. P. Perkins, *J. Amer. Chem. Soc.*, *51*, 3511 (1929).

44. W. J. Doran and E. M. VanHeyningen, U. S. Patent 2,561,689 (1951).

45. J. Y. Bogue and H. C. Carrington, *Brit. J. Pharmacol.*, *8*, 230 (1953).

46. S. Kushner, H. Dallian, J. L. Sanjuro, F. L. Bach, S. R. Safir, V. K. Smith, and J. H. Williams, *J. Amer. Chem. Soc.*, *74*, 3617 (1952).

47. E. Felder and U. Tiepolo, German Patent 1,129,492 (1962).

48. E. J. Cragoe, Belgian Patent 639,386 (1964).
49. S. Kushner, L. M. Brancone, R. I. Hewitt, W. L. McEwen, Y. Subbarow, H. W. Steward, R. J. Turner, and J. J. Denton, *J. Org. Chem., 13*, 144 (1948).
50. P. A. J. Janssen, U. S. Patent 2,997,472 (1961).
51. P. A. J. Janssen, Netherland Application 6,507,312 (1965).
52. A. R. Surrey, W. G. Webb, and R. M. Gesler, *J. Amer. Chem. Soc., 80*, 3469 (1958).
53. E. J. Modest, *J. Org. Chem., 2*, 1 (1956).
54. O. Clauder and G. Bulsu, *Magy. Kem. Foly., 57*, 68 (1951).
55. R. Stolle, *Chem. Ber., 63*, 1032 (1930).
56. R. A. Maxwell, R. P. Mulland, and A. J. Plummer, *Experientia, 15*, 267 (1959).
57. R. Hardie and J. E. Aaron, U. S. Patent 3,547,951.

CHAPTER 15

Derivatives of Morphine, Morphinan, and Benzomorphan 4-Phenylpiperidines

The sensation of pain is at one and the same time the salvation and bane of all sentient living organisms. In teleologic terms, the function of pain is to alert the organism to the fact that something is amiss in its relation to the environment. Put more simply, pain is an alert signal to injury or malfunction of some organ system. On the other hand, the signal does not terminate once the injury has been noted. Rather, pain often persists past the point at which the causal stimulus has been removed. Pain, too, can often be so intense as to greatly impair normal functions. The relief of pain has therefore figured prominently in many mythologies as one of mankind's aspirations.

Opium, the crude dried sap of the immature fruit of the poppy, *Papaver somniferum*, had some folkloric use as a means of inducing euphoria. The beginning of the nineteenth century saw an increasing interest in systematic study of plant materials that seemed to possess pharmacologic activity. It was in the course of one of these studies that the major alkaloid contained in opium, *morphine (1)*, was isolated and identified. Recognition of its analgesic properties followed the isolation. Although the mechanism of action of this drug and its host of congeners are not known in any detail to this day, their mode of action is usually classed as narcotic. Most of the drugs in this class tend to show very similar pharmacologic response; in cases of dependence the compounds can often be substituted for each other.

It is generally accepted that the narcotic analgesics do not in fact interfere with the pain as such; rather, these compounds change the perception of the pain. In other words, the patient may come to regard pain with detachment. This very mechanism may be responsible for one of the major drawbacks of the narcotic
286

1

analgesics as a class; since not all pain is physical, there are
always a sizeable number of individuals who like nothing better
than to gain a sense of detachment from their psychic pain. The
euphoriant properties exhibited by some of the narcotics, of
course, aggravate this problem. Thus, the prone individual will
develop psychic dependence to these drugs. The phenomenon of
physical dependence adds an ominous note to this cycle of addiction. As an individual keeps ingesting these drugs, he develops
tolerance, that is, he needs ever larger amounts to achieve the
desired effect. In addition, the addict develops a true physiologic need for the narcotic. Sudden cessation of drug administration leads to severe physical illness. There has therefore been
a major effort of some duration to develop analgesics without
this addiction potential.

1. MORPHINE

Although *morphine* has been prepared by total synthesis,[1] the complexity of the molecule makes such an approach unattractive on a
commercial scale. The drug in fact is obtained by fractionation
of opium obtained from the poppy; *morphine* in turn is used as
starting material for various derivatives. If it were not
for the importance of these drugs in the clinic, some progress
might have been made in eradication of the plant.
　　　Initial synthetic work was aimed at decreasing side effects
such as addiction potential and respiratory depression, as well
as at increasing potency and oral activity. Methylation of the
phenolic group at 3 affords *codeine (2)*, a weaker analgesic than
morphine, which has been used as an antitussive agent. The homolog, *ethylmorphine (3)*,[1] obtained by alkylation of *morphine* with
ethyl sulfate, shows somewhat greater potency than codeine; its
chief use has been in ophthalmology. Alkylation of *1* with *N*(2-
chloroethyl)morpholine yields *pholcodeine (4)*. Continuing in the

vein of simple modification, acetylation of *morphine* leads to the
diacetyl compound *heroin (5)*.   This drug, much favored by
addicts for its potent euphoriant action on intravenous injection,
has been outlawed in the United States for a good many years.
Acetylation of *codeine (2)* by means of acetic anhydride affords
thebacon (6).[3]

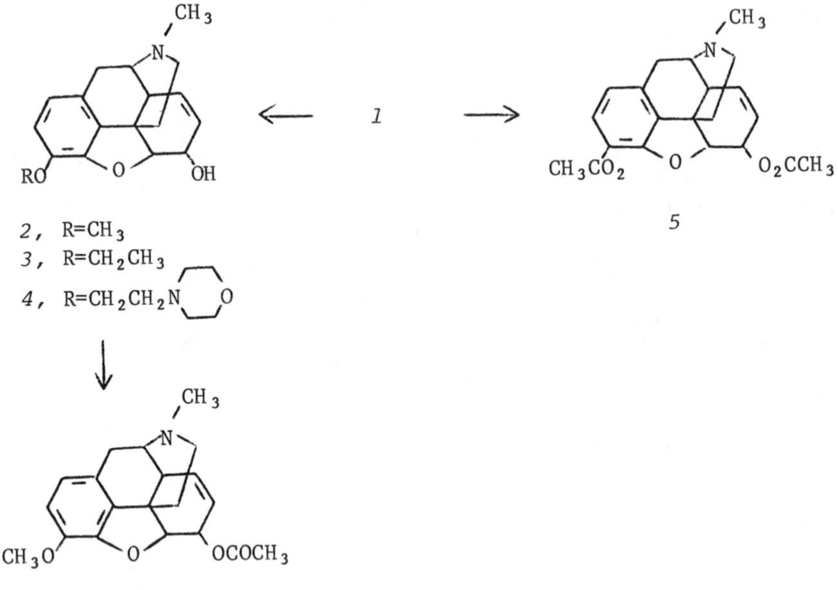

2, R=CH$_3$
3, R=CH$_2$CH$_3$
4, R=CH$_2$CH$_2$N O

5

6

Catalytic reduction of *codeine (2)* affords the analgesic
dihydrocodeine (7).[4] Oxidation of the alcohol at 6 by means of
the Oppenauer reaction gives *hydrocodone (9)*,[5] an agent once
used extensively as an antitussive. It is of note that treatment
of *codeine* under strongly acidic conditions similarly affords
hydrocodone by a very unusual rearrangement of an allyl alcohol
to the corresponding enol, followed by ketonization.
     When morphine is subjected to a similar reduction-oxidation
sequence *(1→10)*, there is obtained *hydromorphone (10)*.[6]
     An invariant feature in the molecules discussed thus far has
been the presence of a methyl group on nitrogen. Replacement of
this group by allyl produces a drug with a markedly different
pharmacologic profile. *Nalorphine (13)*, while possessing some
analgesic effect in its own right, is used mainly as narcotic
antagonist. That is, the agent will prevent many of the side
effects of *morphine* or its congeners such as respiratory depres-

| 1, R=H | 7, R=CH$_3$ | 9, R=CH$_3$ |
| 2, R=CH$_3$ | 8, R=H | 10, R=H |

sion, euphoria, nausea, and drowsiness, particularly in cases of narcotic overdoses. It is of interest that the narcotic antagonists may in fact precipitate withdrawal symptoms on administration to addicts. Pure antagonists devoid of significant analgesic activity have a rather limited role in the practice of medicine. It should be noted, however, that a mixture of a pure antagonist, *naloxone*, and an analgesic, *methadone*, has recently been proposed for use in humans. In theory the antagonist will tend to block the euphoria or "rush" on intravenous administration sought by the addict, without interfering with the analgesic effect. Some of the more recent narcotic antagonists may find use beyond the treatment of overdosage because they show some analgesic activity in their own right. These antagonist-analgesics promise agents with reduced abuse and addiction potential in part because of the low euphoriant effect. As might be inferred from the close structural similarity of agonists and antagonists, there is good biochemical evidence that the latter may act by competing for receptor sites with true agonists.

The prototype of this series is synthesized by first reacting *morphine* with cyanogen bromide. This reagent in effect serves to replace the methyl group by cyano. Hydrolysis of the intermediate *(11)* affords desmethylmorphine *(12)*. Alkylation of the last with allyl bromide affords *nalorphine (13)*.[7]

As in the case of the steroids, introduction of additional nuclear substituents yields *morphine* analogs of increased potency. The more important of these are derived from one of the minor alkaloids that occur in opium. Thebaine *(14)*, present in crude opium in about one-tenth the amount of *morphine*, exhibits a reactive internal diene system that is well known to undergo various addition reactions in a 1,4 manner (e.g., bromination). Thus, reaction with hydrogen peroxide in acid may be visualized to afford first the 14-hydroxy-6-hemiketal *(15)*. Hydrolysis yields the isolated unsaturated ketone *(16)*.[8] Catalytic reduction

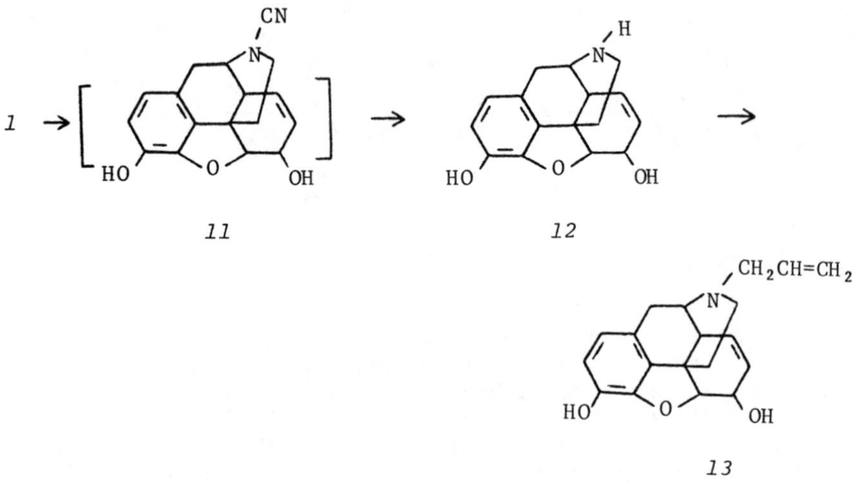

11   12

13

affords *oxycodone (17)*, a relatively potent analgesic. Removal
of the aromatic methyl group by means of hydrobromic acid leads
to *oxymorphone (18)*,[9] an analgesic about ten times as potent as
morphine in man, but with high addiction potential.

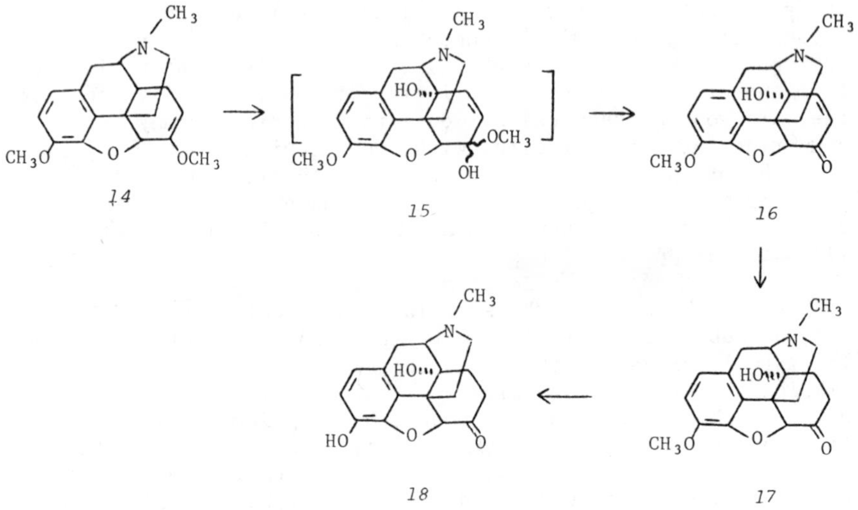

14   15   16

18   17

The 14-hydroxy analog of nalorphine constitutes one of the

most potent pure narcotic antagonists available. The synthesis
of this agent begins with the acetylation of *oxymorphone* by means
of acetic anhydride to afford the 3,6-diacetate (19). Treatment
with cyanogen bromide followed by hydrolysis gives the corresponding desmethyl compound (20). Removal of the acetate groups
by hydrolysis followed by alkylation of the secondary amine with
bromide affords *naloxone* (21).[10]

most potent pure narcotic antagonists

18 →

19   20

21

Displacement at carbon by Grignard reagents has been not
infrequently observed in allylic systems possessing a good leaving group. One need only bring to mind the coupling by-products
observed during the formation of Grignard reagents from allylic
or benzylic halides. Thus, treatment of dihydrothebaine (22),
obtained by catalytic reduction of thebaine, with methylmagnesium
iodide results in displacement of the allylic oxygen at 5 with
consequent cleavage of the furan ring. The fact that the leaving
group in this case is a phenoxide ion no doubt favors this reaction course. Hydrolysis of the enol ether during the workup
affords the intermediate methylated ketone (26).[11] Subsequent
work revealed that the same product could be obtained more con-
veniently by analogous reaction on the enol acetate from *hydrocodone* (23).[12] In order to reform the furan ring, the ketone is
first brominated to afford a dibromoketone formulated as 27.
Treatment of this with base results first in formation of the
phenoxide ion at 4. Displacement of the halogen at 5 affords the
recyclized product, 28. The remaining superfluous halogen is

removed by catalytic reduction *(29)*. Removal of the methyl group at 3 by one of the usual methods affords *methyldihydromorphinone (30)*.[11,12] This agent is a very potent narcotic analgesic, notable particularly for its good oral activity.

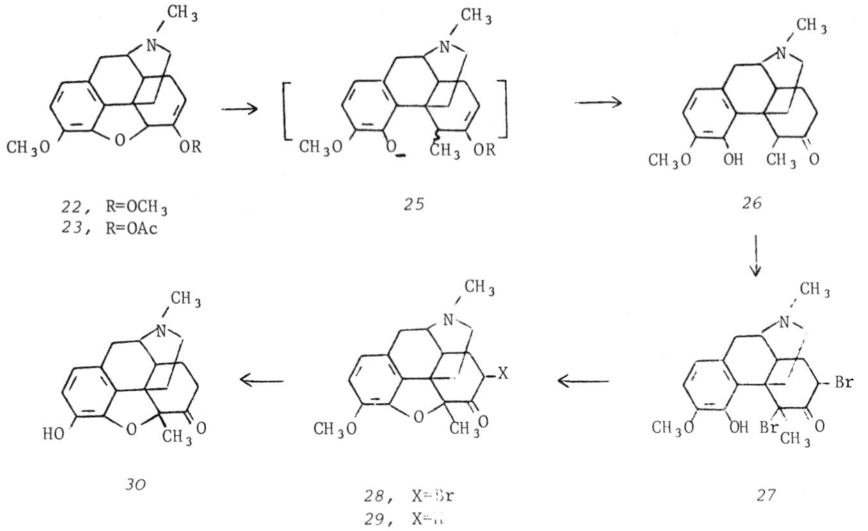

22, R=OCH₃
23, R=OAc

25

26

30

28, X=Br
29, X=ᵢᵢ

27

2. MORPHINANS

Research towards modulation of the pharmacologic profile of narcotic analgesics and their antagonists for quite some time consisted in modification performed on the natural product such as outlined above. This of necessity precluded deep-seated chemical changes that might profoundly alter the pharmacologic properties. The discovery that many highly simplified molecules that possessed some of the structural features of *morphine* still showed analgesic activity opened the door to just such chemical manipulations. Although a great many structurally diverse drugs resulted from these researches, the salient problem of the narcotics, addiction liability, seems to go hand in hand with activity in all but a few of these agents. (It should be noted that the following discussion is cast on the lines of progressive structural simplification; no attempt is made to present chronology.)

The researches of Grewe and Mondon opened the way to the

preparation of the morphinans—morphine analogs lacking the furan
ring—by total synthesis.[13] Modified Knoevnagel condensation of
carbethoxycyclohexanone with ethyl cyanoacetate gives the unsaturated cyanoester, 31. Saponification followed by decarboxylation gives the corresponding dicarboxylic acid; migration of the
double bond is a consequence of the mechanism of decarboxylation.
Reaction with ammonium carbonate affords the corresponding cyclic
imide. This dihydroxypyridine (33) is but a tautomer of the
initial product. Treatment with phosphorus oxychloride leads to
the dihalo compound (34), which affords the tetrahydroisoquino-
line, 35, on reduction. Reaction with methyl iodide gives the
methiodide (36). Since this ring system now carried a positive
charge, there is present in the ring what is in effect a ternary
imminium function, a group known to add organometallic reagents.
Thus, exposure of the salt to benzylmagnesium chloride affords
the adduct (37). Catalytic reduction in the presence of acid
results in selective removal of that double bond which is in
effect part of an enamine. Treatment of the olefin thus obtained
(38) with phosphoric acid leads to Friedel-Crafts-type cyclization into the aromatic ring and formation of the unsubstituted
morphinan (39). Although cyclization at the alternate terminal
of the double bond is possible in theory, the known preference
for six-membered ring formation in this reaction assures regio-
selectivity.

In an extension of this work, Schnider and his colleagues
condensed the salt (36) with the Grignard reagent from p-methoxybenzyl chloride. The product (40), on reduction (41) and cyclization, affords the methoxylated morphinan (41). Removal of the
methyl ether affords the narcotic analgesic racemorphan (43).[14]

As an alternate route to functionalized morphinans, the
intermediate, 38, is first nitrated, the group entering para to
the methylene bridge (44). Reduction of the nitro to the aniline
(45) followed then by diazotization and replacement by hydroxyl
gives intermediate, 46. Cyclization as above again gives racemorphan.[14]

Resolution of racemorphan via the tartrate salt affords a
very potent analgesic. The (-) isomer, [(-)43],[15] is a narcotic
analgesic showing six to eight times the potency of morphine in
man. The methyl ether of the epimer [(+)42], dextromorphan, on
the other hand, shows little if any analgesic activity; this compound, however, is quite effective in suppressing the cough
reflex. As such it is used extensively in cough remedies.

Demethylation of the acetyl derivative (47) of levorphanol
affords desmethyl compound, 48. Hydrolytic removal of the acetate (49) followed by alkylation with allyl bromide affords the
narcotic antagonist levallorphan (50),[15] an agent with properties

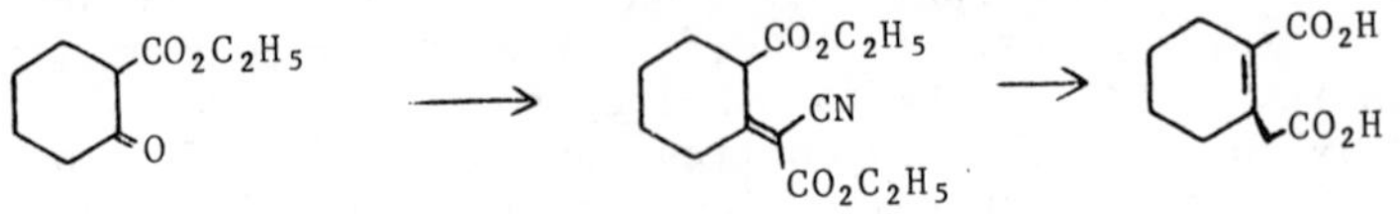

31   32

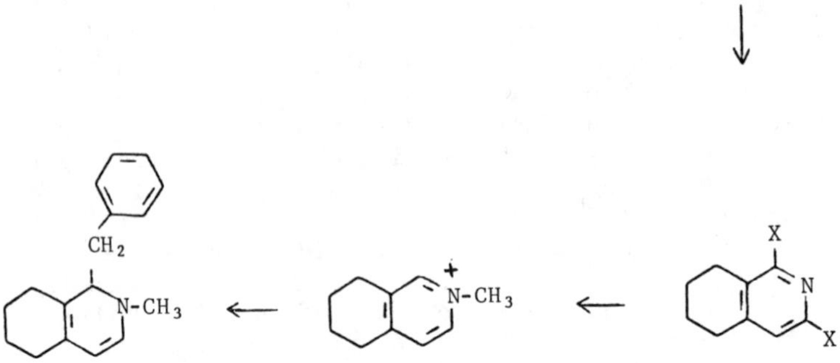

37   36   33, X=OH
                                      34, X=Cl
                                      35, X=H

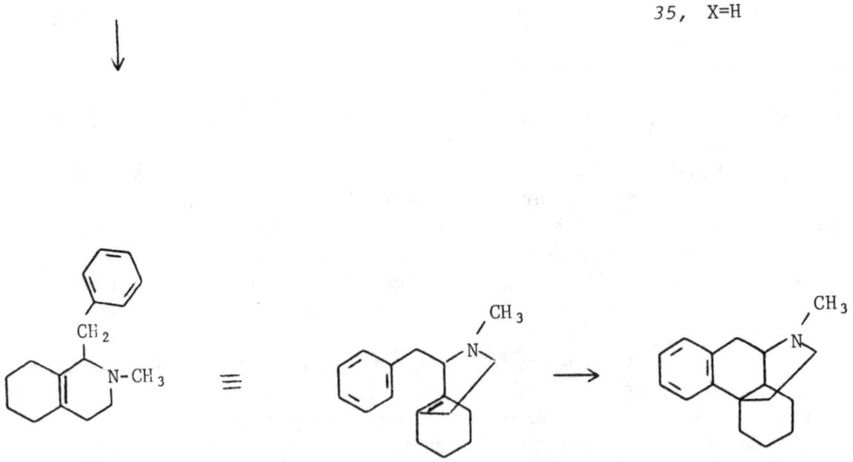

38   38   39

quite similar to *nalorphine (13)*. Alternately, alkylation of *49*
with 2-phenethyl bromide gives the antagonist *phenomorphan (51)*;
in a similar manner alkylation by means of phenacyl bromide
affords the antagonist *levophenacylmorphan (52)*.[16]

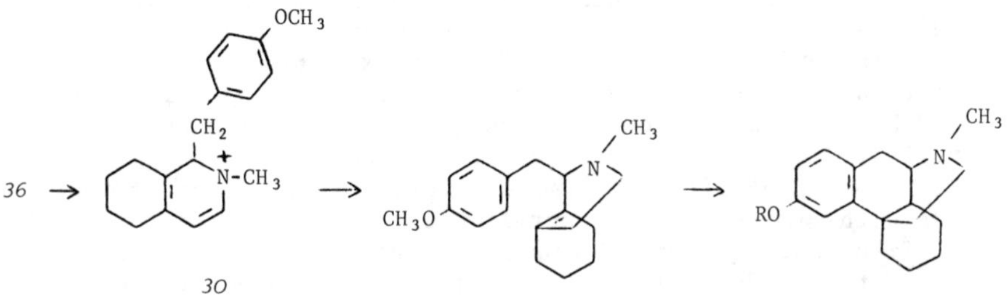

$36 \rightarrow$

30

41

$42,\quad R=CH_3$
$43,\quad R=H$

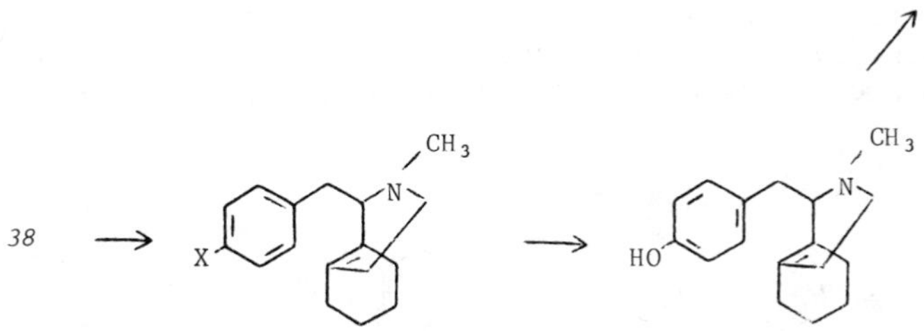

$38 \rightarrow$

$44,\quad X=NO_2$
$45,\quad X=NH_2$

46

$(-)43 \rightarrow$

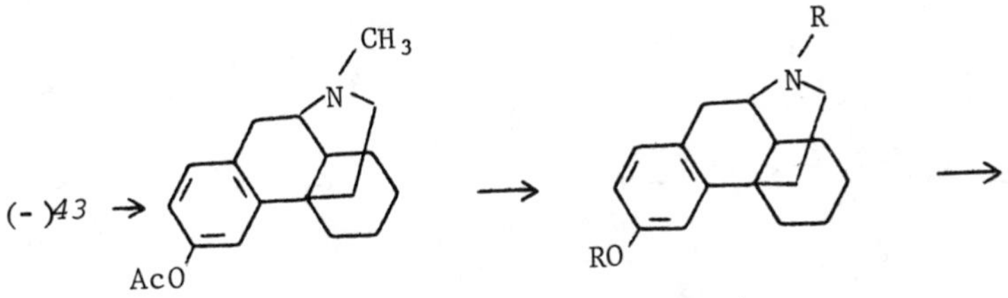

47

$48,\quad R=Ac$
$49,\quad R=H$

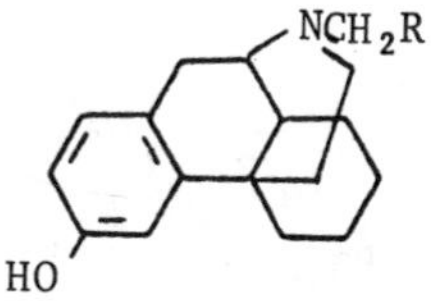

$50,\quad R=CH=CH_2$
$51,\quad R=CH_2C_6H_5$
$52,\quad R=COC_6H_5$

The narcotic antagonists in the morphinan series are more readily available by an alternate synthesis that avoids the demethylation step. Reaction of cyclohexanone with ethyl cyano-acetate affords the condensation product (53). Hydrolysis followed by decarboxylation leads to the unconjugation unsaturated nitrile (54). This is then reduced to the corresponding amine (55) by means of lithium aluminum hydride. Formation of the amide with p-methoxyphenylacetyl chloride gives the intermediate, 56. Treatment with phosphorus oxychloride brings about condensation of the amide—as its enolate—with the isolated cyclohexane double bond, and thus cyclization. The resulting imine double bond is then selectively reduced to afford the isoquinoline derivative (57).[17] Demethylation followed by resolution yields a key intermediate to compounds 50-52. N-alkylation with an appropriate side chain affords 58; cyclization in a manner analogous to that used to prepare levorphanol (43) gives the desired product.[18]

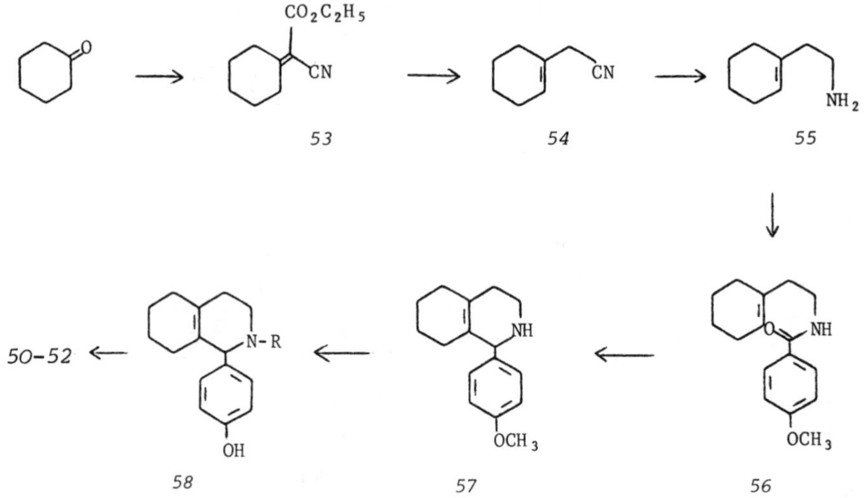

3. BENZOMORPHANS

In a continuation of the theme of simplification of the morphine ring, it was found that one of the carbocyclic rings (that which contained the allyl alcohol in morphine proper) can be dispensed with as well, to give compounds that show the full activity of the natural prototype. These agents, the benzomorphans, are of unusual clinical significance, since one of these compounds, *pentazocine (67)*, seems to show greatly diminished addiction potential when compared to the classic narcotic analgesics. Pharmacologic research in this series pointed up the importance of narcotic antagonist activity in the search for nonaddictive analgesics. It is now considered that analgesics with low addiction potential may well come from those agents which show varying mixtures of agonist and antagonist activity in test animals. It is clear that the search for pure analgesics among compounds bearing some of the structural features of the narcotics have more often than not led to highly addictive agents.

The prototype, benzomorphan *(63)*, can be obtained by a variation of the morphinan synthesis. Thus, reaction of the Grignard reagent from p-methoxybenzyl chloride with the lutidine methiodide *(59)* affords the benzylated dihydropyridine *60*. (The addition to the most highly hindered position is rather puzzling.) Reduction of the enamine double bond leads to the tetrahydropyridine *(61)*. Cyclization by means of acid leads directly into the benzomorphan ring system *(62)*. Demethylation of the aromatic ether affords the phenol, *63*.[19] Although this last compound is in fact a relatively potent analgesic, it is not available commercially as a drug.

The key to clinical agents in this series, the secondary amine, *65*, is obtained by a sequence analogous to that used to obtain desmethymorphine. Thus, the phenol *(63)* is first acetylated *(64)*, and then demethylated by treatment with cyanogen bromide; hydrolysis gives the desired aminophenol *(65)*. Alkylation

with 2-phenethyl bromide affords the potent analgesic agent,
phenazocine (66),[20] a compound used briefly in the clinic. Alkylation by means of 3,3-dimethylallyl chloride yields *pentazocine
(67)*,[21] the analgesic alluded to above. Finally, alkylation with
cyclopropylmethyl bromide gives *cyclazocine (68)*,[22] a potent narcotic antagonist that has shown analgesic activity in man. This
last would be an analgesic agent of choice but for its halucino-
genic propensity.

63 $\longrightarrow$

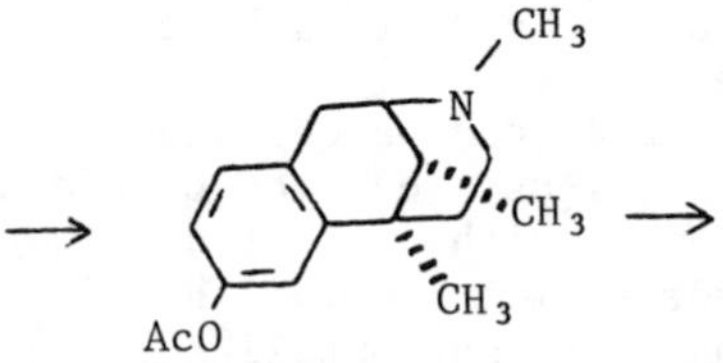

64

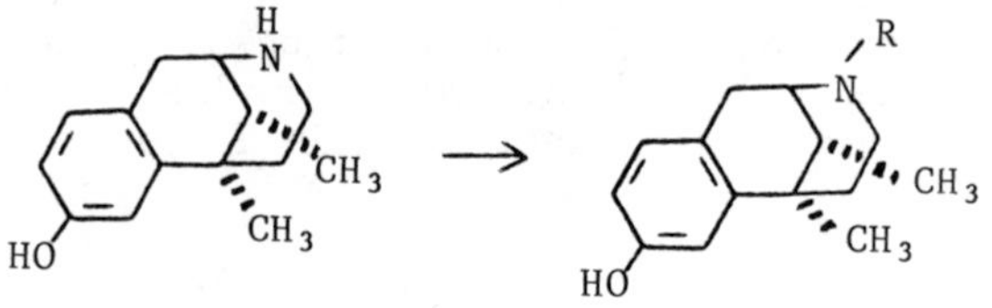

65 $\longrightarrow$

66, $R=CH_2CH_2C_6H_5$

67, $R=CH_2CH=C\begin{smallmatrix} CH_3 \\ CH_3 \end{smallmatrix}$

68, $R=CH_2$◁

4.   4-PHENYLPIPERIDINES

More radical dissection of the morphine molecule was in progress
concurrently with the work above. The chemistry of the series of
analgesics that rely on an acyclic skeleton, the compounds related
to *methadone*, is discussed earlier. Suffice it to say that this
series of agents, with the possible exception of *propoxyphene*,
seem to share abuse and addiction potential with their polycyclic
counterparts.
        Examination of the morphine molecule reveals the presence of
a 4-phenylpiperidine fragment within the molecule (A). It was

presumably this line of reasoning that led to yet another extensive series of synthetic analgesics. The great diversity of
structural types that have exhibited analgesic activity has led
medicinal chemists to seek the thread common to these various
molecules. The so-called "morphine rule" represents one formulation of the elements shared by the large majority of analgesics.
Briefly, activity seems to require an aromatic ring (a) attached
to a quaternary center (b) and a tertiary nitrogen atom (c)
removed at a distance of two carbon atoms from (a). Like most
such generalizations, this rule has its exceptions; *fentanyl
(141)*, for example, does not fit the rule very well.

CH$_3$

R   R
N(c)

HO   OH

(a)

A   *B*

The prototype for the phenylpiperidine analgesics (*meperidine*, also known as *pethidine, 75*) was discovered by Eisleb in
Germany on the very eve of World War II. The consequent blackout
on international scientific communications led to work on these
molecules being pursued in parallel in both warring camps; it
goes without saying that analgesics are at a premium in time of
war. The dislocation in Germany following the war meant that the
majority of publications on these molecules originated outside
Germany.

One of the early syntheses of *meperidine (75)* starts with
the double alkylation of phenylacetonitrile with the bischloroethyl amine, *72*.[23] The highly lachrimatory nature of this material led to the development of an alternate synthesis for the
intermediate piperidine *(73)*. Alkylation of phenylacetonitrile
with two moles of 2-chloroethylvinyl ether leads to the intermediate *(69)*. This is then hydrolyzed without prior isolation to
the diol, *70*. Treatment with thionyl chloride affords the corresponding dichloro compound *(71)*. This last is then used to effect
a bis alkylation on methylamine, in effect forming the piperidine
(73) by cyclization at the opposite end from the original scheme.
Saponification to the acid *(74)* followed by esterification with
ethanol affords the widely used analgesic *meperidine (75)*[24]; substitution of isopropanol for ethanol in the esterification affords
properidine (76).[24]

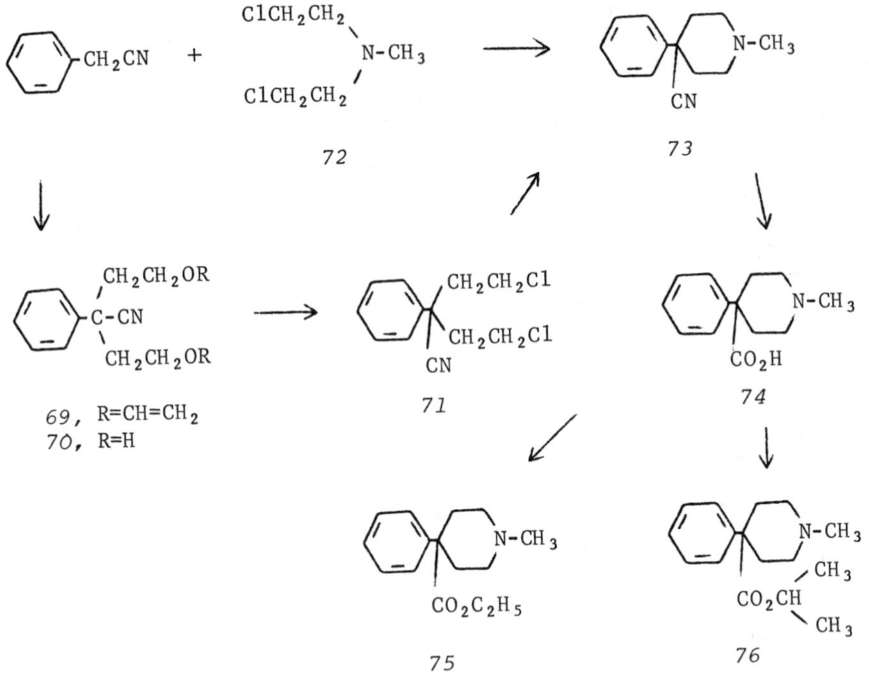

69, R=CH=CH$_2$
70, R=H

71

72

73

74

75

76

Much work has been carried out in this series on changing the substitution on nitrogen in the hopes of producing compounds with some degree of narcotic antagonist activity in analogy to the agents more closely related to *morphine* While that goal has not been met, such substitution has afforded agents with enhanced potency relative to *meperidine*.

The key intermediate, *normeperidine (81)*, is obtained by a scheme closely akin to that used for the parent molecule. Thus, alkylation of phenylacetonitrile with the tosyl analog of the bischloroethyl amine *(78)* leads to the substituted piperidine *(79)*. Basic hydrolysis serves to convert the nitrile to the acid *(80)*. Treatment of this last with sulfuric acid in ethanol serves both to esterify the acid and to remove the toluenesulfonyl group to yield the secondary amine *(81)*.[25]

Alkylation of that amine with *p*-(2-chloroethyl)aniline affords *anileridine (82)*,[26] an analgesic similar to the parent compound but somewhat more potent. In similar fashion alkylation by means of *N*-(2-chloroethyl)morpholine gives *morpheridine (83)*,[27] while the use of 2-(chloroethyl)-ethanol yields *carbethi-*

dine (84).[28] Use of halide, *87* (obtained by reaction of furfuryl alcohol with ethylene oxide, followed by formation of the chloride from the condensation product *(86)*, in this reaction affords the analgesic *furethidine (85).*[29]

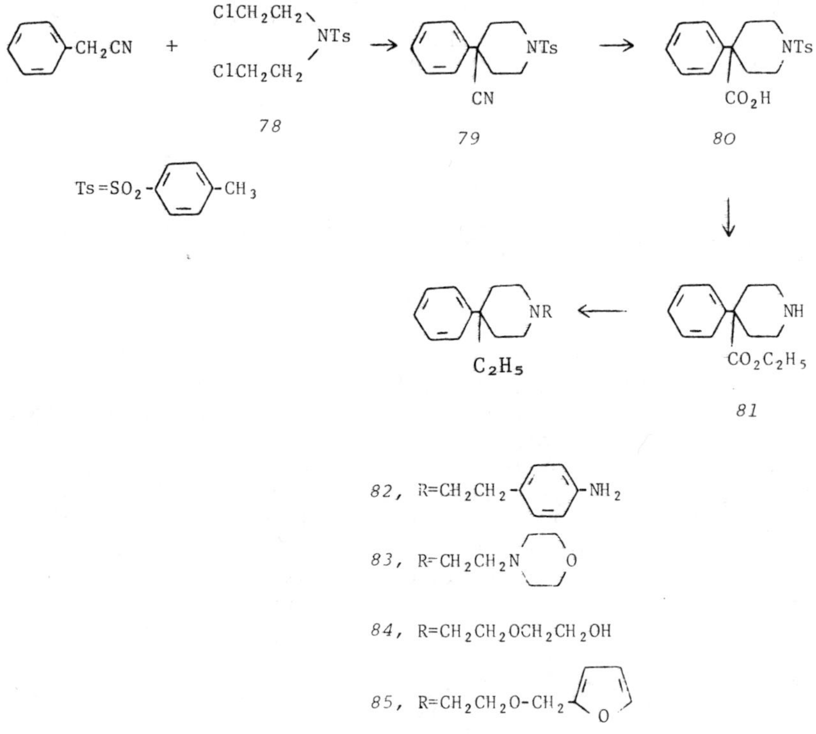

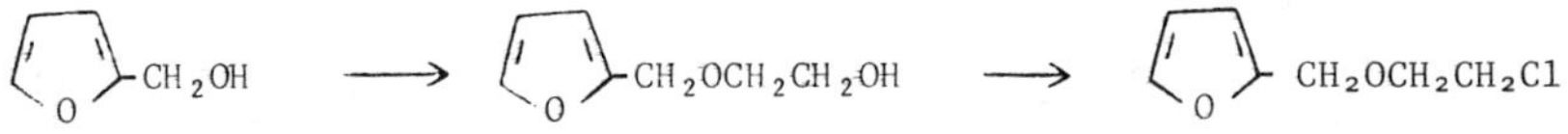

Condensation of *normeperidine (81)* with 3-chloropropan-1-ol affords the compound possessing the alcohol side chain *(88).* The hydroxyl is then converted to chlorine by means of thionyl chloride *(89);* displacement of the halogen by aniline yields *piminodine (90).*[30] Condensation of the secondary amine, *81,* with styrene oxide affords the alcohol, *91;* removal of the benzyllic hydroxyl group by hydrogenolysis leads to *pheneridine (92).*[31]

Conjugate addition of norpethidine *(81)* to benzoylethylene gives
the ketone, *93*. Reduction of the carbonyl group to the alcohol
affords the potent analgesic *phenoperidine (94)*.[32]

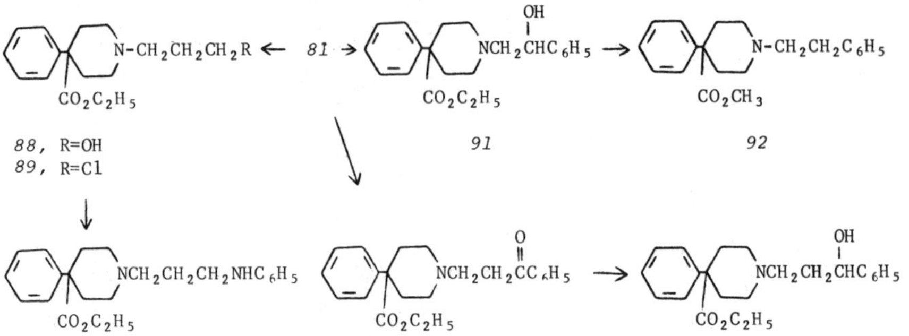

A not uncommon side effect observed with *morphine* and some
of the other narcotic analgesics is constipation due to decreased
motility of the gastrointestinal tract. It proved possible to
so modify *pethidine* as to retain the side effect at the expense
of analgesic activity. Relief of diarrhea, it will be realized,
is a far from trivial indication. Alkylation of the anion from
diphenylacetonitrile *(95)* with ethylene dibromide gives the intermediate, *96*.[33] Alkylation of normeperidine *(81)* with that halide
affords *diphenoxylate (97)*,[34] an antidiarrheal agent.

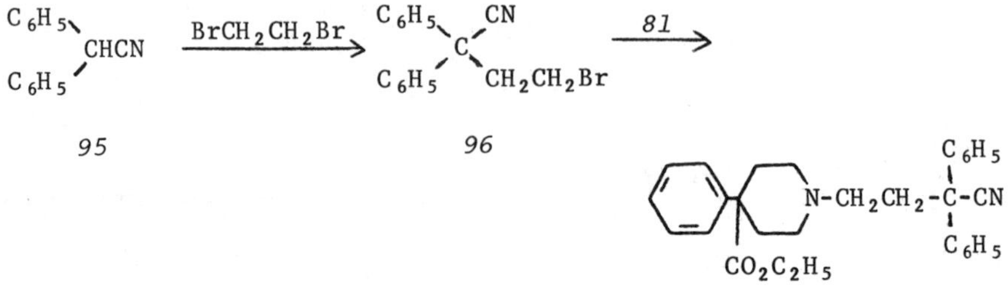

In an effort to more closely mimic the aromatic substitution
pattern found in *morphine* (see A) the pethidine analog containing
the *m*-hydroxy group was prepared as well. Thus, in a synthesis
analogous to that used to prepare the parent compound, double
alkylation of *m*-methoxyphenylacetonitrile with the chloroamine,

72, affords the piperidine *(98)*. Treatment with hydrogen bromide
effects both demethylation of the phenolic ether and hydrolysis
of the nitrile *(99)*; esterification with ethanol affords *bemidone*
(100).[35] Alternately, reaction of the nitrile of *98* with ethylmagnesium bromide gives, on acidic workup, the ketone *(101)*;
demethylation affords *ketobemidone (102)*.[36] Both these agents
are effective analgesics.

Ring expansion of the nitrogen-containing ring has proven
compatible with retention of analgesic activity. Phenylacetonitrile is again the starting material. Alkylation with one
equivalent of *N*-(2-chloroethyl)dimethylamine gives the aminonitrile *(103)*; alkylation of this with bromochloropropane yields the
molecule containing the requisite carbon atoms *(104)*. Simply
heating the free base leads to cyclization by means of formation
of the internal quaternary salt *(105)*; pyrolysis of that salt at
225°C results in elimination of one of the methyl groups, possibly by displacement on carbon by the chloride gegenion. Saponification of the product *(106)* followed by esterification with
ethanol gives *ethoheptazine (107)*,[37] an orally effective analgesic
used largely in the treatment of mild pain.

Exploratory research on structure activity relationships in
the *meperidine* series revealed the interesting fact that the
oxygen atom and carbonyl group of this molecule could often be
interchanged. That is, the so-called "reversed *meperidine*" (C)
still exhibits analgesic activity in experimental animals. (Note
that, except for the interchange, the rest of the molecule is
unchanged.)

An analog of the above "reversed" *pethidine, alphaprodine*
(114), has found application as an analgesic in the clinic.
Michael addition of methylamine to methyl methacrylate *(108)*

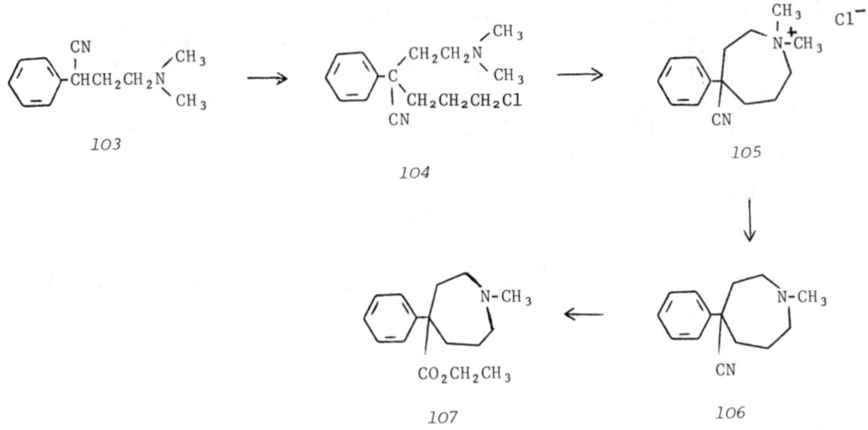

103 → 104 → 105

↓

107 ← 106

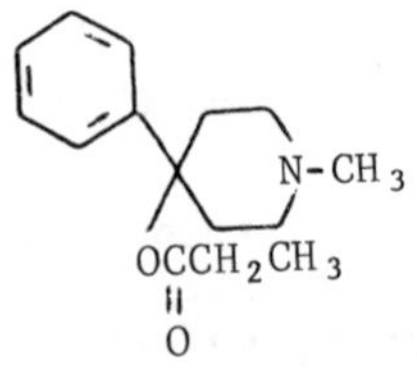

C

gives the amino ester, 109. Addition of ethyl acrylate in a
second conjugate addition leads to the diester (110). Treatment
of this last with base affords via Dieckmann cyclization, the
carbomethoxy piperidone (111). The direction of cyclization is
probably controlled by formation of the enolate obtained by
removal of the most acidic proton (i.e., that on the tertiary
carbon atom). Hydrolysis of the ester followed by decarboxylation gives the piperidone (112). It is highly likely that the
methyl group in this ketone occupies the equatorial position.
Reaction with phenylmagnesium bromide gives the corresponding
tertiary alcohol, 113, which affords alphaprodine (114)[38] on
acylation with propionic anhydride. Stereochemical assignment by
x-ray crystallography showed that the phenyl and methyl groups
bear a trans relation.[39] It is of note that this isomer is that
which would be produced from attack of the organometallic reagent
on 112 from the less-hindered side.

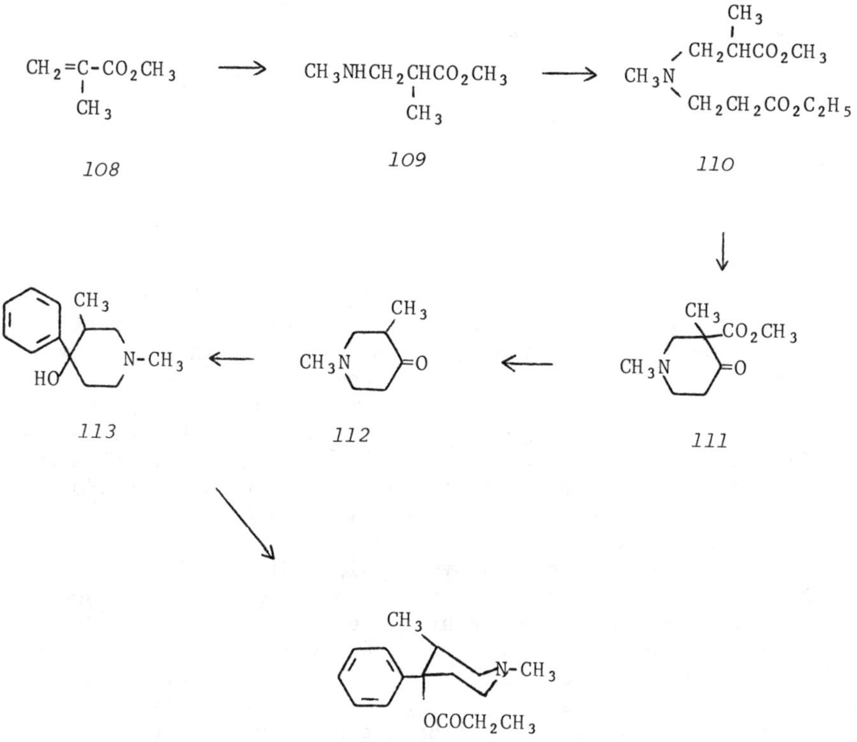

$$CH_2=C-CO_2CH_3 \longrightarrow CH_3NHCH_2CHCO_2CH_3 \longrightarrow$$

with CH_3 substituents below.

108 — 109 — 110

$$CH_3N \overset{CH_2CHCO_2CH_3}{\underset{CH_2CH_2CO_2C_2H_5}{\diagdown}}$$

110

113 ← 112 ← 111

114

The ring-contracted analog of alphaprodine is prepared by a variation of the scheme above. Alkylation of *109* with ethyl bromoacetate affords the lower homolog diester *(115)*. Dieckmann cyclization followed by saponification-decarboxylation yields the pyrrolidine *(116)*. Reaction with phenylmagnesium bromide leads to the condensation product *(117)*; acylation with propionic anhydride gives the analgesic agent *prolidine (118)*.[40]

Further chemical modification of the phenylpiperidine moiety has proven unusually fruitful in producing medicinal agents that affect the central nervous system. First, a series of compounds loosely related to the reversed meperidines produced several drugs with important antipsychotic activity. Further discussion of this pharmacologic activity, often referred to as major tranquilizer activity, will be found in the section on phenothiazines. The group led by Janssen took advantage of the chemistry of the

$109 \rightarrow$ $CH_3N \overset{\overset{\displaystyle CH_3}{\underset{\displaystyle |}{CH_2CH-CO_2CH_3}}}{\underset{\displaystyle CH_2CO_2C_2H_5}{}}$ $\rightarrow$ $CH_3N \overset{CH_3}{\underset{O}{\bigcirc}}$ $\rightarrow$ $CH_3N \overset{CH_3}{\underset{RO}{\bigcirc}}$

115   116

117, R=H
118, $R=\overset{O}{\overset{\|}{C}}CH_2CH_3$

ketone of 4-piperidone to produce several major tranqulizers that
bear only the slightest relation to *meperidine*. The circle was
finally closed with the finding that one of the agents developed
by this route—*fentanyl (141)*—is an extremely potent analgesic
agent in man. It would almost seem that informed chemical manipulation in the hands of chemists well versed in medicinal agents
on some molecule of known activity more often than not produces
compounds with biologic activity in some related areas.

The initial series of major tranquilizers consists of alkylated derivatives of 4-aryl-4-hydroxypiperidines. Construction
of this ring system is accomplished by a set of rather unusual
reactions. Condensation of methylstyrenes with formaldehyde and
ammonium chloride afford the corresponding hexahydro-1,3-oxazines
(119). Heating these oxazines in the presence of acid leads to
rearrangement with loss of water to the tetrahydropyridines.
Scheme 1 shows a possible reaction pathway for these transformations. Addition of hydrogen bromide affords the expected 4-bromo
compound *(121)*. This last is easily displaced by water to lead
to the desired alcohol *(122)*.[41] The side chain *(123)* is obtained
by Friedel-Crafts acylation of *p*-fluorobenzene with 4-chloro-
butyryl chloride. Alkylation of the appropriate arylpiperidinol
with *123* affords the desired butyrophenone derivative. Thus,
122a gives the important antipsychotic agent *haloperidol (124a)*.[42]
Similar reaction on *122b* leads to *trifluoperidol (124b)*,[43] while
122c gives *chlofluperidol (124c)*.

In a departure from the prototype molecule, the benzylpiperi-
done is first converted to the corresponding aminonitrile (a
derivative closely akin to a cyanohydrin) by treatment with aniline hydrochloride and potassium cyanide *(126)*. Acid hydrolysis
of the nitrile affords the corresponding amide *(127)*. Treatment
with formamide followed by reduction affords the spiro oxazinone
(128). The synthesis of the tranquilizer, *spiroperone (130)*,[44]
is completed by removal of the benzyl group by hydrogenolysis
(129), followed by alkylation with the butyrophenone side chain

(123).

Scheme 1

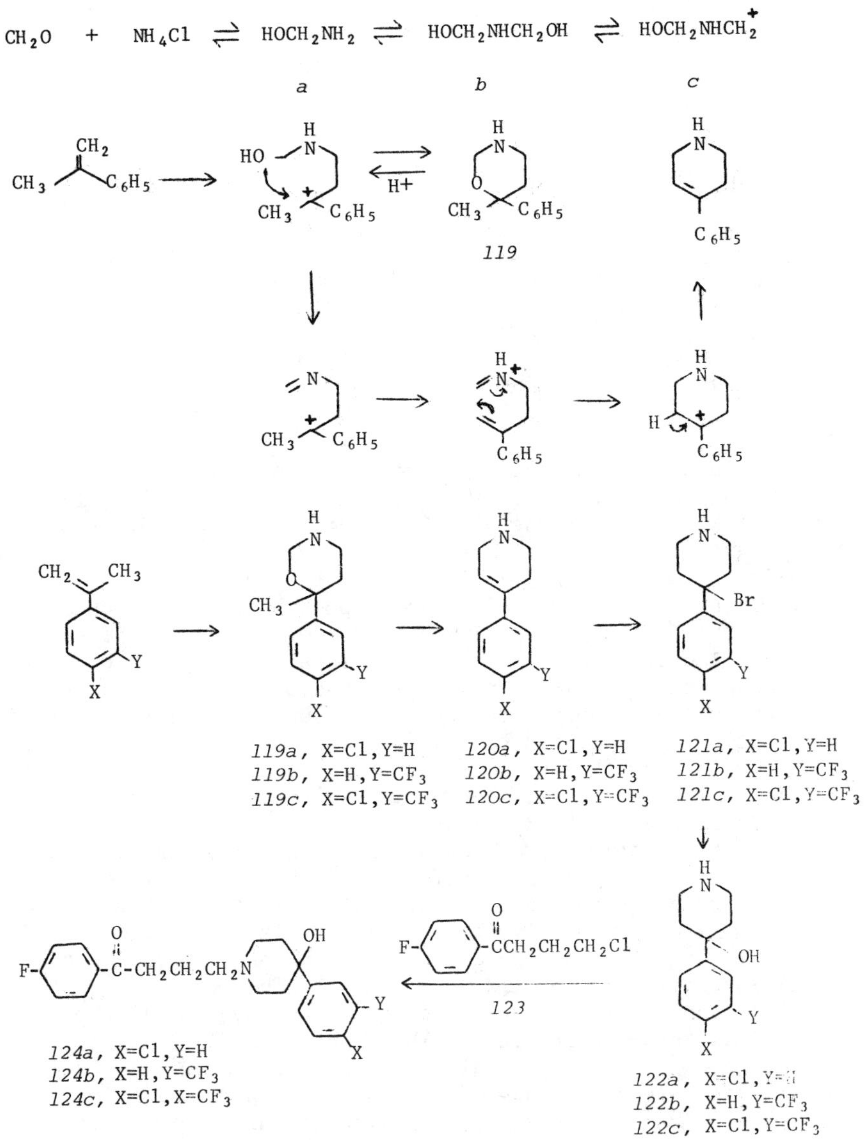

CH2O + NH4Cl ⇌ HOCH2NH2 ⇌ HOCH2NHCH2OH ⇌ HOCH2NHCH2+
a
b
c
H+
119
119a, X=Cl,Y=H
119b, X=H,Y=CF3
119c, X=Cl,Y=CF3
120a, X=Cl,Y=H
120b, X=H,Y=CF3
120c, X=Cl,Y=CF3
121a, X=Cl,Y=H
121b, X=H,Y=CF3
121c, X=Cl,Y=CF3
123
124a, X=Cl,Y=H
124b, X=H,Y=CF3
124c, X=Cl,X=CF3
122a, X=Cl,Y=H
122b, X=H,Y=CF3
122c, X=Cl,Y=CF3

In another essay in heterocyclic chemistry, the ketoester, *131* (an intermediate in the preparation of *125*), is allowed to react with *o*-phenylene diamine. While the transformations involved in formation of the isolated product *(132)* can be rationalized (decarbomethoxylation, enamine formation, and finally cyclization to a benzimidazolone, possibly with the carbon derived from the decarboxylation), the order of these reactions is far from clear. Catalytic reduction, interestingly, selectively cleaves the benzyl group. It is possible that the bulky substituent on the enamine protects this usually readily reducible function. Alkylation by means of the familiar side chain completes the synthesis of *droperidol (134)*.[45] This tranquilizer finds important use in conjunction with the analgetic *fentanyl* *(141)* in preanesthetic sedation.

Aminonitrile formation on *125* with potassium cyanide and piperidine hydrochloride affords the derivative, *135*. Hydrolysis as above gives the corresponding amide *(136)*. Debenzylation is accomplished by catalytic reduction. Alkylation of the secondary amine with the side chain *(96)* used in the preparation of diphenoxylate affords *pirintramide (138)* [46] This compound, interestingly enough, is an analgetic agent, although still one that follows the *morphine* rule, albeit in the side chain.

Finally, this general approach produced one of the most potent analgesics known, a compound that paradoxically does not fit the *morphine* rule at first sight. While details of the preparation are not readily available, in theory at least, treatment of piperidone, *139*, with aniline would be expected to give the

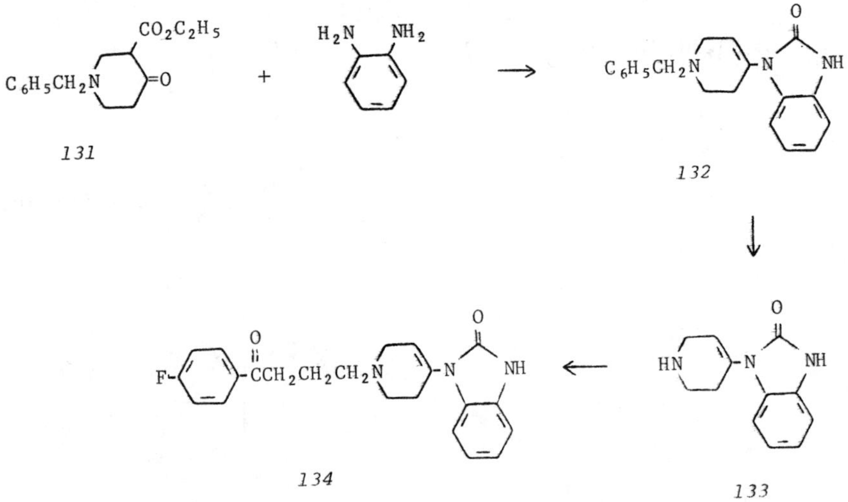

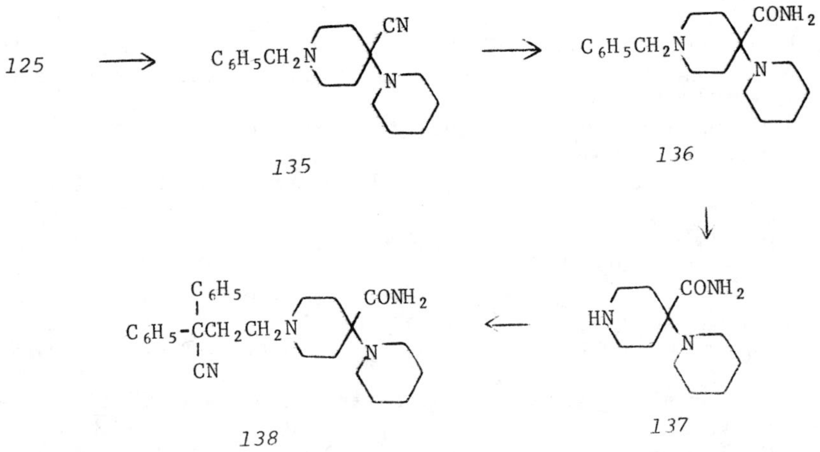

corresponding Shiff base *(140)*. Reduction then would afford the diamine *(141)*. Acylation with propionic anhydride would afford *fentanyl (142)*, an analgetic that shows some 50 times the potency of *morphine* in man.

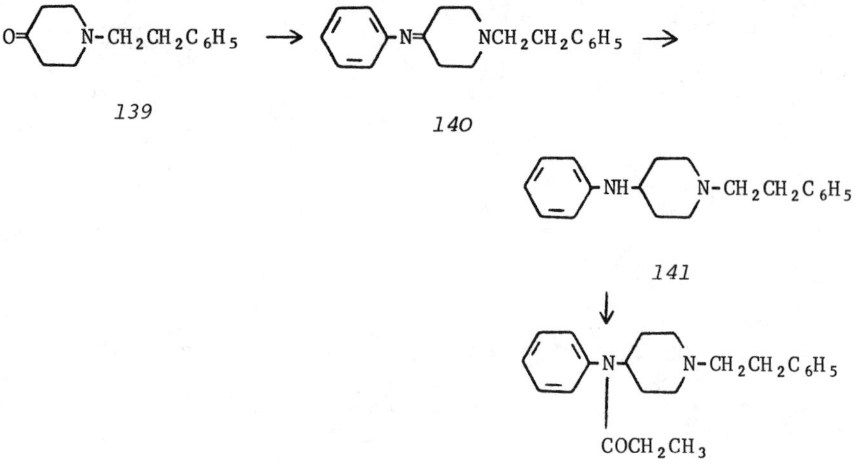

REFERENCES

1. (a) M. Gates and M. Tschudi, *J. Amer. Chem. Soc.*, *78*, 1380 (1956). (b) D. Elad and D. Ginsburg, *J. Amer. Chem. Soc.*, *76*, 312 (1954).
2. P. Chabrier, P. R. L. Ciuclicelly, and C. H. Genot, U. S. Patent 2,619,485 (1952).
3. L. Small, S. G. Turnbull, and H. M. Fitch, *J. Org. Chem.*, *3*, 204 (1939).
4. H. Wieland and E. Koralek, *Ann.*, *433*, 269 (1923).
5. K. Pfister and M. Tishler, U. S. Patent 2,715,626 (1955).
6. H. Rapoport, R. Nauman, E. R. Bissell, and R. M. Bouner, *J. Org. Chem.*, *15*, 1103 (1956).
7. J. Weijland and A. E. Erickson, *J. Amer. Chem. Soc.*, *69*, 869 (1942).
8. M. Freund and E. Speyer, *J. Prakt. Chem.*, *94*, 135 (1916).
9. U. Weiss, *J. Amer. Chem. Soc.*, *77*, 5891 (1955).
10. M. J. Lowenstein, British Patent 955,493 (1964).
11. L. Small and H. M. Fitch, *J. Amer. Chem. Soc.*, *58*, 1457 (1936).
12. L. Small, S. G. Turnbull, and H. M. Fitch, *J. Org. Chem.*, *3*, 204 (1939).
13. A. Grewe and A. Mondon, *Chem. Ber.*, *81*, 279 (1948).

14. O. Schider and A. Gussner, *Helv. Chim. Acta, 32*, 821 (1949).
15. O. Schider and A. Gussner, *Helv. Chim. Acta, 34*, 2211 (1951).
16. A. Grussner, J. Hellerbach, and O. Schider, *Helv. Chim. Acta, 40*, 1232 (1957).
17. O. Schider and J. Hellerbach, *Helv. Chim. Acta, 33*, 1437 (1950).
18. J. Hellerbach, A. Gussner, and O. Schnider, *Helv. Chim. Acta, 39*, 429 (1956).
19. E. L. May and J. H. Ager, *J. Org. Chem., 24*, 1432 (1959).
20. E. L. May and N. B. Eddy, *J. Org. Chem., 24*, 295 (1959).
21. S. Archer, N. F. Albertson, L. S. Harris, A. K. Pierson, and J. G. Bird, *J. Med. Chem., 7*, 123 (1964).
22. S. Archer, Belgian Patent 611,000 (1962).
23. O. Eisleb, *Chem. Ber., 74*, 1433 (1941).
24. A. L. Morrisson and H. Rinderknecht, *J. Chem. Soc.*, 1469 (1950).
25. R. H. Thorp and E. Walton, *J. Chem. Soc.*, 559 (1948).
26. J. Weijlard, P. Dorahovats, A. P. Sullivan, G. Purdue, F. K. Heath, and K. Pfister, *J. Amer. Chem. Soc., 78*, 2342 (1956).
27. R. J. Anderson, P. M. Frearson, and E. S. Stern, *J. Chem. Soc.*, 4088 (1956).
28. H. Morren, U. S. Patent 2,858,316 (1958).
29. P. M. Frearson, D. G. Hardy, and E. S. Stern, *J. Chem. Soc.*, 2103 (1960).
30. B. Elpern, P. Carabateas, A. E. Soria, L. N. Gardner, and L. Grumbach, *J. Amer. Chem. Soc., 81*, 3784 (1959).
31. T. D. Perine and N. B. Eddy, *J. Org. Chem., 21*, 125 (1956).
32. P. A. J. Janssen and N. B. Eddy, *J. Med. Chem., 2*, 31 (1960).
33. D. J. Dupre, J. Elks, B. Attems, K. N. Speyer, and R. M. Evans, *J. Chem. Soc.*, 500 (1949).
34. P. A. J. Janssen, A. H. Jagenau, and J. Huygens, *J. Med. Chem., 1*, 299 (1959).
35. A. L. Morrison and H. Rinderknecht, *J. Chem. Soc.*, 1469 (1950).
36. A. W. D. Aridon and A. L. Morison, *J. Chem. Soc.*, 1471 (1950).
37. J. Diamond, W. F. Bruce, and F. T. Tyson, *J. Org. Chem., 22*, 399 (1957).
38. A. Ziering, A. Motchane, and J. Lee, *J. Org. Chem., 22*, 1521 (1957).
39. F. R. Ahmed, W. H. Barnes, and G. Kartha, *Chem. Ind.*, 485 (1959).
40. J. F. Caralla, J. Daroll, M. J. Dean, C. S. Franklin, D. M. Temple, J. Wax, and C. V. Winder, *J. Med. Chem., 4*, 1 (1961).
41. C. S. Schmiddle and R. C. Mansfield, *J. Amer. Chem. Soc., 78*, 1702 (1956).

42. P. A. J. Janssen, C. VanDeWesteringhe, A. H. M. Jageneau, P.
    J. A. Demoen, B. F. K. Hermans, G. H. P. VanDaele, K. H. L.
    Schellekens, C. A. M. VanDerEycken, and C. J. E. Niemegeer,
    J. Med. Chem., *1*, 281 (1959).
43. P. A. J. Janssen, British Patent 895,309 (1962).
44. P. A. J. Janssen, U. S. Patent 3,125,578 (1964).
45. P. A. J. Janssen, Belgian Patent 626,307 (1963).
46. P. A. J. Janssen, Belgian Patent 606,856 (1961).

CHAPTER 16

Five-Membered Heterocycles
Fused to One Benzene Ring

1. BENZOFURANS

The spasmolytic agents described previously have in common substitution by basic nitrogen. Recently there has been developed a series of antispasmodic drugs that have as a common structural feature an oxygen-containing heterocyclic ring fused to a benzene ring. Two of the more important drugs, *khelin* and *chromoglycic acid*, possess six-membered heterocyclic rings and are discussed in the next section. The five-membered counterpart of these agents, *benziodarone (4)*, has found use as a coronary vasodilator.

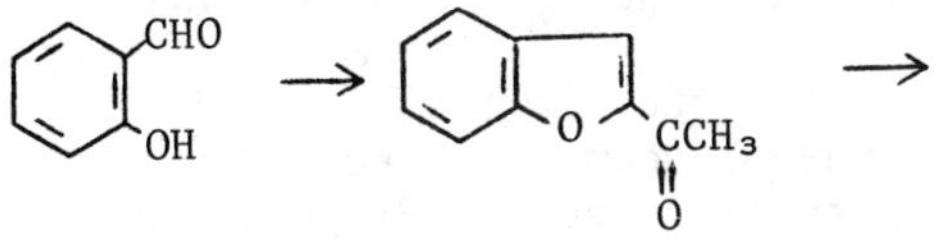

1

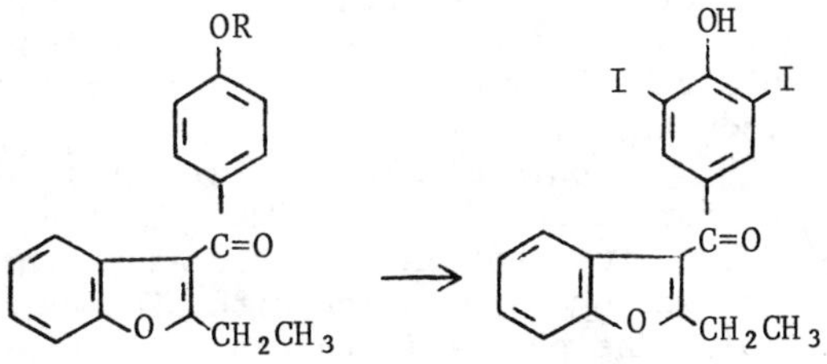

2, R=CH₃
3, R=H

4

313

Reaction of the potassium salt of salicylaldehyde with chloroacetone affords first the corresponding phenolic ether; aldol cyclization of the aldehyde with the ketonic side chain affords the benzofuran (1). Reduction of the carbonyl group by means of the Wolf-Kischner reaction affords 2-ethyl-benzofuran. Friedel-Crafts acylation with anisoyl chloride proceeds on the remaining unsubstituted position on the furan ring (2). The methyl ether is then cleaved by means of pyridine hydrochloride (3). Iodination of the phenol is accomplished by means of an alkaline solution of iodine and potassium iodide. There is thus obtained *benziodarone (4).*[1]

Research on novel fungal secondary metabolites resulted in the isolation of an interesting spiran, *griseofulvin (15)*, from fermentation beers of the mold *Penicillium griseofulvum*. This compound was eventually found to have activity against a series of pathogenic fungi rather than bacteria. Diseases such as ringworm of the body, scalp, feet, and nails constitute a group of fungal infections limited to the outer cutaneous layers known as superficial mycoses. These infections are unusually tenacious and even successful cures are often quickly followed by reinfection. *Griseofulvin* owes much of its effectiveness to the fact that the drug binds to the keratin cells which will eventually differentiate to form skin, hair, and so forth. These cells consequently become resistant to infection by the fungus. This mode of action also means that therapy is very slow; weeks to months are required for complete cure.

Although *griseofulvin* is probably still prepared commercially by extraction from fermentation beers, numerous total syntheses of the drug have been reported.

In the first of these,[2] the key step in the synthetic sequence involves an oxidative phenol coupling reaction patterned after the biosynthesis of the natural product. Preparation of the moiety that is to become the aromatic ring starts by methylation of phloroglucinol (5) with methanolic hydrogen chloride to give the dimethyl ether (6). Treatment of that intermediate with sulfuryl chloride introduces the chlorine atom needed in the final product (7).

Synthesis of the remaining half of the molecule starts with the formation of the monomethyl ether (9) from orcinol (8). The carbon atom that is to serve as the bridge is introduced as an aldehyde by formylation with zinc cyanide and hydrochloric acid (10). The phenol is then protected as the acetate. Successive oxidation and treatment with thionyl chloride affords the protected acid chloride (11). Acylation of the free phenol group in 7 by means of 11 affords the ester, 12. The ester is then rearranged by an ortho-Fries reaction (catalyzed by either titanium

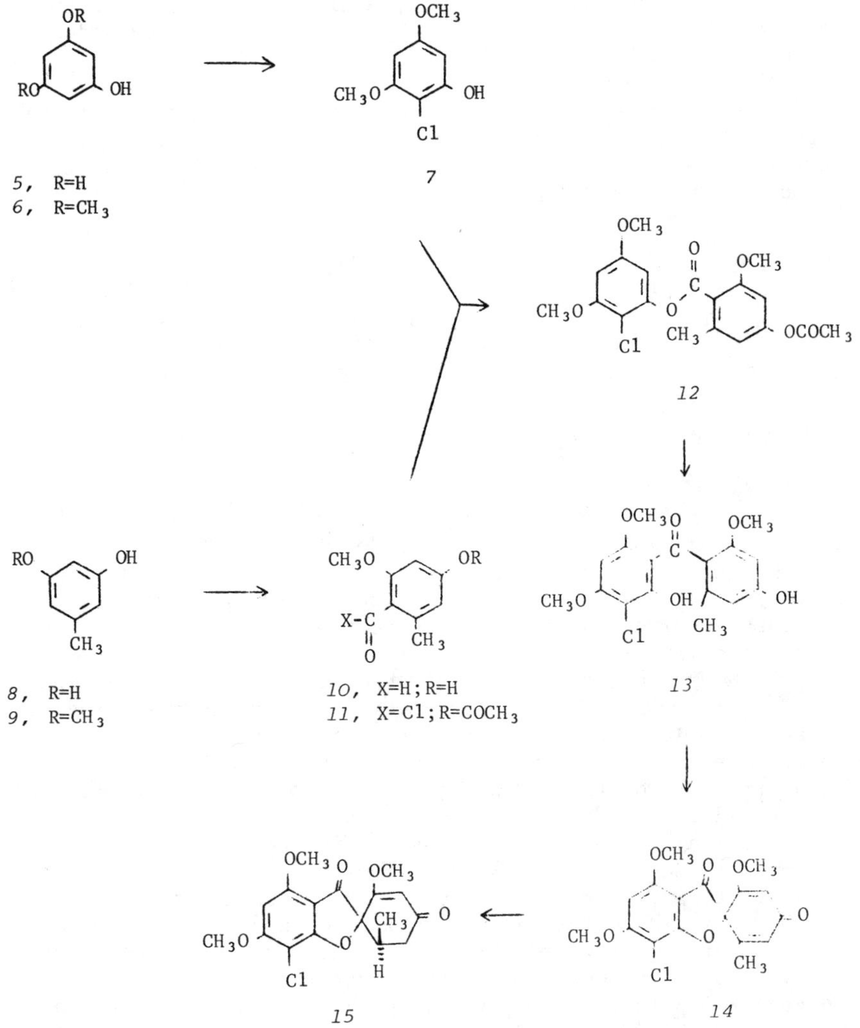

tetrachloride or ultraviolet irradiation) to give the hydroxy-
benzophenone, *13*, which contains, in their proper arrangement, all
the carbon atoms of the final product. Treatment with alkaline
ferricyanide produces the diradical (presumably on the phenol oxygen and the carbon bearing the carbonyl group); coupling leads to

the spiro compound, dehydrogriseofulvin *(14)*. Catalytic hydrogenation produces predominantly *d,l-griseofulvin (15)*, as the
other diastereoisomeric pair is apparently not favored under the
conditions used.

The second synthesis follows an entirely different synthetic
plan—one dependent upon a double-Michael reaction to establish
the spiran junction. Chlorophenol, *7*, is reacted with chloro-
acetylchloride to give coumaranone, *16*. This is treated with
methoxyethynyl propenyl ketone *(17)* (itself prepared by 1,2-

7   16   17

addition of lithium ethoxyacetylene to crotonaldehyde followed by
manganese dioxide oxidation of the doubly activated secondary carbinol function) in the presence of K *tert*-butoxide catalyst. The
ensuing double-Michael reaction is surprisingly stereospecific;
the enantiomeric diastereoisomers representing *d,l-griseofulvin*
(15) predominate.

Although well known to most chemists as an acid-base indica-
tor, *phenolphthalein (19)* in fact has a venerable history as a
laxative. (An apocryphal tale has it that it was at one time
added to some rather expensive white wines in order to foil
counterfeiters of that product; that is, only the authentic product would turn red on addition of caustic. One may imagine that
the medicinal use was thus discovered inadvertently to the discomfort of many a tastevin.) The biologic effect of this compound is irritation of the bowel of sufficient intensity to start
the peristalsis that leads eventually to evacuation. The low
toxicity of the drug as well as its otherwise innocuous nature
has led to its extensive over-the-counter use as a laxative.
Reaction of phthalic anhydride with phenol in the presence of any
one of a number of acid catalysts affords phenolphthalein *(19)*;
as an example, the reaction can be catalyzed by a mixture of zinc
chloride and thionyl chloride.[4] The acid base indicating properties depends on the opening of the phthalide to quinone, *20*,
above pH 9. Under some circumstances the drug is excreted as
the highly colored quinoid form. The resulting red feces and/or
urine can alarm the unprepared.

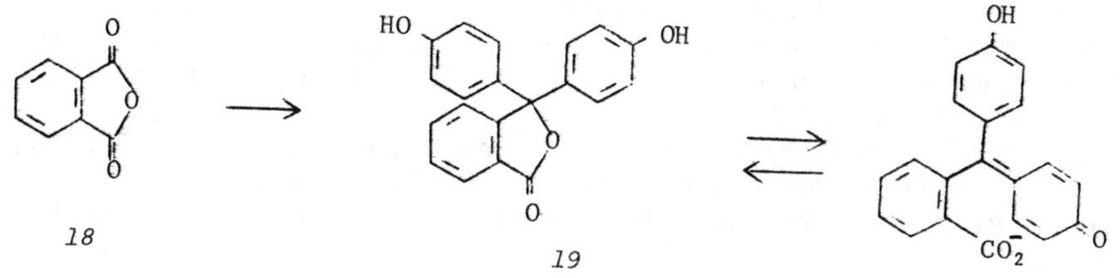

18

19

20

2. INDOLES

The presence of the indole moiety in many biologically active
alkaloids has long held out the promise that simpler compounds
built around this nucleus would provide useful drugs. Although
a great many such compounds have in fact shown biological activity, relatively few of these agents have found clinical use. It
is perhaps of note in this connection that the indole nucleus does
not confer on molecules any unique set of biological properties;
activities of indole seem to depend more on the nature of the
substituents.

Etryptamine (23) is a tryptamine derivative which has been
used as an antidepressant. Its synthesis involves the condensation of indole-3-carboxaldehyde (21) with the active methylene
group of 1-nitropropane to form the inner nitronium salt of the
substituted nitrovinyl indole (22). This then is readily reduced
to etryptamine (23).[5]

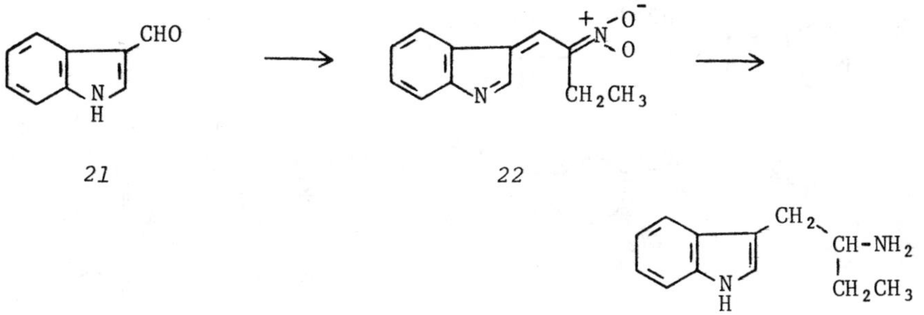

21   22

23

Iprindol (25) is yet another antidepressant drug that differs structurally from the classical tricyclic antidepressants. Condensation of phenylhydrazine and cyclooctanone by the Rogers-Corson modification of the Fischer indole synthesis affords the tricyclic intermediate, 24. The active hydrogen of 6,7,8,9,10-hexahydro-5H-cyclooct[b]indole (24) is removed by reaction with sodium metal in DMF and the resulting salt condensed with 3-dimethylaminopropyl chloride. There is thus obtained iprindol (25).[6]

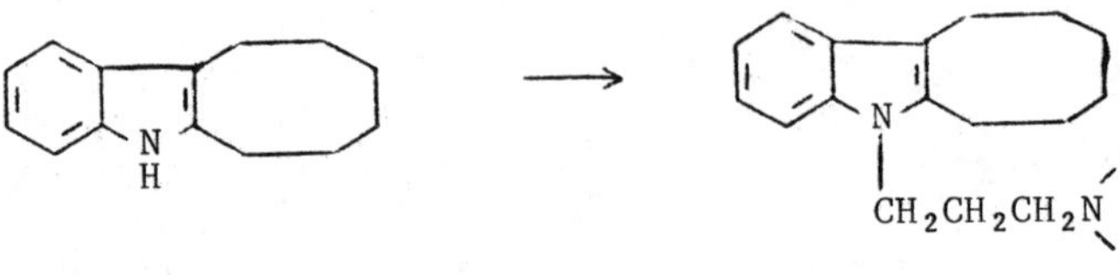

24

25

The pharmacologic activity of indomethacin (28) has occasioned much interest because it is one of the most potent of the nonsteroidal antiinflammatory agents. Its reported synthesis starts by conversion of 2-methyl-5-methoxyindoleacetic acid (26) to its tert-butyl ester (27) by means of dicyclohexylcarbodiimide and tert-butanol in the presence of zinc chloride. With the carboxyl group thus protected, the amine function of 27 is acylated with p-chlorobenzoyl chloride. The tert-butyl ester protecting group is then removed pyrolytically to give indomethacin (28). Although such esters are usually removed by treatment with acid, the instability of N-acyl indoles toward acid and base hydrolysis requires pyrolytic scision.

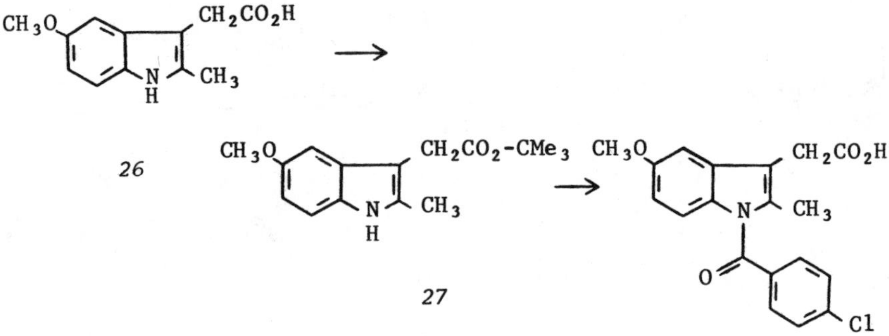

26

27

28

Fischer indole condensation of N_1-benzylphenyl-hydrazine and 1-methyl-4-piperidone under the usual acid conditions affords *mebhydroline (29)*,[8] an indole used as an antihistaminic agent.

29

3. INDOLE ALKALOIDS

Reserpine (30) is the most important of the related alkaloids found in extracts of the Indian Snakeroot, *Rawaulfia serpentina*. This root, which had been in use in folkloric medicine in the foothills of the Himalayas, was prescribed for treatment of ills ranging from snakebite through insomnia to insanity. Such diverse claims for natural product mixtures frequently turn out to be groundless when examined by the procedures of modern pharmacology. However, a sufficient number of these have provided leads for new drugs; therefore they cannot be lightly dismissed. In the case of *reserpine*, authentic reports on the pharmacology of the extracts were published in journals accessible to western scientists in 1949. By 1954 the alkaloid *reserpine* had been isolated and purified; its value as a medicinal agent was established soon after. This development was followed by the chemical structure determination. Initially, *reserpine* was used for the treatment of both hypertension and psychoses. The latter indication nearly coincided with the discovery of the tranquilizer *chlorpromazine*. It is of note that the two drugs ushered in the new era of psychopharmacology. The advent of a host of synthetic antipsychotic agents has diminished the importance of *reserpine* for this indication. The agent is still frequently prescribed in the treatment of hypertension, as are its closely related congener, *rescinnamine (31)*, and the semisynthetic compound *syrosingopine (32)*.

The preparation of *reserpine* by an ingenious and elegant total synthesis was completed astonishingly soon after completion of the structure determination.[9] The great demand for this drug coupled with shortage of material from natural sources because of overharvesting and embargoes led the group at Roussel-UCLAF to effect improvements on the Woodward synthesis.[10,11] For a time, at least, the synthetic material was competitive with *reserpine* obtained by extraction of the snake root.

Omission of the methoxyl group on the aromatic ring of the parent alkaloid affords *deserpidine (40)*, a drug that closely mimics the activity of *reserpine* itself. Total synthetic preparation of this agent has the important advantage of using tryptamine rather than the difficultly accessible 6-methoxy analog as starting material. A Czech group developed a total synthesis for *deserpidine* starting with the key intermediate in the Woodward synthesis *(33)*.[9] Reaction of that compound with zinc and acetic acid simultaneously effects elimination of the cyclic bromoether to the unsaturated ketone and reductively cleaves the lactone initially fused to the carbonyl group. In a single stage there is thus established both the substitution and stereochemistry of substituents for the future E ring. Acetylation gives the intermediate, *34*. Hydroxylation of the double bond with a trace of osmium tetroxide in the presence of potassium perchlorate leads to the glycol, *35*. Treatment of that compound with periodic acid first cleaves the glycol to the corresponding dialdehyde. The aldehyde adjacent the carbonyl group is cleaved again with loss of one carbon atom under the reaction conditions. Esterification of the crude product then affords the highly functionalized cyclohexane, *36*. Condensation of the aldehyde of *36* with the amine group of tryptamine serves to join ring E with the fragment that will form the remaining rings *(37)*.

Reduction of the imine with sodium borohydride leads to an intermediate amino-ester that cyclizes spontaneously to the δ-lactam function. Solvolysis of the acetyl group with methoxide followed by acylation of the hydroxyl group thus liberated with trimethoxybenzoyl chloride leads to *38*. Bischler-Napieralski cyclodehydration (phosphorus oxychloride) effects closure of the remaining ring. Reduction of the imine thus formed with sodium borohydride gives *39*. This, it should be noted, leads to the

30, R=OMe,X=-,R'=OMe
31, R=OMe,X=CH=CH,R'=OMe
32, R=OMe,X=-,R'=CO$_2$Et

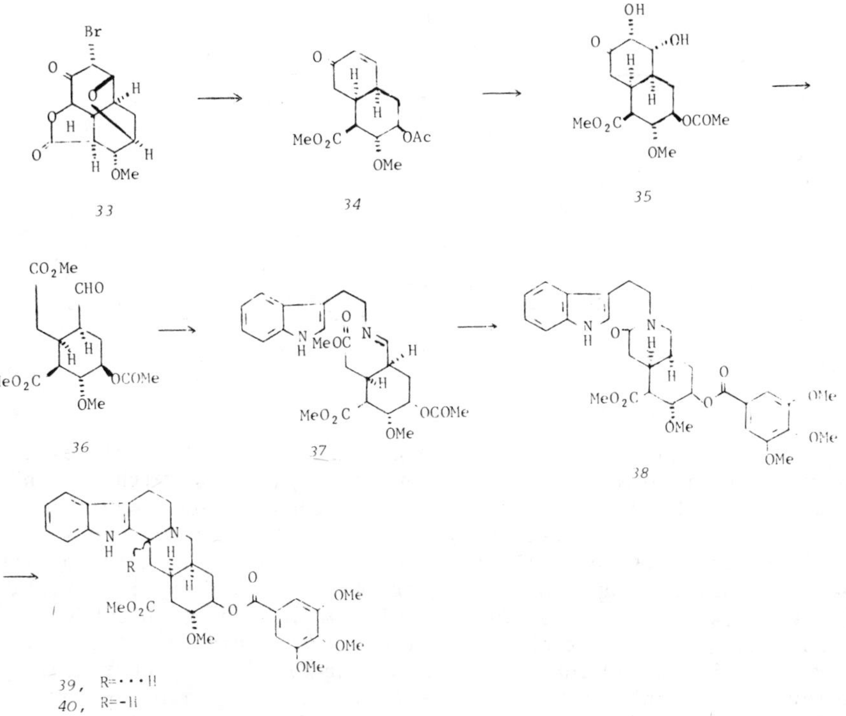

33   34   35

36   37   38

39, R=···H
40, R=-H

"wrong" stereochemistry at C_3, affording nearly inactive iso-deserpidine *(39)*. Formation of the iminoperchlorate salt followed by reduction with zinc-perchloric acid, however, leads to a mixture sufficiently rich in the natural stereoisomer that fractional crystallization gives satisfactory yields of *d,l-deserpidine (40)*. This is then resolved by crystallization of the *d*-camphor-sulfonic acid salt to complete the synthesis.

4.   ISOINDOLES

Chlorexolone (46) was apparently synthesized in following up the structural lead represented by *chlorothiazide*. It was felt, correctly, that significant alterations in pharmacologic profile would follow changes in the heterocyclic ring rather than the ring bearing the sulfonamide group. *Chlorexolone* was the best of a series of analogs prepared by this rationale.

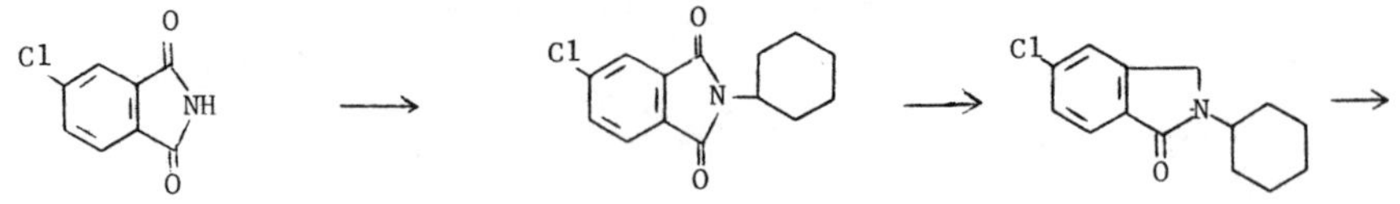

41   42   43

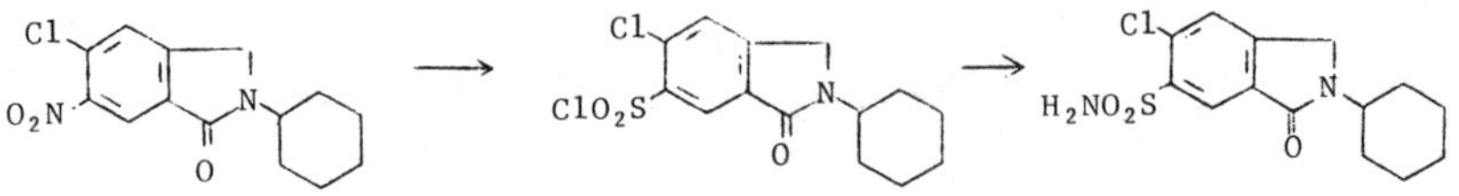

44   45   46

Imine exchange of 4-chlorophthalimide *(41)* with cyclohexyl-
amine gives intermediate, *42*. Reduction by heating with tin and
a mixture of hydrochloric-acetic acids leads to the *1*-oxoisoin-
dole system *(43)*. Nitration by means of potassium nitrate in
sulfuric acid mixture follows normal directing influences to give
44. The nitro group can then be transformed to a chlorosulfonyl
function *(45)* by successively reducing with stannic chloride,
diazotizing the resulting amine with nitrous acid, and then per-
forming a Sandmeyer reaction with sulfur dioxide and cuprous
chloride in acetic acid. Treatment with liquid ammonia gives
chlorexolone (46),[13] a diuretic agent used in treatment of hypertension.

Chlorthalidone (49) is another thiazide-like diuretic agent
that formally contains an isoindole ring. Transformation of the
amine in benzophenone, *47*, to a sulfonamide group by essentially
the same process as was outlined for chlorexolone *(46)* affords
intermediate *48*. This product cyclizes to the desired pseudo-
acid 1-ketoisoindole *(49)* on successive treatments with thionyl

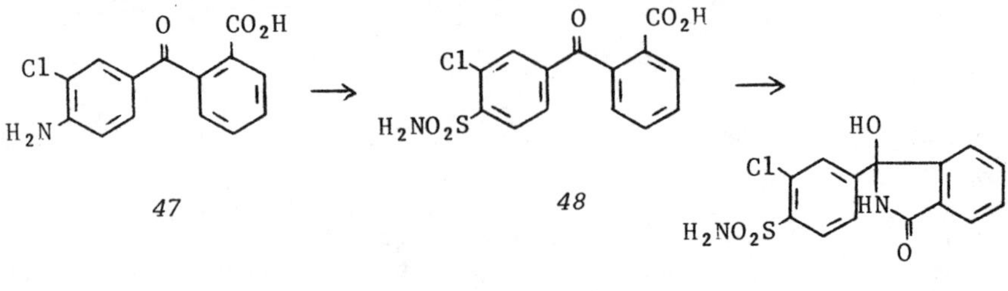

47   48

49

chloride and ammonia in aqueous ethanol.[14] Pseudoacids of this
general type are well known in organic chemistry; such acid-base
interactions of orthocarboxybenzophenones (50-51) have been
studied in some detail.

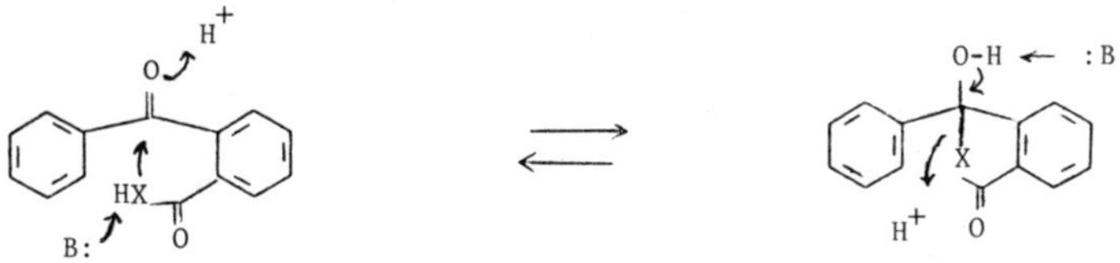

50, X=O,S or NH

51

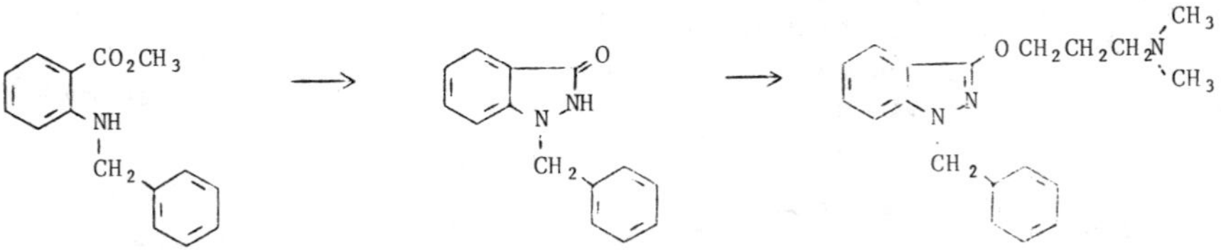

52

53

54

5. INDAZOLES

Indazoles can be considered as either azaindoles or azaisoindoles
depending on the reader's prejudice. Benzydamine (54) represents
a drug with this heterocyclic nucleus. Alkylation of the amine
of anthranilic acid methyl ester with benzyl chloride in the
presence of sodium acetate gives 52. Treatment with nitrous acid
leads to the nitrosoamine, which cyclizes spontaneously to the 3-
ketoindazole system, 53. This intermediate forms an ether of its
enol form on heating the sodium salt with 3-dimethylaminopropyl
chloride. There is thus obtained benzydamine (54),[15] a fairly
potent nonsteroidal antiinflammatory agent with significant antipyretic and analgesic properties.

6. BENZOXAZOLES

The antispasmodic agent, chlorzoxazone (56),[16] is obtained by
cyclization of the o-hydroxybenzformamide (55), a general method

for preparation of this ring system.

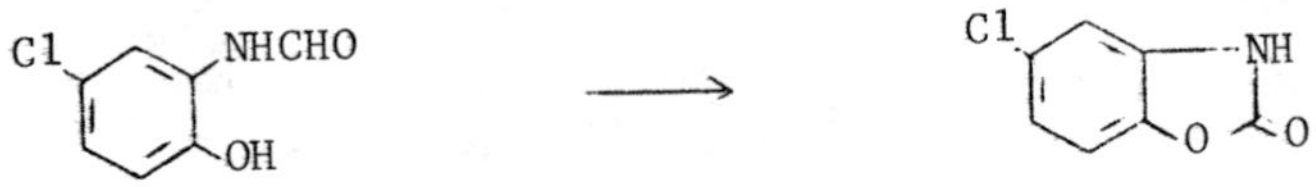

                          55   56

7. BENZIMIDAZOLES

Benzimidazoles are generally synthesized from *ortho*-diamino-ben-
zenes and carboxylic acid derivatives. The antihistaminic agent,
clemizole (60), for example, can be prepared by first reacting
ortho-diaminobenzene *(57)* with chloroacetic acid to form 2-chloro-
methylbenzimidazole *(58)*. Displacement of the halogen with pyro-

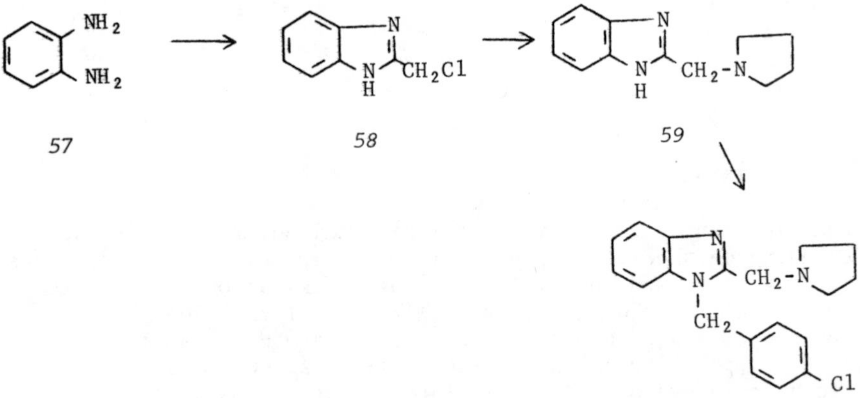

     57   58   59

                                    60

lidine leads to *59*; this is then converted to *clemizole (60)*[17]
by reacting its silver salt with *p*-chlorobenzylchloride. Although
chlormidazole (62)[18] is structurally very similar, it is used as
a spasmolytic and antifungal agent. It is prepared from 2-methyl-
benzimidazole *(61)* by treatment with sodium amide followed by *p*-
chlorobenzyl chloride.
     As shown previously, most strong analgesics incorporate some
portion of the *morphine* molecule; put another way, these agents

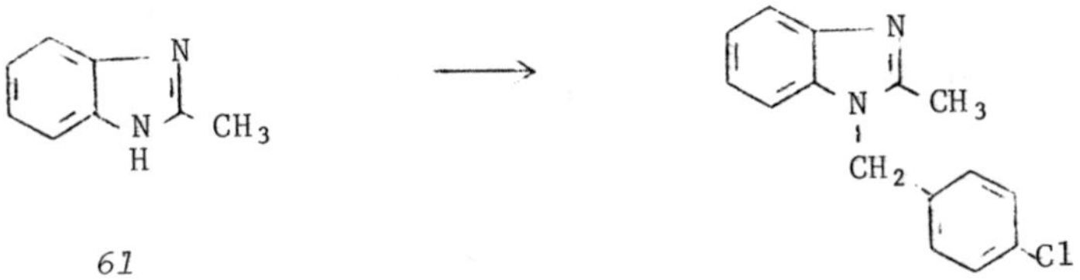

61   62

tend to conform to the *morphine* rule. Analgesics are known that
deviate from these structural requirements. Paradoxically, these
drugs, such as, for example, *fentanyl*, are often far more potent
than *morphine* itself as analgesics. A pair of closely related
benzimidazoles similarly show analgesic activity far in excess
of the natural prototype; at the same time these drugs also show
far higher addictive liability than *morphine*. Nucleophilic aromatic substitution of 2-diethylaminoethylamine on 2,4-dinitro-
chlorobenzene affords the corresponding amine; reduction with
ammonium sulfide selectively converts the nitro group adjacent to
the amine to the aniline *(64)*. Condensation of that ortho diamine
with the iminoether *(65)* from *p*-chlorophenylacetonitrile affords
clonitazine (66a).[19] Condensation with the iminoether containing
the para ethoxy group *(65b)* leads to *etonitazine (66b)*.[19]

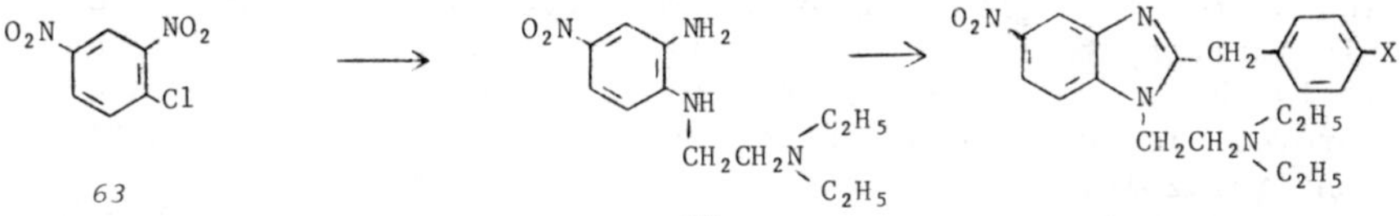

63   64

66a, X=Cl
66b, X=OC$_2$H$_5$

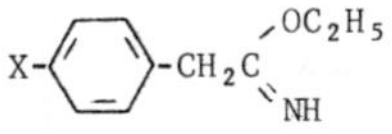

65a, X=Cl
65b, X=OC$_2$H$_5$

Changing the substitution pattern on the benzimidazole
greatly alters the biologic activity. Thus, inclusion of a thiazole ring affords *thiabendazole (70)*, a drug used for the treatment of helminthiasis.

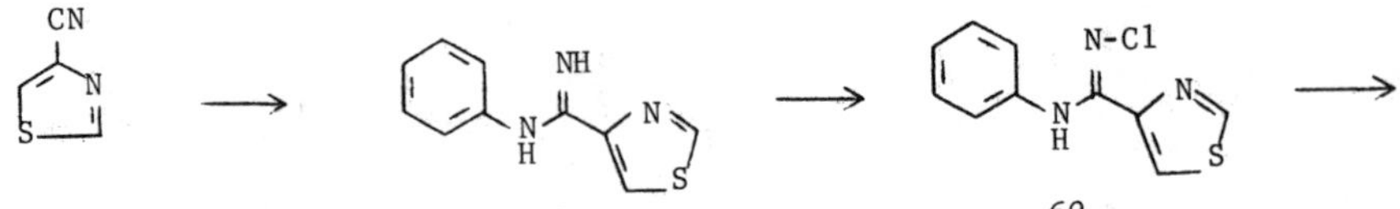

67   68   69

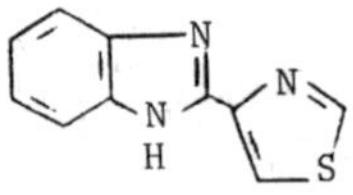

70

Intermediate arylamidine, 68, is prepared by the aluminum chloride-catalyzed addition of aniline to the nitrile function of 4-cyanothiazole (67). Amidine, 68, is then converted to its *N*-chloro analog (69) by means of sodium hypochlorite. On base treatment, this apparently undergoes a nitrene insertion reaction to produce *thiabendazole (70)*.[20]

8.   BENZOTHIAZOLES

The sulfonamide group has been used successfully to confer diuretic activity to both aromatic and simple heterocyclic compounds. It is therefore not unexpected to find a similar effect in a heterocycle fused to a benzene ring. Reaction of the substituted benzothiazole, 71, with sodium hypochlorite in a mixture of sodium hydroxide and ammonia affords the sulfenamide, 72, probably by the intermediacy of the sulfenyl chloride.

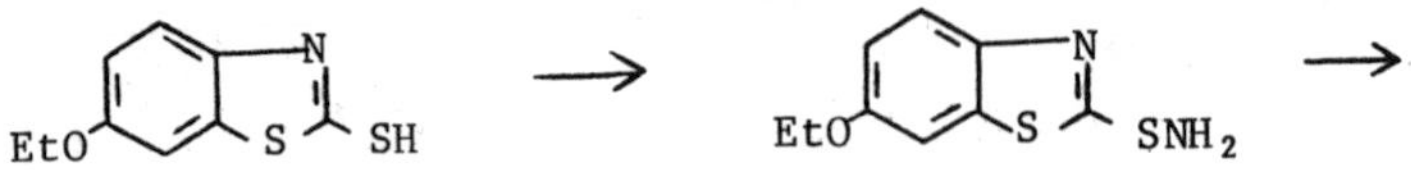

71   72

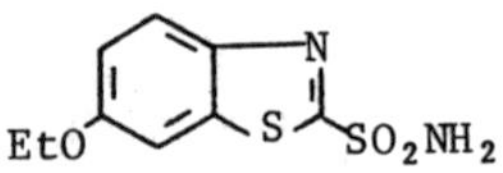

73

In the key step, oxidation with permanganate in acetone leads from the sulfenamide to the sulfonamide. There is thus obtained *ethoxysolamide (73)*.[21]

The antifungal agent, *dianithazole (76)*,[22] is prepared by cleaving the ether function of 2-dimethylamino-6-ethoxybenzothiazole *(74)* with aluminum chloride in chlorobenzene and then alkylating the sodium salt of the resulting phenol *(75)* with 2-diethylaminoethyl chloride.

A dicarbocyanine dye, *dithiazinine (79)*,[23] is used as a broad-spectrum anthelmentic agent, although, interestingly, it seems to have been prepared initially for use in photographic emulsions. It is made by heating 2-methylbenzothiazole ethiodide *(77)* with the malondialdehyde equivalent, β(ethylmercapto)-acrolein diethylacetal *(78)* in the presence of pyridine. There apparently ensues a sequence of addition-elimination reactions; quenching the reaction mixture with potassium iodide solution results in separation of green crystals of *dithiazanine* iodide *(79)*.

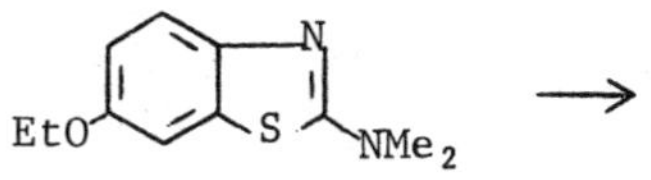

74

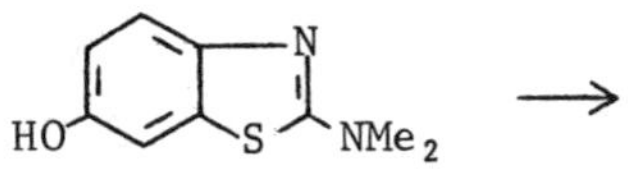

75

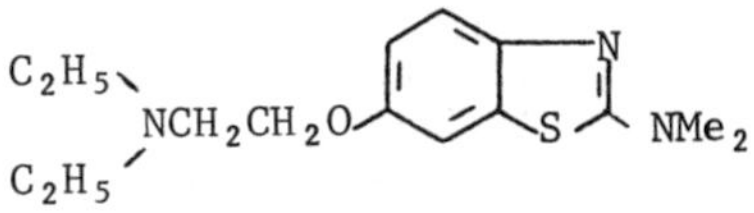

76

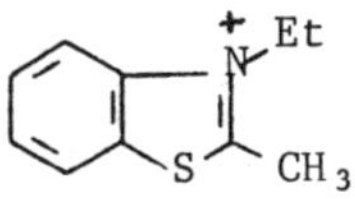

77

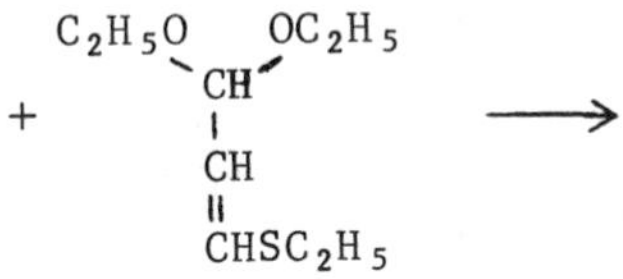

78

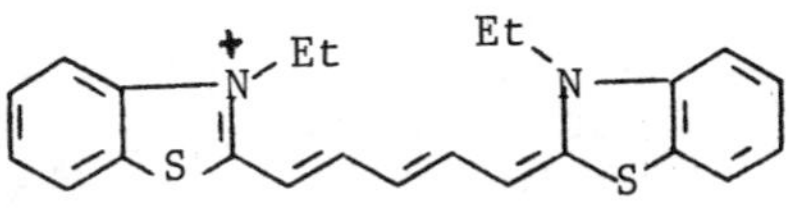

79

REFERENCES

1. N. P. Buu Hoi and C. Beaudet, U. S. Patent 3,021,042 (1971).
2. D. Taub, C. H. Kuo, H. L. Slates, and N. L. Wendler, *Tetrahedron, 12*, 1 (1963).
3. G. Stork and M. Tomasz, *J. Amer. Chem. Soc., 86*, 471 (1964).
4. H. R. Beaudet, U. S. Patent 2,527,939 (1950).
5. R. V. Heinzelman, W. C. Anthony, D. A. Little, and J. Szmuszkovicz, *J. Org. Chem., 25*, 1548 (1960).
6. L. M. Rice, E. Hertz, and M. E. Freed, *J. Med. Chem., 7*, 313 (1964).
7. T. Y. Shen, R. L. Ellis, T. B. Windholz, A. R. Matzuk, A. Rosegay, S. Lucas, B. E. Witzel, C. H. Stammer, A. N. Wilson, F. W. Holly, J. D. Willet, L. H. Sarett, W. J. Holtz, E. A. Rislay, G. W. Nuss, and C. A. Winter, *J. Amer. Chem. Soc., 85*, 488 (1963).
8. U. Horlein, *Chem. Ber., 87*, 463 (1954).
9. R. B. Woodward, F. E. Bader, H. Bickel, A. J. Frey, and R. W. Kierstead, *J. Amer. Chem. Soc., 78*, 2023; 2657 (1956); *Tetrahedron, 2*, 1 (1958).
10. L. Velluz, G. Muller, R. Joly, G. Nomine, A. Allais, J. Warnant, R. Bucort, and J. Jolly, *Bull. Soc. Chim. Fr.,* 145 (1958).
11. L. Velluz, G. Muller, R. Joly, G. Nomine, J. Mathieu, A. Allais, J. Warnant, J. Valls, R. Bucort, and J. Jolly, *Bull. Soc. Chim. Fr.,* 673 (1958).
12. E. Adlerova, L. Blaha, M. Borovicka, I. Ernest, J. O. Jilek, B. Kakac, L. Novak, M. Rajsner, and M. Protiva, *Coll. Czech. Chem. Commun., 25*, 221 (1960); L. Blaha, J. Weichet, J. Zvacek, S. Smolik, and B. Kakac, *Coll. Czech. Chem. Commun., 25*, 237 (1960).
13. E. V. Cornish, G. E. Lee, and W. R. Wragg, *Nature, 197*, 1296 (1963).
14. W. Graf, E. Girod, E. Schmid, and W. G. Stoll, *Helv. Chim. Acta, 42*, 1085 (1959).
15. Anon., French Patent 1,382,855 (1964). *Chem. Abstr., 62*, 13,155a (1965).
16. D. F. Marsh, U. S. Patent 2,895,877 (1950).
17. D. Jerchee, H. Fischer, and M. Kracht, *Ann., 575*, 173 (1952).
18. S. Herring, H. Keller, and H. M. Muckier, U. S. Patent 2,876,233 (1959).
19. A. Hunger, J. Kebrle, A. Rossi, and K. Hoffman, *Experientia, 13*, 400 (1957).
20. V. J. Grenda, R. E. Jones, G. Gae, and M. Sletzinger, *J. Org. Chem., 30*, 259 (1965).
21. Anon., British Patent 795,194 (1958); *Chem. Abstr., 52*,

20,212a (1958).
22. N. Steiger and O. Keller, U. S. Patent 2,578,757 (1951).
23. J. Kendall and H. D. Edwards, U. S. Patent 2,412,815 (1946).

CHAPTER 17

Six-Membered Heterocycles
Fused to One Benzene Ring

1. COUMARINS AND CHROMONES

Clotting of blood is the body's first line of defense against
injuries that compromise the integrity of the vasculature. The
process of clotting, or coagulation, in essence consists in the
polymerization and cross linking of a soluble serum protein, pro-
thrombin, to a hard insoluble polypeptide known as fibrin. Situations do obtain in which it is desirable to retard or even sus-
pend the clotting mechanism. Major surgery is often accompanied
by a state known as hypercoagulability; coagulation occurs even
within apparently sound vessels to form clots that can block the
blood supply to vital organs. Diseases of the circulation such
as thrombosis and phlebitis can be controlled by lowering the
coaguability of blood. Although still subject to some controversy, anticoagulant therapy has been used in the treatment of
stroke.

The development of anticoagulant drugs owed its start to an
investigation of a disease of cattle characterized by massive
hemorrhages. An epidimiologic study revealed that the disease
was in fact caused by a factor in the animal's diet; specifically,
the affected cattle had fed on spoiled sweet clover. Isolation
of the active compound led to its identification as the hydroxycoumarin derivative, 3. The degradative structural assignment
was then confirmed by total synthesis. Acylation of methyl sali-
cylate with acetic anhydride affords the intermediate, 1. Strong
base forms the carbanion on the acetyl methyl group; this then
adds to the carbonyl group of the adjacent ester. Elimination of
methanol affords the coumarin (2). Condensation of that product
with formaldehyde leads to the addition of two molecules of the
heterocycle to the aldehyde in a well-known reaction of enols.

There is thus obtained *bishydroxycoumarin (3)*.[1] Subsequent pharmacologic and clinical work revealed this compound to be an effective anticoagulant drug in humans.   It is of note that none of
the synthetic anticoagulants shows in vitro activity. Rather,
these compounds owe their effect to inhibition of synthesis by
the liver of one of the co-factors necessary for coagulation.

Further work in this area showed that only one of the coumarin rings was needed for biologic activity. Condensation of
the hydroxyacetophenone, *4*, with diethyl carbonate affords 4-
hydroxycoumarin *(2)*. The reaction may involve the β-ketoester
(5); cyclization of this would afford 2. Alternately, the reagent
may first give the O-acyl derivative; cyclization as above will
give the same product. Michael condensation of the coumarin with
benzalacetone *(6)* affords the anticoagulant *warfarin* (named
after its place of origin: Wisconsin Alumni Research Foundation,
WARF) *(7)*.[2] The same reaction with *p*-nitrobenzalacetone
(8) affords *acenocoumarole (9)*.[3] It might be mentioned in passing
that one of the largest uses of *warfarin* is in fact as a rat poi-
son; animals that ingest the drug in large amounts simply bleed
to death.
      A change in the pK of the molecule by elimination of the
acidic enol function and inclusion of basic nitrogen leads to a
marked change in biologic activity. That agent, *chromonar (13)*,[4]
shows activity as a coronary vasodilator. Alkylation of ethyl
acetoacetate with 2-chlorotriethylamine affords the substituted
ketoester *(10)*. Condensation with resorcinol in the presence of
sulfuric acid affords directly the substituted coumarin *(11)*.
The first step in the sequence may involve Friedel-Crafts-type
condensation of resorcinol with the enolate of *10* to afford the
unsaturated ester, *11*. Alkylation of the free phenol on *12* by
means of ethyl bromoacetate affords *chromonar (13)*.[4]

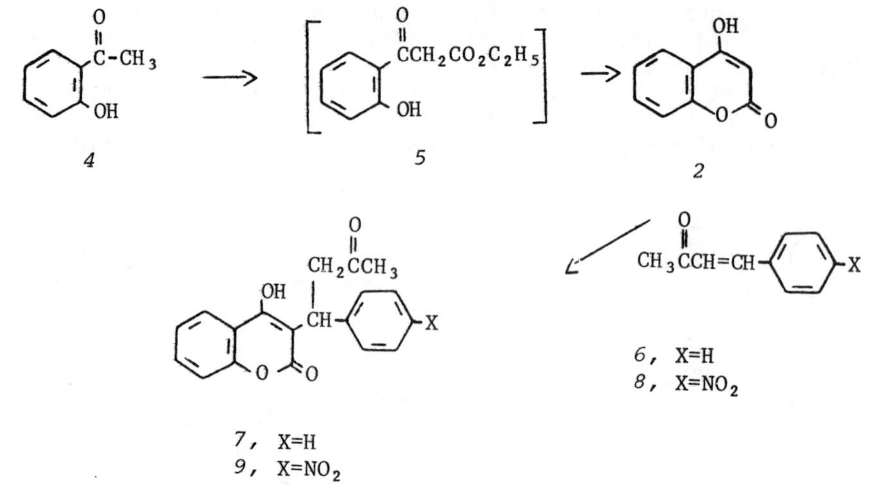

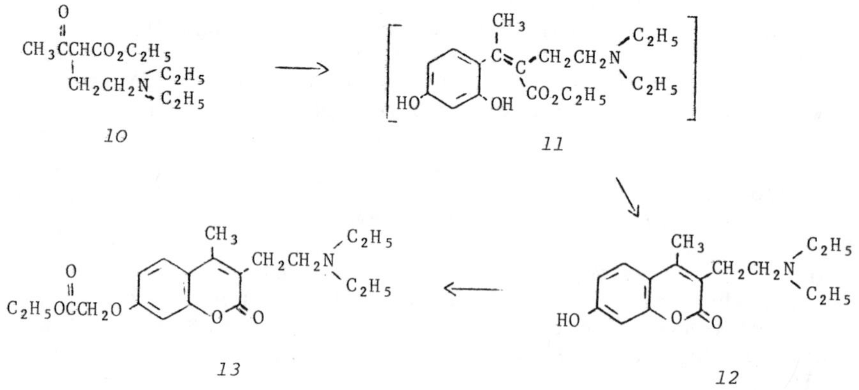

4   5   2

7, X=H
9, X=NO₂

6, X=H
8, X=NO₂

10   11

13   12

The psoralens are a family of naturally occurring furocou-
marins widely distributed in nature. The crude plant products
have a long folkloric history as agents that promote the development of suntans. These products are distinguished from the cos-
metic tanning agents in that they are orally active. These drugs
have clinical utility in allowing extremely fair-skinned individuals to develop tolerance to sunshine.
    Preparation of one of the natural products starts with
Friedel-Crafts acylation of pyrocatechol with chloroacetic acid
by means of phosphorus oxychloride (14). Treatment of the result-

ing haloketone with sodium ethoxide leads to cyclization with the
adjacent phenol (15). Catalytic hydrogenation serves to reduce
the carbonyl to a methylene group (16). Condensation of the product with malic acid in sulfuric acid serves to build the coumarin ring in a single step (18). The initial step in this
sequence may involve decarboxylation to malonic acid-aldehyde;
reaction of the enolate of that product with the aromatic ring
would afford an intermediate such as 17. Cyclization with the
phenolic hydroxyl followed by decarboxylation would then give
18.) Etherification of the remaining phenol is accomplished by
means of diazomethane (19). Dehydrogenation with palladium on
carbon in diphenyl ether completes the synthesis of methoxsalen
(20).[5]

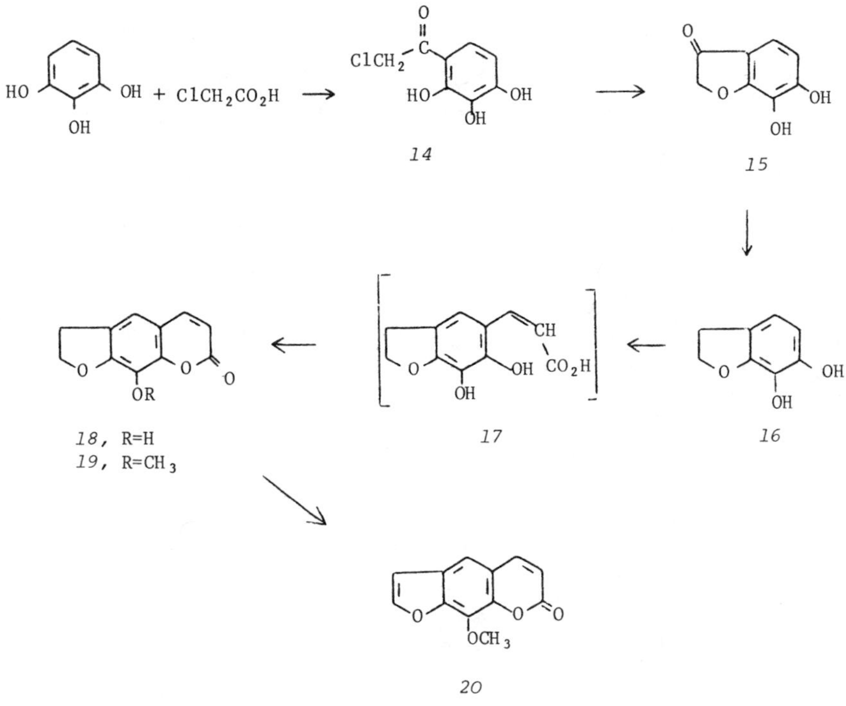

18, R=H
19, R=CH$_3$

14

15

17

16

20

The synthesis of the psoralen containing a methyl rather
than methoxy group on the aromatic ring starts with construction
of the coumarin ring. Knoevenagel-like condensation of malonic
acid with the substituted salicylaldehyde, 21, affords initially

the unsaturated acid (22). This is then cyclized to the coumarin (23) without prior purification. Decarboxylation completes preparation of the coumarin ring (24). Alkylation of the phenol by means of allyl bromide gives the allyl ether (25). This is converted to the C-allyl compound (26) by the thermal Claisen rearrangement; acetylation with acetic anhydride affords 27. Bromination followed by saponification of the acetate leads to the dibromophenol (28). Solvolysis of this compound in base leads to displacement of halogen by phenoxide to give the dihydrofuran (29). Elimination of the remaining bromine presumably first gives the exocyclic methylene compound. This presumed intermediate is in fact not observed. The overall product from the last reaction is the fully conjugated isomer trioxsalen (30).[6]

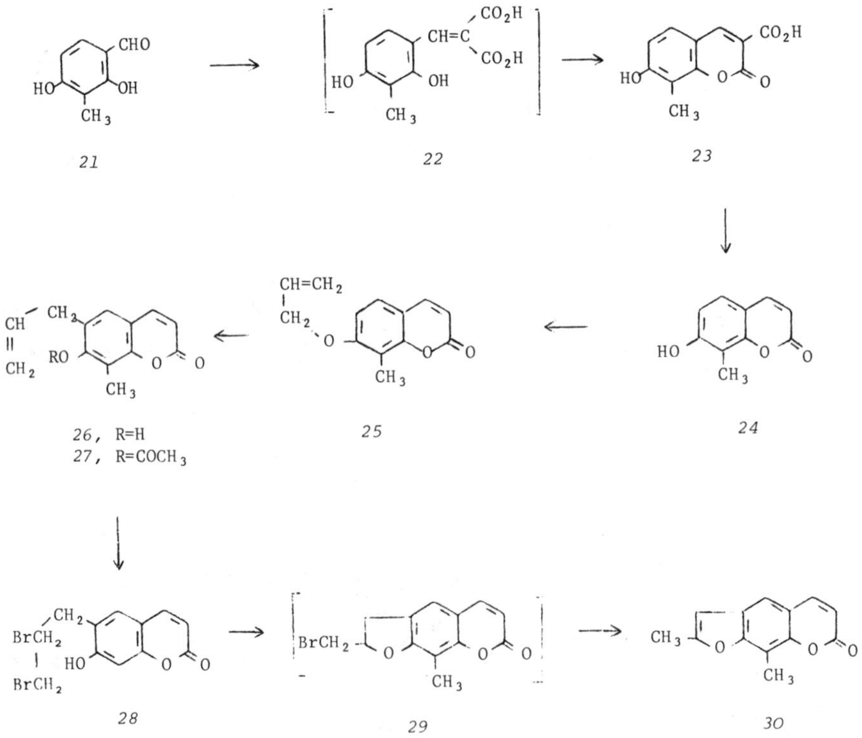

One of the few nonnitrogenous compounds to show spasmolytic activity is a rather simple chromone. Acylation of the phenolic ketone, 31, with the half ester-half acid chloride from oxalic

acid presumably first gives the C-acylated derivative (*32*, shown
as the enol). This cyclizes to the chromone under the reaction
conditions (*33*). An alternate path of course involves O-acyla-
tion followed by aldol cyclization. Saponification (*34*) followed
by decarboxylation affords *methylchromone (35).*[7]

31

32

33, R=CO$_2$C$_2$H$_5$
34, R=CO$_2$H
35, R=H

    Khellin is a natural product closely related to the psora-
lens in which a chromone ring has been substituted for the coumarin. The plant material has been used since ancient times as a
folk remedy; modern pharmacologic work has confirmed the bronchiodilating and antispasmodic activity of *khellin*. The synthesis
outlined below, it should be noted, is selected from a half-dozen
or so reported within the last quarter century.
    Acylation of the hydroquinone derivative, *35*, affords the
only possible product, acetophenone, *36*. The less-hindered phenol
is then preferentially converted to its allyl ether (*37*) and the
remaining phenolic function converted to the *p*-toluenesulfonyl
ester (*38*). In an operation similar to one employed in psoralen
synthesis above, the ether is then heated so as to bring about
the electrocyclic rearrangement to the C-allylated phenol (*39*).
Ozonization of the double bond gives the corresponding phenylacet-
aldehyde (*40*). This is then cyclized without prior isolation to
the furan and the tosylate removed by saponification (*41*). This
is an interesting reminder that a benzofuran is formally a
cyclized form of an *o*-hydroxyphenylacetaldehyde. Condensation of
41 with ethyl acetate at the acetyl methyl group affords the
corresponding acetoacetate (*42*). Cyclization of this last product
affords *khellin (43).*[8]

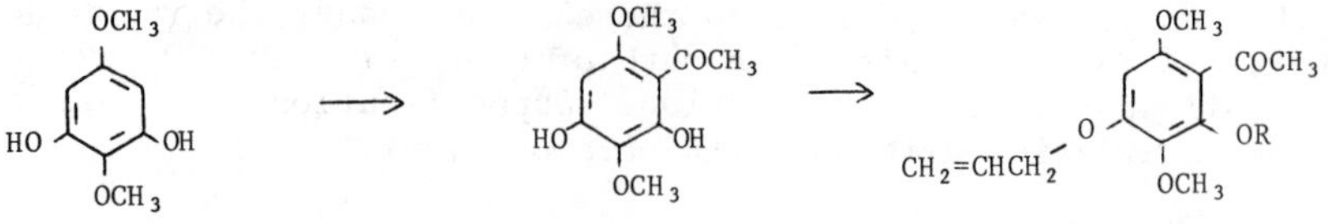

35   36   37, R=H
                                                        38, R=p-SO$_2$C$_6$H$_4$CH$_3$

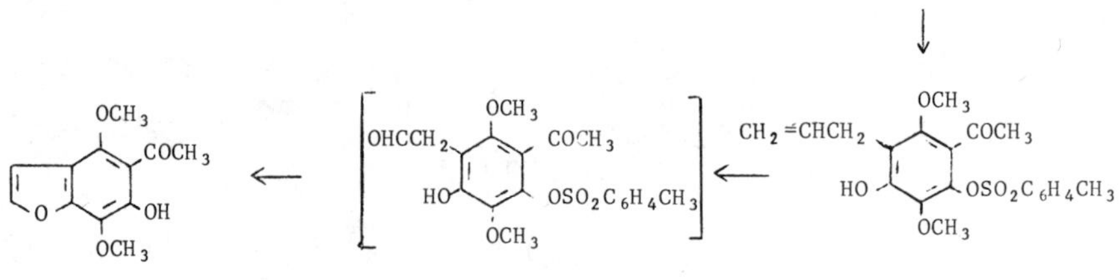

41   40   39

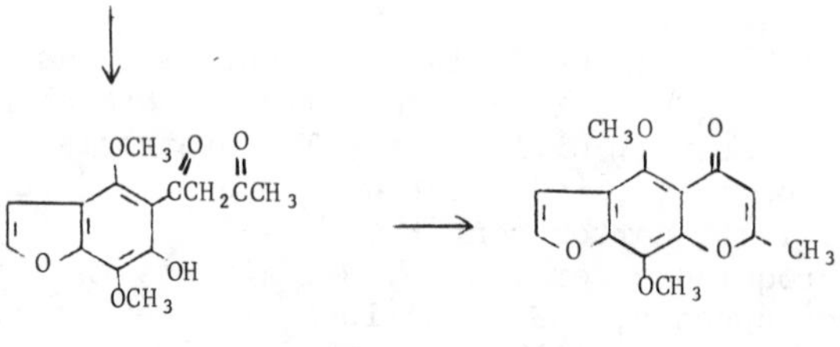

42   43

Perhaps one of the most effective agents currently available for the treatment of the bronchial spasms attendant to asthma is a synthetic agent that incorporates the chromone moiety.

Alkylation of the dihydroxyacetophenone, 44, with epichlorohydrin results in condensation of two molecules of the phenol with the latent glycerol (45). Reaction of the intermediate with ethyl oxalate affords the chromone ester, 46. Saponification leads to the bronchiodilator *cromoglycic acid* (47). The agent is usually administered by oral insufflation as its extremely insoluble disodium salt.

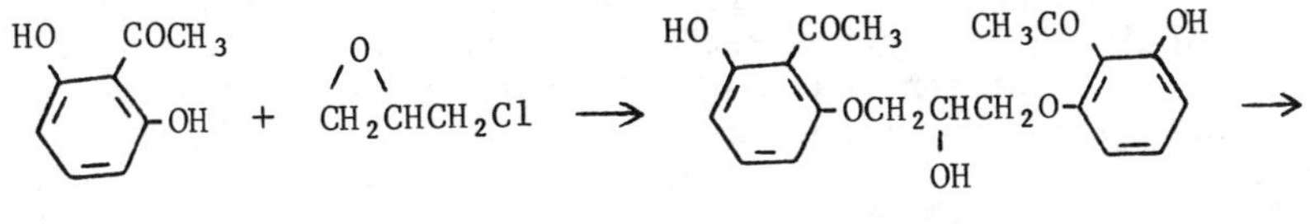

44   45

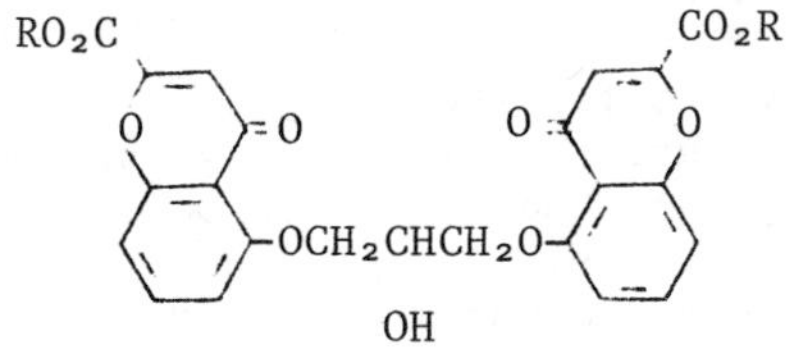

46, R=C$_2$H$_5$
47, R=H

2. QUINOLINES

One of the world's most widespread diseases is malaria. Although virtually completely eradicated in the United States, almost one-third of the world's population is exposed to the ravages of this disease. Malaria in man is caused by several species of proto-zoan parasites known as *plasmodia*. The organism has an extremely complex life cycle requiring dwelling times in both a mosquito and a vertebrate for multiplication. The multiplicity of forms through which the parasite progresses in these hosts means dif-ferences in drug sensitivity at various stages in the life cycle of a plasmodium. This in part explains the wide structural var-iations found among antimalarial agents, since different drugs are effective against plasmodia at different times in their life cycle. It is of note that antibiotics are of limited value in the treatment of malaria.

The oldest effective drug for the treatment of this disease is indisputably *quinine*. Although the antipyretic activity of cinchona bark was known to the Incas, it remained for the Jesuit missionaries to uncover its antimalarial properties in the early seventeenth century. The advance of organic chemistry led to the isolation and identification of the alkaloid, *quinine*, as the active compound at the turn of this century. The emerging clini-cal importance of this drug led up to the establishment of cin-chona plantations in the Dutch East Indies. This very circum-

stance brought on major efforts towards the development of synthetic antimalarial agents with each World War. In the first
such conflict, Germany was cut off from its supplies of *quinine*
and sought eagerly for some synthetic substitute. This effort
continued into the 1920s and was eventually rewarded with clinically useful antimalarial drugs. The Second World War saw the
United States deeply involved in a war in a fertile breeding
ground for malaria—the jungles of the South Pacific—and the
Japanese in control of the quinine plantations. A major program
was mounted in this country that resulted in the preparation of
numerous effective antimalarial agents. The war in Vietnam was
fought in malaria country. Although synthetic drugs were by now
readily available, they had lost some part of their efficacy due
to the development of resistant strains of plasmodia. Considerable interest was again devoted to the development of novel antimalarial drugs. At the same time a new effort was launched for
the development of commercially feasible routes for the total
synthesis of the oldest of these drugs, *quinine*.

Woodward achieved his first signal success of a lifetime
devoted to the preparation of increasingly complex natural products by total synthesis by the successful preparation of *quinine*.[9]
Despite its elegance, this synthesis did not provide a commercially viable alternative to isolation of the drug from chincona
bark. A rather short synthesis for this drug from readily available starting materials has been only recently developed by the
group at Hoffmann-LaRoche. (The economics of this synthesis are,
however, not known.) The first step consists in carbethoxylation
of the anion obtained from 2-ethyl-3-methylpyridine and lithium
diisopropyl amide by means of dimethyl carbonate *(49)*. Catalytic
reduction of the ester affords the piperidine *(50)* in which the
two side chains are fixed in the cis configuration. Treatment of
the piperidine with sodium hypochlorite yields the corresponding
N-chloro derivative *(51)*. Photolysis of that active halogen
intermediate in the presence of acid leads to the Leffler-Freytag
rearrangement, that is, the 1,5-transfer of halogen, and in
effect terminal chlorination of the ethyl side chain *(52)*. (This
reaction, probably free radical in nature, is thought to involve
a five-membered ring transition state, hence the observed regiospecificity.) The secondary amine is then acylated. Dehydrogenation of *52* by means of tertiary butoxide in DMSO provides the
vinyl side chain crucial to *quinine (53)*. Esterification gives
the intermediate *(54)* needed for addition of the quinoline moiety.[10] (An alternate scheme for the preparation of this intermediate was devised by the same group as well.[11])

Assembly of the carbon atoms of the natural product is completed by acylation of the lithio derivative obtained from the

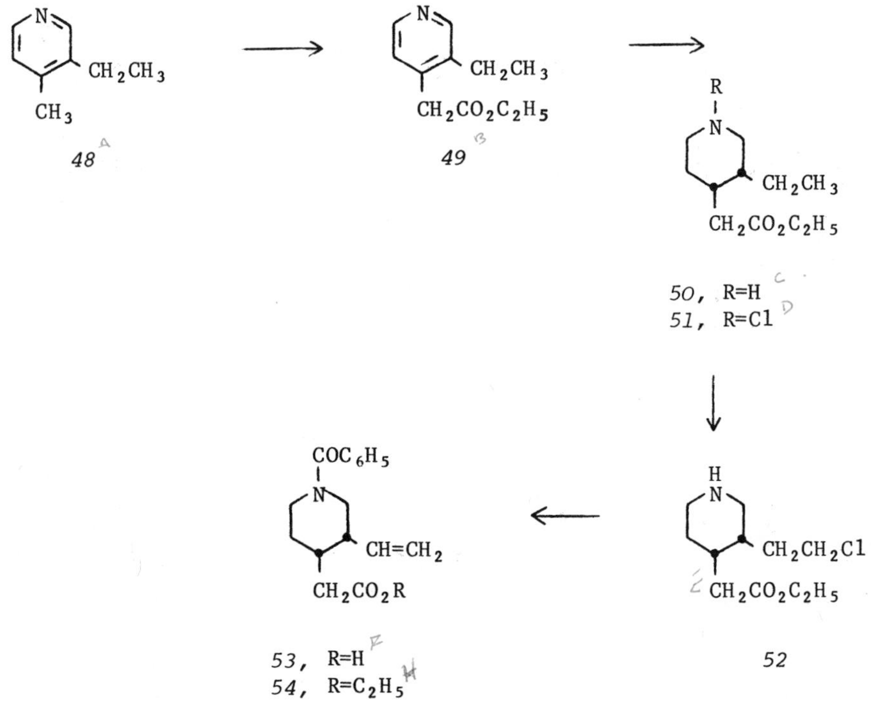

quinoline, 55, with 54 to afford the ketone (56). The carbonyl
group is then reduced by means of a metal hydride and the base
deacylated (58). Resolution of this base into its optical isomers
affords the starting material of proper configuration for completion of the synthesis. Thus, cyclization of the base by SN_2 displacement of the hydroxyl group by nitrogen gives the quinucli-
dine-containing structure 59. Oxygenation of the carbanion of
59 unfortunately proves to be sterically nonselective; there are
obtained in equal amounts quinine (60) and quinidine (61).[12]
Although separation of these diastereomers adds a step, this is
one of the interesting cases in which the by-product is an important drug in its own right. Although it has some activity as
an antimalarial agent, quinidine is one of the more effective
drugs available for the treatment of cardiac arrythmias.

      A variation on the Wittig reaction provides an interesting
alternate method for construction of the desoxy compound (59).
In work carried out in Taylor's laboratory, it was found that
reaction of the chloroquinoline, 62, with excess methylenetri-

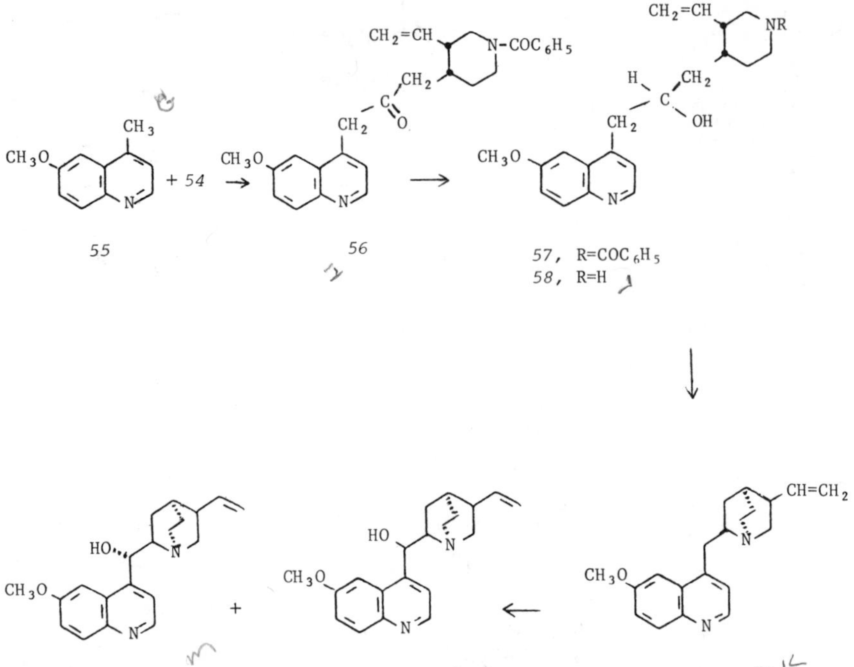

phenylphosphorane affords the ylide, 63. (The first equivalent
of ylide presumably displaces the halogen on the heterocycle to
give the methyl-phosphonium salt, now attached to the 4 position
by a C-C bond; this then reacts with a second mole of methylene
ylide to form the less basic 63.) Condensation of 63 with the
aldehyde, 64 (obtained by a variation of the scheme used to prepare 54), yields the olefin (65). Treatment of that olefin with
base serves to first hydrolyze the acetyl group; the basic nitrogen then adds conjugatively to the reactive vinyl quinoline
double bond to form the quinuclidine ring and thus, 59.

The pioneering work carried out in Germany in the 1920s
showed that appropriately substituted aminoquinolines and amino-
acridines afforded a series of synthetic compounds that exhibited
antimalarial activity.[14] The exigencies of the Second World War
led to a massive program aimed at the same goal in this country.
This work led to the development of two distinct structural
classes of quinoline antimalarials: the 4-amino-7-chloroquino-
lines and the 8-amino-6-methoxyquinolines. These will be consi-

dered without regard to chronology.

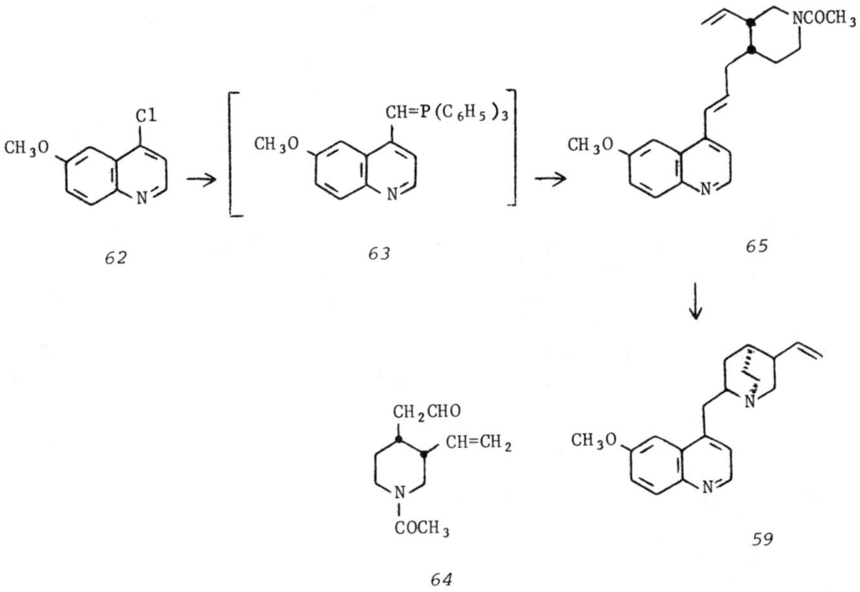

62   63   65

59

64

Preparation of the key intermediate for the chloroquinoline series starts with Shiff base formation of metachloroaniline with ethyl oxaloacetate (66). Heating of the intermediate leads to cyclization into the aromatic ring and consequent formation of the quinoline ring (67). Saponification of the ester to the acid (68) followed by decarboxylation gives the 4-hydroxy quinoline (69). The hydroxyl group is then replaced by chlorine by means of phosphorus oxychloride (70). Displacement of the reactive halogen at the 4 position by means of the aliphatic diamine, 71, yields the synthetic antimalarial agent chloroquine (72).[15]

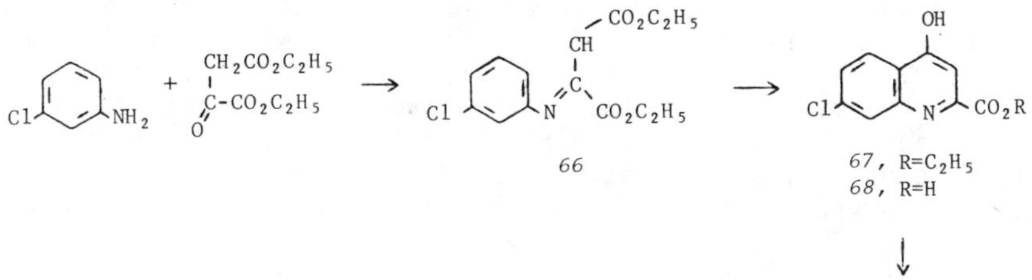

66   67, R=C_2H_5
                       68, R=H

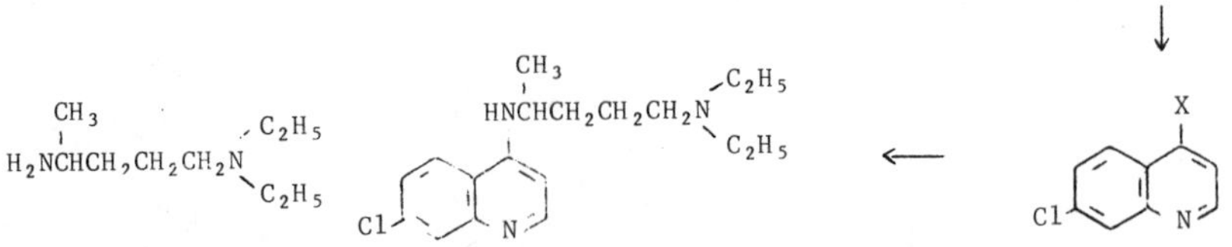

One scheme for preparation of the diamine side chain consists in first reducing the carbonyl group of the haloketone, 73.
Displacement of the halogen with diethylamine gives the amino
alcohol (74). Treatment of that intermediate with thionyl bromide serves to replace the hydroxyl by bromine (75). The synthesis is completed by displacement of the bromine with ammonia.[16]

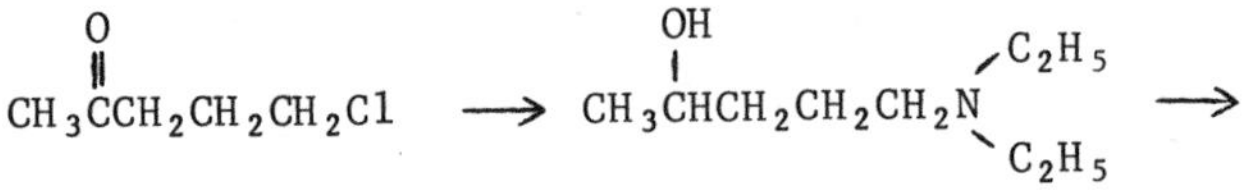

A variation on this theme consists in first displacement of
the chlorine in 73 with ethylaminoethanol. Reductive amination
of the ketone by means of ammonia in the presence of hydrogen
gives the hydroxylated diamine (77). Use of this intermediate to
effect displacement of the halogen at the 4 position of 70 affords
hydroxychloroquine (78).[17]

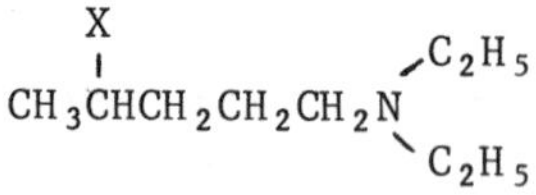

Inclusion of the carbon atoms of an aromatic ring in the side
chain sequence is apparently quite consistent with antimalarial
activity. Thus, reaction of p-acetamidophenol with formaldehyde
and diethylamine affords the Mannich product, 79. This is then
converted to the diamine (80) by saponification. Alkylation with
the chloroquinoline, 70, affords amidoquine (81).[18] The same
sequence starting with the Mannich product in which pyrrolidine
has been used as the amine (82) gives amopyroquine (83).

Deletion of the basic nitrogen atom remote from the quinoline
ring serves to abolish antimalarial activity. Thus, glaphenine

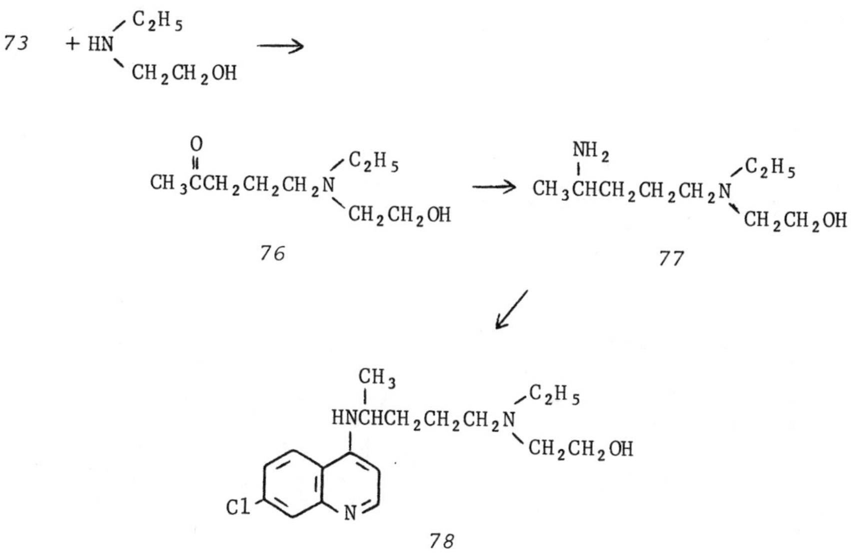

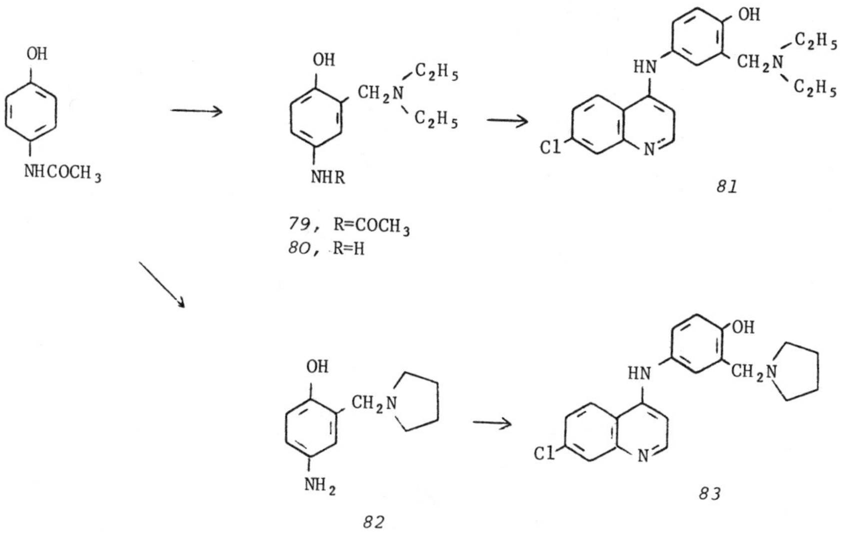

$73 + HN\overset{C_2H_5}{\underset{CH_2CH_2OH}{}}\longrightarrow$

76: $CH_3\overset{O}{\overset{\|}{C}}CH_2CH_2CH_2N\overset{C_2H_5}{\underset{CH_2CH_2OH}{}}$

77: $CH_3\overset{NH_2}{\underset{|}{C}}HCH_2CH_2CH_2N\overset{C_2H_5}{\underset{CH_2CH_2OH}{}}$

78

79, R=COCH$_3$
80, R=H

81

82

83

(85)[19] exhibits antiinflammatory activity. It should be noted
that this agent in essence is a fenamic acid in which quinoline
replaces one of the benzene rings of the prototype. The compound
is prepared by condensation of the glycerol ester of anthranilic

acid with the chloroquinoline, 70.

$$70 \quad + \quad 84 \quad \rightarrow \quad 85$$

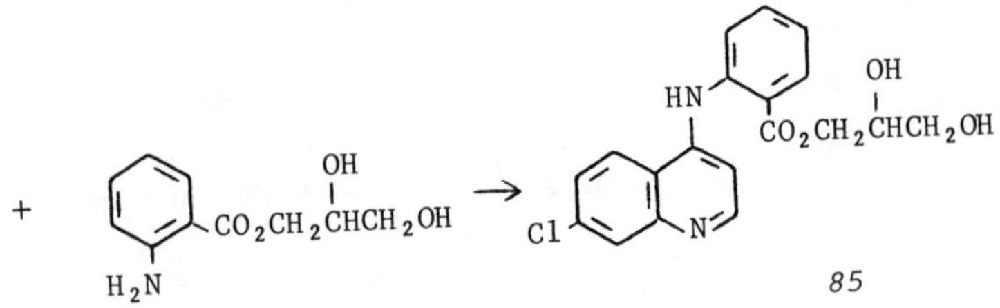

Finally, the quinoline ring can be methylated at the 3 position with retention of biologic activity. The starting quinoline is prepared by the same scheme as that used for the desmethyl compound by substituting the methylated oxosuccinate ester, 86, in the sequence. The initial quinoline carboxylate (87) is taken on to the dichloro compound (88) by the standard reactions. Condensation with the ubiquitous diamine (76) affords *sontoquine* (89).[20]

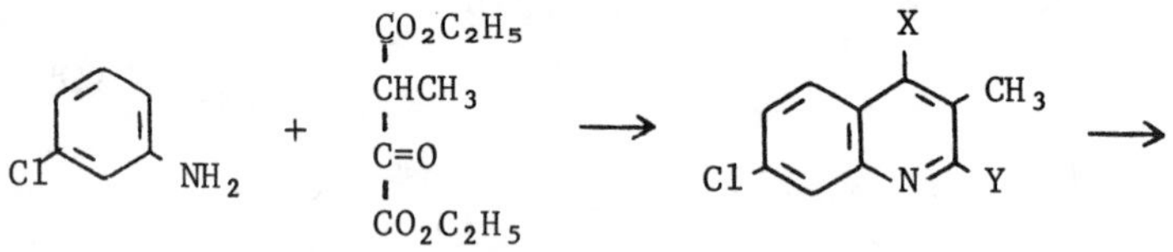

86

87, X=OH, Y=$CO_2C_2H_5$
88, X=Cl, Y=H

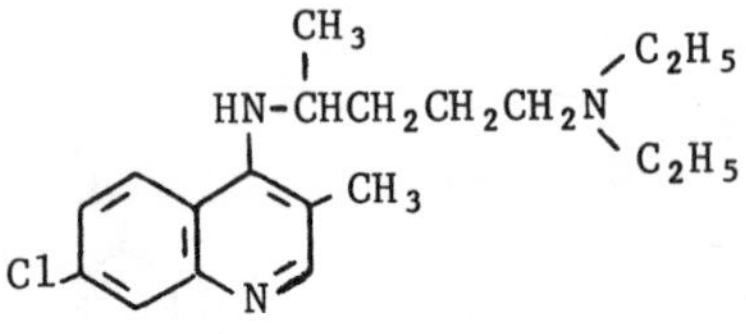

89

The key intermediate for the preparation of the 8-aminoquinoline antimalarial agents is obtained by condensation of the substituted aniline, 90, with "dynamite-grade" glycerol in concentrated sulfuric acid. (The reaction may well follow some scheme such as that depicted below.) The nitroquinoline obtained from this reaction *(91)* is reduced to the amine *(92)* as needed, since that base is an unstable compound. Alkylation with haloamine *(75)* affords *pamaquine (93)*.[16] (This compound was, in fact, developed in Germany in the 1930s; since the process then used for preparation of the side chain gave a pair of regioisomers, the drug at that time was usually sold as a mixture.)

$$[HOCH_2\overset{\overset{\displaystyle OH}{\displaystyle |}}{C}HCH_2OH] \longrightarrow [OHC-CH_2CH_2OH] \longrightarrow OHC-CH=CH_2$$

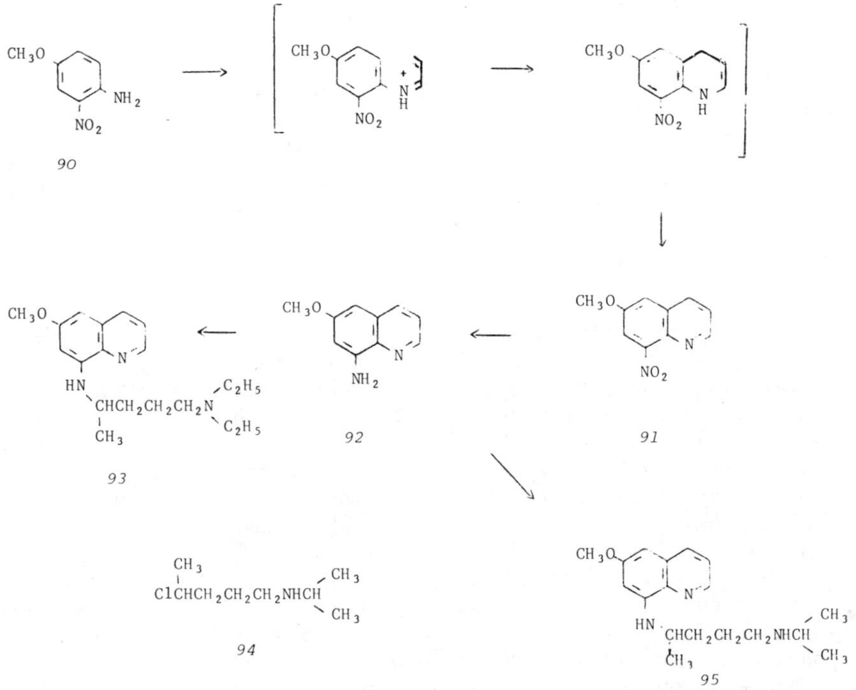

Modification of the synthesis of the side chain by reaction of *73* with isopropyl amine rather than diethylamine gives eventually the haloamine, *94*. Alkylation of the aminoquinoline *(92)*

with this halide gives *isopentaquine (95)*.[21]

Reductive amination of dihydropyran (which may be regarded as the dehydration product of the cyclic acetal of 5-hydroxy-pentanal) in the presence of isopropylamine and a trace of acid affords the aminoalcohol, *96*. Treatment of this compound with thionyl chloride affords the haloamine, *97*. Alkylation of the quinoline, *92*, with this halide yields *pentaquine (98)*.[22]

$$\text{(pyran)} \longrightarrow XCH_2CH_2CH_2CH_2CH_2NHCH \begin{smallmatrix} \diagup CH_3 \\ \diagdown CH_3 \end{smallmatrix} \longrightarrow$$

96, X=OH
97, X=Cl

$$CH_3O\text{(quinoline)}$$
$$HN{\diagdown}CH_2CH_2CH_2CH_2CH_2NHCH\begin{smallmatrix} \diagup CH_3 \\ \diagdown CH_3 \end{smallmatrix}$$

98

Finally the aminoquinoline bearing a primary amine at the terminal carbon atom of the side chain is itself an effective antimalarial drug. Ring opening of 2-methyltetrahydrofuran by bromine gives the dibromide, *99*. The primary halide is suffi-ciently less hindered so that reaction with potassium phthalimide affords exclusively the product of displacement of that halogen *(100)*. Alkylation of the aminoquinoline with *100* affords the secondary amine, *101*. Removal of the phthalimide group by means of hydrazine yields *primaquine (102)*.[23]

The quinoline nucleus has also provided the basis for an effective poultry coccidiostat. Hydrogenation of the bisisobuty-ryl ether of 3,4-dihydroxynitrobenzene *(103)* affords the corre-sponding aniline *(104)*. Reaction of this compound with ethoxy-methylene malonate leads to an addition elimination reaction in which the amine in effect displaces the ethoxy group *(105)*. Cyclization of the ester group onto the highly activated aroma-tic ring is accomplished by heating in Dowtherm. There is thus obtained *buquinolate (106)*.[24]

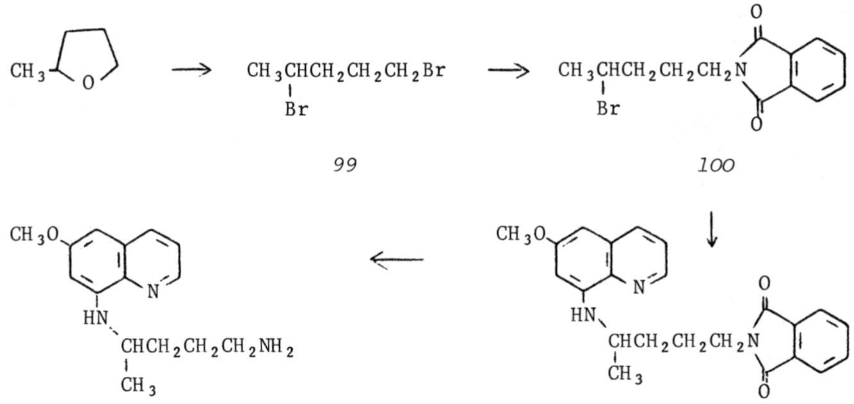

99   100

102   103

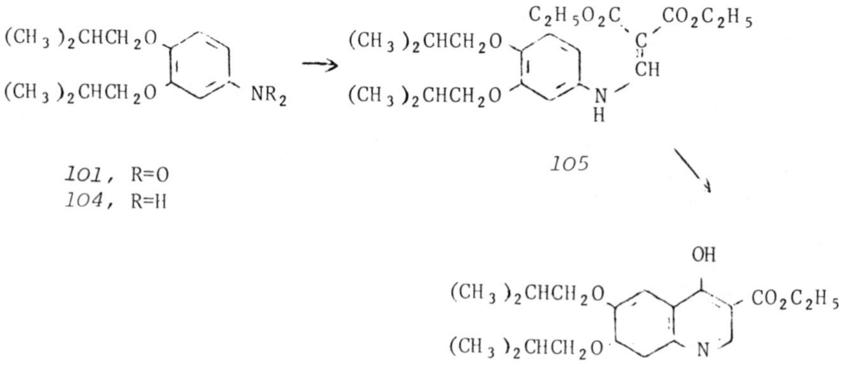

101, R=O
104, R=H

105

106

3. ISOQUINOLINES

Papaverine (107) is among the host of minor alkaloids that have been isolated from opium. The compound is distinct in its biologic activity from many of the other opium constituents in that it does not exhibit any analgesic activity. Instead, *papaverine* acts as a nonspecific spasmolytic agent. As such, it has found

considerable use in the treatment of spasms of the vascular, gastrointestinal, and bronchial tracts.

Although this isoquinoline at first bears little structural
resemblance to *morphine (108)*, careful rearrangement of the structure (A) shows the narcotic to possess the benzylisoquinoline
fragment within its framework. Indeed, research on the biogenesis of *morphine* has shown that the molecule is formed by oxidative
coupling of a phenol closely related to *papaverine*.

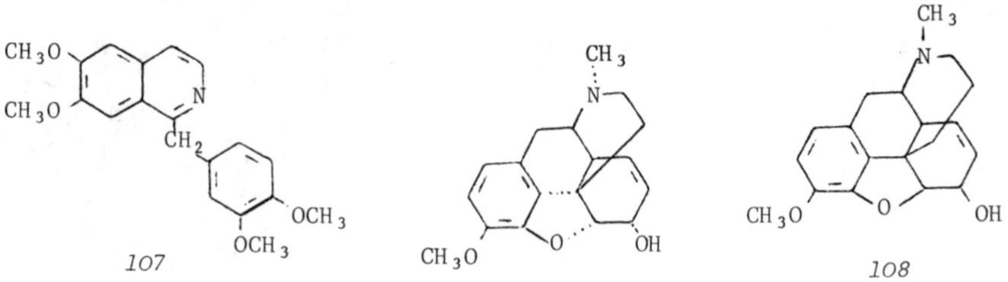

The initial synthesis of *papaverine* is due to Pictet, and
fittingly enough involved as its key step the name reaction.
Acylation of veratrylamine *(109)* with dimethoxyphenylacetylchlo-
ride affords the amide *(110)*. Cyclization by means of phosphorus
oxychloride constitutes the same reaction and affords the dihydroisoquinoline *(111)*. Dehydrogenation by means of a noble
metal catalyst affords *papaverine (107)*.[25]

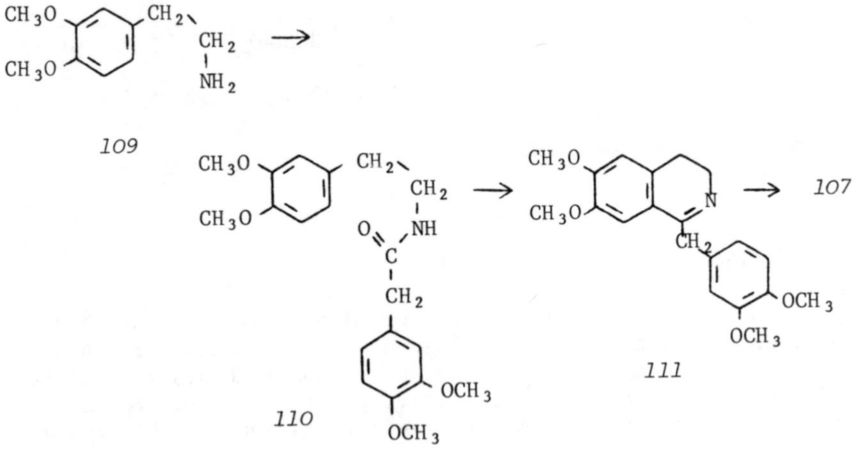

A variant on this structure, *dioxyline*, has much the same activity as the natural product but shows a better therapeutic ratio. Reduction of the oxime *(113)* from 3,4-dimethoxyphenyl-acetone *(112)* affords the veratrylamine homolog bearing a methyl group on the amine carbon atom *(114)*. Acylation of this with 4-ethoxy-3-methoxyphenyl acetyl chloride gives the corresponding amide *(115)*. Cyclization by means of phosphorus oxychloride followed by dehydrogenation over palladium yields *dioxyline (116)*.[26]

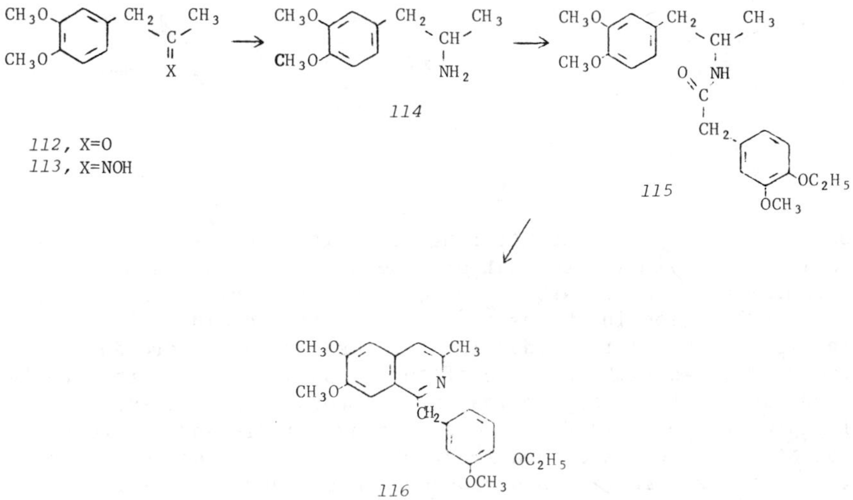

112, X=O
113, X=NOH

Reduction of the heterocyclic ring and extension of the side chain bearing the phenyl ring affords a compound with analgesic and antitussive activity. Cyclization of the acetamide of vera-trylamine gives the dihydroisoquinoline, *117*. Treatment of this compound with acetic anhydride leads to N-acylation with a con-comitant shift of the double bond to the exocyclic position *(118)*. Acid hydrolysis of that intermediate opens the heterocyclic ring to afford the acetophenone *(119)*. Aldol condensation of the ketone with *p*-chlorobenzaldehyde gives the corresponding chalcone *(120)*. Treatment with strong acid serves to deacylate the amide to the amine *(121)*; this condenses to the cyclic Shiff base under the reaction conditions to give a new dihydroisoquinoline *(122)*. Catalytic reduction of both the double bonds followed by methylation of the resulting secondary amine *(123)* by means of methyl iodide yields *methopholine (124)*.[27]

Tetrahydroisoquinolines, in which nitrogen occupies a bridge-

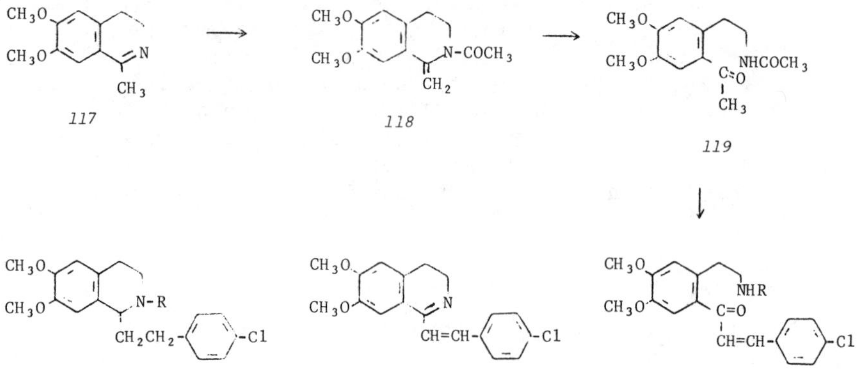

117   →   118   →   119

123, R=H
124, R=CH₃

122

120, R=COCH₃
121, R=H

head position to yet another ring, exhibit tranquilizing activity
qualitatively similar to that of reserpine. Acylation of vera-
trylamine with the 2-carbethoxyacetyl chloride gives the amide,
125. Cyclization in the usual way leads to the dihydroisoquinoline *(126)*. Catalytic reduction affords the tetrahydro derivative *(127)*. Mannich reaction of the secondary amine with formaldehyde and diethyl isopropylmalonate affords the corresponding N-
alkylated compound *(128)*. Successive hydrolysis and decarboxylation of the diacid and then reesterification affords the diester,
129. The last ring is then closed by Dieckmann cyclization;
decarboxylative hydrolysis of that intermediate affords the atar-
actic *tetrabenazine (130)*.[28]

A similar scheme involving reaction of the intermediate,
127, with diethyl malonate proper affords the ketoester, *131*,
following the cyclization step. Reaction of the ester with
diethylamine gives the amide, *132*. Catalytic reduction leads to
the alcohol *(133)*; acetylation completes the synthesis of the
tranquilizer *benzquinamide (134)*.[29]

As we have had occasion to note more than a few times previously, the guanidine function forms the basis of a family of
hypotensive agents active by reason of their activity as blockers
of the peripheral sympathetic system. Condensation of tetra-
hydroisoquinoline with the S-methyl ether of thiourea affords the
antihypertensive drug *debrisoquin (135)*.[30]

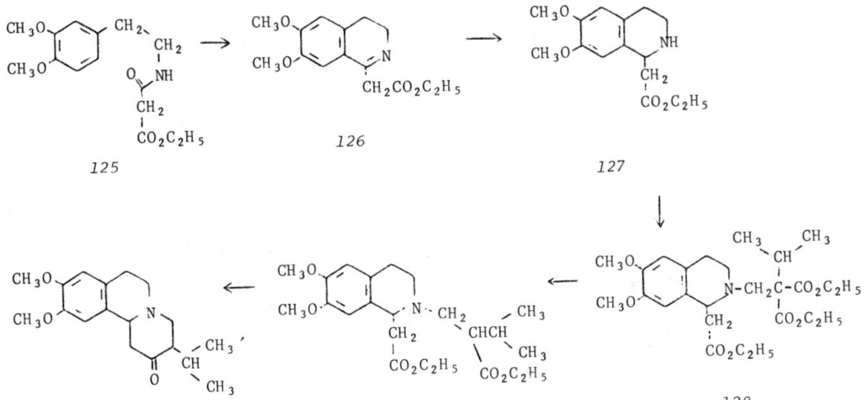

125 → 126 → 127 → 128 → 129 → 130

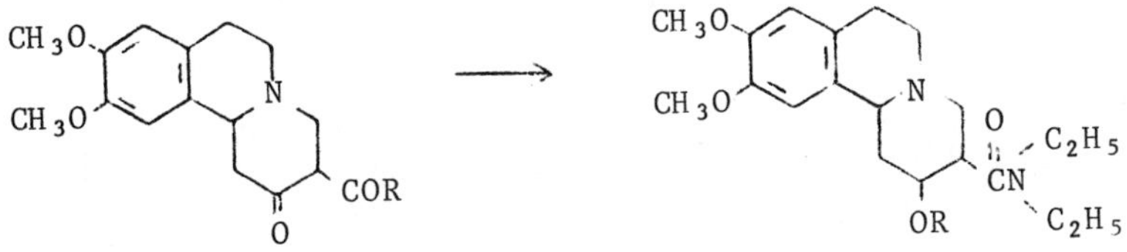

131, R=OC$_2$H$_5$
132, R=N(C$_2$H$_5$)$_2$

133, R=H
134, R=COCH$_3$

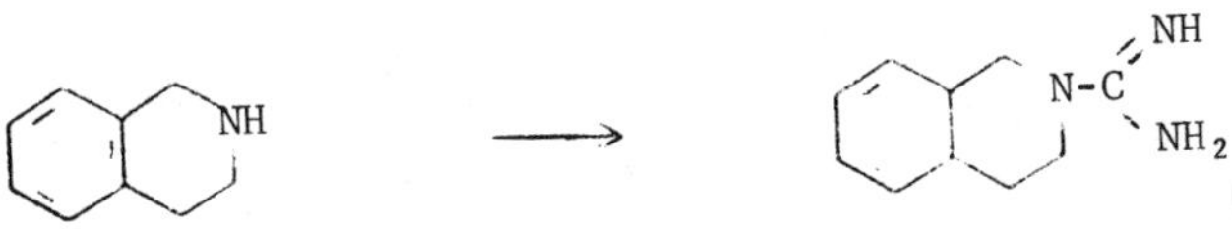

135

4. SIX-MEMBERED RINGS CONTAINING TWO HETERO ATOMS FUSED TO ONE BENZENE RING

A miscellany of medicinal agents are based on heterocyclic systems that contain two hetero atoms. Unlike their counterparts unfused to an aromatic ring, these drugs do not show any unifying biologic activity. It is therefore likely that in most cases the

nucleus simply acts as a carrier for the pharmacophoric groups.
     Reaction of pyrocatechol with epichlorohydrin in the pre-
sence of base affords the benzodioxan derivative, *136*. (The
reaction may well involve initial displacement of halogen by
phenoxide followed by opening of the oxirane by the anion from
the second phenolic group.) Treatment of the alcohol with thionyl chloride gives the corresponding chloro compound *(137)*.[31]
Displacement of halogen by means of diethylamine affords *piperoxan (138)*,[32] a compound with α-sympathetic blocking activity.
     Esterification of *136* with *p*-toluenesulfonyl chloride leads
to the tosylate *(139)*. Displacement of the ester with guanidine
affords *guanoxane (140)*.[33] This drug, not surprisingly, shows
peripheral sympathetic blocking activity and is therefore used in
control of hypertension.

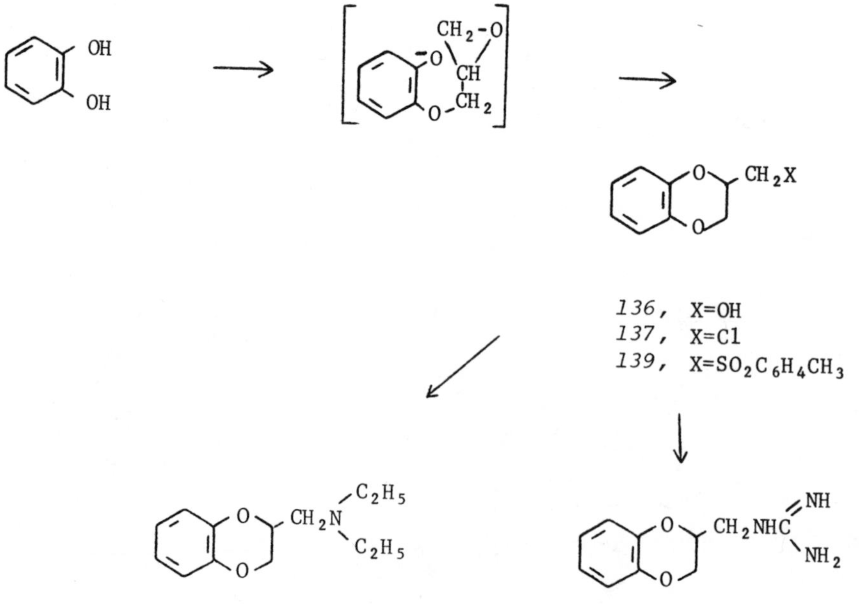

136, X=OH
137, X=Cl
139, X=SO$_2$C$_6$H$_4$CH$_3$

138   *140*

     The phthalazine ring system has yielded a pair of quite
effective antihypertensive agents. Both these drugs are believed
to act as vasodilators; they would owe much of their effectiveness to the consequent decrease in resistance to blood flow in
the periphery. Condensation of the half-aldehyde corresponding

to phthalic acid *(141)* with hydrazine affords the internal hydra-
zone-hydrazide *(142)*. Reaction of that intermediate with phosphorus oxychloride gives the chloro compound *(143)*, probably by
the intermediacy of the enol. Displacement of halogen with
hydrazine yields *hydralazine (144)*.[34]

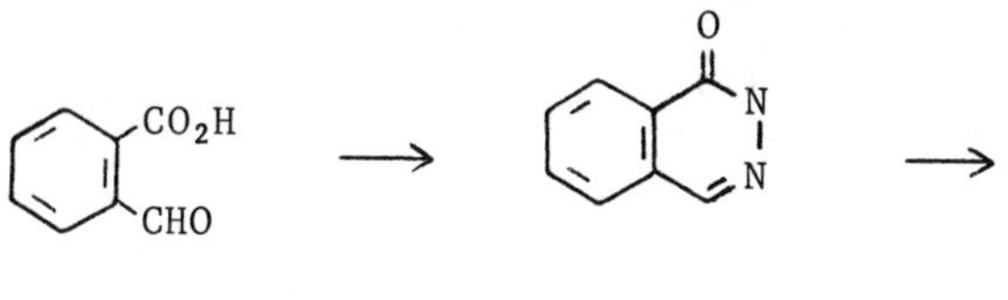

141   142

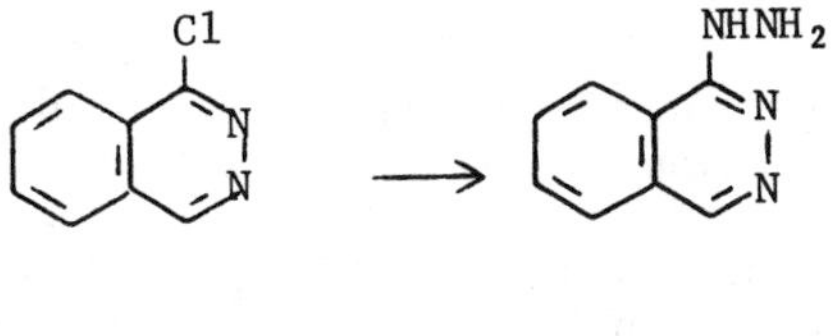

143   144

In much the same vein, reaction of the heterocycle, *145*
(obtainable from phthalic acid and hydrazine), with phosphorus
oxychloride gives the dichloride, *146*. Double displacement of
halogen by means of hydrazine leads to *dihydralazine (147)*.[34]

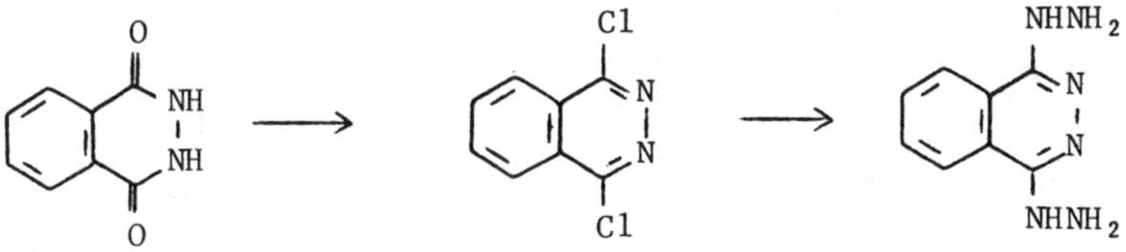

145   146   147

The lack of structural specificity among sedative-hypnotic
drugs has been alluded to before. It is perhaps not too surprising that quinazolones, too, show this activity. The prototype,
methaqualone (149), is obtained in a single step from the condensation of the anthranilamide, *148*, with *o*-toluidine.[35] (The
reaction may well involve first formation of the bisamide; cyclization will then give the quinazolone ring system.) Condensation

of the same starting amide with *o*-chloroaniline yields *mequoqua-lone (150)*.[36]

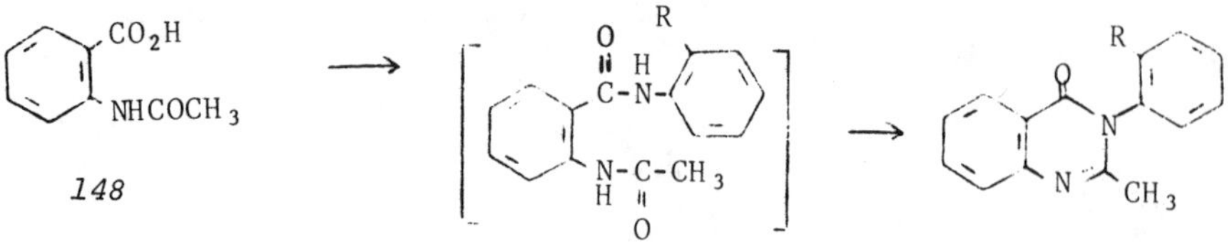

149, R=CH$_3$
150, R=Cl

Sulfonamide groups are often associated with diuretic activity, as shown in the section devoted to that functionality; the section immediately following deals with heterocyclic variants of this function. It is of interest in connection with the present discussion that the sulfonamide grouping affords a diuretic agent when substituted onto a properly constituted quinazolone. Chlorosulfonation of the substituted acetanilide, *151*, followed by ammonolysis of the intermediate sulfonyl chloride *(152)* serves to introduce the sulfonamide function *(153)*. Oxidation of the methyl group gives the corresponding anthranilamide *(154)*; the acetyl group is then removed by hydrolysis *(155)*. Fusion of the amino acid with propionamide leads directly to the quinazoline ring system *(156)*. (One scheme for formation of the product involves formation of a diacylated amide.) Catalytic reduction then gives *quinethazone (157)*.[37]

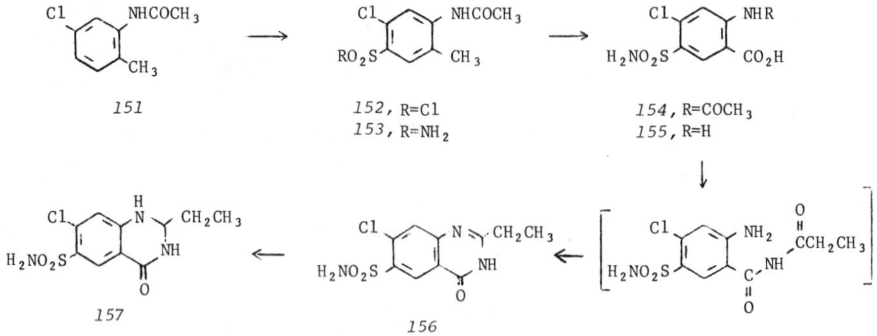

151

152, R=Cl
153, R=NH$_2$

154, R=COCH$_3$
155, R=H

157

156

5.   1,2,4-BENZOTHIADIAZINES AND THEIR REDUCTION PRODUCTS

The development of the so-called thiazide diuretics represents
perhaps the most fruitful application of the theory of rigid
analogs to medicinal chemistry.   At the inception of this work,
there were available to clinicians the bissulfonamide carbonic
anhydrase inhibitors.   Although these descendants of the antibacterial sulfonamides were effective drugs, their use was limited
by, among other reasons, their low potency.   One route chosen in
an effort aimed at improving these drugs consisted in the interposition of an additional atom between the adjacent nitrogen
atoms in a drug such as *chlorophenamide (158)* to form a heterocyclic ring.   This new ring is in effect a rigid analog, since
one of the nitrogen atoms of one of the amides is now fixed in
space.

158

The efficacy of these diuretics led to their extensive use
in the clinic, particularly in treatment of hypertension.   In
theory at least, reduction of the blood volume by diuresis should
lead to a lowering of pressure (PV=RT).   This expectation was in
fact met in actual practice.   Recent research does, however, seem
to indicate that the thiazides have an antihypertensive effect
beyond that explainable by a simple lowering of blood volume.
    Preparation of the first compound in this series, *chloro-
thiazide (162)*, starts with the high-temperature chlorosulfonation of *m*-chloroaniline.   Ammonolysis of the resulting bissulfonyl
chloride *(159)* leads to the corresponding bissulfonamide *(160)*.
Acetylation of the amine gives the amide *(161)*.   Formation of the
heterocycle is achieved by a reaction analogous to the formation
of the quinazolone ring system (*161* may be viewed simplistically
as the sulfur analog of an anthralic acid diamide).   Thus, treatment of *161* with anthranillic acid leads to the benzothiadiazine
ring system and consequently to *chlorothiazide (162)*.[38]   The
analogous scheme starting with *m*-trifluoromethylaniline affords
flumethazide (163).[39]
    Replacement of the sulfonamide group at the 7 position by
chlorine markedly diminishes the diuretic effect in this series.
One such compound, *diazoxide (169)*, exhibits instead potent anti-

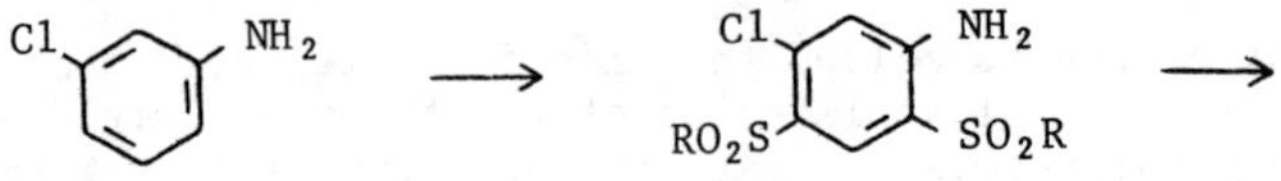

159, R=Cl
160, R=NH$_2$

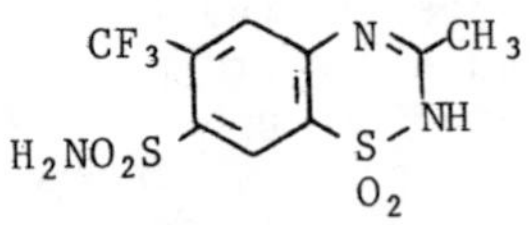

163

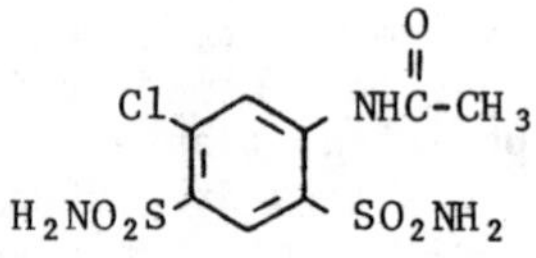

161

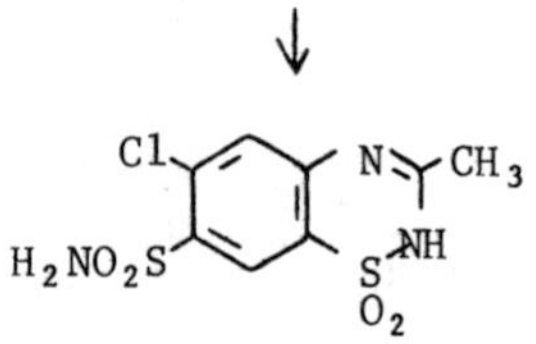

162

hypertensive activity.   It is likely that this drug exerts its
blood pressure-lowering activity by means of vasodilitation.
Preparation starts with the aromatic nucleophilic displacement of
one of the halogens of 164 by the anion from benzylthiol.   (It is
not clear why displacement occurs at the ortho position in preference to the less-hindered para chlorine.)   Debenzylation with
concomitant oxidation is achieved with aqueous chlorine.   Reaction of the resulting sulfonyl chloride (166) with ammonia gives
the corresponding sulfonamide (167).   Reduction of the nitro
group to the amine (168) followed by insertion of the 3 carbon by
means of ethyl orthoacetate affords diazoxide (169).[40]

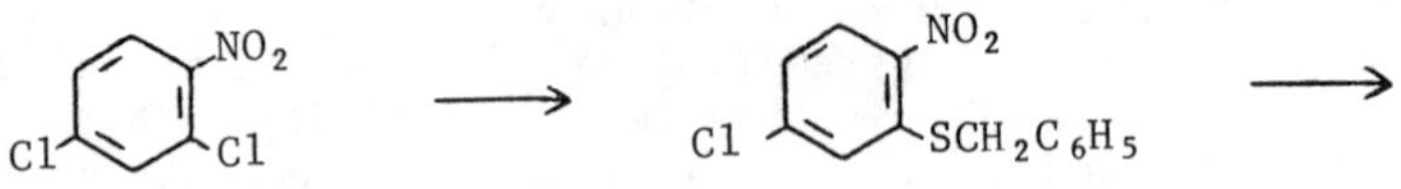

164   165

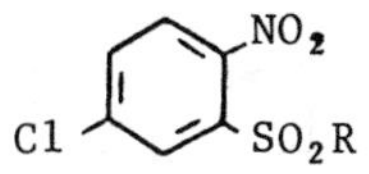

$$\begin{array}{c}\text{Cl}\underset{}{\overset{\text{NO}_2}{\bigcirc}}\text{SO}_2\text{R}\end{array}$$

166, R=Cl
167, R=NH$_2$

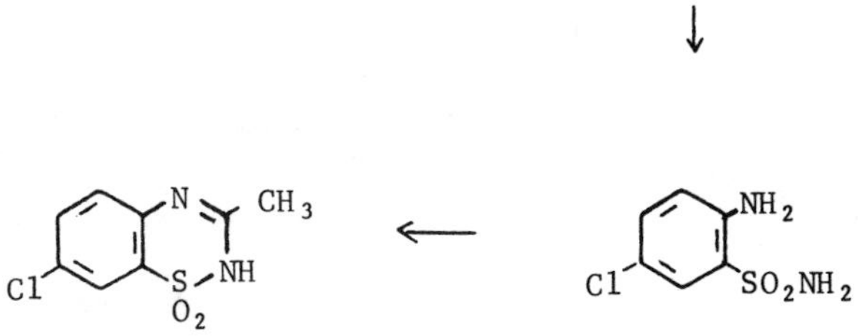

↓

$$169 \qquad\qquad 168$$

Analogs of 162 and 163 in which the heterocyclic ring is fully reduced show a marked increase in potency over the prototypes as well as a more favorable pharmacologic ratio. In practice, however, such compounds are not prepared by reduction of their unsaturated counterparts. Instead, cyclization of the orthoaminosulfonamide is performed with a carbonyl component in a lower oxidation state (e.g., aldehydes rather than acids). In the formal sense at least the products are quite analogous to aminal derivatives of aldehydes. The aromatic component is usually 160. An alternate preparation of the trifluoromethyl analog starts with nucleophilic displacement on 170 by sodium sulfide. Chlorolysis and aminolysis of the product (171) yields the corresponding sulfonamide (173). Reduction of the nitro group followed by reaction with chlorosulfonic acid leads then to the sulfonyl chloride (174). This is then converted to the bissulfonamide by treatment with ammonia. Table 1 lists the plethora of diuretic agents that have been prepared by the basic reaction scheme for forming the heterocyclic ring (A-B).

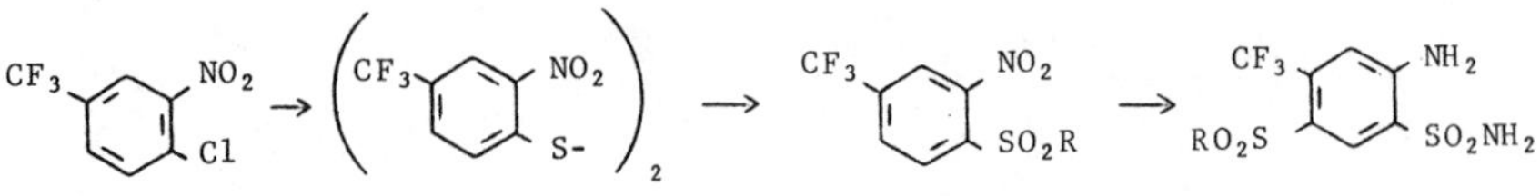

$$170 \qquad 171$$

$$172, \ R=Cl \qquad 174, \ R=Cl$$
$$173, \ R=NH_2 \qquad 175, \ R=NH_2$$

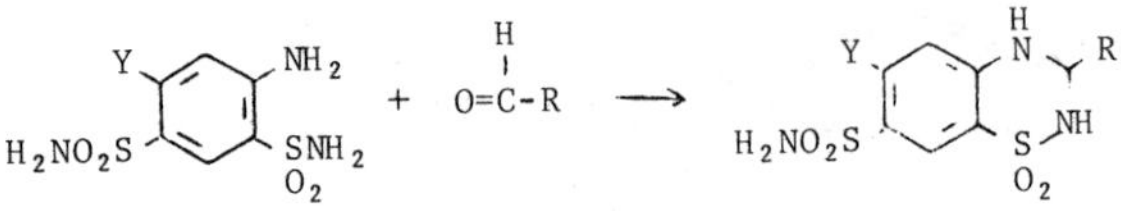

$$A \qquad\qquad B$$

Table 1. 3,4-Dihydro-2H-1,2,4-benzothiadiazines

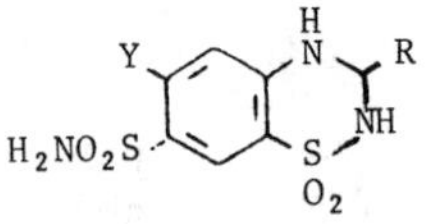

Compd. No.	Y	R	Generic Name	Reference
176	Cl	H	hydrochlorothiazide	41
177	CF_3	H	hydrofluamethiazide	42
178	CF_3	$CH_2C_6H_5$	bendroflumethiazide	42
179	Cl	C_2H_5	ethithiazide	43
180	Cl	$CH_2CH(CH_3)_2$	thiabutazide	43
181	Cl	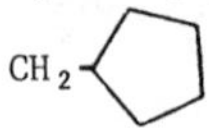 CH_2—⬠	cyclopenthiazide	44
182	Cl	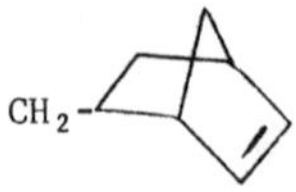 CH_2—	cyclothiazide	44

Table 1, continued

183	Cl	CHCl$_2$	*trichlomethiazide*	45
184	Cl	CH$_2$SCH$_2$CH=CH$_2$	*althizide*	46
185	Cl	CH$_2$SCH$_2$CF$_3$	*epithiazide*	47

Preparation of the aldehyde required for the synthesis of *cyclothiazide (182)* starts by carbonation of the Grignard reagent obtained from the Diels-Alder adduct *(186)* from allyl bromide and cyclopentadiene.[49] The resulting acid *(187)* is then converted to the aldehyde *(189)* by reduction of the corresponding diethyl amide *(188)* with a metal hydride.

186   *187,* R=OH
                         188, R=N(C$_2$H$_5$)$_2$

189

In the preparation of the thiazides containing more highly functionalized side chains *(183-185)*, an acetal of the aldehyde is usually used rather than the free carbonyl compound. Thus, *trichlomethiazide (183)* is prepared by reaction of *160* with the dimethyl acetal from dichloroacetaldehyde. In a similar vein, alkylation of the acetalthiol, *190*, with allyl bromide affords *191*. This yields *altizide (184)* on condensation with *160*. Alkylation of *190* with 2,2,2-trifluoroethyl iodide gives *192*. This leads to *epithiazide (185)* on condensation with *160*.

Methylation of nitrogen at the 2 position also proves to be consistent with diuretic activity. Condensation of *160* with urea affords the heterocycle, *193*. Treatment of this compound with methyl iodide and base effects alkylation on the more acidic ring nitrogen *(194)*. Basic hydrolysis then gives the N-methylated aminosulfonamide *(195)*. Condensation of this with chloroacetaldehyde leads to *methyclothiazide (196)*[48]; condensation with the acetal, *192*, affords *polythiazide (197)*.[47]

$$CH_2=CHCH_2SCH_2CH(OCH_3)_2 \longleftarrow HSCH_2CH(OCH_3)_2 \longrightarrow$$

191   *190*

$$CF_3CH_2SCH_2CH(OCH_3)_2$$

192

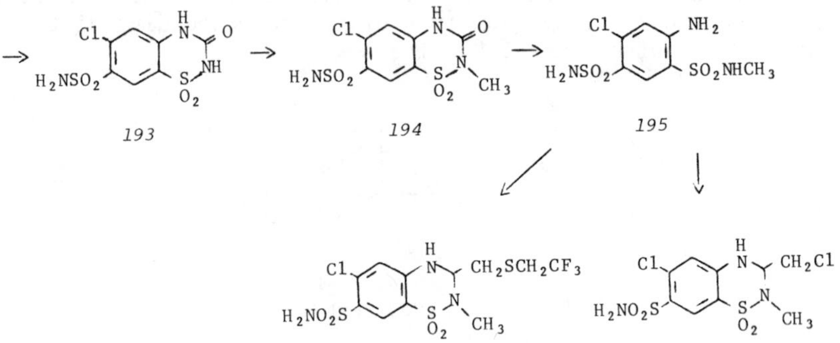

193   *194*   *195*

197   *196*

REFERENCES

1. M. A. Stahman, C. F. Huebner, and K. P. Link, *J. Biol. Chem.,* *138*, 513 (1941).
2. M. I. Kawa, M. A. Stahmann, and K. P. Link, *J. Amer. Chem. Soc.,* *66*, 902 (1944).
3. W. Stoll and F. Litvan, U. S. Patent 2,648,682 (1953).
4. R. E. Nitz and E. Potzch, *Arzneimittel Forsch.,* *13*, 243 (1963).
5. C. Lagercrants, *Acta Chem. Scand.,* *10*, 647 (1956).
6. K. D. Kaufman, *J. Org. Chem.,* *26*, 117 (1961).
7. M. Clerc-Bory, H. Pacheco, and C. Mentzer, *Bull. Soc. Chim. Fr.,* 1083 (1955).
8. R. Aneja, S. K. Mukerjee, and T. S. Seshadri, *Chem. Ber.,* *97*, 297 (1960).
9. R. B. Woodward and W. E. Doering, *J. Amer. Chem. Soc.,* *67*, 860 (1945).

10. M. Uskokovic, C. Reese, H. L. Lee, G. Grethe, and J. Gulzwiller, *J. Amer. Chem. Soc.*, *93*, 5902 (1971).
11. M. Uskokovic, J. Gutzwiller, and T. Henderson, *J. Amer. Chem. Soc.*, *92*, 203 (1970).
12. J. Gutzwiller and M. Uskokovic, *J. Amer. Chem. Soc.*, *92*, 204 (1970).
13. E. C. Taylor and S. F. Martin, *J. Amer. Chem. Soc.*, *94*, 6218 (1972).
14. W. Schulemann, F. Schonhofer, and A. Wingler, German Patent 486,079 (1930).
15. A. R. Surrey and H. F. Hammer, *J. Amer. Chem. Soc.*, *68*, 113 (1946).
16. R. C. Elderfield, et al., *J. Amer. Chem. Soc.*, *68*, 1579 (1946).
17. A. R. Surrey and H. F. Hammer, *J. Amer. Chem. Soc.*, *72*, 1814 (1950).
18. J. H. Burckhalter, F. H. Tendrick, E. M. Jones, W. F. Holcomb, and A. L. Rawling, *J. Amer. Chem. Soc.*, *70*, 1363 (1948).
19. Anon., Belgian Patent 636,381 (1964).
20. E. A. Steck, L. L. Hallock, and A. J. Holland, *J. Amer. Chem. Soc.*, *68*, 380 (1946).
21. R. C. Elderfield, et al., *J. Amer. Chem. Soc.*, *68*, 1524 (1946).
22. N. L. Drake, J. VanHook, J. A. Garman, R. Hayer, R. Johnson, S. Melamea, and R. M. Peck, *J. Amer. Chem. Soc.*, *68*, 1529 (1946).
23. R. C. Elderfield, H. E. Mertel, R. T. Mitch, I. M. Wempen, and E. Werble, *J. Amer. Chem. Soc.*, *77*, 4816 (1955).
24. J. Watson, U. S. Patent 3,267,106 (1966).
25. A. Pictet and M. Finklestein, *Chem. Ber.*, *42*, 1979 (1909).
26. E. R. Shepard, U. S. Patent 2,728,769 (1958).
27. A. Brossi, H. Besendorf, B. Pellmont, M. Walter, and O. Schnider, *Helv. Chim. Acta*, *43*, 1459 (1960).
28. A. Brossi, H. Lindlar, M. Walter, and O. Schnider, *Helv. Chim. Acta*, *41*, 119 (1958).
29. J. R. Tretter, U. S. Patent 3,053,845 (1962).
30. W. Wenner, Belgian Patent 629,007 (1963).
31. A. Grun, U. S. Patent 2,366,102 (1944).
32. E. Fourneau, U. S. Patent 2,056,046 (1936).
33. A. M. Monro, *Chem. Ind.*, 1806 (1964).
34. J. Druey and B. H. Ringler, *Helv. Chim. Acta.*, *34*, 195 (1951).
35. I. K. Kacker and S. H. Zanner, *J. Indian Chem. Soc.*, *28*, 344 (1951).
36. G. B. Jackman, V. Petrow, and O. Stephenson, *J. Pharm.*

Pharmacol., 28, 344 (1960).

37. E. Cohen, B. Karberg, and J. R. Vaughan, *J. Amer. Chem. Soc., 82,* 2731 (1968).

38. F. C. Novello and J. M. Sprague, *J. Amer. Chem. Soc., 79,* 2028 (1957).

39. H. L. Yale, K. Losee, and J. Bernstein, *J. Amer. Chem. Soc., 82,* 2042 (1960).

40. A. A. Rubin, F. E. Roth, M. W. Winburg, J. G. Topliss, M. H. Sherlock, N. Sperber, and J. Black, *Science, 133,* 2067 (1961).

41. G. DeStevens, L. H. Werner, A. Halamandavis, and S. Ricca, *Experientia, 14,* 463 (1950).

42. C. T. Hodvege, R. Babel, and L. C. Cheney, *J. Amer. Chem. Soc., 81,* 4807 (1959).

43. J. G. Topliss, M. H. Sherlock, F. H. Clark, M. C. Daly, B. W. Pettersen, J. Lipski, and N. Sperber, *J. Org. Chem., 26,* 3842 (1961).

44. C. W. Whitehead, J. J. Traverso, H. R. Sullivan, and F. J. Marshall, *J. Org. Chem., 26,* 2814 (1961).

45. G. DeStevens, L. H. Werner, W. E. Barrett, and A. H. Renzi, *Experientia, 16,* 113 (1960).

46. J. M. McMannus, British Patent 902,658 (1962).

47. J. M. McMannus, U. S. Patent 3,009,911 (1961).

48. W. J. Close, L. R. Swett, L. E. Brady, J. H. Short, and M. Vernstein, *J. Amer. Chem. Soc., 82,* 1132 (1960).

CHAPTER 18

Benzodiazepines

Each era of medicinal chemistry has been marked by intensive concentration on some structural type in a large number of laboratories. One need only look back in this book to the tables of sulfonamides, barbiturates, and thiazide diuretics, noting the small time span covered by the references to each list. The benzodiazepines have provided such a focus for the past decade.

The pace of life in the highly developed industrial nations leads many to become anxious and depressed in view of the high demands placed on them by their peers and society at large. The success ethic and the high price of failure contribute in no small way to this malaise. There thus seemed to exist a need for some anxiolytic agent that would enable the individual to continue functioning in spite of his angst. Such an agent should be without the frank sedation of the barbiturates or the side effects of the major tranquilizers. To anticipate, the benzodiazepines seem to fulfill exactly this role. This, in fact, accounts both for their enormous sales and the efforts of so many pharmaceutical companies to enter this market.

This class of medicinal agents was uncovered quite adventitiously in a chemical study, although due credit must be given for the acute pharmacologic studies that uncovered this novel type of activity.

The original objective of the synthetic work was the preparation of basic derivatives of the 3,1,4-benzoxadiazepine system *(2)* for animal testing. The basic ring system had been reported previously in the literature as the dehydration products of 2-acylaminobenzophenone oximes *(1)*. Repetition of the work quickly cast doubt on the earlier structural assignment. Both the chemistry of the products and their spectral data suggested that the products were in fact quinazoline-3-oxides *(3)*.

A preparation of authentic *3a* was then undertaken. Reaction of *p*-chloroaniline with benzoyl chloride in the presence of zinc

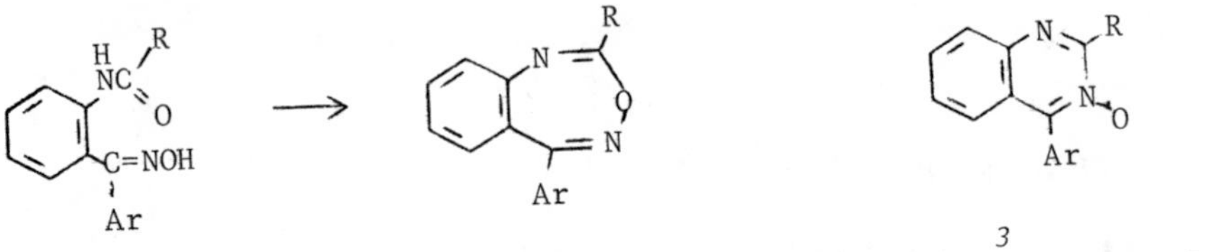

1 → 2 → 3

3a, R=CH$_2$Cl

chloride initially affords a dimer of the orthoacylation product (5). Hydrolysis gives the orthoaminobenzophenone (6). Reaction with hydroxylamine converts the ketone to the oxime (7); acylation of the aniline by means of chloroacetyl chloride affords the desired intermediate, 8. Cyclodehydration by means of hydrogen chloride then gives the quinoxaline N-oxide (9).

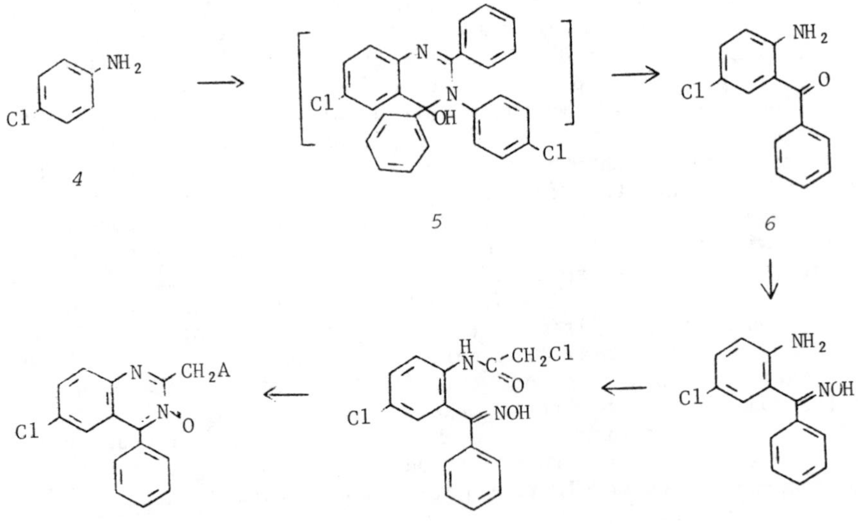

4 → 5 → 6

9, A=Cl
10, A=NHCH$_3$ 8   7

Displacement of the activated halogen in 9 led to a series of compounds with marked anxiolytic activity in laboratory animals. It soon became apparent that fate had intervened a second time in the chemistry of this series: the compounds were not simple products of displacement of halogen (10) but new hetero-

cycles from a ring expansion reaction. The rearrangement is
visualized as involving first addition of methylamine to the
amidine-like function on the quinoxaline ring (the electron with-
drawing effect of the N-oxide group may favor this process).
Ring opening will then lead to intermediate, 12. Internal displacement of halogen by the oxime nitrogen affords the benzodiazepine, 13.[1] This compound, *chlordiazepoxide*, is better known by
its trademark, Librium®. Both this drug and its successors are
widely used as minor tranquilizers and muscle relaxants. Several
of the more recent drugs of this class show somewhat differing
profiles, with some agents exhibiting marked hypnotic activity.

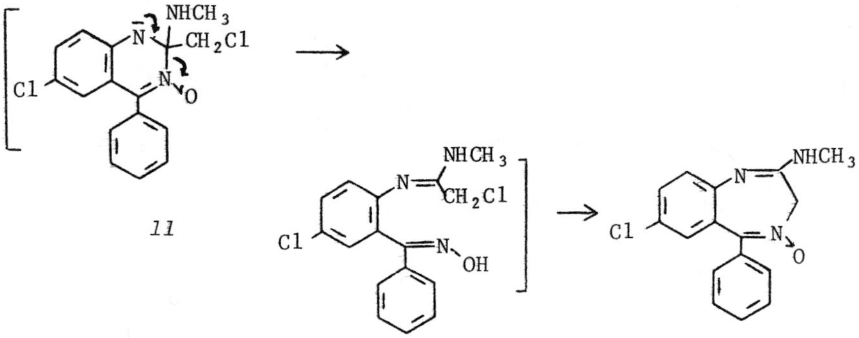

11   12   13

        Neither the oxide nor the amidine function are in fact
required for activity. Treatment of the oxime, 7, with chloroacetyl chloride in the presence of sodium hydroxide proceeds
directly to the benzodiazepine ring system *(14)*(the hydroxyl
ion presumably fulfills a role analogous to methylamine in the
above rearrangement). Reduction of the N-oxide function of 14
leads to *diazepam (15)*.[1]

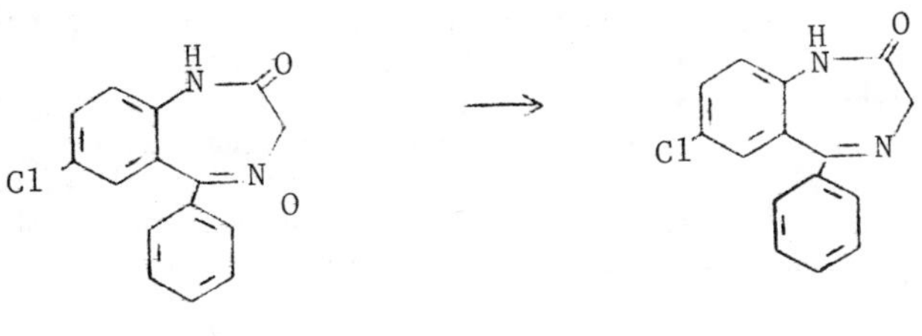

        14   15

Careful study of the metabolic disposition of these compounds led to the realization that active metabolites were quickly
formed following administration; it was even suggested that the
"real" active agent might be one of these. One of the metabolites, *oxazepam (18)*, was soon prepared and in fact proved to
have anxiolytic activity. This drug, too, has found wide acceptance. Treatment of *diazepam* intermediate *14* with acetic acid
results in a reaction analogous to the well-known Polonovski
rearrangement (perhaps via *16*) to give ester *17*. Treatment with
an equivalent of base gives *oxazepam (18)*.[2] This minor tranquilizer is more potent than *diazepam*, which is in turn more active
than *chlordiazepoxide*.

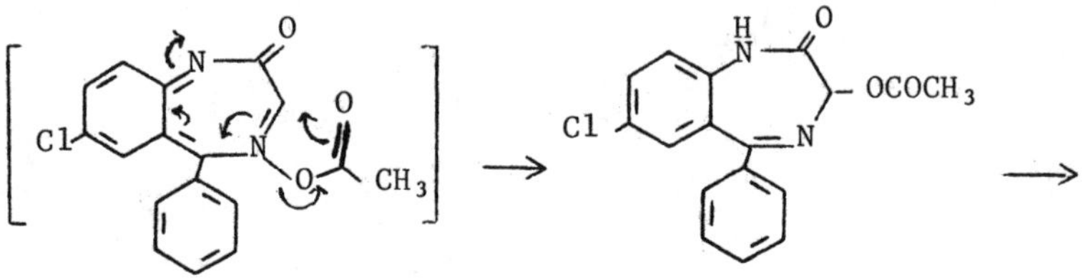

16   17

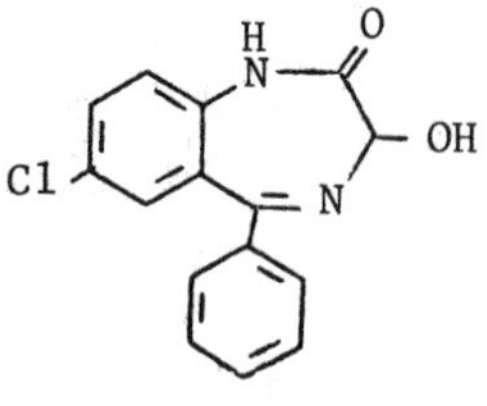

18

A more recent derivative with activities typical of the
class is *nitrazepam (21)*. Reaction of 2-amino-5-nitrobenzophe-
none *(19)* with bromoacetylbromide affords the amide, *20*. Ring
closure in liquid ammonia gives *nitrazepam (21)*.[3] More simply,
diazepinone, *22*, can be nitrated directly at the more reactive C_7
position with potassium nitrate in sulfuric acid.

Inclusion of fluorine on the pendant aromatic ring and the
basic side chain seems to emphasize the anticonvulsant and hypnotic effects of this class of drugs. Thus alkylation of the
benzodiazepinone, *24* (prepared from the corresponding substituted
aminobenzophenone), with 2-chlorotriethylamine via its sodium
salt affords *fluazepam*.[4]

The orthochloro analog of oxazepam is in fact prepared by a

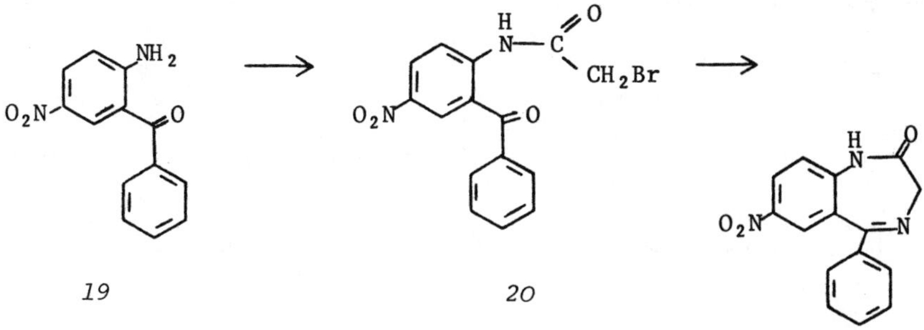

19

20

21

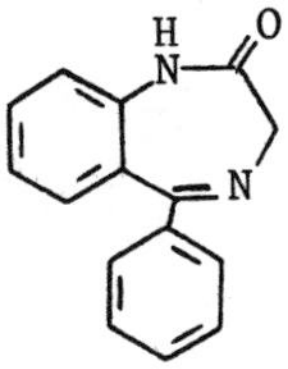

22

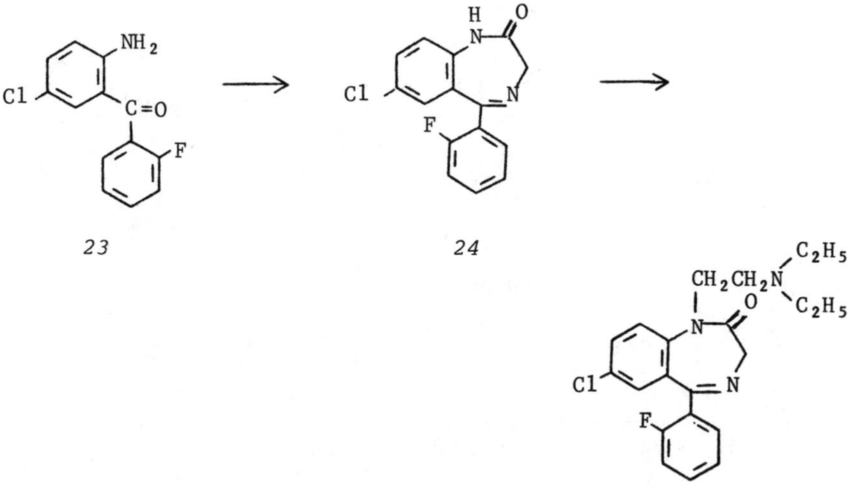

23

24

25

somewhat more circuitous route than the prototype. Condensation
of the aminobenzophenone, 26, with diethyl aminomalonate leads
directly to the benzodiazpine containing a carbethoxy group at the
3 position (27). Bromination proceeds at the carbon atom activated by two carbonyl groups (28). Solvolysis of the halogen in
methanol leads to the corresponding methyl ether (29). Saponification of the ester followed by decarboxylation of the ketoacid
affords the methyl ether of the desired product (30). Cleavage
of the ether by means of boron tribromide gives lorazepam (31).[5,6]

26   27

                                                          28, X=Br
                                                          29, X=OCH$_3$

                                                          30, R=CH$_3$
                                                          31, R=H

     The benzodiazepine ring system is also accessible by some of
the more traditional methods for forming benzoheterocycles, such
as, for example, cyclodehydration reactions. Reaction of 1-
benzoylaziridine (33) with the aniline, 32, results in ring opening of the aziridine to produce the amide, 34. This undergoes
cyclization into the aromatic ring on heating with either polyphosphoric acid or polyphosphoric acid ethyl ester. There is
thus obtained medazepam (35).[7,8]
     Fusion of an additional heterocyclic ring onto that already
present in the benzodiazepines has led to some medicinal agents
with considerable activity. Treatment of an intermediate like
15 with phosphorus pentasulfide affords the corresponding thioamide (37). Condensation of this intermediate with acetyl hydrazide affords triazolam)37).[9] The same agent can be prepared by
reaction of the amidine, 38,[10] with acetylhydrazide.[11]
     The N-methylated analog of intermediate, 15, contains a

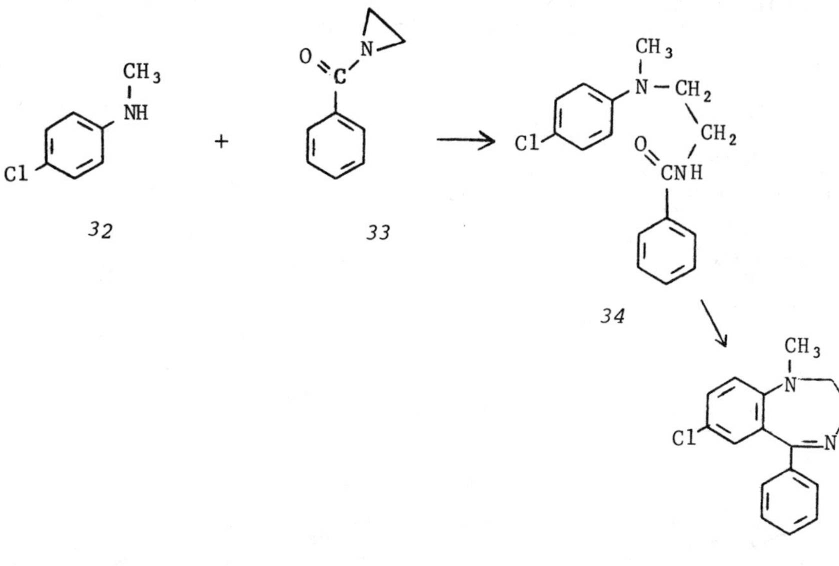

reactive imine function at the 4-5 position *(39)*. This imine in
fact readily adds diketene (an acetoacetate equivalent) to afford
ketazolam (40).[12]

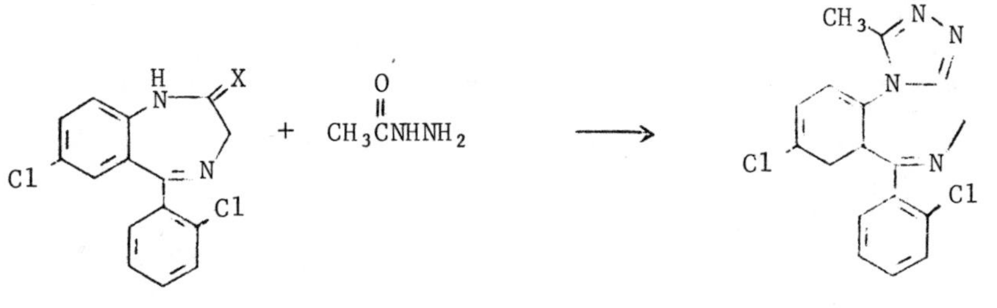

In an alternate approach to the preparation of compounds containing the additional ring, haloamide, *41*[13] (obtained from the
aminobenzophenone and bromoacetylbromide) is alkylated with ethanolamine to afford *42*. Treatment of the amino alcohol in acetic
acid affords the carbonyl addition product, *43*, at the same time

resulting in the formation of two rings. The product, *cloxaze-*
pam (43),[14] is an active anxiolytic agent.

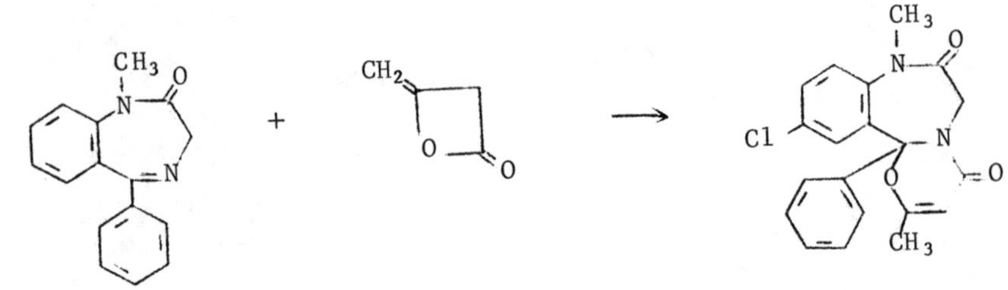

39

40

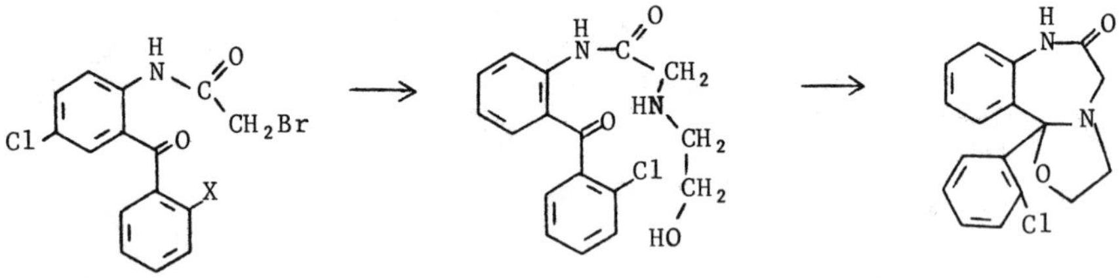

41, X=Cl
44, X=H

42

43

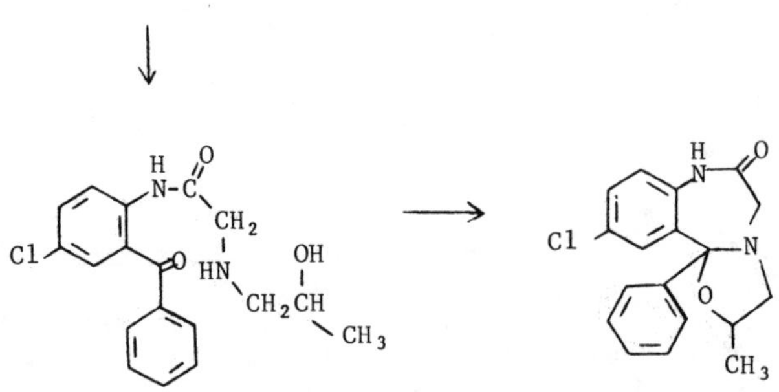

45

46

In much the same manner, alkylation of the deschloro intermediate *(44)* with 2-hydroxypropylamine, followed by cyclization of
the resulting amino alcohol *(45)* affords *oxazolapam (46)*.

REFERENCES

1. L. H. Sternbach and E. Reeder, *J. Org. Chem.*, *26*, 4936 (1961).
2. S. C. Bell and S. J. Childress, *J. Org. Chem.*, *27*, 1691 (1962).
3. L. H. Sternbach, R. I. Fryer, O. Keller, W. Metlesics, G. Sachs, and N. Steiger, *J. Med. Chem.*, *6*, 261 (1963).
4. L. H. Sternbach, G. A. Archer, J. V. Early, R. I. Fryer, E. Reeder, N. Wasyliw, L. D. Randall, and R. Banziger, *J. Med. Chem.*, *8*, 815 (1965).
5. S. C. Bell, R. J. McCaully, C. Gochman, S. C. Childress, and M. I. Gluckman, *J. Med. Chem.*, *11*, 457 (1968).
6. S. C. Bell and S. C. Childress, *J. Org. Chem.*, *33*, 216 (1968).
7. K. H. Wünsch, H. Dettmann, and S. Schönberg, *Chem. Ber.*, *102*, 3891 (1969).
8. G. F. Field, L. H. Sternbach, and W. J. Szally, U. S. Patent 3,624,073 (1971).
9. J. B. Hester, C. G. Chidester, D. J. Duchamp, F. A. MacKellar, and J. Slomp, *Tetrahedron Lett.*, 3665 (1971).
10. G. A. Archer and L. H. Sternbach, *J. Org. Chem.*, *29*, 231 (1964).
11. R. Nakajima, C. Hattori, and Y. Nagawa, *Jap. J. Pharmacol.*, *21*, 489 (1971).
12. J. Szmuszkovicz, C. G. Chidester, D. J. Duchamp, F. A. MacKellar, and G. Slomp, *Tetrahedron Lett.*, 3665 (1971).
13. L. H. Sternbach, R. I. Fryer, W. Metlesics, E. Reeder, G. Sach, G. Saucy, and A. Stempel, *J. Org. Chem.*, *27*, 3788 (1962).
14. T. Miyadera, A. Terada, M. Fukunaga, Y. Kawano, T. Kamioka, C. Tamura, H. Takagi, and R. Tachikawa, *J. Med. Chem.*, *14*, 520 (1971).
15. T. L. Lemke and A. R. Hanze, *J. Heterocycl. Chem.*, *8*, 125 (1971).

CHAPTER 19

Phenothiazines

Compounds containing the benzhydryl grouping are prominent among the antihistamines; they are represented in this class by both derivatives of benzhydrol and benzhydrylamines. It will be recalled further that the latter usually incorporate some version of an ethylenediamine side chain. It was therefore logical that synthetic work on these agents turn to derivatives in which one of the nitrogens of the side chain replaced the benzhydryl carbon. This line of work, in fact, met with initial success when an additional heteroatom was included to bridge the two aromatic ring. The phenothiazines, in which the additional bridge is represented by sulfur, have in fact proven a particularly fertile ground for the development of compounds with varying pharmacologic activities. As we see below, simple two-carbon side chains generally afford antihistamines; several of these had sufficient sedative effects to be proposed for treatment of Parkinson's disease. Inclusion of a methyl group on the side chain adjacent the nitrogen remote from the ring led to potent antihistamines, many of which possess sedative activities.

The most dramatic changes in pharmacologic activity involved extension of the side chain so as to separate the nitrogens by three carbon atoms. The initial biologic observations suggested that these compounds had increased sedative activity and diminished antihistamine potency. It remained for an astute pharmacologist to discover that an entirely new biologic activity was displayed by these compounds. That is, these agents were uniquely useful in treatment of various neuroses and psychoses. Administration of chlorpromazine, although not curative, made previously hopelessly ill patients amenable to treatment. The effects of the availability of these drugs on therapy of mental illness have been no less than revolutionary. Synthetic work subsequent to the discovery of the first of the so-called neuroleptic phenothiazines has produced a series of drugs with subtly differing

biologic profiles; we consider the synthesis of these agents at
the expense of the pharmacology.

Of the several syntheses available for the phenothiazine
ring system, perhaps the simplest is the sulfuration reaction.
This consists of treating the corresponding diphenylamine
with a mixture of sulfur and iodine to afford directly the
desired heterocycle. Since the proton on the nitrogen of the
resultant molecule is but weakly acidic, strong bases are
required to form the corresponding anion in order to carry out
subsequent alkylation reactions. In practice such diverse bases
as ethylmagnesium bromide, sodium amide, and sodium hydride have
all been used. Alkylation with N-(chloroethyl)diethylamine
affords *diethazine (1)*, a compound that exhibits both antihistaminic and antiParkinsonian activity.[1] Substitution of N-(2-
chloroethyl)pyrrolidine in this sequence leads to *pyrathiazine
(2)*,[2] an antihistamine of moderate potency.

As noted above, methylation of the side chain leads to an
increase in antihistaminic potency. Alkylation of phenothiazine
with the halide *3* using sodium amide as a base leads to *promethazine (4)*.[1] Interestingly, an attempt to prepare the isomeric
side chain, as in *6*, by use of the secondary chloride *5*, again
results in formation of the *promethazine*.[1] As in the case of the
problem concerning the structure of *methadon*, this finding has
been attributed to intervention of the internal alkylation product *(7)* in the course of reaction.[3] Alkylation of phenothiazine
with the N,N-diethyl analog of *3* by means of methylmagnesium
iodide leads to *ethopropazine (8)*.[4] This compound, which is of
course the methyl analog of *3*, has also found some use in the
treatment of Parkinsonianism.

Extensive work on the effects of substitution on the aromatic rings of the phenothiazines on both antihistamine and neuroleptic activity seems to have shown fairly clearly that maximum changes are obtained by inclusion of a substituent at the 2 position. *Methopromazine (13)* represents an antihistamine bearing such a substituent. Aromatic nucleophilic substitution on o-chloronitrobenzene by means of a salt of the thiophenol, *10*, affords the corresponding sulfide *(11)*. Reduction of the nitro group followed by cyclization of the resulting amine leads to the substituted phenothiazine, *12*. Alkylation of the latter at the 10 position with the aminohalide, *3*, by means of sodium amide in xylene gives the desired product *(13)*.[5]

In a similar vein, the amino group in sulfide *14* (obtained presumably by an aromatic displacement reaction) is first converted to the bromide by Sandmeyer reaction to give *15*. Reduction of the nitro group *(16)* followed by cyclization gives the substituted phenothiazine. Alkylation with the familiar halide *(3)* affords *dimethothiazine (18)*.[6]

Electrophilic aromatic substitution affords yet another route to ring-substituted phenothiazines. Conversion of the parent phenothiazine to the propionamide (via the magnesium salt) serves both as a protecting group for the amine and as a means of allowing the para-directing effect of the sulfide to prevail. Acylation with propionyl chloride and aluminum chloride thus affords, after saponification of the amide, the ketone *(20)*. This is then treated with phosgene to give *21*, and this last esterified with the aminoalcohol (a) to yield the corresponding urethane *(22)*.

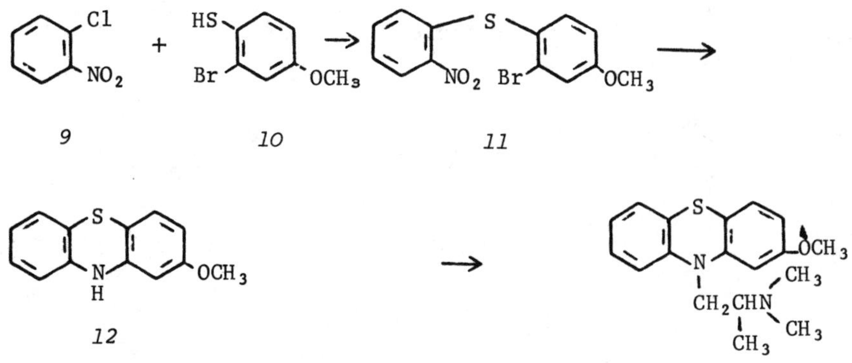

9 *10* *11*

12 *13*

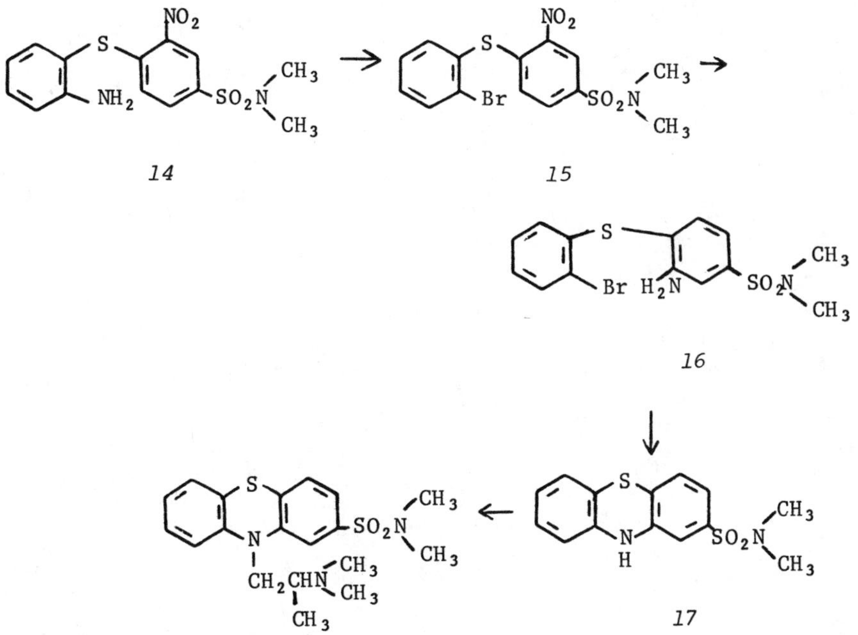

14 *15*

16

17

18

In an interesting reaction, pyrrolysis of the urethane leads to extrusion of carbon dioxide and formation of *23*, *propiomazine*.[7] Although this agent contains the ethylenediamine side chain, its main use is as a sedative.

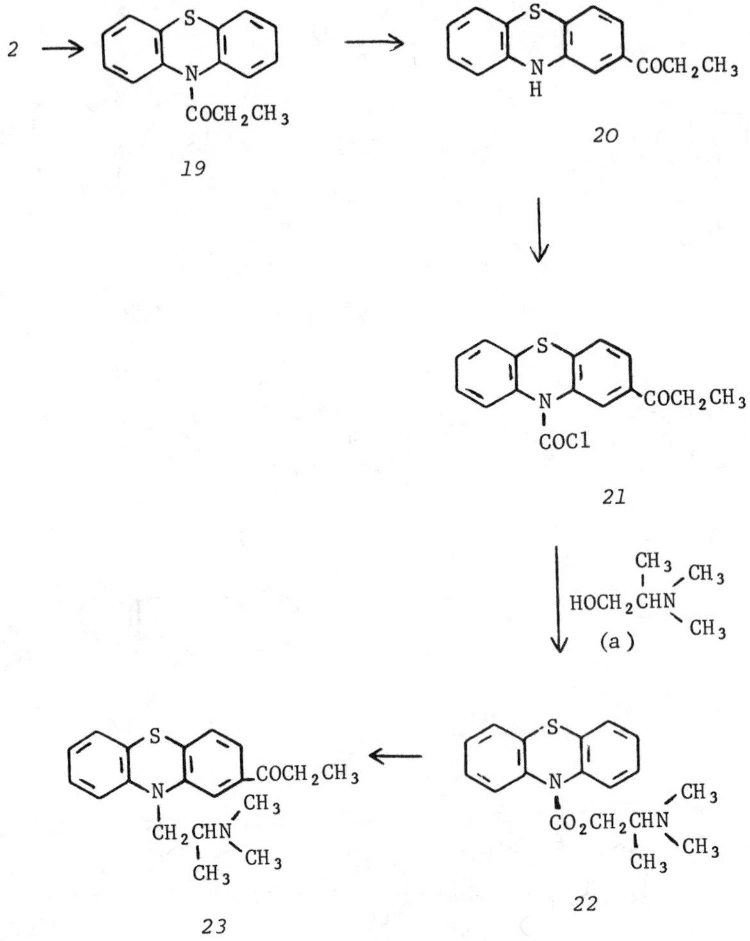

The most prominent pharmacologic activity exhibited by phenothiazines bearing the 1,3-propyldiamine side chain is, of course, that of a neuroleptic agent. Treatment of psychoses and severe neuroses constitutes the largest single use of these so-called

major tranquilizers. In addition, however, many of these drugs
have useful activity as sedatives and antiemetics. It should be
noted that one of the more potent 1,2 diamines, *promethazine*, is
occasionally used for these indications as well. Extensive synthetic work has been devoted to attempts to isolate these various
activities with the result that specific phenothiazine drugs vary
greatly in their clinical profile. Discussion of these profiles
is beyond the scope of this book; compounds that are indicated
for use other than neuroleptics are, however, identified.

The parent drug of this series, *promazine (24)*, was prepared
originally as an antihistamine. Following the identification of
the more potent chloro analog as an antipsychotic, it too came
into use for that indication. The drug is prepared by straightforward alkylation of phenothiazine with *N*-(3-chloropropyl)di-
methylamine by means of sodium hydride in xylene.[8]

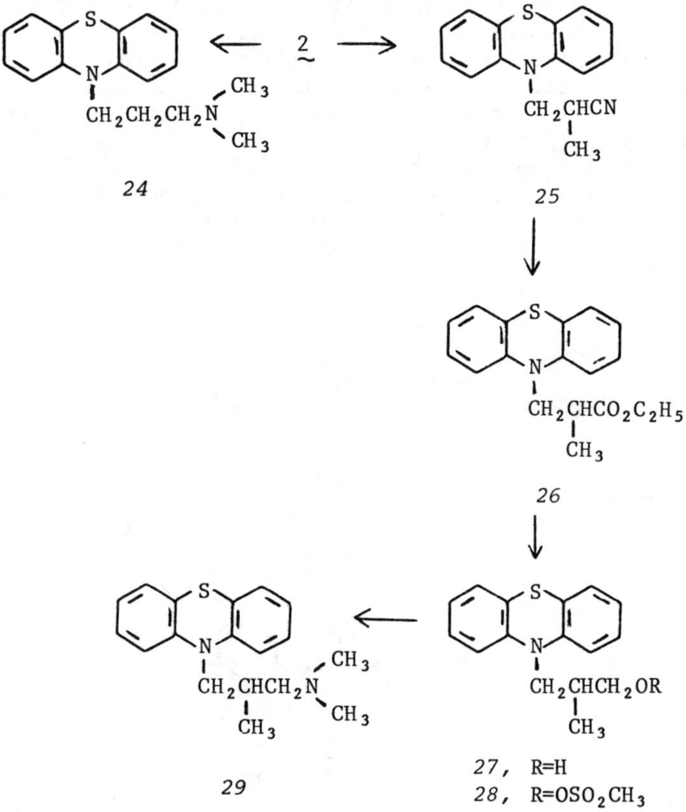

Alkylation of phenothiazine with the homologous *N*-(3-chloro-2-methylpropyl)dimethylamine leads to *trimeprazine (29)*. An interesting alternate synthesis to this agent begins with the Michael addition of phenothiazine to methacrylonitrile. Alcoholysis of the nitrile gives the ester *(26)*. The carbonyl group is then reduced by means of lithium aluminum hydride and the resulting alcohol *(27)* converted to the corresponding mesylate. Displacement with dimethylamine gives *trimeprazine (29)*,[5] a major tranquilizer that retains some antihistaminic properties.

Chlorpromazine (33) can probably be considered the prototype of the phenothiazine major tranquilizers. The antipsychotic potential of the phenothiazines was in fact discovered in the course of research with this agent. It is of note that, despite the great number of alternate analogs now available to clinicians, the original agent still finds considerable use. The first recorded preparation of this compound relies on the sulfuration reaction. Thus, heating 3-chlorodiphenylamine *(30)* with sulfur and iodine affords the desired phenothiazine *(31)* as well as a lesser amount of the isomeric product *(32)* produced by reaction at the 2 position. The predominance of reaction at 6 is perhaps due to the sterically hindered nature of the 2 position. Alkylation with *N*-(3-chloropropyl)dimethylamine by means of sodium amide affords *chlorpromazine (33)*.[9]

Sulfuration of the methoxy analog of *30* similarly gives a mixture of the desired 2-substituted phenothiazine *(35)* and byproduct *(36)*. Alkylation of *35* as above affords *methoxypromazine (37)*.[9]

30, R=Cl
34, R=OCH$_3$

31, R=Cl
35, R=OCH$_3$

32, R=Cl
36, R=OCH$_3$

33, R=Cl
37, R=OCH$_3$

Alkylation of the parent compound *(30)* with *N*-(3-chloropro-
pyl)diethylamine rather than the lower homolog affords *chlorproethazine (43)*. This same compound is available by an alternate
route that bypasses the sulfuration reaction. Aromatic nucleo-
phylic substitution on 2,4-dichloronitrobenzene *(38)* with 2-bro-
mothiophenoxide *(39)* affords the sulfide *(40)*. Reduction of the
nitro group followed by alkylation of the resulting amine *(41)*
with *N*-(3-chloropropyl)diethylamine gives the intermediate, *42*.
This is then cyclized by heating in dimethylformamide to give the
desired product *(43)*.[10]

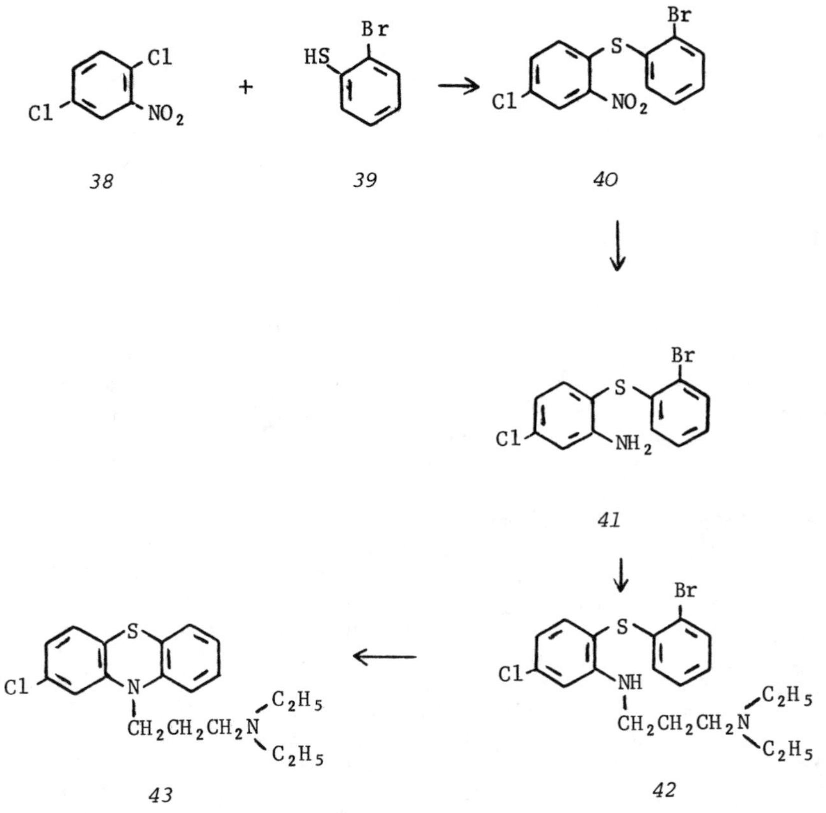

An intermediate used in the preparation of the antihistamine, *propiomazine*, serves as starting material for a 2-substi-
tuted major tranquilizer as well. Thus, reaction of the phosgene

adduct *(21)* with amino alcohol *44* affords the carbamate *(45)*. As in the case of the two-carbon side chain, pyrrolysis of this urethane leads, after loss of carbon dioxide, to *propiomazine (46)*.[11]

21 $\xrightarrow[\quad\quad 44 \quad\quad]{\text{HOCH}_2\text{CH}_2\text{CH}_2\text{N} \overset{\text{CH}_3}{\underset{\text{CH}_3}{}}}$

45

46

    It has often been observed in medicinal chemistry that, in those series in which substitution of halogen on an aromatic ring results in increased potency, a yet greater increase can be achieved by inclusion of the trifluoromethyl group. The phenothiazines have proved to be such a series. The requisite starting material can be obtained by the sulfuration reaction of the substituted diphenylamine, *53*, with the usual mixture of isomers resulting.[13] The Smiles rearrangement offers a regioselective, albeit longer, route to this compound. Displacement on the nitrobenzene, *47*, by means of the thiophenoxide from *48* yields the corresponding sulfide. Treatment with base presumably generates an anion on the formamide nitrogen; this negatively charged species then adds to the aromatic ring at the carbon bearing the sulfur *(50)*. Ring opening results in the loss of the better leaving group to give the thiophenoxide, *51*. This last then again undergoes an addition-elimination reaction *(52)* to give finally the desired product *(54)* (the strongly basic conditions lead to hydrolysis of the amide).[12] Alkylation of that phenothiazine with *N*-(3-chloropropyl)dimethylamine affords the very potent major tranquilizer *triflupromazine (55)*.[13]

    Incorporation of a second nitrogen atom in the side chain, particularly when that atom is part of a piperazine ring, was found to give a series of major tranquilizers similar in biologic activity to chlorpromazine, but of much increased potency. Alky-

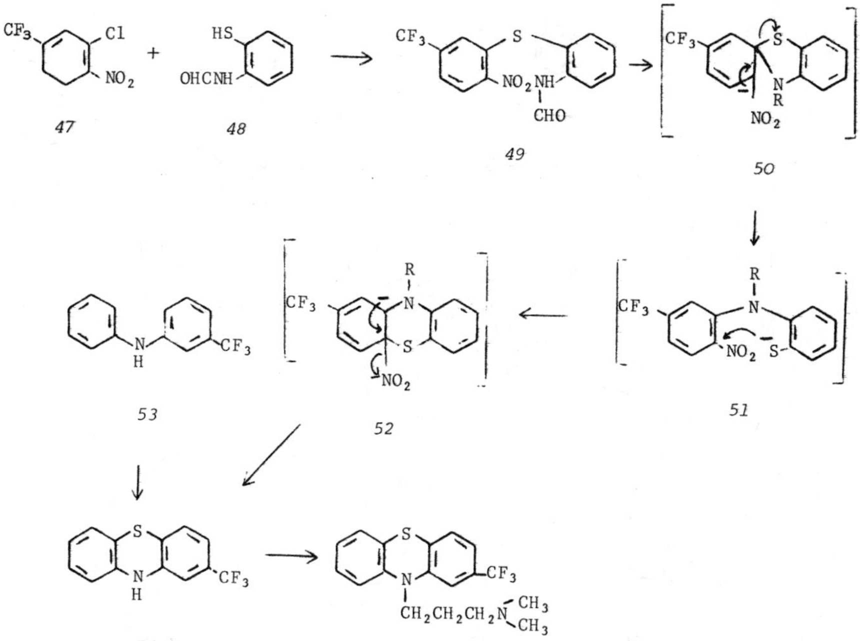

lation of the lithium salt of phenothiazine by means of 3-
bromo-1-propanol toluenesulfonate affords the intermediate containing the bromopropyl side chain *(63)*. Condensation of this
with the monocarbethoxy derivative of piperazine gives the urethane *(64)*. Reduction of the last by means of lithium aluminum
hydride yields *perazine (62)*.[14] In an analogous approach, 2-
chlorophenothiazine *(31)* is first alkylated by means of 3-bromo-
1-chloropropane to afford the compound containing the chloropropyl side chain *(58)*. Alkylation of 4-methylpiperazine with that
halide affords *prochlorperazine (60)*.[15] In much the same manner,
the trifluromethyl analog *(54)* is first converted to the chloropropyl compound *(59)*, and this then used to alkylate 4-methyl-
piperazine; the product obtained in this case is *triflupromazine*
(61).[16] The synthesis of *butaperazine (66)* involves yet another
variation on this theme. Thus, alkylation of the substituted
phenothiazine *(56)* (obtained by a reaction sequence similar to
that used to prepare *20*) with the complete preformed side chain
(65) (obtainable from 3-bromo-1-chloropropane and methylpipera-
zine) affords the desired product in a single step.[17]

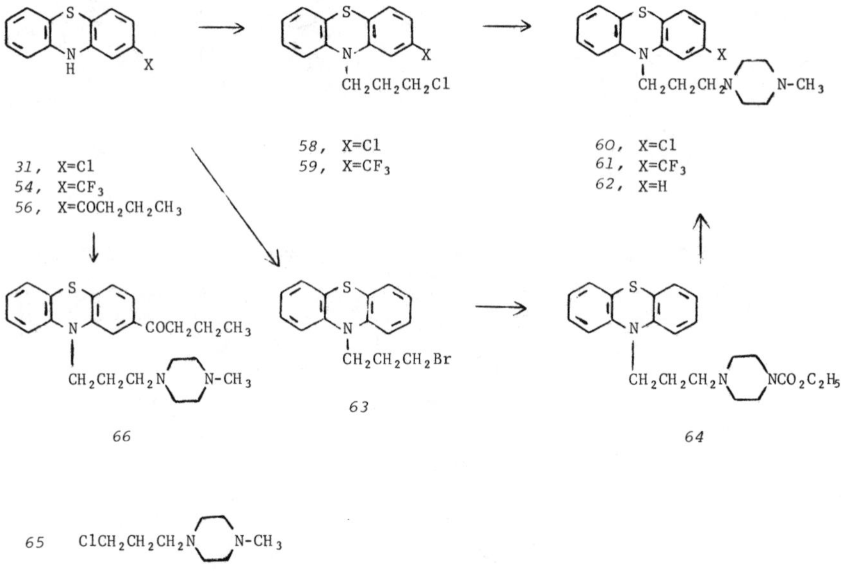

31, X=Cl
54, X=CF$_3$
56, X=COCH$_2$CH$_2$CH$_3$

58, X=Cl
59, X=CF$_3$

60, X=Cl
61, X=CF$_3$
62, X=H

66

63

64

65   ClCH$_2$CH$_2$CH$_2$N$\diagup$N-CH$_3$

Preparation of the phenothiazine containing a sulfur substituent at the 2 position involves a modification of the schemes reviewed thus far. In essence, the initial step depends on activation of aromatic chlorine towards nucleophilic aromatic substitution by a group that can be easily removed later; a carboxyl group is found to fulfill this need. Thus, treatment of o-chlorobenzoic acid with the substituted aniline (68) affords the corresponding anthranilic acid (69). Decarboxylation removes the activating group. Heating of diphenylamine (70) thus produced with sulfur and iodine gives the desired phenothiazine 71 as well as some of the 4-ethylthio isomer.[18] Alkylation of the former (71) with the side chain, 65, affords thiethylperazine (72).[19]

Replacement of the methyl group of the piperazine-substituted phenothiazines by some more polar group such as hydroxyethyl fragment leads to a further small increase in potency. It should be noted at this point that all phenothiazines manifest a series of side effects. The given set of these varies, however, with the side chains. The availability of the great variety of such structural variations makes it more likely that some drug will be found that a given individual will tolerate.

Key to this series is hydroxyethylpiperazine. This intermediate is attainable from the monocarbamate of piperazine

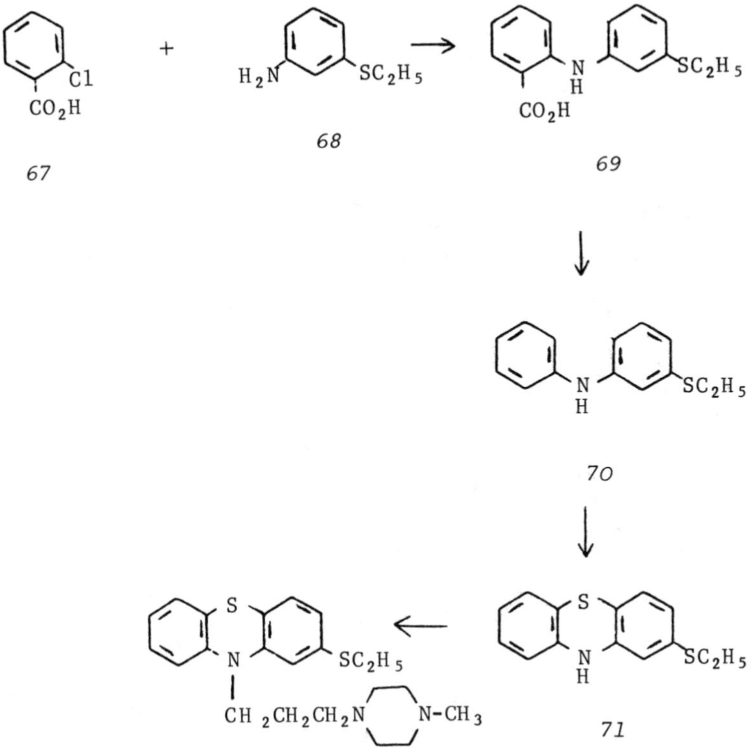

by several routes such as, for example, with ethylene oxide followed by hydrolysis of the urethane. Alkylation of the piperazine derivative with the chloropropyl derivative, *58*, affords
perphenazine (75)[20]; the trifluoromethyl derivative, *59*, gives
fluphenazine (76).[21] The 2-acetyl compound *(73)*, prepared in a
manner analogous to *56*, gives *acetophenazine (77)*,[22] and finally
use of *74* (obtained by alkylation of *20* with bromochloropropane)
in the alkylation reaction gives *carphenazine (78)*.[23] Acetylation of *perphenazine* with acetic anhydride yields *thiopropazate*
(79).[24]

Alkylation of phenothiazine with 1-chloro-2-methyl-3-
bromopropane affords the methylated analog *(80)* of the intermediate above. Use of this halide to alkylate the piperazine

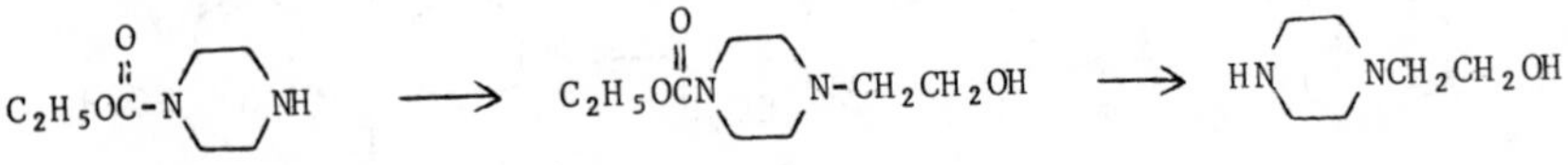

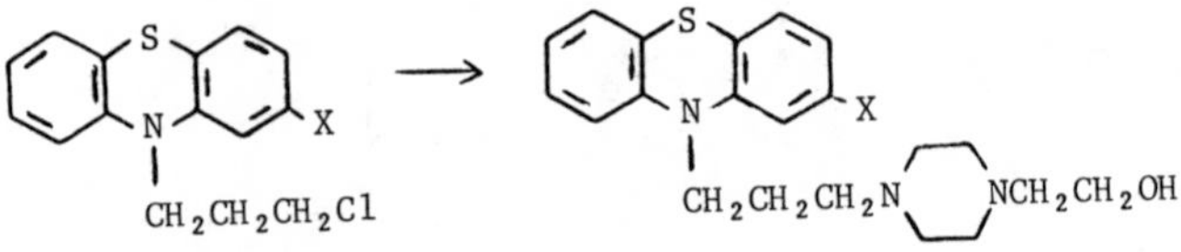

58, X=Cl
59, X=CF$_3$
73, X=CH$_3$CO
74, X=CH$_3$CH$_2$CO

75, X=Cl
76, X=CF$_3$
77, X=CH$_3$CO
78, X=CH$_3$CH$_2$CO

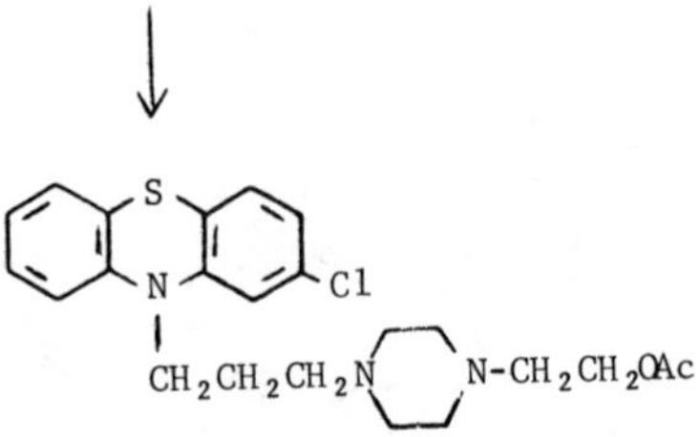

79

derivative, *81*, affords the tranquilizer *dixyrazine (82)*.[25]

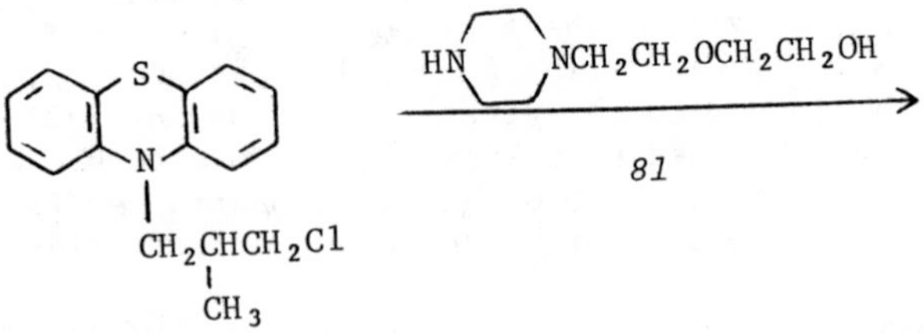

80

81

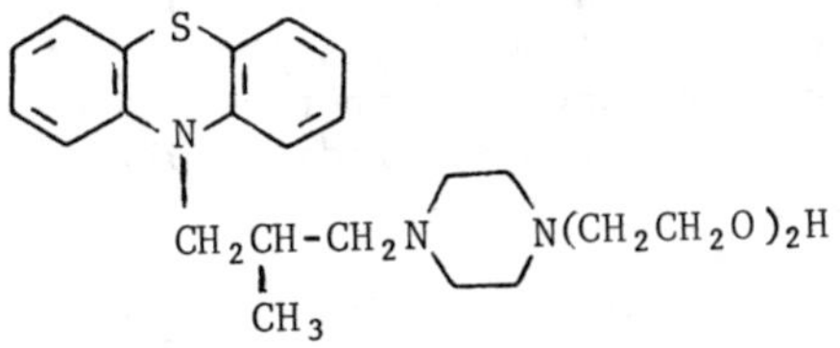

$$CH_2CH-CH_2N \quad N(CH_2CH_2O)_2H$$
$$\qquad\qquad CH_3$$

82

The most complex side chain of the piperazine phenothiazines is to be found on *chlorimpiphenine (86)*. The side chain is prepared by first alkylating monocarbethoxypiperazine with the chlorobenzimidazole *83* (itself attainable by alkylation of methylbenzimidazole with a dihalide). Removal of the carbethoxy group affords the substituted piperazine, *85*. Alkylation of this base with the chloropropyl phenothiazine, *58*, affords finally the desired compound *(86)*.[26]

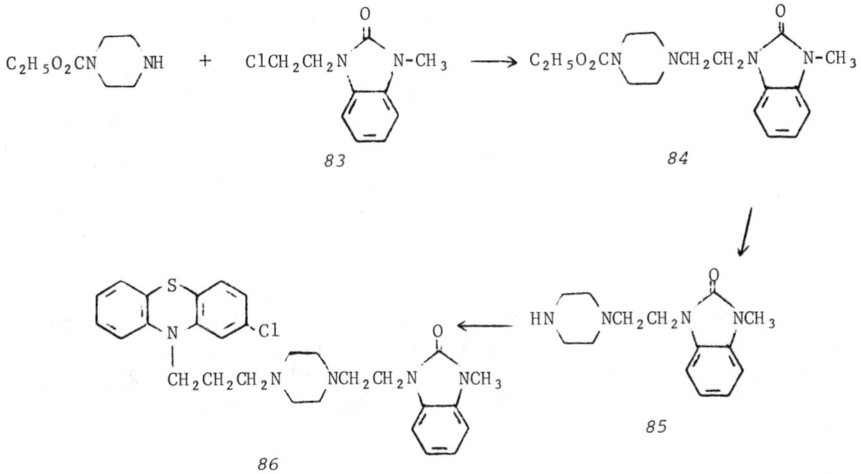

$$C_2H_5O_2CN \quad NH \quad + \quad ClCH_2CH_2N \quad N-CH_3 \quad \longrightarrow \quad C_2H_5O_2CN \quad NCH_2CH_2N \quad N-CH_3$$

83   *84*

$$CH_2CH_2CH_2N \quad NCH_2CH_2N \quad NCH_3 \quad \longleftarrow \quad HN \quad NCH_2CH_2N \quad NCH_3$$

86   *85*

Replacement of the terminal nitrogen of the piperazine by carbon is said to enhance the antiemetic activity of the phenothiazines at the expense of the other pharmacologic effects. The simplest compound in this series, *pipamazine (88)*, is prepared by alkylation of nipecotamide *(87)* with the chloropropyl phenothiazine *(58)*.[27] Preparation of the analogous sulfoxide begins with acetylation of the thiomethyl compound, *89* (prepared by a route analogous to that used to obtain 71). Oxidation of the product with peracid followed by saponification gives the sulfone (91). This is then converted to the chloropropyl derivative (92). Treatment with the piperidine (87) affords metopimazine (93).[28]

58 + HN⟨⟩—CONH₂ ⟶

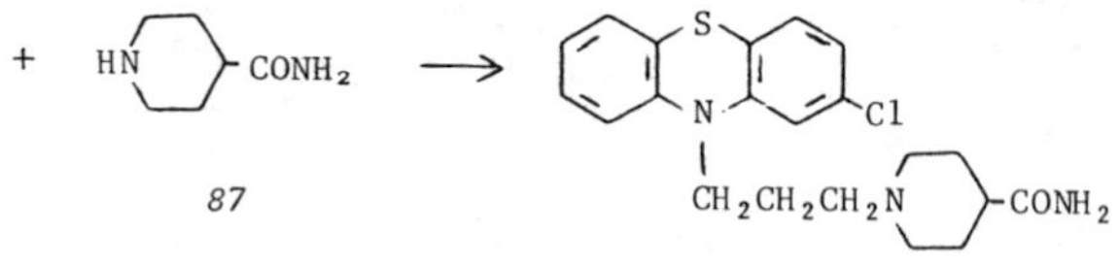

87

CH₂CH₂CH₂N⟨⟩—CONH₂

88

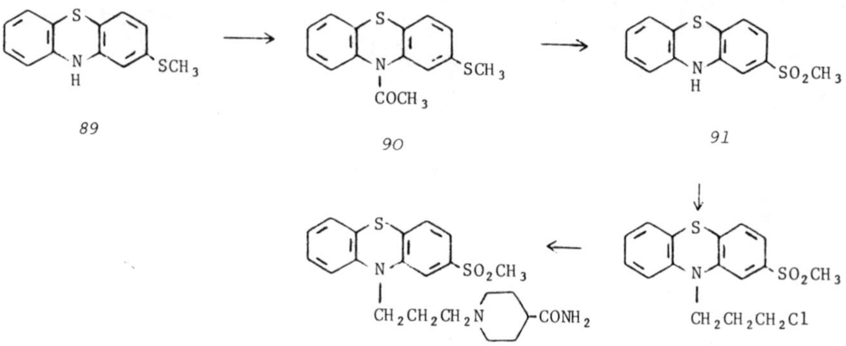

89 ⟶ 90 ⟶ 91

93 ← 92

That this is not a general observation is indicated by the fact that piperactizine (95), in which carbon again replaced nitrogen, obtained by alkylation of amino alcohol, 94, with the halide (73) is used mainly as a major tranquilizer.

73 + HN⟨⟩—CH₂CH₂OH ⟶

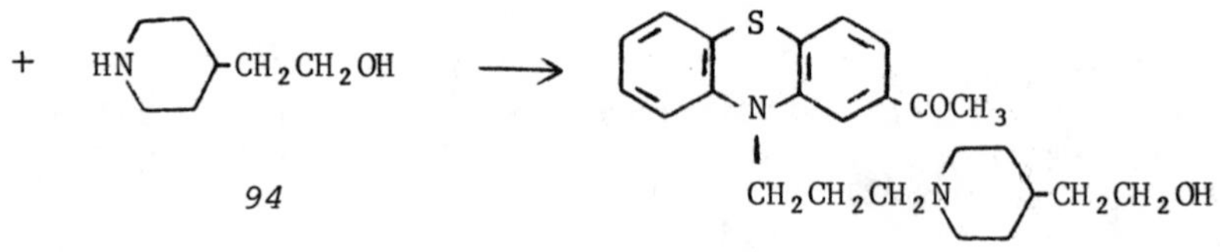

94

CH₂CH₂CH₂N⟨⟩—CH₂CH₂OH

95

Rigid analogs have met with some success in medicinal chemistry. In brief, it is first assumed that some particular steric
orientation of a given grouping within a molecule is required to
give the best possible interaction with the hypothetical receptor
site. A loose floppy side chain, of course, has the best chance
of assuming the required orientation. That very process, however, must pay the cost of an entropy factor. If, on the other
hand, the group is locked into the proper configuration before-
hand, an energetically more favorable situation, and hopefully
greater potency, will result. The most common way of achieving
such rigidity is the inclusion of the group in question into a
ring system. It should, however, be added that, during the synthetic work involved in drug development, rigid analogs have been
known more than once to lock a group into a configuration that
gives no fit whatever with the receptors (i.e., inactive compounds).

It will be at once appreciated that the propyl side chain
interposed between the two nitrogens in the prototype phenothiazines constitutes a rather flexible arrangement with a large
number of possible conformations. One approach towards restrict-
ing the degree of freedom of the side chain incorporates the aliphatic nitrogen in a piperidine, with that heterocycle attached
to the phenothiazine by a methylene bridge. Construction of the
piperidine starts with a double Michael condensation of ethyl
acrylate on methylamine. Dieckmann cyclization of the resulting
diester (96) gives the piperidine (97). Catalytic reduction over
Raney nickel gives the corresponding hydroxymethyl compound (98)
(possibly by hydrogenolysis of the intermediate β-hydroxy ester),
which is then converted to the bromo compound (99). Alkylation
of phenothiazine with that halide affords the relatively potent
major tranquilizer *pecazine (100)*.[29]

The ring-contracted analog of *100, methdilazine (106)*, interestingly enough shows only very weak activity as a tranquilizer;
instead, that agent constitutes an important antihistamine. Preparation of the side chain in this case starts with the condensation of N-methylpyrrolidone (101) with ethyl oxalate. The condensation product is then reduced catalytically to remove the
double bond and interrupt the conjugated system. Subsequent
reduction with lithium aluminum hydride serves to reduce the lactam to the amine and the ester to the corresponding alcohol (103).
Cleavage of the diol with sodium periodate to the aldehyde followed by catalytic reduction yield the carbinol (104). This last
is then converted to the chloride (105) with thionyl chloride.[30]
Alkylation of phenothiazine with the cyclic side chain affords
methdilazine (106).[31]

The 2-piperidinoethyl side chain leads to some very potent

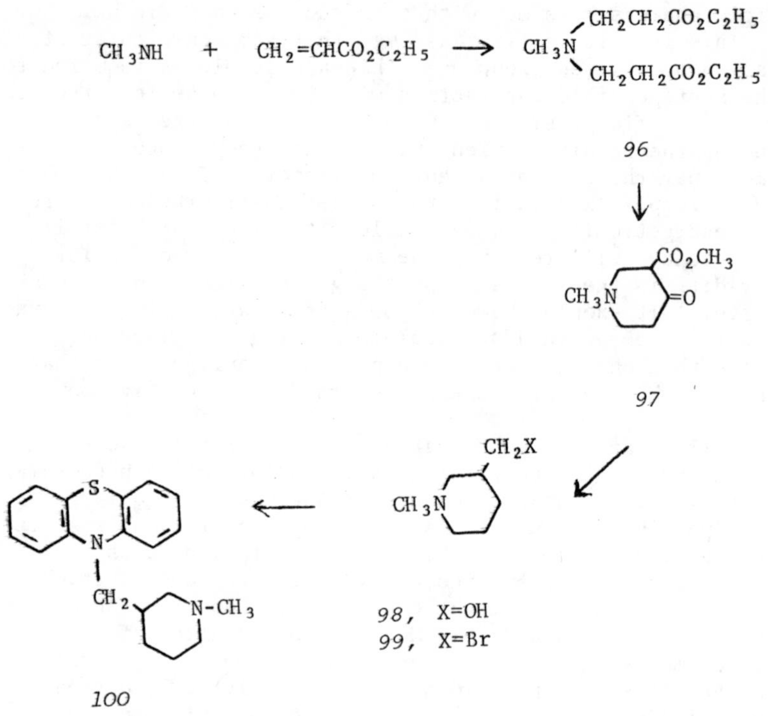
CH3NH
+
CH2=CHCO2C2H5
CH3N
CH2CH2CO2C2H5
CH2CH2CO2C2H5
96
CO2CH3
CH3N
=O
97
CH2X
CH3N
98, X=OH
99, X=Br
S
N
CH2
N-CH3
100

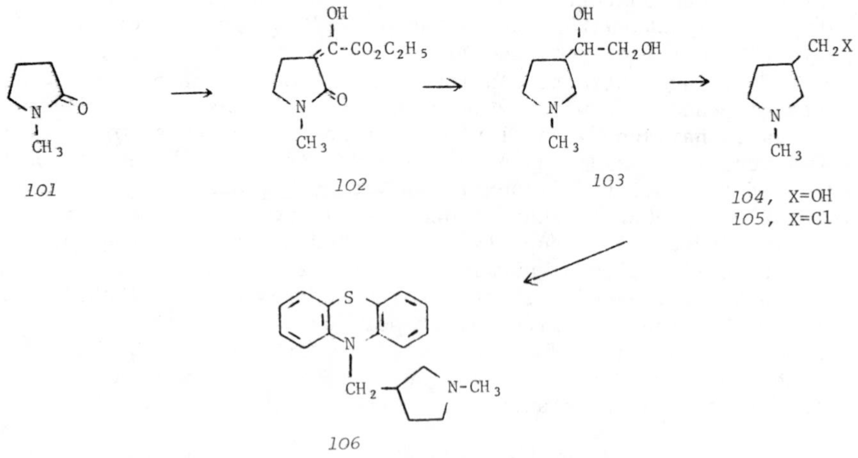
N
O
CH3
101
OH
C-CO2C2H5
N
O
CH3
102
OH
CH-CH2OH
N
CH3
103
CH2X
N
CH3
104, X=OH
105, X=Cl
S
N
CH2
N-CH3
106

major tranquilizers that are said to be unusually free of the
side effects characteristic of the phenothiazines. Preparation
of the side chain in this case involves first conversion of 2-
picoline (107) to the homologated alcohol, 108, by treatment of
the lithium salt of the former with formaldehyde. Reaction with
methyl iodide followed by catalytic reduction of the pyridinium
salt (109) affords the piperidine (110). This is then converted
to the chloro compound (111).[32] Alkylation of the methylthio-
substituted phenothiazine with this side chain affords mesoridazine (115).[19]

Alternately, the N-acylated derivative of the substituted
phenothiazine (112) is oxidized to the corresponding sulfoxide
by means of periodic acid. Saponification (113) followed by
alkylation with the above side chain affords thioridazine (114).[19]

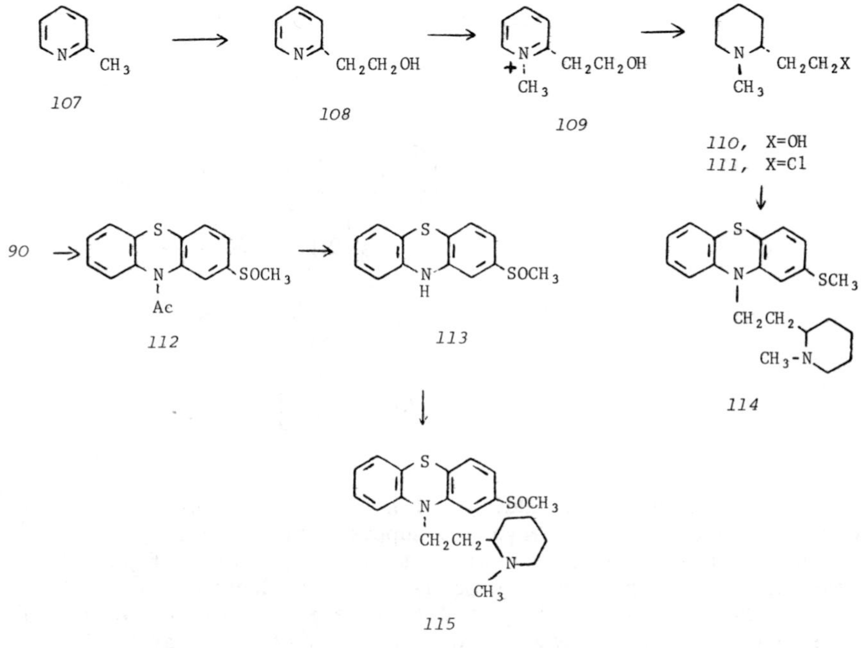

The use of urethanes of phenothiazines involving the heterocyclic nitrogen (22, 45) as a means of attaching the side chain
is discussed above. Although these intermediates apparently do
not possess antipsychotic activity, two compounds of this general
class, endowed with somewhat more complex appendages, do exhibit

antispasmodic activity. Both these compounds have found some use
as antitussive agents. Alkylation of the condensation product of
diethylaminoethanol and ethylene oxide (117) with the carbamoyl
chloride from phosgene and phenothiazine (116) affords *dimethoxanate* (119).[33] Analogous reaction of the pyrrolidyl alcohol
(118) yields *pipazethate* (120).[34]

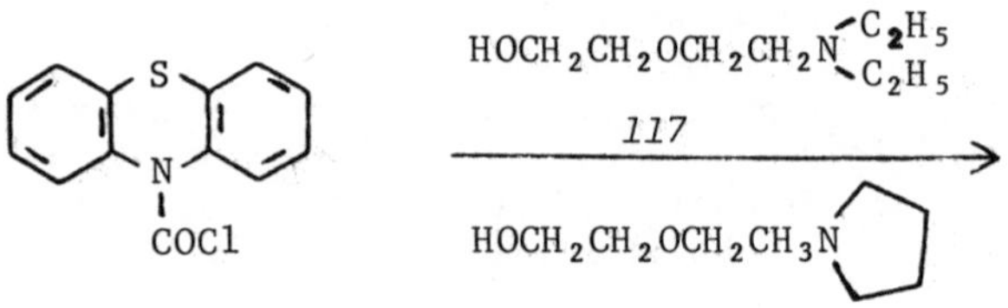

$$HOCH_2CH_2OCH_2CH_2N\begin{smallmatrix}C_2H_5\\C_2H_5\end{smallmatrix}$$

117

$$HOCH_2CH_2OCH_2CH_3N\bigcirc$$

116   118

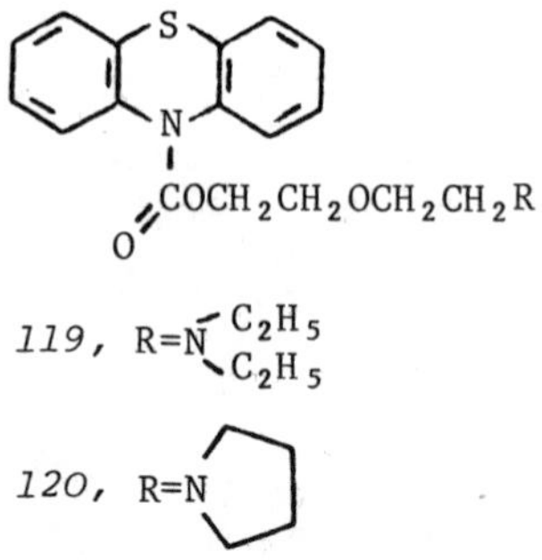

119, $R=N\begin{smallmatrix}C_2H_5\\C_2H_5\end{smallmatrix}$

$COCH_2CH_2OCH_2CH_2R$

120, $R=N\bigcirc$

Substitution of an additional nitrogen atom onto the three-
carbon side chain also serves to suppress tranquilizing activity
at the expense of antispasmodic activity. Reaction of phenothiazine with epichlorohydrin by means of sodium hydride gives the
epoxide *121*. It should be noted that, even if initial attack in
this reaction is on the epoxide, the alkoxide ion that would
result from this nucleophilic addition can readily displace the
adjacent chlorine to give the observed product. Opening of the
oxirane with dimethylamine proceeds at the terminal position to
afford the amino alcohol, *122*. The amino alcohol is then converted to the halide (123). A displacement reaction with
dimethylamine gives *aminopromazine* (124).[35]

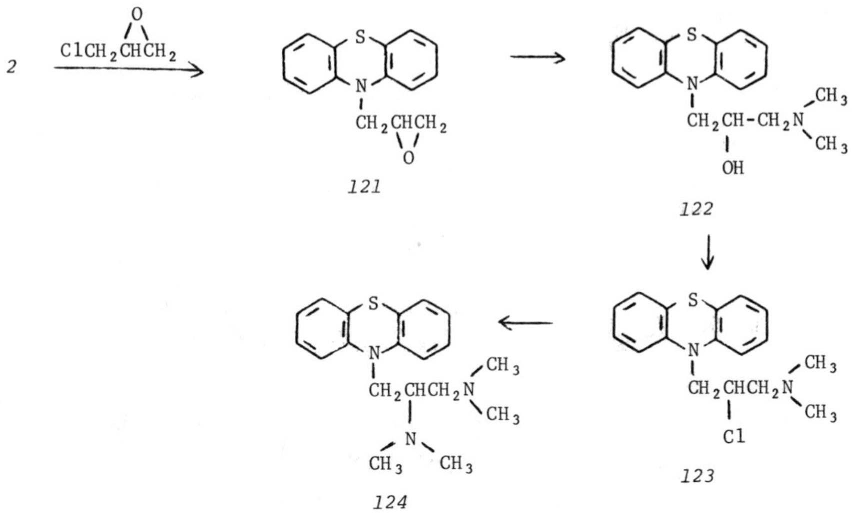

$$2 \xrightarrow{\text{ClCH}_2\overset{\text{O}}{\overset{/\backslash}{\text{CH}}}\text{CH}_2}$$

121

122

123

124

REFERENCES

1. P. Charpentier, *Compt. Rend.*, *225*, 306 (1947).
2. W. B. Reid, J. B. Wright, H. G. Kolloff, and J. H. Hunter, *J. Amer. Chem. Soc.*, *70*, 3100 (1948).
3. E. M. Schultz, C. M. Robb, and J. M. Sprague, *J. Amer. Chem. Soc.*, *69*, 188 (1947).
4. S. S. Berg and J. N. Ashley, U. S. Patent 2,607,773 (1952).
5. R. M. Jacob and J. G. Robert, U. S. Patent 2,837,518 (1958).
6. Authors unknown, British Patent 814,512 (1959).
7. J. Schmitt, A. Halot, P. Comoy, M. Susquet, R. Fallard, and J. Boitard, *Bull. Soc. Chim. France*, 1474 (1957).
8. P. Charpentier, U. S. Patent 2,159,886 (1950).
9. P. Charpentier, P. Gailliot, R. Jacob, J. Gaudechon, and P. Buisson, *Compt. Rend.*, *235*, 59 (1952).
10. P. J. C. Buisson and P. Gailliot, U. S. Patent 2,769,002 (1956).
11. J. Schmitt, J. Boitard, P. Comoy, A. Hallot, and M. Susquet, *Bull. Soc. Chim. France*, 938 (1957).
12. A. Roe and W. F. Little, *J. Org. Chem.*, *20*, 1577 (1955).
13. H. L. Yale, F. Sowinsky, and J. Bernstein, *J. Amer. Chem. Soc.*, *79*, 4375 (1957).
14. O. Hromotka, G. Stehlik, and F. Sauter, *Monatsh.*, *91*, 107

(1960).

15. R. J. Herclois, U. S. Patent 2,902,484 (1959).
16. P. N. Craig, E. A. Nodiff, J. J. Lafferty, and G. E. Ullyot, *J. Org. Chem., 22,* 709 (1957).
17. U. Hoerlein, K. H. Risse, and W. Wirth, German Patent 1,120,451 (1956).
18. J. P. Bourquin, G. Schwarb, G. Gamboni, R. Fischer, L. Ruesch, S. G. Uldimann, U. Theuss, E. Schenke, and J. Renz, *Helv. Chim. Acta, 41,* 1061 (1958).
19. J. P. Bourquin, G. Schwarb, G. Gamboni, R. Rischer, L. Ruesch, S. G. Uldimann, U. Theuss, E. Schenke, and J. Renz, *Helv. Chim. Acta, 41,* 1072 (1958).
20. M. H. Sherlock and N. Sperber, U. S. Patent 2,860,138 (1958).
21. H. L. Yale and F. Sowinski, *J. Amer. Chem. Soc., 82,* 2039 (1960).
22. M. H. Sherlock and N. Sperber, U. S. Patent 2,985,659 (1961).
23. R. F. Tislow, W. F. Bruce, and J. A. Page, U. S. Patent 3,023,146 (1962).
24. E. L. Anderson, G. B. Bellizona, P. N. Craig, G. E. Jaffe, K. P. Janeway, C. Kaizer, B. M. Lester, E. J. Nikawitz, A. M. Parloff, H. E. Reiff, and C. Zirkle, *Arzneimittel Forsch., 12,* 937 (1962).
25. H. G. Moren, British Patent 861,420 (1961).
26. Author unknown, Belgian Patent 668,927 (1965).
27. J. W. Cusic and H. W. Sause, U. S. Patent 2,957,870 (1960).
28. R. M. Jacob and J. G. Robert, German Patent 1,092,476 (1959).
29. W. A. Schuler, U. S. Patent 2,784,185 (1957).
30. L. W. Marsch and R. Peterson, *Arzneimittel Forsch., 9,* 715 (1959).
31. R. F. Feldkamp and Y. H. Wu, U. S. Patent 2,945,855 (1960).
32. T. R. Narton, R. A. Seibert, A. A. Benson, and F. W. Bergstrom, *J. Amer. Chem. Soc., 68,* 1573 (1946).
33. C. vonSeeman, U. S. Patent 2,778,824 (1957).
34. R. M. Jacob, R. Herlclois, R. Vaupre, and M. Messer, *Compt. Rend., 243,* 1637 (1956).

CHAPTER 20

Additional Heterocycles
Fused to Two Benzene Rings

1. DIBENZOPYRANS

A great many organic quaternary bases can inhibit the action of acetyl choline in organ systems activated by that neurotransmitter and thus possess anticholinergic-antispasmodic activity. One such agent is *methantheline bromide (4)*, used in the treatment of peptic ulcer and as an antispasmodic agent in intestinal disorders. Its synthesis involves Friedel-Crafts cyclization of o-

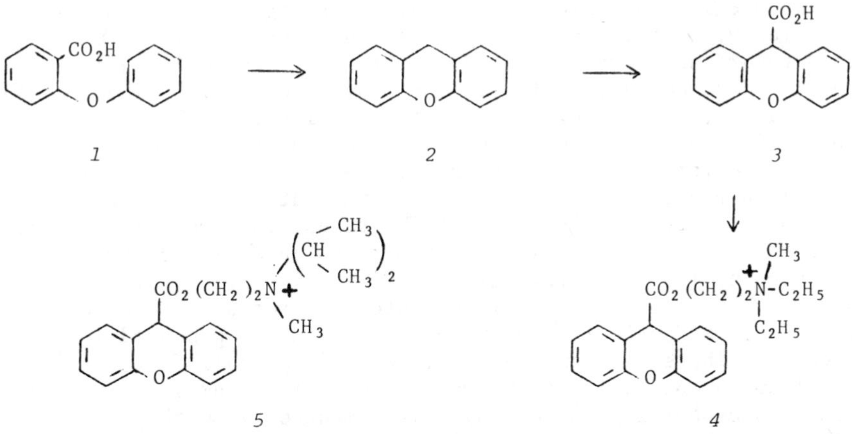

phenoxybenzoic acid *(1)* followed by hydrogenolysis with sodium and alcohol of the xanthone carbonyl group to form dibenzopyran, *2*. Formation of the requisite acid *(3)* is accomplished by car-

bonation of the lithium salt obtained by ionization of the acidic
proton on 2 by treatment with butyl lithium. Esterification is
accomplished by heating the sodium salt of 3 with 2-diethylamino-
ethyl chloride. Quaternization with methyl bromide gives *methantheline bromide (4)*.[1] The closely related analog, *propantheline bromide (5)*, is rather more potent than 4.

Cannabis is essentially the dried resinous mixture obtained
from the leaves and flowering tops of varieties of the Indian
hemp plant, *Cannabis sativa*, a hardy weed that grows in large
areas of the inhabited world. This preparation has long been
used in many lands as an inhaled sedative and, in the proper
surroundings and mental conditions, as a psychotropic agent.
Marihuana, tea, Mary Jane, pot, bhang, ganja, Acapulco gold, and
grass are but a few of the colorful nicknames for various grades
of cannabis. It is thought that the properties of cannabis are
largely attributable to the presence of Δ^1-*tetrahydrocannabinol*
(8). The content of 8 in cannabis is quite variable, depending
not only on the variety of plant and the conditions of its culti-
vation but also, since Δ^1-THC is unstable to acid and heat, the
methods used for harvesting, processing, storage, and administration. There is, of course, no quality control for this street
drug. Because of these objective factors and the substantial
subjective component regarding its effects, a raging controversy
surrounds this drug; the danger, efficacy, and potential value in
clinical medicine are all hotly disputed.

The availability of pure Δ^1-THC for carefully controlled
pharmacologic and toxicologic studies has begun to sort out fact
from fancy. Total chemical syntheses have been very useful in
this regard and largely depend on carefully controlled acid-
catalyzed condensation of selected monoterpenes with olivetol *(7)*.
For example, citral *(6)* and olivetol cyclize to Δ^1-THC *(8)* in
about 12% yield when condensed in ethanol containing 0.0005 N
hydrogen chloride. This process gives somewhat better yields
when 1% boron trifluoride is used as the catalyst. Since isomerization to virtually inactive Δ^6-THC takes place readily in acid
or upon heating, the cyclizations must be carefully controlled.
The mechanism of the cyclization reaction is not certain, but the
scheme shown below *(9)* may illustrate the process. Because
citral *(6)* is optically inactive, the Δ^1-THC so produced is also
racemic. The subsequent synthesis [4-6] of optically active Δ^1-
THC from an optically active monoterpene, for example, verbenol
(10), is especially noteworthy. Treatment of *10* with boron trifluoride in the presence of olivetol *(7)* leads to optically
active Δ^6-THC *(12)*, possibly via *11*. Double-bond isomerization
is then accomplished by addition of hydrogen chloride catalyzed
by zinc chloride. Treatment of the resulting halide *(13)* with

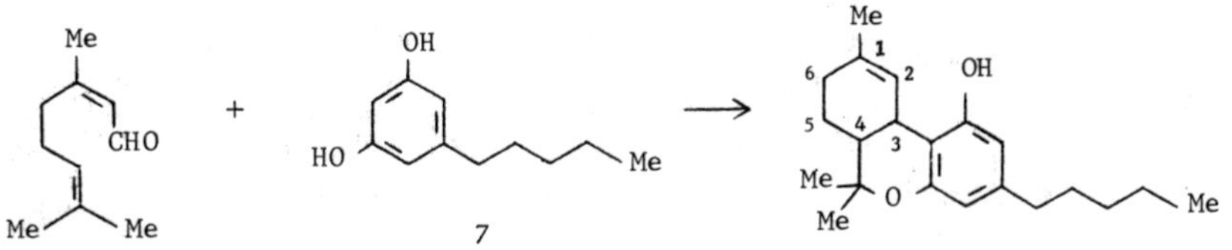

potassium tertiary amylate leads to elimination of hydrogen chloride from the 1,2 position, thus affording 8 in good yield.[7]

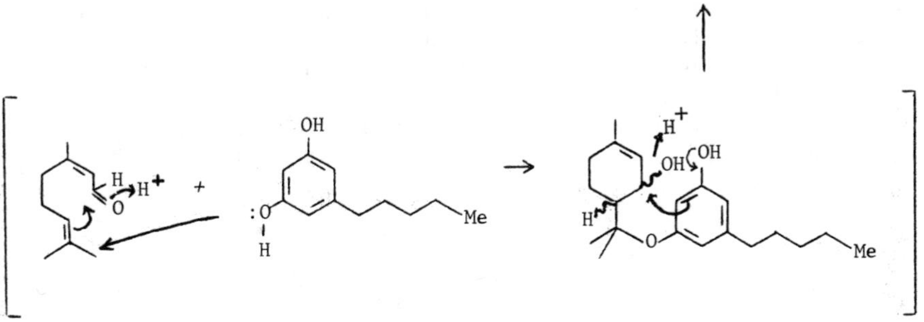

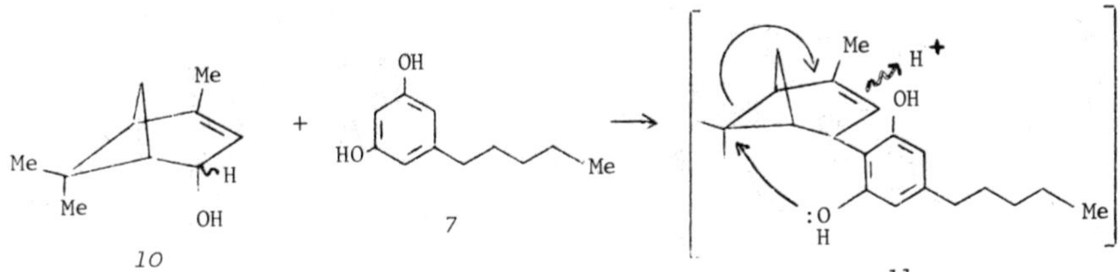

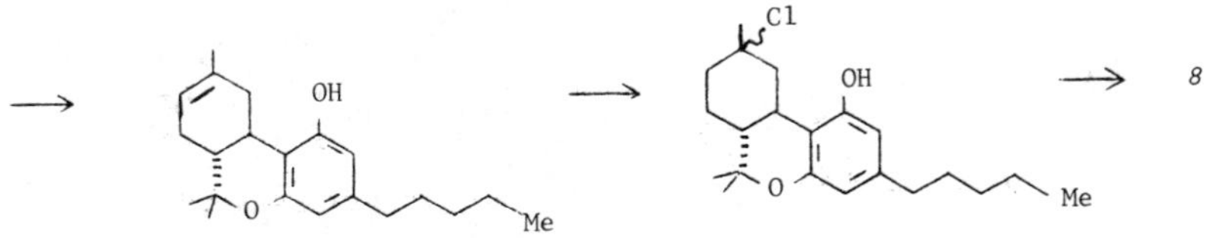

2. ACRIDINES

Malaria and the development of synthetic antimalarial drugs are
discussed in some detail in the section covering quinolines. The
organization of this book unfortunately sometimes distorts the
chronology involved in drug development. A series of acridine
antimalarial compounds were in fact developed almost simultaneously with the quinolines. One of these, *quinacrine (18)*, was
used extensively in World War II under the trade name of Ata-
brine®. Nucleophilic aromatic displacement of the ortho halogen
in *14* by *para*-anisidine affords the aminobenzoic acid, *16*.
Cyclization of this intermediate by means of phosphorus oxychloride affords initially the acridone; the presence of excess reagent serves to convert the carbonyl group to the halide *(17)*.
Displacement of that halogen by 1-diethylamino-4-aminopentane
yields *quinacrine (18)*.[8]

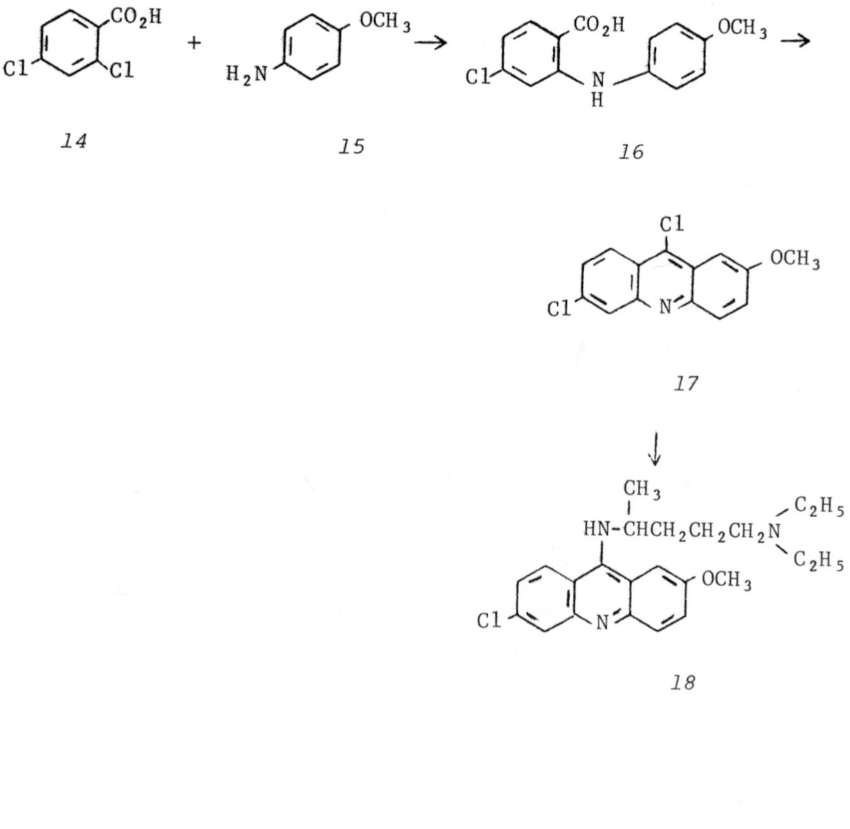

14   *15*   *16*

17

18

An acridine with a radically different substitution pattern, interestingly, still exhibits antimalarial activity. Condensation of acetone with diphenylamine in the presence of strong acid affords the partly reduced acridine, 20. Alkylation with 3-chloro-dimethylaminopropane (via the sodium salt of 20) affords *dimethacrine (21)*.[9]

19   20

21

3.   THIOXANTHENES

Lucanthone is one of the few orally effective drugs available for treatment of the dread tropical disease schistosomiasis, an infestation of blood flukes of the genus *Schistosoma*. This drug is paradoxically much better tolerated by children than adults; the relatively high incidence of side effects in the latter means that the agent is used mainly in treating the young. One route to this drug starts with the acid-catalyzed condensation of thiosalicylic acid *(22)* with p-chlorotoluene *(23)*.[10] There is obtained a difficultly separable mixture of isomeric thioxanthones *(24,25)*. Resort is therefore made to the differing reactivities of the halogen in these isomers towards nucleophilic aromatic displacement. The chlorine in 25 is activated by the ortho carbonyl group, while that in 24 should be relatively inert to this reaction. Heating the mixture of isomeric thioxanthones in the presence of 2-diethylaminoethylamine thus leads to an easily separable mixture of *lucanthone (26)* and recovered 24. Subsequent syntheses were reported that avoid the isomer problem. One of these starts with conversion of p-chlorotoluene to the sulfonyl chloride *(27)* by reaction with chlorosulfonic acid.

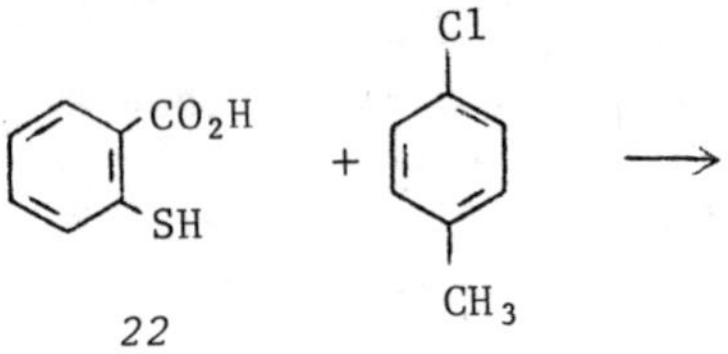

22

23

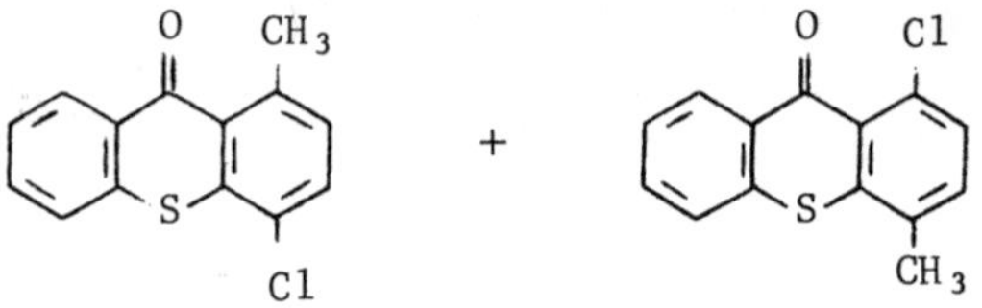

24   25

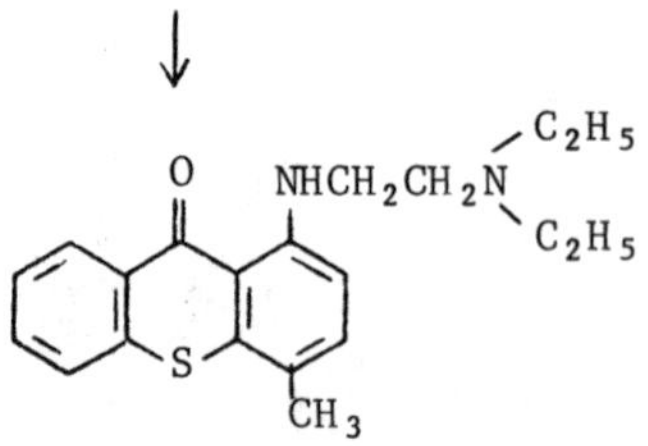

26

Reduction with zinc dust in aqueous sulfuric acid gives 2-methyl-4-aminothiophenol *(28)*. Condensation with 2-chlorobenzoic acid (Ullmann reaction) leads to *29*, which can close to but one thioxanthone *(25)* on treatment with sulfuric acid. Although this procedure is longer than the original, the yields are good and the sequence is regioselective.[11]

It was subsequently discovered that *lucanthone* is metabolized in the body in part to *hycanthone (30)*, a compound with enhanced schistomacidal activity. The relatively high biologic activity of *lucanthone* in experimental animals compared to man was subsequently attributed to the inefficient hydroxylating system present in man for this biochemical conversion.[12] Microbiologic oxidation of *lucanthone* by fermentation with the fungus *Aspergillus scelorotium* affords *hycanthone*.[13]

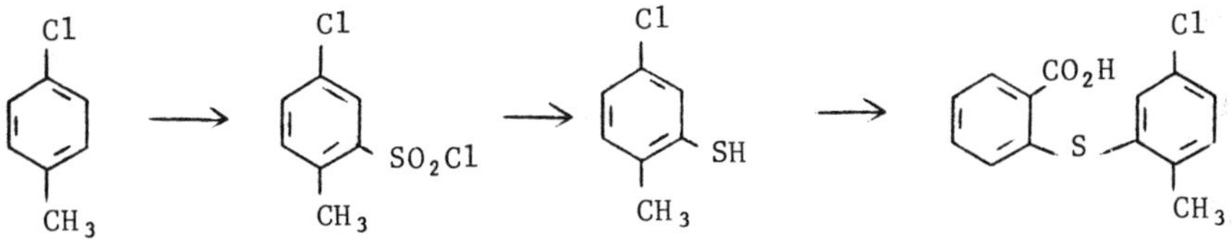

23   27   28

29

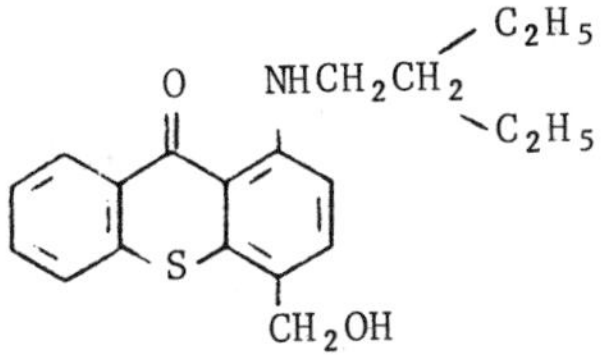

30

The efficacy of the phenothiazines for the treatment of various psychoses led to extensive synthetic programs aimed at modulation of the biologic spectrum of these molecules. As seen
elsewhere, much of this work has centered on changes of the
nature of the atoms that constitute the center ring. Thus, for
example, it has proven possible to replace the nitrogen atom of
the phenothiazine by carbon while maintaining neuroleptic activity.

Ullmann condensation of the sodium salt of p-chlorothiophe-
nol (31) with 2-iodobenzoic (32) acid gives 33. Cyclization by
means of sulfuric acid affords the thioxanthone, 34. Reaction
with the Grignard reagent from 3-dimethylaminopropyl chloride
affords the tertiary carbinol (35). Dehydration by means of
acetic anhydride affords chlorprothixene as a mixture of geomet-
ric isomers, 36.[14] (Subsequent work showed the Z isomer—chlorine
and amine on the same side—to be the more potent compound.)
Chlorprothixene is said to cause less sedation than the phenothiazines.

Appropriate modification of the last few steps affords clo-
penthixol (37).[15] It is of note that this compound approaches
the potency of one of the most active phenothiazines, perphenazine, an agent that has a very similar side chain.

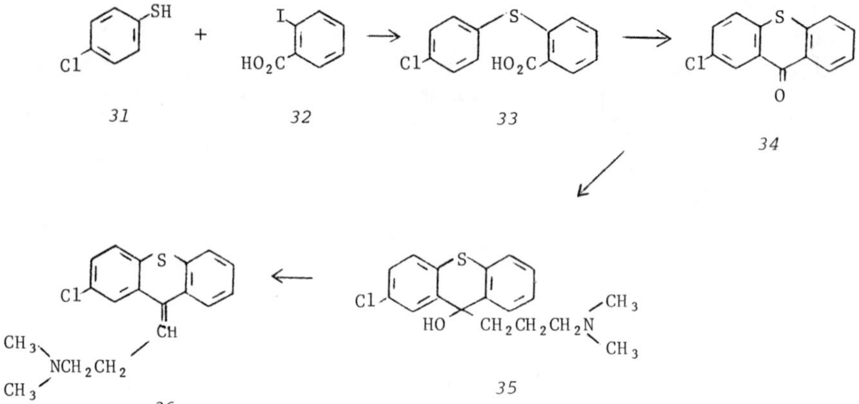

31   32   33

34

36   35

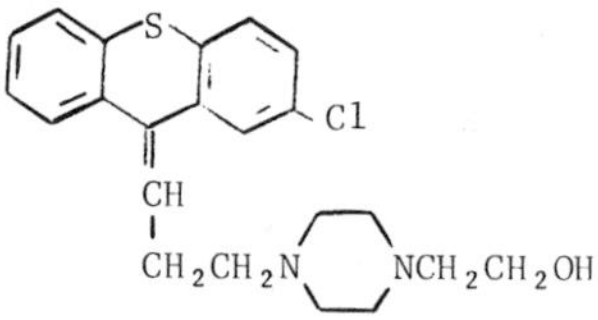

37

Alkylated sulfonamide groups have proven useful additions to the phenothiazine nucleus. The same seems to hold true in the thioxanthene series. Chlorosulfonation of the benzoic acid, *38*, followed by displacement with dimethylamine affords the sulfonamide, *39*. This is then taken on to the substituted thioxanthone *(41)* by the sequence of steps shown above; Grignard condensation followed by dehydration gives *thiothixine (42)*.[16]

Reduction of the exocyclic double bond generally decreases neuroleptic activity in this series. Some of these compounds, however, show other activities. *Methixene (44)*, for example, is used as an antispasmodic agent. It is prepared by alkylation of the sodium salt of thioxanthene *(43)* with *N*-methyl-3-chloromethyl-piperidine.[17]

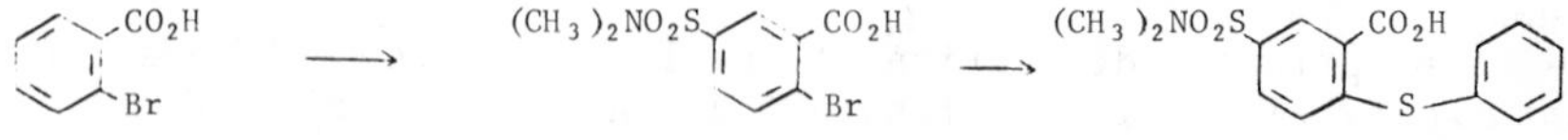

38   39   40

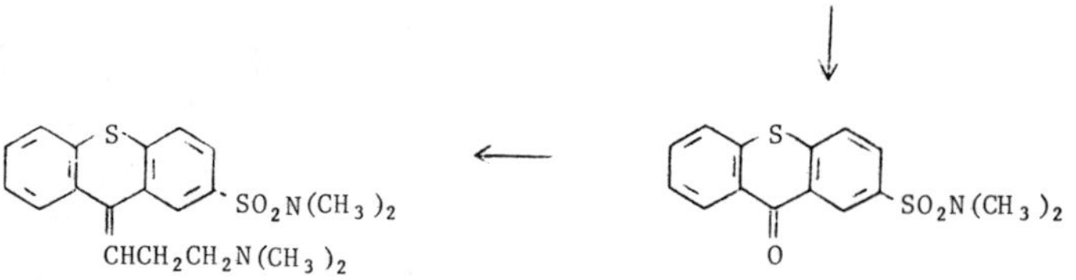

4. DIBENZAZEPINES

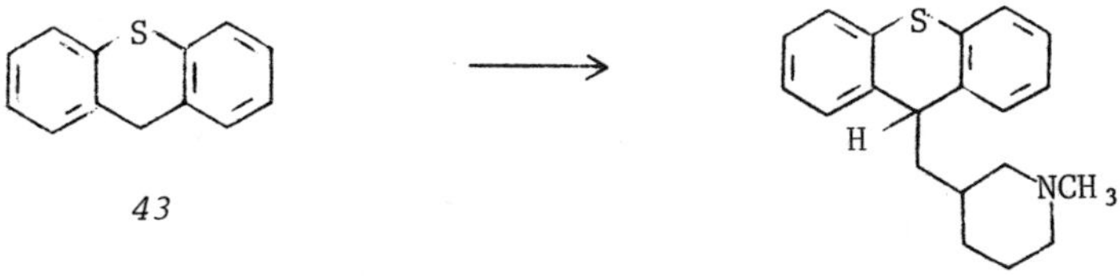

a. Dihydrodibenzazepines

Although these compounds, too, are structurally closely related
to the phenothiazines with which they may be considered isosteric,
their main activity tends to be as antidepressant agents. The
dibenzazepines do themselves enjoy a considerable vogue in the
treatment of endogenous depression. Together with the dibenzo-
cycloheptadiene derivatives, they are often referred to collectively as the tricyclic antidepressants. Although this basic
ring system has been known since 1899, its pharmacology is of
much more recent origin. The synthesis of *imipramine (50)*[18] is
typical of the chemistry of this series. 2-Chloromethylnitro-
benzene *(45)* self-condenses to styrene *(46)* under alkaline conditions (see, for example, *stilbestrol*). The nitro groups are then
reduced to give diamine, *47*. Reaction with sodium in amyl alcohol serves to reduce the double bond *(48)*. Strong heating results
in cyclization to 10,11-dihydro-5*H*-dibenz[b,f]azepine *(49)*, the
parent nucleus for the series. *Imipramine (50)* is prepared from
49 by forming the sodium salt on nitrogen with sodium amide and
alkylating this with 3-dimethylaminopropyl chloride. Metabolic
disposition of *imipramine* involves, among other processes, N-

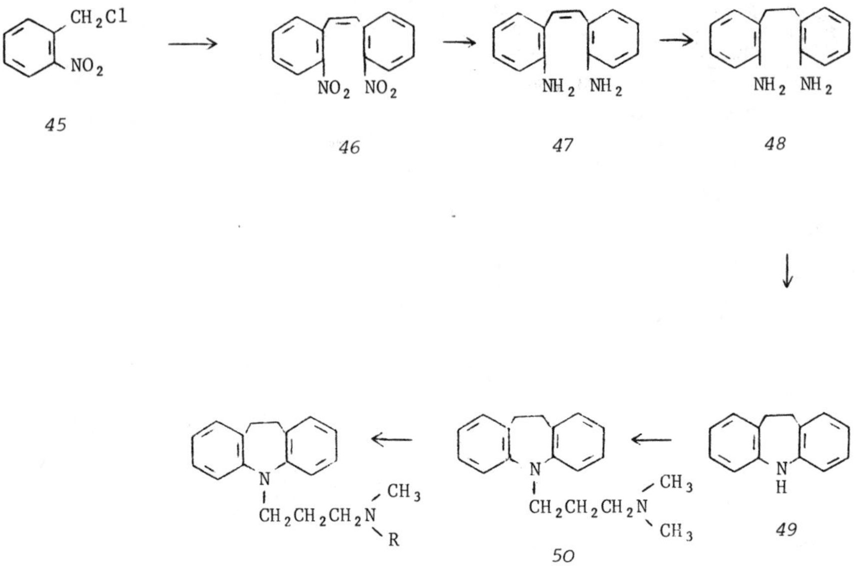

demethylation. This metabolic transformation product, *desipra-*
mine (52), is an antidepressant agent in its own right. It is
thought by some to be the authentic active agent on administration of *imipramine*. It may be synthesized chemically from *50* by
heating the compound with ethylchlorocarbonate to give the urethane *(51)*; saponification gives the secondary amine.[19] This
technique for monodealkylation of a tertiary amine has largely
supplanted the classic von Braun reaction.

The synthetic scheme used to obtain *49* is, of course, not
suitable for compounds containing substituents on only one aromatic ring. An interesting ring enlargement has been used to
obtain starting materials for such substituted dibenzazepines.
Displacement of the benzhydryl chlorine in *53* by cyanide affords
the corresponding nitrile *(54)*; hydrolysis to the acid *(55)* followed by metal hydride reduction gives the primary alcohol *(56)*.
Treatment with phosphorus pentoxide leads to dehydration with
phenyl migration to afford the ring-enlarged product *(57)*. Catalytic reduction of the stilbene double bond affords the desired
halogenated starting material. This dihydrodibenzazepine *(58)*
is then N-alkylated by means of 3-dimethylaminopropyl chloride to
give *chloripramine (59)*.[20]

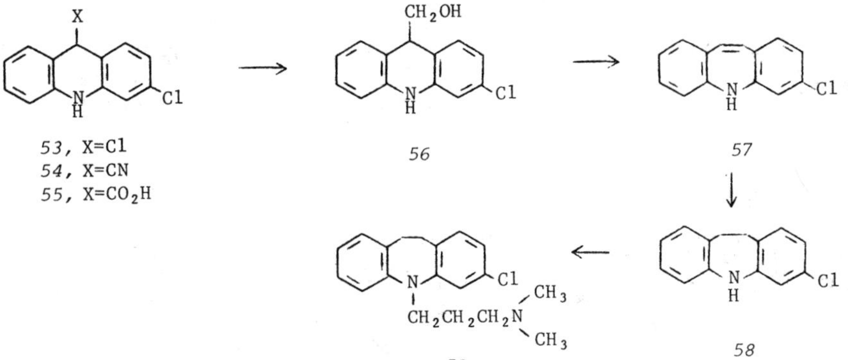

53, X=Cl
54, X=CN
55, X=CO$_2$H

56

57

59

58

b. Dibenzazepines

The fully unsaturated tricyclic compounds are also used clinically as antidepressants. *Carbamazepine (62)*,[21] for example, is
prepared from 10,11-dihydro-5*H*-dibenz[b,f]azepine *(49)* by *N*-
acetylation followed by bromination with *N*-bromosuccinimide to
give *60*. Dehydrohalogenation by heating in collidine introduces
the double bond. Saponification with potassium hydroxide in
ethanol leads to dibenz[b,f]azepine *(61)*, the parent substance
for the fully unsaturated analogs. Treatment of the secondary

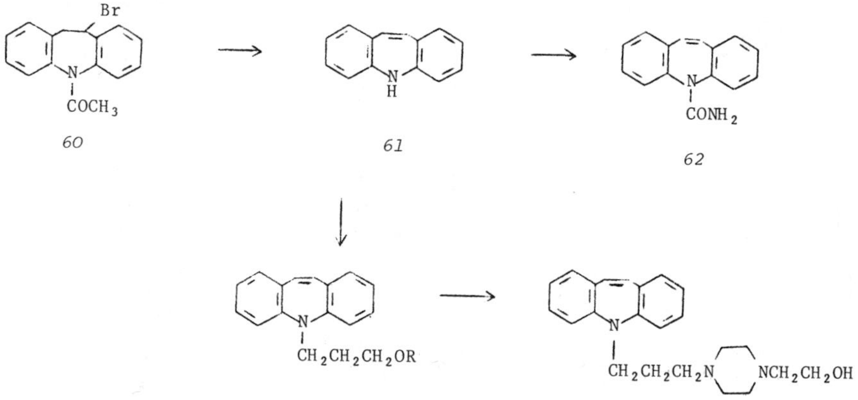

60

61

62

63, R=H
64, R=p-SO$_2$C$_6$H$_4$CH$_3$

65

amine *(61)* with phosgene followed by heating of the carbamoyl
chloride thus obtained with ammonia affords *carbamazepine (62)*.[21]
Alkylation of the sodium salt of *61* with 3-chloropropan-1-ol followed by reaction of the intermediate *(63)* with tosyl chloride
gives the tosylate, *64*. Displacement by 1-(2-hydroxyethyl)piper-
azine gives *opipramol (65)*.[22]

5. DIBENZOXEPINS

One of the two carbon atoms of the ethylene bridge of the antidepressants may be replaced by oxygen. Attachment of the side
chain via the olefinic linkage found in *amytriptyline* affords
antidepressants with a biologic profile similar to the carbocyclic prototype.

Cyclization of 2-benzyloxybenzoic acid *(66)* by means of polyphosphoric acid affords the dibenzoxepinone, *67*. Condensation
with the Grignard reagent from 3-dimethylaminopropyl chloride,
followed by dehydration of the alcohol thus produced affords
doxepin (68),[23] presumably as a mixture of geometrical isomers.

In an alternate synthesis of the intermediate ketone, the
benzylic halide, *69*, is used to alkylate sodium phenoxide.
Cyclization of the acid *(70)* obtained on hydrolysis of the ester
by means of trifluoroacetic anhydride again gives *67*.[24]

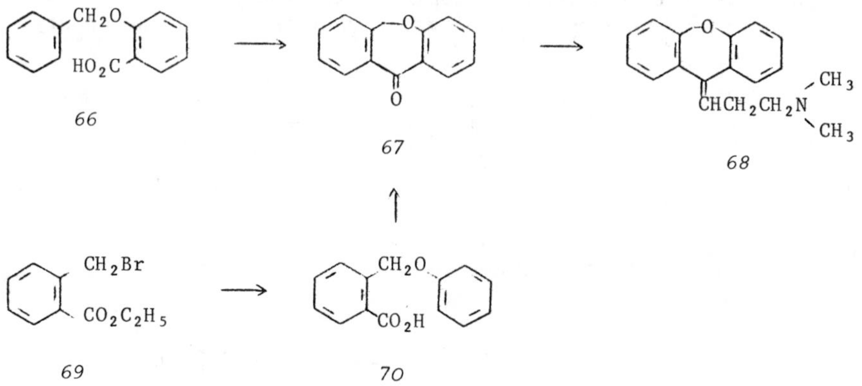

6. DIBENZODIAZEPINES

Fusion of an additional aromatic ring onto the diazepine ring system markedly alters the activity of the resulting compound; this imaginary transformation serves to convert an anxiolytic into an antidepressant agent.

Nucleophilic aromatic substitution of the anthranilic acid derivatives, *72*, on *ortho*-bromonitrobenzene affords the diphenylamine, *73*. The ester is then saponified and the nitro group reduced to the amine *(74)*. Cyclization of the resulting amino acid by heat affords the lactam *(75)*. Alkylation on the amide nitrogen with 2-dimethylaminoethyl chloride by means of sodium amide affords *dibenzepine (76)*.[25]

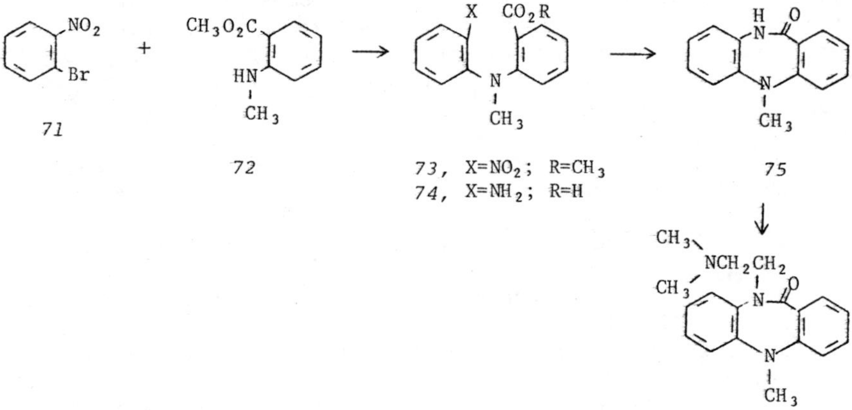

71   *72*   *73*, X=NO$_2$; R=CH$_3$ *75*
                                                74, X=NH$_2$; R=H

7. DIBENZOTHIAZEPINES

An interesting additional example of the interchangeability of the bridging atoms in the neuroleptic series comes from the finding that the biologic activity of the phenothiazines is maintained in a compound that contains an extra atom on the nitrogen

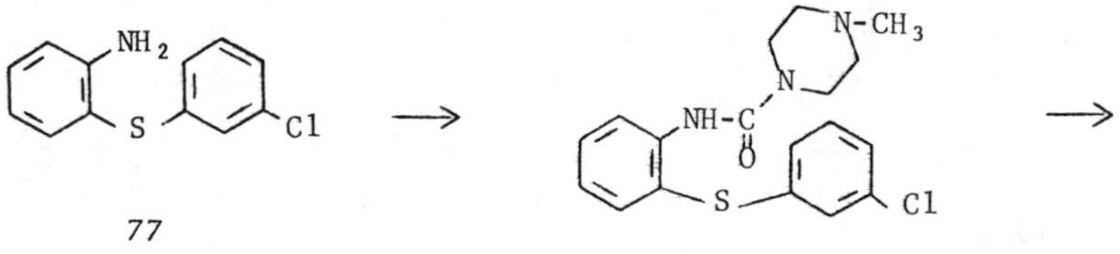

77   *78*

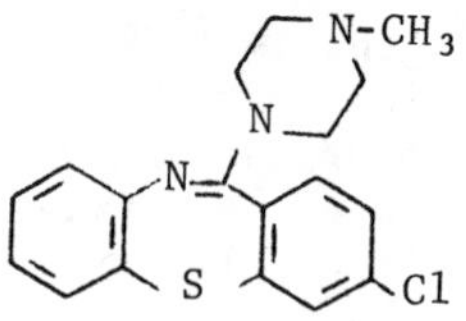

79

bridge. Acylation of the amine, 77, by means of the carbamoyl
chloride obtained by treatment of *N*-methylpiperazine with phosgene gives the unsymmetrical urea, 78. Cyclization with phosphorus oxychloride in DMF leads to the major tranquilizer *clothiapine (79)*.[26]

REFERENCES

1. J. W. Cusic and R. A. Robinson, *J. Org. Chem.*, *16*, 1921
    (1951).
2. E. C. Taylor, K. Leonard, and Y. Shro, *J. Amer. Chem. Soc.*,
    88, 367 (1966).
3. R. Mechoulam, P. Braun, and Y. Gaoni, *J. Amer. Chem. Soc.*,
    94, 6159 (1972).
4. R. K. Radzan and G. R. Handrick, *J. Amer. Chem. Soc.*, *92*,
    6061 (1970).
5. T. Petrzilka, W. Haefliger, and C. Sikemeier, *Helv. Chim.
    Acta*, *52*, 1102 (1969).
6. T. Y. Jen, G. A. Hughes, and H. Smith, *J. Amer. Chem. Soc.*,
    89, 4551 (1967).
7. T. Petrzilka and C. Sikemeyer, *Helv. Chim. Acta*, *50*, 2111
    (1967).
8. F. Mietzsch and H. Mauss, U. S. Patent 2,113,357 (1938);
    Chem. Abstr., *32*, 4287 (1938).
9. T. Holm, British Patent 933,875 (1963); *Chem. Abstr.*, *60*,
    510a (1964).
10. H. Mauss, *Chem. Ber.*, *81*, 19 (1948).
11. S. Archer and C. M. Suter, *J. Amer. Chem. Soc.*, *74*, 4296
    (1952).
12. D. A. Berberian, E. W. Dennis, M. Freele, D. Rosi, T. R.
    Lewis, R. Lorenz, and S. Archer, *J. Med. Chem.*, *12*, 607
    (1969).
13. D. Rosi, G. Peruzzotti, E. W. Dennis, D. A. Berberian, H.
    Freele, and S. Archer, *J. Med. Chem.*, *10*, 867 (1967).

14. J. M. Sprague and E. L. Englehardt, U. S. Patent 2,951,082 (1960).
15. P. V. Petersen, N. O. Lassen, and T. O. Holm, U. S. Patent 3,149,103 (1964).
16. B. M. Bloom and J. F. Muren, Belgian Patent 647,066 (1964); *Chem. Abstr., 63,* 11 512a (1965).
17. J. Schmutz, U. S. Patent 2,905,590 (1959).
18. W. Schindler and F. Hafliger, *Helv. Chim. Acta, 37,* 472 (1954).
19. Anon., Belgian Patent 614,616 (1962); *Chem. Abstr., 58,* 11338c (1963).
20. P. N. Craig, B. M. Lester, A. J. Suggiomo, C. Kaiser, and C. M. Zirkle, *J. Org. Chem., 26,* 135 (1961).
21. W. Schindler, U. S. Patent 2,948,718 (1960).
22. W. Schindler, French Patent M209 (1961); *Chem. Abstr., 58,* 3442f (1963).
23. K. Stach and F. Bickelhaupt, *Montash, 93,* 896 (1962).
24. B. M. Bloom and J. R. Tretter, Belgian Patent 641,498 (1968); *Chem. Abstr., 64,* 719c (1966).
25. F. Hunziker, H. Lauener, and J. Schmutz, *Arzneimittel Forsch., 13,* 324 (1963).
26. Anon., French Patent CAM51 (1964); *Chem. Abstr., 61,* 8328h (1964).

β-Lactam Antibiotics

1. PENICILLINS

It is well known even to segments of the general public that the penicillin story began with the adventitious discovery of the lysis of pathogenic *Staphylococcus aureus* by *Penicillium notatum* in Sir Alexander Fleming's laboratory in 1929. The initial work led to extensive and ultimately successful chemical studies that were greatly facilitated by an international cooperative effort which included participation of industrial and governmental laboratories in the United States. During this technology-sharing and transfer phase, it was learned that the natural penicillins (those produced by fermentation on complex natural media) were mixtures of closely related compounds and that the product composition could be profoundly affected by the presence of certain compounds in the growth media. Addition of phenylacetic acid to the fermentation led to predominance of *benzylpenicillin*, known also as *penicillin G*. Long after the antibiotic was an established clinical success the structure of *penicillin G* was determined to be *1*. The strain in the fused thiazolidine-β-lactam system results in enormously more pronounced hydrolytic susceptibility of the β-lactam bond than is characteristic of amides in general and nonstrained β-lactams in particular. This structural feature hindered early progress in working with these compounds and must be borne uppermost in mind in any consideration of the chemistry of these substances.

The β-lactam antibiotics are cell-wall inhibitors toward susceptible bacteria. To survive in a hostile environment with ionic strengths often quite different from the interior of the cell, bacteria have evolved a rigid, quite complex cell wall. This wall, which has no counterpart in mammals, does differ somewhat among different species of bacteria. Differences in chemical composition lead to variations in their reactions to various staining procedures. The terms, gram-negative and gram-positive, which are often used to denote differences in sensitivities to various classes of antibiotics, merely denote reaction or lack thereof to the gram stain procedure.

The cell walls of bacteria, which consist of cross-linked peptidoglycans, are elaborated by a specialized series of enzymes. Interference with this process insults the integrity of the protective coating and thus leads eventually to the death of the organism. It has been established that one of the final steps in the cell wall-forming sequence is a cross-linking reaction between peptide chains that gives the polymer three-dimensional character. It is generally accepted that the penicillins and cephalosporins bear a topographical resemblance to the natural substrate for a transamidase essential to this biochemical sequence and that they irreversibly inhibit the enzyme by acylation of the active site. The lack of a counterpart to this process in mammals obviates toxic reactions from this inhibitory process.

The penicillins isolated from the beers resulting from fermentation of the molds, Penicillium notatum and Penicillium chrysogenum, were in fact complex mixtures of closely related compounds—a rather common occurrence in antibiotic research. The active compounds proved to be amides of 6-aminopenicillanic acid (2, 6-APA) with differing acyl groups attached to the amine of the β-lactam ring. 6-APA possesses weak but definite antibacterial properties, and its structure represents the minimum structural requirements for the characteristic bioactivity of the penicillins. The incorporation of an acyl side chain, particularly one containing an aryl residue, increases potency by 50 to 200-fold. Thus 6-APA (2) is the penicillin pharmacophore, and the amide function serves to modulate the kind and intensity of antimicrobial activity. All the clinically useful analogs that have reached the marketplace have flowed from this basic fact or have resulted from the adventitious discovery of analogous substances from natural sources.

Penicillin G has a fairly narrow antibacterial spectrum. In particular, fungi and many gram-negative bacteria are relatively insensitive to this agent. A number of strains of bacteria that were once sensitive to penicillins elaborate enzymes, known collectively as penicillinases, that hydrolyze the β-lactam bond to produce the microbiologically inactive penicilloic acids. Such organisms are resistant to the drug. In addition to this enzymatic destruction, benzyl penicillin hydrolyzes readily in water at all but neutral pH. This leads to storage problems and, because the acid milleau of the stomach and the alkaline conditions extant in the duodenum are too extreme for the antibiotics, leads to substantial loss of drug on oral administration. This requires injection for the treatment of severe infections. Finally, a significant percentage of patients are allergic to the penicillins and cephalosporins.

These defects have spurred attempts to prepare analogs. The techniques used have been: (1) natural fermentation (in which the penicillin-producing fungus is allowed to grow on a variety of complex natural nutrients from which it selects acids for incorporation into the side chain), (2) biosynthetic production (in which the fermentation medium is deliberately supplemented with unnatural precursors from which the fungus selects components for the synthesis of "unnatural" penicillins), (3) semisynthetic production (in which 6-aminopenicillanic acid *(2)* is obtained by a process involving fermentation, and suitably activated acids are subsequently reacted chemically with 6-APA to form penicillins with new side chains) and (4) total synthesis (potentially the most powerful method for making deep-seated structural modifications but which is at present unable to compete economically with the other methods).

Following the realization that the presence of phenylacetic acid in the fermentation led to a simplification of the mixture of penicillins produced by the fungus due to preferential uptake of this acid and its incorporation into *benzylpenicillin (4)*, a wide variety of other acids were added to the growing culture. Inclusion of the appropriate acids in the culture medium thus afforded, respectively, *phenoxymethylpenicillin (5, penicillin V)*, *phenethicillin (6)*,[2,3] *propicillin (7)*, and *phenbencillin (8)*. These modifications served to increase stability of the lactam bond towards hydrolysis and thus conferred some degree of oral activity.

The nature of the penicillin derivatives accessible by this "feeding" route was severely limited by the fact that the acylating enzyme of the *Penicillium* molds would accept only those carboxylic acids which bore at least some resemblance to its natural substrates. A breakthrough in this field was achieved by the finding that rigid exclusion of all possible side-chain substrates from the culture medium afforded 6-APA as the main fermentation

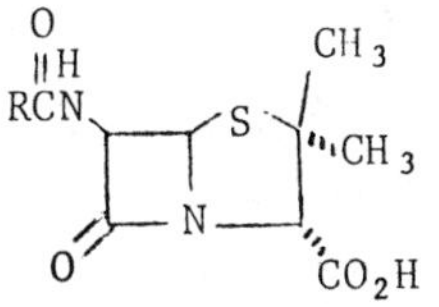

$$\begin{array}{c} O \\ \| H \\ RCN \end{array} \quad \text{(β-lactam structure)} \quad \begin{array}{c} CH_3 \\ \text{''}CH_3 \\ CO_2H \end{array}$$

4,   R= ⟨benzene⟩-CH$_2$

5,   R= ⟨benzene⟩-OCH$_2$

6,   R= ⟨benzene⟩-O$\overset{CH_3}{\underset{}{CH}}$-

7,   R= ⟨benzene⟩-O$\overset{CH_2CH_3}{\underset{}{CH}}$-

8,   R= ⟨cyclohexadiene⟩-OCH-

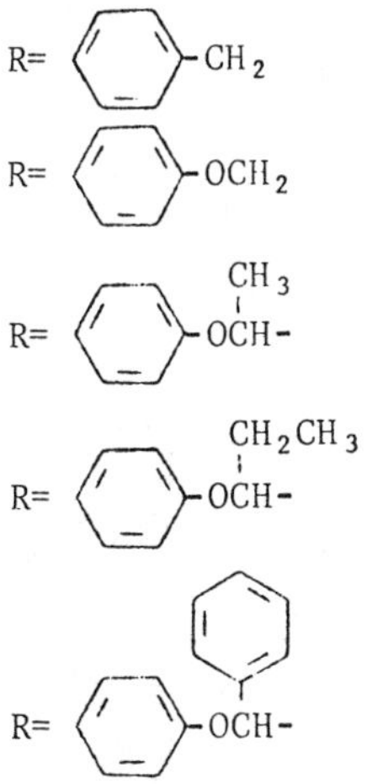

product.[4] It was subsequently found that certain Gram-negative bacteria and some fungi elaborated amidase enzymes that would selectively remove the acyl groups from penicillins produced by natural fermentation, thus again yielding 6-APA.[5-8] The availability of this nucleus permitted free reign on the part of the medicinal chemist in the design of side chains to be included in the penicillin antibiotics. It is of note that 6-APA is today classed as a bulk chemical.

The proper design of the side chains thus accessible has served not only to overcome many of the shortcomings of the early penicillins, such as acid lability, lack of oral activity, and ready destruction by bacterial penicillinase enzymes, but has provided antibiotics with broadened antibacterial spectra.

Although the last step in the preparation of a semisynthetic penicillin may appear to be a straightforward acylation of 6-APA, the wealth of functionality and reactivity of the β-lactam requires highly specialized conditions for achieving this transformation.

Attachment of an aromatic or heterocyclic ring directly to

to the amide carbonyl affords antibiotics with increased resistance to bacterial penicillinases. Thus, acylation of 6-APA with
2,6-dimethoxybenzoic acid (9) affords methicillin (10).[9] The
isomeric lactam, 12, which lacks one of the ortho substituents,
interestingly lacks this resistance.[10]

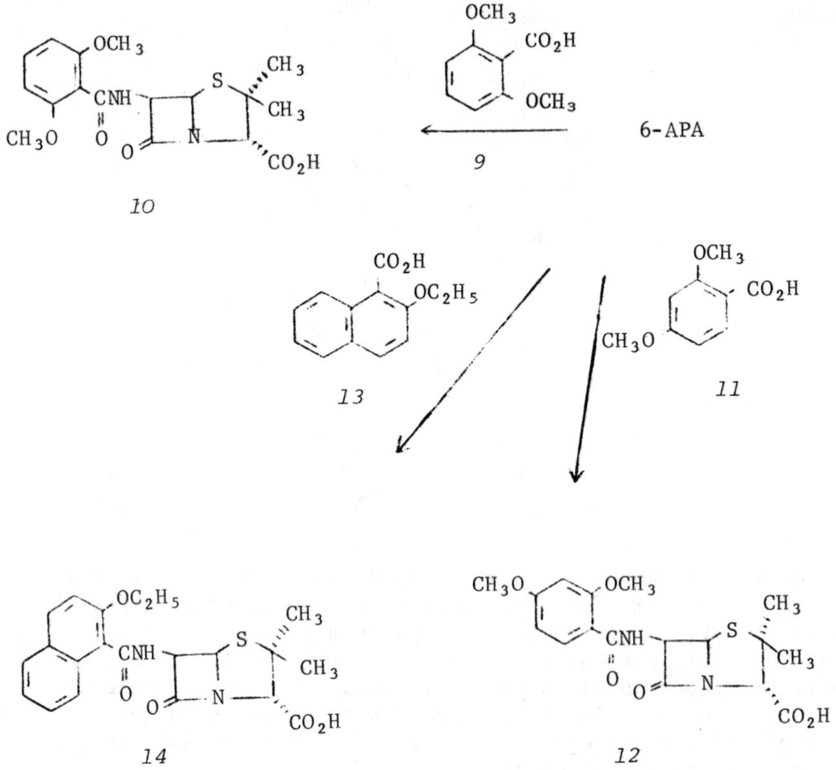

Acylation of 6-APA by the naphthoic acid, 13, again affords
an agent with considerable steric hindrance about the amide function. There is thus obtained the antibiotic nafcillin (14).[11],[12]
a compound with good resistance to penicillinases.

Sterically hindered derivatives of isoxazole carboxylic
acids have yielded a goodly number of antibiotics. Chlorination
of the oxime of the appropriately substituted benzaldehydes (15)
leads to the intermediates, (16). Condensation of the chloro
oximes with ethyl acetoacetate in base gives the esters (17) of
the desired isoxazole carboxylic acids. Alternately, the esters

may be obtained directly by reaction of the aroylated acetoacetates (19) with hydroxylamine. Condensation of the free acids
(18) with 6-APA affords, respectively, oxacillin (20),[13] cloxacillin (21),[14] dicloxacillin (22),[15] and floxacillin (23).

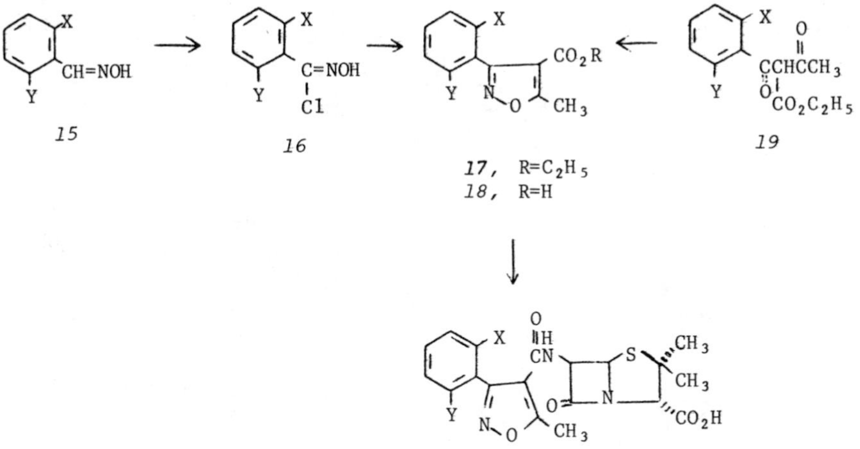

17, R=C₂H₅
18, R=H

20, X=Y=H
21, X=H; Y=Cl
22, X=Y=Cl
23, X=Cl; Y=F

It was observed in some of the early research on penicillin
that drugs acylated by amino acids had somewhat greater oral
activity than those compounds with neutral side chains. Addition
of an amino group to benzyl-penicillin, interestingly, also leads
to antibiotics with a broadened antibacterial spectrum. One
synthesis of this agent begins by protection of the amino group
of phenylglycine (24) as its carbobenzyloxy derivative (25). The
intermediate is then converted to the mixed carbonic anhydride
(26) by means of ethyl chloroformate. Condensation with 6-APA
affords the amide (27). Catalytic hydrogenation removes the protecting group to afford ampicillin (28).[16]

An alternate route to ampicillin not only circumvents the
need for 6-APA but also has the advantage of providing a prodrug
form of ampicillin as well as the parent compound. Reaction of
benzylpenicillin (4) with the acid protecting group, 29, gives
the formol ester, 30. Reaction of the product with phosphorus
pentachloride leads to the corresponding imino chloride (31).

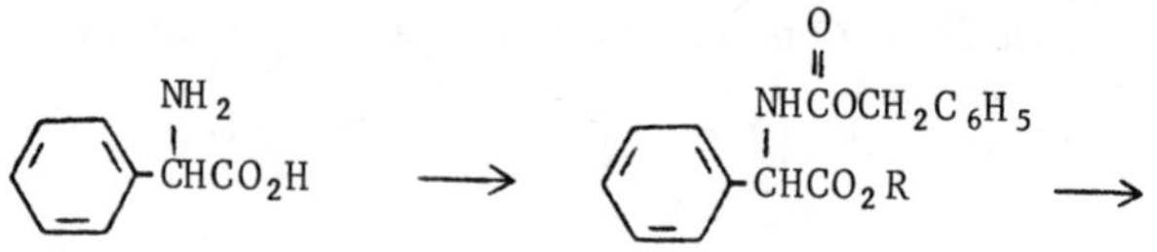

24

25,   R=H
26,   R=COC$_2$H$_5$
        ‖
        O

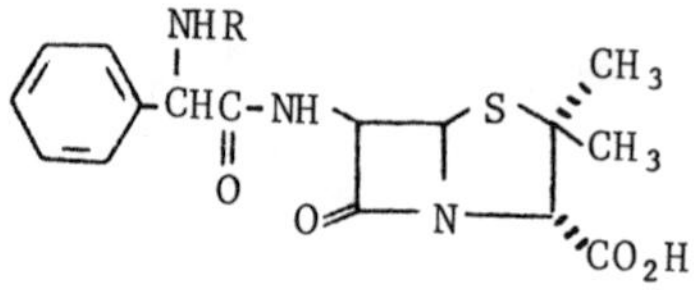

27,   R=CO$_2$CH$_2$C$_6$H$_5$
28,   R=H

Successive treatment with propanol and then acid serves in effect
to hydrolyze the amide linkage. (Note particularly that this
sequence is selective for the exocyclic amide over the azetidone.)
Reaction of the protected 6-APA derivative *(32)* with the acid
chloride from *24* affords the pivaloylmethylenedioxy derivative,
pivampicillin (33).[17,18] This last is a drug in its own right,
presumably undergoing hydrolysis to ampicillin *(28)* after administration. The same transformation can be carried out in vitro
by mild acid treatment.

Latentiation of *ampicillin* can also be achieved by tying up
the proximate amino and amide functions as an acetone aminal.
Inclusion of acetone in the reaction mixture allows 6-APA to be
condensed directly with the acid chloride from *24*. There is thus
obtained directly the prodrug *hetacillin (34)*.[19a] Although this
compound has little antibiotic activity in its own right, it
hydrolyzes to *ampicillin* in the body. The *p*-hydroxy derivative
amoxycillin (35)[19b] shows somewhat better oral activity. A
similar sequence using formaldehyde gives *metampicillin (36)*.[20]

Replacement of the primary amine in *ampicillin* by a carboxylic acid group significantly changes the biologic spectrum of
the product. There is obtained the antibiotic *carbencillin (37)*,[21]
an agent with significant activity against the Gram-negative
Pseudomonas genus. The compound is attainable by chemistry simi-

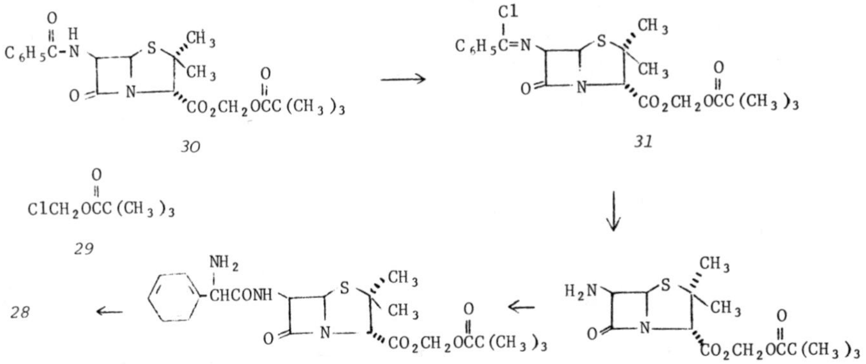

30

29

28 ←

33

32

6-APA + R—⟨benzene⟩—CHCOCl → (structures)

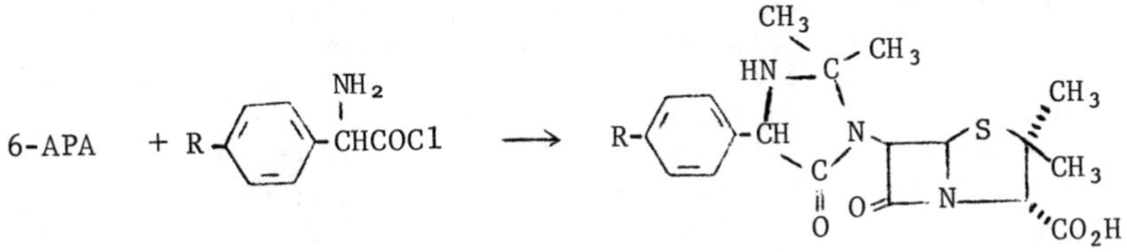

34, R=H
35, R=OH

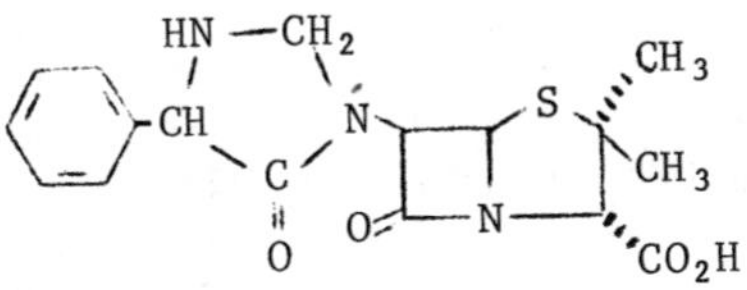

36

lar to that above, using a suitably half-protected ester of
phenylmalonic acid.

6-APA   +   [structure: benzene ring with CH bearing CO$_2$R and CO$_2$H]   →   [structure: benzene ring with CHC-N, CO$_2$H, H, O, β-lactam fused bicyclic ring with S, CH$_3$, CH$_3$, CO$_2$H]

37

2.   CEPHALOSPORINS

The existence of fungi that produce antibiotics when present in milieus replete with pathogenic organism makes good teleologic sense; this is, after all, the first line of defense for the fungus against its neighbors. The observation that such antibiotic-producing fungi do in fact occur in soils and other environments rich in bacteria initiated a worldwide examination of soils, sewage sludges, and related offal for new antibiotics. This program, which has met with some signal successes, continues to this day. It might be added that one of the most troublesome aspects of such programs consists in the constant rediscovery of known antibiotics; the profligacy of nature is apparently not limitless.

Considerable interest was generated by the finding that a *Penicillium* from Sardinian sewage outfall elbatorated a mixture of antibiotics, cephalosporin C, effective against Gram negative bacteria. Structural elucidation of one component, penicillin N, showed the compound to have many features in common with penicillin *(38)*.[11] Indeed, the agent is related formally to the earlier antibiotic by cleaving the carbon sulfur bond and then recyclizing onto one of the geminal methyl groups. (A transformation akin to this has in fact been achieved in the laboratory.)

The low potency of cephalosporin C soon made it clear that the natural product itself was unsuitable as a clinical antibiotic. The structure would have to be modified in the laboratory to give a more potent semisynthetic analog.

Despite much research, no method has yet been found to culture cephalosporin C in such a way as to afford the bare nucleus. This intermediate, 7-ACA *(42)*, is to an analog program in this series what 6-APA is to any penicillin program. Fortunately, several ingenious schemes were elaborated for regioselective cleavage of the side-chain amide. Treatment of cephalosporin with nitrosyl chloride presumably first nitrosates the primary amine on the adipyl side chain; this then goes in the usual way

to the diazonium salt (40). Displacement of this excellent leaving group by oxygen from the enol form of the amide gives the
iminopyran (41). The latter undergoes facile hydrolysis with
dilute acid to give 7-ACA (42).[22]

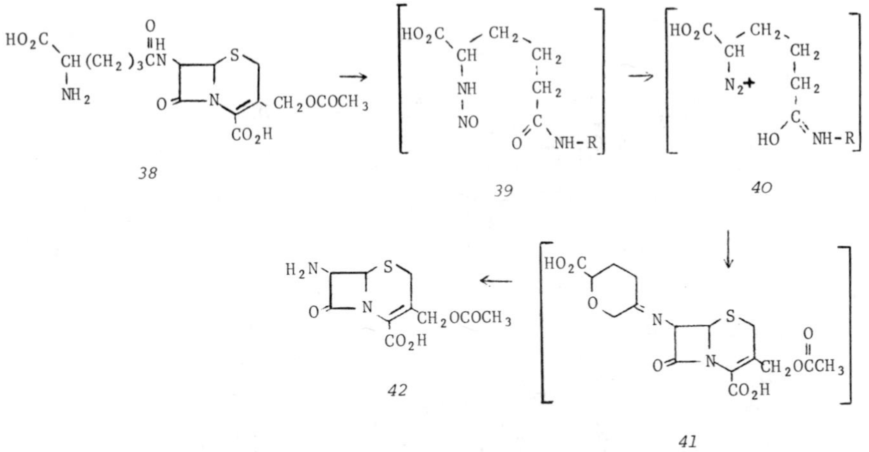

The alternate schemes that have been developed for achieving
removal of the side chain similarly depend on intramolecular
interaction of some derivative of the amine with the amide oxygen
to afford some easily hydrolyzed intermediate at an oxidation
stage analogous to 41.[23]

Acylation of 7-ACA with 2-thienylacetylchloride gives the
amide cephalothin (43). Displacement of the allylic acetyl group
by pyridine affords the corresponding pyridinium salt cephalori-
dine (44).[25] Both these compounds constitute useful injectable
antibiotics with some activity against bacteria resistant to
penicillin by reason of penicillinase production.

In an interesting analogy to the penicillin series, acylation of 7-ACA with the phenylglycine moiety affords a compound
with oral activity. Thus, phenylglycine is first protected as
the carbo tertiary butyloxy derivative (45). Reaction of this
with isobutyloxy chloroformate affords the mixed anhydride (46).
Condensation of that with 7-ACA gives the intermediate, 47.
Treatment with either trifluoroacetic or formic acid provides the
free amine cephaloglycin (48).[26]

The allylic acetoxy group is apparently not necessary for
antibiotic activity. Hydrogenolysis of that group in 48 affords
cephalexin (49),[27] a drug with enhanced oral activity.

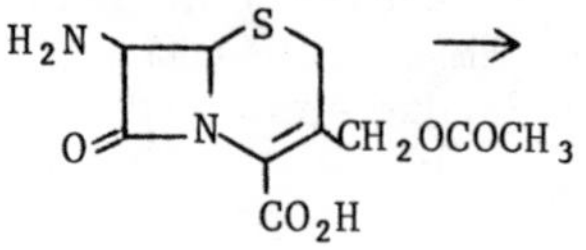

42

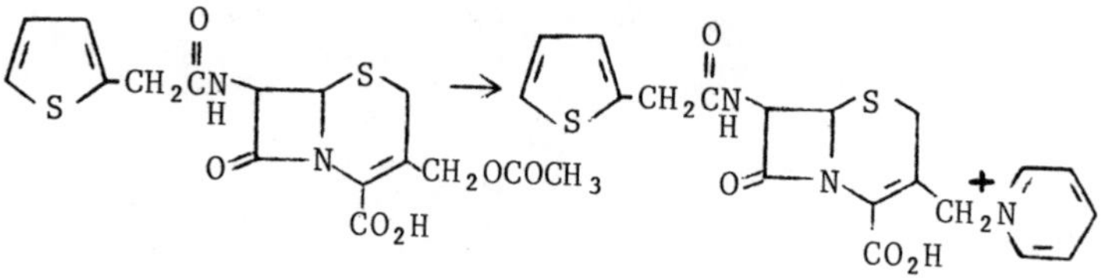

43   44

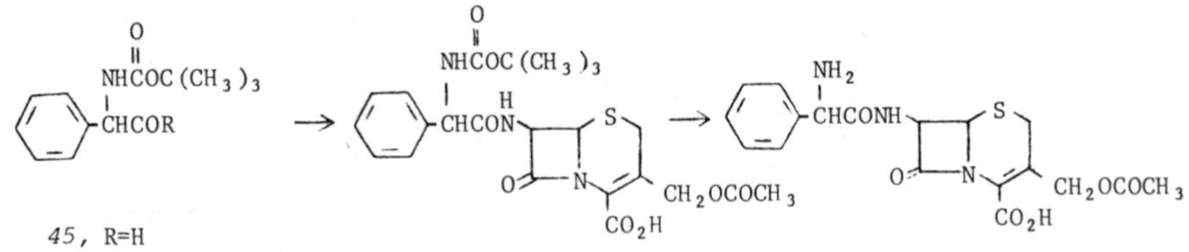

45, R=H
46, R=OCOCH(CH₃)₂

47

48

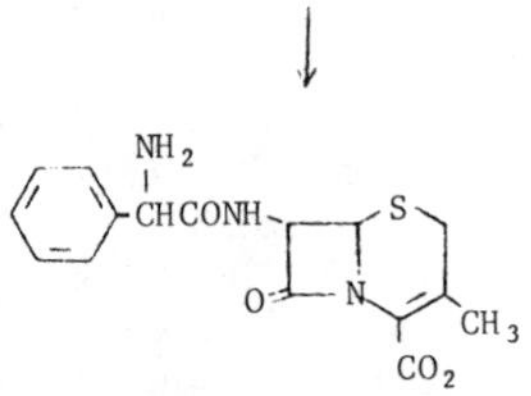

49

    The total syntheses of penicillin[28] and cephalosporin[29] represent elegant tours de force that demonstrated once again the power of synthetic organic chemistry. These syntheses, however, had little effect on the course of drug development in the respective fields, since they failed to provide access to analogs that could not be prepared by modification of either the side chains or, as in the case of more recent work, modification of 6-APA and 7-ACA themselves. In order to have an impact on drug development, a total synthesis must provide means for preparing

analogs not accessible from natural product starting materials;
cases in point are the Torgov synthesis for steroids, which
allowed preparation of the 19-ethyl analogs, or the various
prostaglandin routes that allow inclusion of "unnatural" substituents.

Very recently total syntheses have been developed for the
cephalosporins that allow replacement of the sulfur in the six-
membered ring by oxygen and carbon.

The synthesis starts by elaboration of a small unit that will
provide the bridgehead nitrogen, the carboxyl group, and a phosphonate unit that will close the six-membered ring by intramolecular ylide condensation. Thus, the amino group of phosphonate,
50, is first protected as the Shiff base by reaction with benzaldehyde (51). Acylation of the lithium derivative with benzyl
chlorocarbonate introduces the future carboxyl group as its
benzyl ester (52). Removal of the benzyl group gives back the
free amine (53). Reaction of that amine with ethyl thionoformate
affords the corresponding formamide derivative of the amine (54).
Alkylation of that formamide goes on sulfur to give the enol thio-
formate (55). This functionality, which represents the eventual
ring fusion, is now set up to act as the acceptor in a 2+2 cyclo-
addition reaction. Thus, exposure of 55 to the ketene obtained
in situ from 2-azidoacetyl chloride and triethylamine affords the
desired azetidone (56).

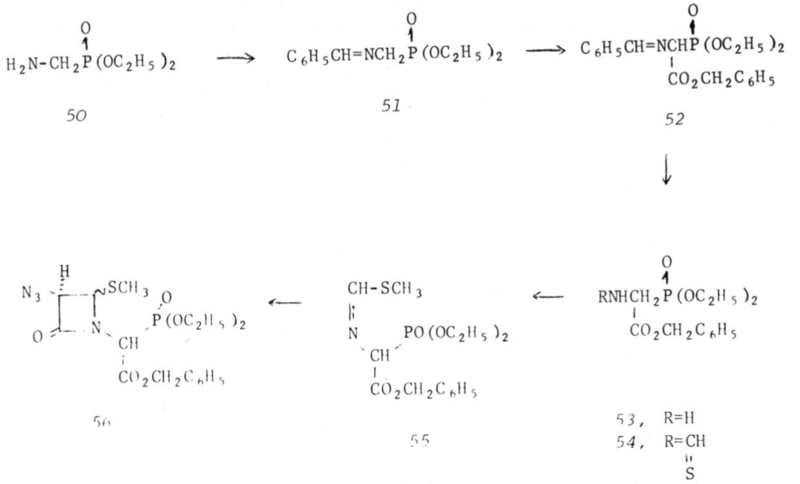

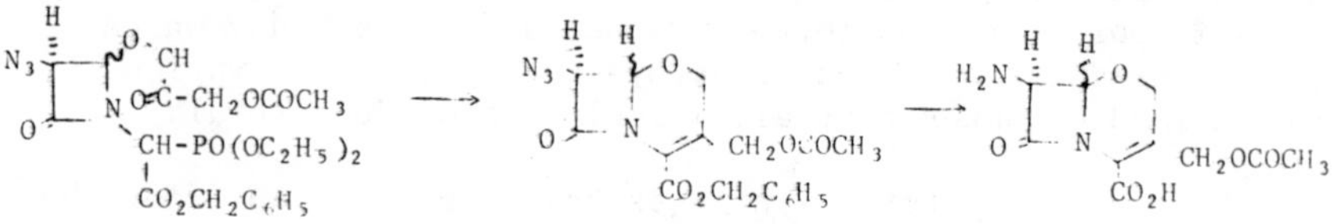

Reaction of the thiomethyl group with chlorine then converts that functionality to the corresponding S-chloronium salt as a mixture of diastereomers (isomers at both carbon and sulfur). Solvolysis of the salt in the monoacetate of dihydroxyacetone in the presence of silver oxide and silver fluoroborate effects net displacement of sulfur by oxygen. The remaining atoms of the six-membered ring are thus incorporated at one fell swoop, albeit with loss of stereochemistry *(57)*. Treatment of that intermediate with sodium hydride forms the ylide on the carbon adjacent to the phosphonate; this condenses with the carbonyl group on the pendant ether side chain to afford the oxacephalosporin nucleus *(58)*. Hydrogenolysis of the intermediate simultaneously removes the benzyl ester and reduces the azide to the primary amine *(59,60)*. Acylation of the cis isomer *(59)* with 2-thienylacetic acid affords ±-1-oxacephalothin *(60)*.[30] Taking into account that the product is racemic, the agent is essentially equipotent with cephalothin *(43)* itself. Appropriate modification of the synthesis from 56 onward followed by the same type of intramolecular ylide reaction affords ±-1-carbacephalothin *(61)*,[31] a compound with very similar antibacterial activity.

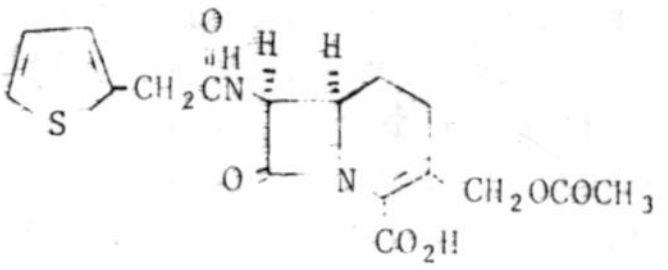

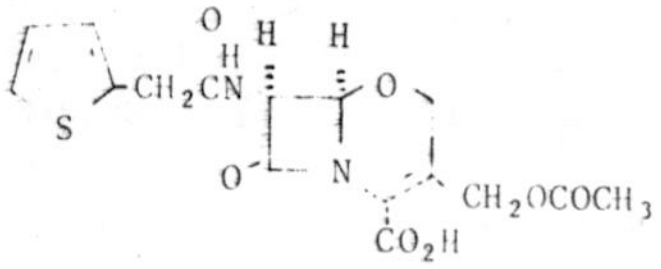

REFERENCES

1. O. K. Behrens, J. Corse, J. P. Edwards, L. Garrison, R. G. Sones, Q. F. Soper, F. R. VanAbeele, and C. W. Whitehead, *J. Biol. Chem.*, 175, 793 (1948).

2. Y. G. Perron, W. F. Minor, C. T. Holdrege, W. J. Gottstein, J. C. Godfrey, L. B. Crast, R. B. Babel, and L. C. Cheney, *J. Amer. Chem. Soc.*, *82*, 3934 (1960).

3. K. W. Glombitza, *Ann.*, *673*, 166 (1964).

4. F. R. Batchelor, F. P. Doyle, J. H. C. Nayler, and G. N. Rolinson, *Nature*, *175*, 793 (1948).

5. K. Kaufmann and K. Bauer, *Naturwissenschaften*, *47*, 474 (1960).

6. G. N. Rolinson, F. R. Batchelor, D. Butterworth, J. Cameron-Wood, M. Cole, G. C. Eustace, M. V. Hart, M. Richards, and E. B. Chain, *Nature*, *187*, 236 (1960).

7. C. A. Claridge, A. Gourevitch, and J. Lein, *Nature*, *187*, 237 (1960).

8. H. T. Huang, A. R. English, T. A. Seto, G. M. Shull, and B. A. Sobin, *J. Amer. Chem. Soc.*, *82*, 3790 (1960).

9. F. P. Doyle, K. Hardy, J. H. C. Nayler, M. J. Soulal, E. R. Stove, and H. R. J. Waddington, *J. Chem. Soc.*, 1453 (1962).

10. K. E. Price, *Advan. Appl. Microbiol.*, *11*, 17 (1969).

11. S. B. Rosenman and G. H. Warren, *Antimicrob. Agents Chemother.*, 611 (1961).

12. E. G. Brain, F. P. Doyle, M. D. Mehta, D. Miller, J. H. C. Nayler, and E. R. Stove, *J. Chem. Soc.*, 491 (1963).

13. F. P. Doyle, A. A. W. Long, J. H. C. Nayler, and E. R. Stove, *Nature*, *192*, 1183 (1961).

14. F. P. Doyle, J. C. Hanson, A. A. W. Long, J. H. C. Nayler, and E. R. Stove, *J. Chem. Soc.*, 5838 (1963).

15. Ch. Gloxhuber, H. A. Offe, E. Rauenbusch, W. Scholtan, and J. Schmid, *Arzneimittel Forsch.*, *15*, 322 (1965).

16. F. P. Doyle, G. R. Fosker, J. H. C. Nayler, and H. Smith, *J. Chem. Soc.*, 1440 (1962).

17. W. vonDaehne, E. Frederiksen, E. Gundersen, F. Lund, P. Morch, H. J. Petersen, K. Roholt, L. Tybring, and E. Ferrero, *Abstr. 5th Int. Congr. Chemother. (Vienna)*, 201 (1967).

18. W. vonDaehne, E. Frederiksen, E. Gundersen, F. Lund, P. Morch, H. J. Petersen, K. Roholt, L. Tybring, and W. O. Gotfredsen, *J. Med. Chem.*, *13*, 607 (1970).

19. (a) G. A. Hardcastle, Jr., D. A. Johnson, C. A. Panetta, A. I. Scott, and S. A. Sutherland, *J. Org. Chem.*, *31*, 897 (1966). (b) A. A. W. Long, J. H. C. Nayler, H. Smith, T. Taylor, and N. Ward, *J. Chem. Soc.*, *Ser. C*, 1920 (1971).

20. E. Ferrero, *Abstr. 5th Int. Congr. Chemother. (Vienna)*, 201 (1967).

21. P. Acred, D. M. Brown, E. T. Knudsen, G. N. Robinson, and R. Sutherland, *Nature*, *215*, 25 (1967).

22. R. B. Morin, B. G. Jackson, E. H. Flynn, and R. W. Roeske, *J. Amer. Chem. Soc.*, *84*, 3400 (1962).

23. B. Fechtig, H. Peter, H. Bickel, and E. Vischer, *Helv. Chim. Acta, 51,* 1108 (1968).

24. R. R. Chauvette, E. H. Flynn, B. G. Jackson, E. R. Lavagino, R. B. Morin, R. A. Mueller, R. P. Pioch, R. W. Roeske, C. W. Ryan, J. L. Spencer, and E. M. VanHeyningen, *J. Amer. Chem. Soc., 84,* 3401 (1962).

25. J. L. Spencer, F. Y. Siu, E. H. Flynn, B. G. Jackson, M. V. Sigal, H. M. Higgins, R. R. Chauvette, S. L. Andrews, and D. E. Bloch, *Antimicrob. Ag. Chemother.,* 573 (1966).

26. J. L. Spencer, E. H. Flynn, R. W. Roeske, F. Y. Siu, and R. R. Chauvette, *J. Med. Chem., 9,* 746 (1966).

27. C. W. Ryan, R. L. Simon, and E. M. VanHeynigen, *J. Med. Chem., 12,* 310 (1969).

28. J. C. Sheehan and K. R. Henery-Logan, *J. Amer. Chem. Soc., 79,* 1262 (1957); *81,* 3089 (1959).

29. R. B. Woodward, K. Henster, J. Gosteli, P. Naegeli, W. Oppolzer, R. Ramage, S. Raganathan, and H. Vorburggen, *J. Amer. Chem. Soc., 88,* 852 (1966).

30. L. D. Cama and B. G. Christensen, *J. Amer. Chem. Soc., 96,* 7582 (1974).

31. R. N. Guthikonda, L. D. Cama, and B. G. Christensen, *J. Amer. Chem. Soc., 96,* 7585 (1974).

CHAPTER 22

Miscellaneous Fused Heterocycles

1. PURINES

It would not be too far fetched to state that life on this planet is totally dependent on two compounds based on the purine nucleus. Two of the bases crucial to the function of DNA and RNA—guanine and adenine—are in fact substituted purines. It is thus paradoxical that the lead for the development of medicinal agents based on this nucleus actually came from observations of the biologic activity of plant alkaloids containing that heterocyclic system, rather than from basic biochemistry.

Xanthines such as *caffeine (1)*, *theophylline (aminophylline) (2)*, and *theobromine (3)* are a class of alkaloids that occur in numerous plants. The CNS stimulant activity of aqueous infusions containing these compounds has been recognized since antiquity. This has, of course, led to widespread consumption of such well-known beverages as coffee *(Coffea arabica)*, tea *(Thea sinesis)*, mate, and cola beverages (in part *Cola acuminata*). The annual consumption of *caffeine* in the United States alone has been estimated to be in excess of a billion kilos. The pure compounds have found some use in the clinic as CNS stimulants. In addition, *caffeine* is widely used in conjunction with aspirin in various headache remedies.

There is some evidence to suggest that these drugs may owe their activity to inhibition of the enzyme that is responsible for hydrolysis of 3',5'-cyclic AMP (itself a guanine derivative) and thus prolong the action of cyclic AMP.

The Traube synthesis represents but one of the many preparations that have been developed for purines. Transesterification of ethyl carboxamidoacetate with methyl urea affords the diamide *(4)*. Treatment with base leads this to cyclize to the pyrimidone *(5)*. Nitrosation on carbon *(6)* followed by reduction of the nitroso group gives the diamine, 7. Condensation with formic

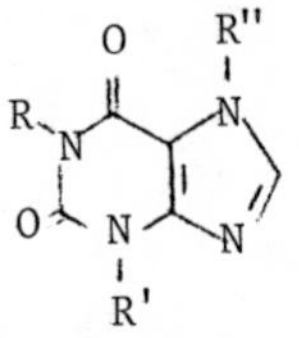

1, R=R'=R''=CH_3
2, R=R'=CH_3; R''=H
3, R=H; R'=R''=CH_3

acid introduces the remaining carbon of the purine nucleus *(8)*. Monomethylation of that compound affords *theobromine (3)*; dimethylation gives *caffeine (1)*. The same sequence using 1,3-dimethylurea as one starting material in this sequence leads to *theophyline (2)*.

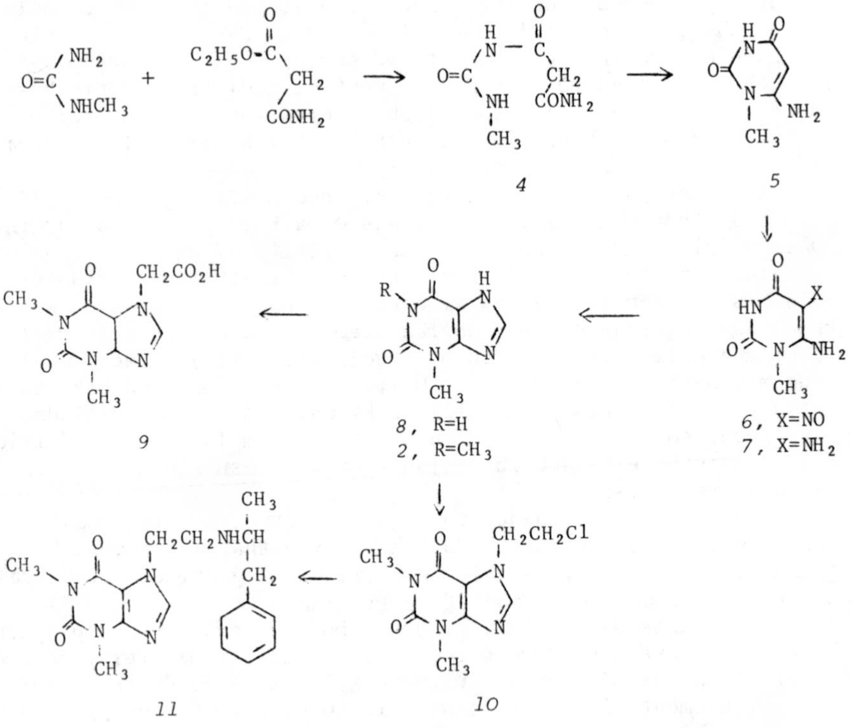

4; *5*; *6*, X=NO; *7*, X=NH_2; *8*, R=H; *2*, R=CH_3; *9*; *10*; *11*

Substitution of somewhat more complex side chains on the imidazole nitrogen of the purines leads to CNS stimulant drugs that have also been used as vasodilators and antispasmodic agents. Thus, alkylation of *theophyline (2)* with ethyl bromoacetate followed by saponification of the product gives *acephylline (9)*.[1] Alkylation with 1-bromo-2-chloroethane gives the 2-chloroethyl derivative *(10)*. Reaction of that intermediate with *amphetamine* yields *fenethylline (11)*.[2]

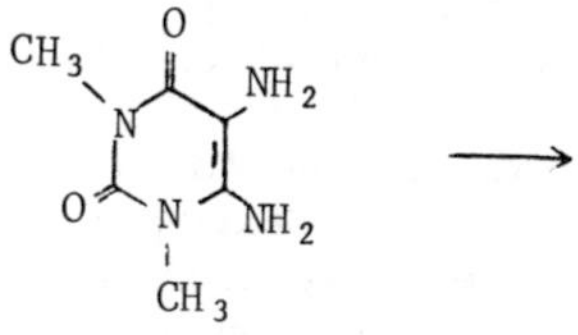

12

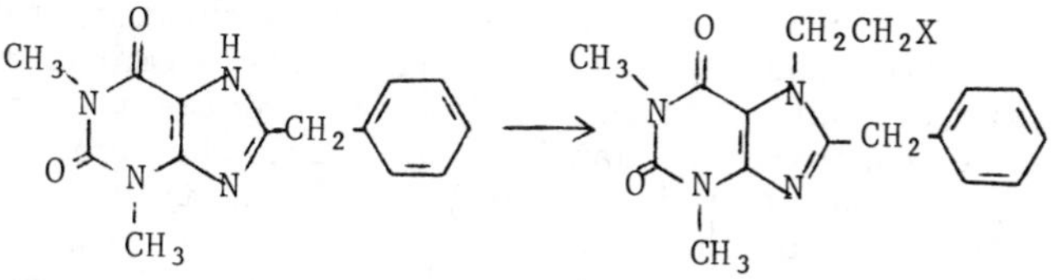

13

14, X=OH
15, X=Cl

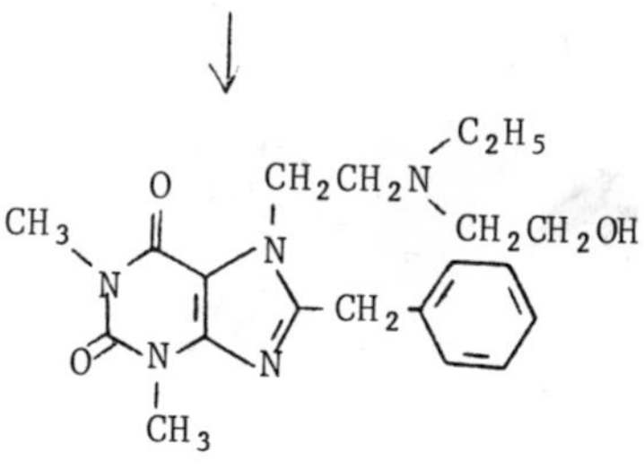

16

Substitution of more complex acids for formic acid in the last step of the purine synthesis will afford intermediates substituted on the imidazole carbon atom. Thus, condensation of diaminouracyl, *12*, with phenylacetic acid gives the benzylated

purine, *13*. Alkylation with 2-chloroethanol *(14)* followed by
treatment with thionyl chloride affords the intermediate, *15*.
Use of that intermediate to alkylate *N*-(2-hydroxyethyl)ethylamine
affords the stimulant *bamiphylline (16)*.[3]

Rational drug design is the ultimate goal of medicinal chemistry. By this is understood the design of medicinal agents on
the basis of knowledge of the intimate biochemistry of the
disease process.

Allopurinol represents one of the first successes towards
this long-term goal. The duration of action of the oncolyltic
agent, 6-mercaptopurine, is limited by its facile oxidation to
inactive 6-thiouric acid by the enzyme xanthine oxidate. The
search for agents that would prolong drug action turned to analogs that contained an extra nitrogen atom—pyrazolo(3,4-d)pyrimi-
dines—in the hopes that these would act as false substrates for
the inactivating enzyme (antimetabolites). One such compound,
allopurinol (20), proved effective in both laboratory animals and
man in inhibiting oxidation of 6-mercaptopurine. In the course
of the trial it was noted that the drug caused a decrease in
excretion of uric acid. Subsequent administration to patients
suffering from gout showed that this well-tolerated drug provided
a useful alternative to *colchicine* for treatment of this disease.

As an inhibitor of xanthine oxidase, *allopurinol* also
markedly decreases oxidation of both hypoxanthine and xanthine
itself to the sole source of uric acid *(19)* in man. This metabolic block thus removes the source of uric acid that in gout
causes the painful crystalline deposits in the joints. It is of
interest that allopurinol itself is oxidized to the somewhat less
effective drug, *oxypurinol (21)*, by xanthine oxidase.

Condensation of hydrazine with ethoxymethylenemalononitrile (22) gives 3-amino-4-cyanopyrazole (23). Hydrolysis with sulfuric acid leads to the amide, 24; heating with formamide inserts

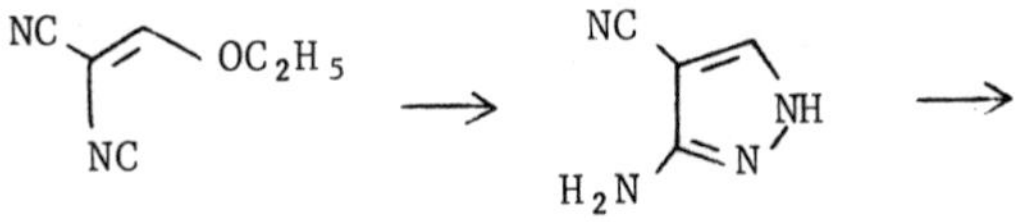

the last carbon atom to afford *allopurinol (20)*.[4] An alternate process starts by reaction of ethyl 2-ethoxymethylene cyanoacetate (25) and hydrazine in an addition-elimination reaction to give 3-carbethoxy-4-aminopyrazole (26). Heating with formamide again results in *allopurinol*.

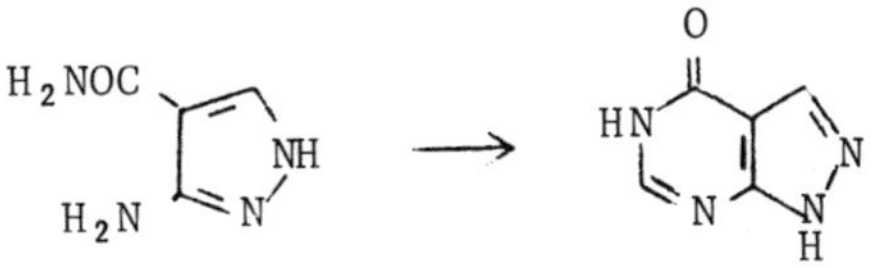

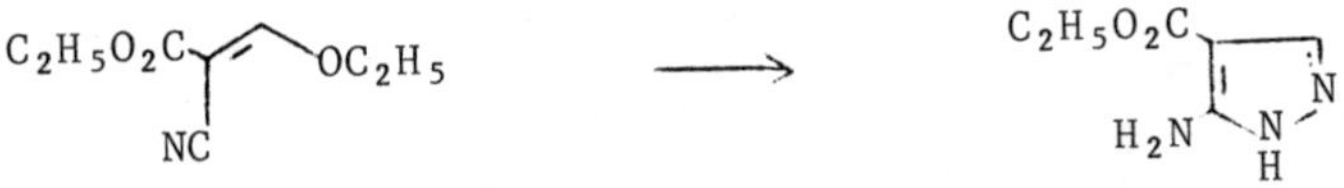

Triamterene (31) is a diuretic that has found acceptance because it results in enhanced sodium ion excretion without serious loss of potassium ion or significant uric acid retention.[5]

Tautomerism of aminopyrimidines (e.g., 27a and 27b) serves to make the "nonenolized" amine at the 5 position more basic than the remaining amines. Thus, condensation of 27 with benzaldehyde goes at the most basic nitrogen to form 28. Addition of hydrogen cyanide gives the α-aminonitrile (29). Treatment of that intermediate with base leads to the cyclized dihydropirazine compound (30). This undergoes spontaneous air oxidation to afford *triamterene (31)*.[6]

Substitution of additional basic groups onto a closely related nucleus affords a compound with muscle relaxant activity with some activity in the treatment of angina. Reaction of the

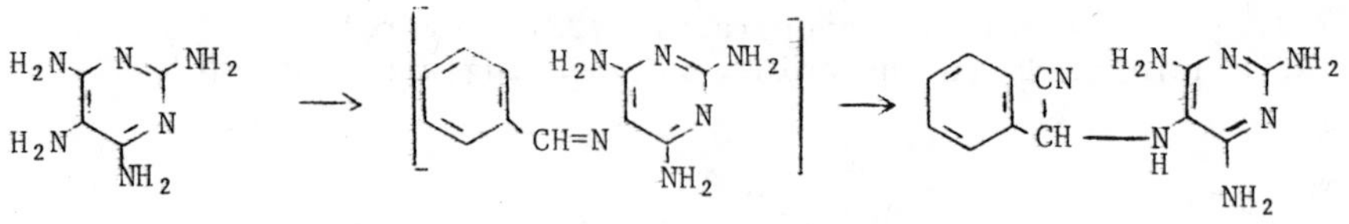

27a   28   29

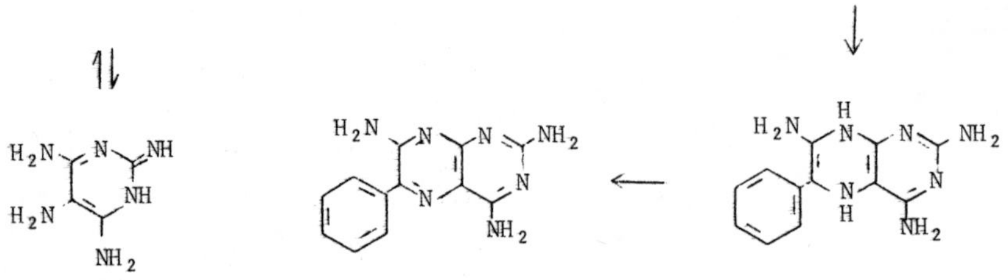

27b   31   30

pyrimidopyrimidine, *32*, with a mixture of phosphorus oxychloride and phosphorus pentachloride gives the tetrachloro derivative, *33*. The halogens at the peri positions (4,8) are more reactive to substitution than the remaining pair, which are in effect at 2 positions of pyrimidines. Thus, reaction with piperidine at ambient temperature gives the diamine, *34*. Subsequent reaction with bis-2-hydroxyethylamine under more strenuous conditions gives *dipyridamole (35)*.[7]

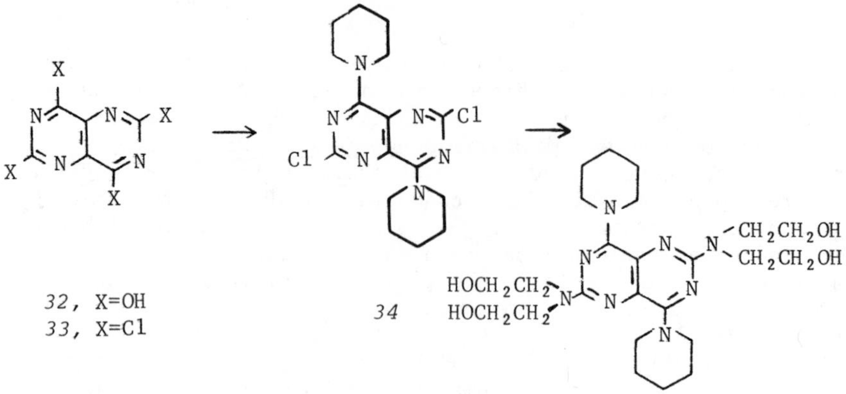

32, X=OH
33, X=Cl

34

35

A 1,8-naphthyridine, *nalidixic acid (39)*, shows clinically useful antibacterial activity against Gram-negative bacteria; as such, the drug is used in the treatment of infections of the urinary tract. Condensation of ethoxymethylenemalonate with 2-amino-6-methylpyridine *(36)* proceeds directly to the naphthyridine *(38)*; the first step in this transformation probably involves an addition-elimination reaction to afford the intermediate, *37*. *N*-Ethylation with ethyl iodide and base followed by saponification then affords *nalidixic acid (39)*.

A benzene ring in a medicinal agent can often be replaced by a pyridine ring with full retention of biologic activity. Some of the more effective antihistamines are in fact products of just such a replacement. Application of this interchange to the phenothiazines affords compounds similar in activity to the parent drugs. The azaphenothiazine nucleus can be prepared by methods quite analogous to those used for the parent ring system. Thus, condensation of 2-chloropyridine with aniline affords the substituted pyridine, *40*; fusion with sulfur in the presence of iodine gives *41*.[9,10] An alternate preparation begins with the aromatic nucleophilic displacement of orthoaminothiophenol *(43)* on the substituted pyridine, *42*, to give the intermediate, *44*; this is then acylated with acetic anhydride *(45)*. Treatment with base leads to the azaphenothiazine, *46*, via the Smiles rearrangement[11] (see section on phenothiazines for a fuller exposition). Hydrolysis of the acyl group gives again *41*. Alkylation of *41* with 3-dimethylaminopropyl chloride gives the tranquilizer, *pro-thipendyl (47)*[10]; reaction of *41* with 2-dimethylaminopropyl chloride leads to *isothipendyl (48)*.[12] As may be inferred from the fact that the latter has in effect an ethylenediamine side chain, its main activity is as an antihistamine.

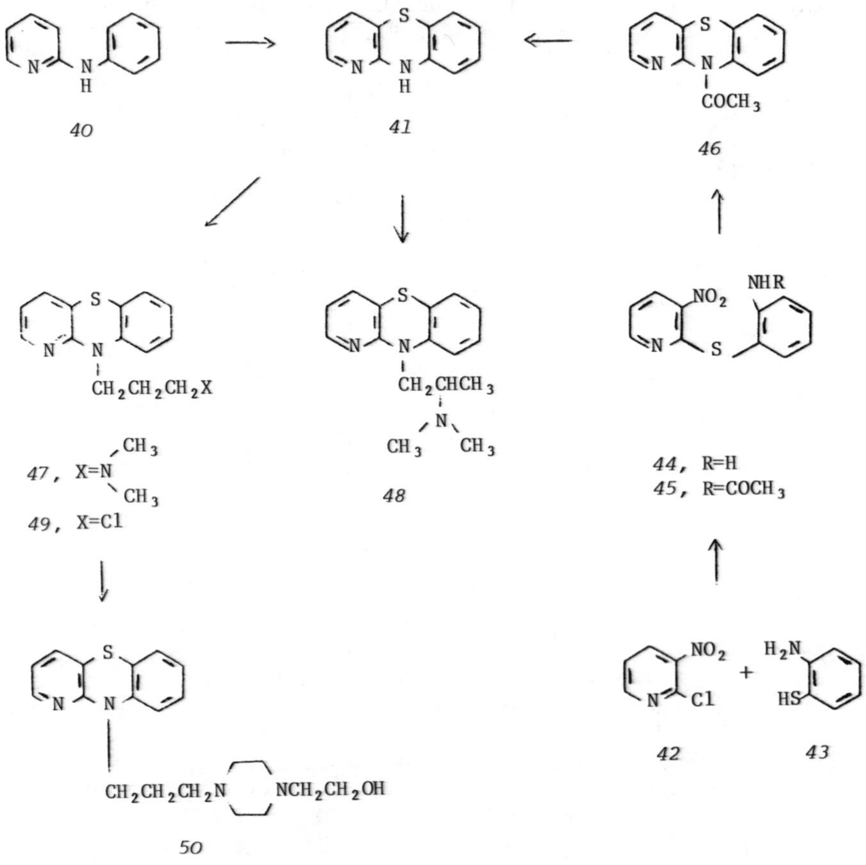

40   41

46

47, X=N(CH_3)_2

49, X=Cl

48

44, R=H
45, R=COCH_3

42   43

50

Alkylation of the intermediate, *41*, with 1-bromo-3-chloroethane affords *49*; the use of this to alkylate *N*-(2-hydroxyethyl) piperazine affords *oxypendyl (50)*,[13] a neuroleptic with good antiemetic and antivertigo properties.

An imidothiazole has proved to be quite active as a broad-spectrum antihelmintic agent. Alkylation of 2-aminothiazoline *(51)*

with phenacyl bromide, interestingly, proceeds on the ring
nitrogen to afford the imino derivative, *52*; acylation of that
intermediate gives *53*. Treatment with sodium borohydride then
effects reduction of the keto group *(54)*. Thionyl chloride
results in cyclodehydration of that alcohol into the heterocyclic
ring to give *tetramisole (55)*.[14]

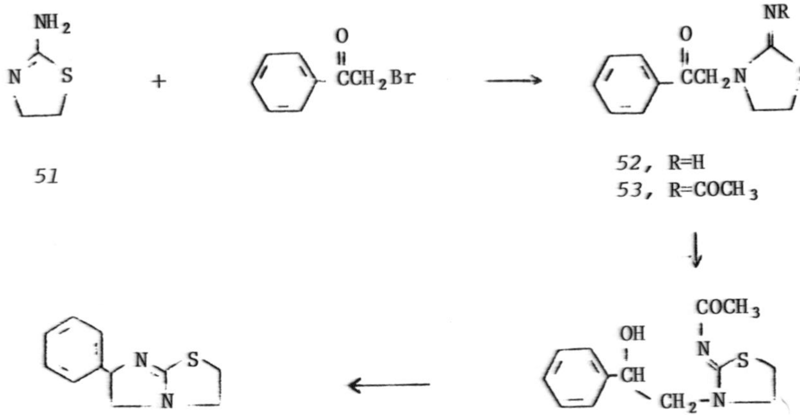

51

52, R=H
53, R=COCH$_3$

55

54

REFERENCES

1. M. Milletti and F. Virgilli, *Chemica (Milan)*, **6**, 394 (1951).
2. E. Kohlstaedt and K. H. Klinger, German Patent 1,123,392
   (1962); *Chem. Abstr.*, **57**, 5,933e (1962).
3. Anon., Belgian Patent 602,888 (1964); *Chem. Abstr.*, **56**,
   5,981c (1962).
4. R. K. Robins, *J. Amer. Chem. Soc.*, **78**, 784 (1956).
5. P. Schmidt and J. Druey, *Helv. Chim. Acta*, **39**, 986 (1956).
6. I. J. Pachter, *J. Org. Chem.*, **28**, 1191 (1963).
7. F. G. Fischer, J. Roch, and A. Kottler, U. S. Patent
   3,031,450 (1962).
8. G. Y. Lesher, E. J. Froelich, M. D. Gruett, J. H. Bailey,
   and R. P. Brundage, *J. Med. Chem.*, **5**, 1063 (1962).
9. A. vonSchlichtegroll, *Arzneimittel Forsch.*, **7**, 237 (1957).
10. A. vonSchlichtegroll, *Arzneimittel Forsch.*, **8**, 489 (1958).
11. H. L. Yale and F. Sowinsky, *J. Amer. Chem. Soc.*, **80**, 1651
    (1958).

12. Anon., French Patent 1,173,134 (1958).
13. W. A. Schuler and H. Klebe, *Ann., 653,* 172 (1962).
14. A. H. M. Raeymaekers, F. T. N. Allewijn, J. Vanderberk, P.
     J. A. Demoen, T. T. Van Offenwert, and P. A. J. Janssen,
     J. Med. Chem., 9, 545 (1966).

Cross Index of Drugs

Adrenergic Agents

Amphetamine
Benzamphetamine
Dextroamphetamine
Ephedrine
ℓ-Epinephrine
Isoproterenol
Levarterenol

Levonordefrine
Mephentermine
Metaraminol
Methamphetamine
ℓ-Norepinephrine
Phenylephrine

α Adrenergic Blocking Agents

Piperoxan

β Adrenergic Blocking Agents

Alprenolol
Butoxamine
Dichloroisoproterenol
Moxysylyt

Oxyprenolol
Propranolol
Pronethalol
Sotalol

Adrenocortical Steroids

Aldosterone
Betamethasone
Cortisone
Cortisone Acetate
Flumethasone
Fluocortolone
Fluorometholone

Hydrocortisone
Hydrocortisone Acetate
Paramethasone
Prednisolone
Prednisone
Triamcinolone

Aldosterone Antagonist

Spironolactone

Anabolic Steroids

Bolasterone
Ethylestrenol
Fluoxymesterone
Metenolone Acetate
Methandrostenolone
Nandrolone
Nandrolone Decanoate
Nandrolone Phenpropionate

Norethandrolone
Normethandrolone
Oxandrolone
Oxymestrone
Oxymetholone
Stanazole
Tiomesterone

Analgesics

Acetaminophen
Acetanilide
Acetylmethadol
Alphaprodine
Aminopropylon
Aminopyrine
Anileridine
Antipyrine
Aspirin
Bemidone
Benzomorphan
Benzydamine
Carbetidine
Clonitazene
Codeine
Cyclazocine
Dextromoramide
Diethylthiambutene
Dimethylthiambutene
Dipipanone
Ethoheptazine
Ethylmorphine
Etonitazene
Fentanyl
Flufenamic Acid
Furethidine
Heroin
Ibufenac
Ibuprofen

Isomethadone
Isopyrine
Ketasone
Ketobemidone
Levorphanol
Meclofenamic Acid
Mefenamic Acid
Meperidine
Methadone
Methopholine
Methyl Dihydromorphinone
Morpheridine
Morphine
Nalorphine
Naloxone
Namoxyrate
Nifenazone
Nifluminic Acid
Normethadone
Norpipanone
Oxycodone
Oxymorphone
Oxyphenbutazone
Pentazocine
Pethidine
Phenacetin
Phenadoxone
Phenazocine
Phenazopyridine

Analgesics (cont.)

Pheneridine
Phenoperidine
Phenylbutazone
Phenramidol
Pholcodine
Piminodine
Pirinitramide
Prolidine

Properidine
Propoxyphene
Racemoramide
Racemorphan
Salicylamide
Thebacon
Tilidine

Androgens

Androstanolone
Dromostanolone Propionate
Ethylestrenol
Fluoxymestrone
Mesteralone

Methyltestosterone
Testosterone
Testosterone Cypionate
Testosterone Decanoate
Testosterone Propionate

Anorexic Agents

Amphetamine
Benzphetamine
Chlorphentermine
Dextroamphetamine
Fenfluramine

Mephentermine
Methamphetamine
Phendimetrazine
Phenmetrazine
Phentermine

Antialcoholic

Disulfiram

Antiallergic Steroids

Betamethasone
Cortisone
Dexamethasone

Dichlorisone
Triamcinolone
Triamcinolone Acetonide

Antiarrhythmic Agents

Lidocaine
Procainamide

Quinidine

Antiasthmatics

Chromoglycic Acid
Epinephrine

Isoproterenol
Khellin

Antiasthmatics (cont.)

Metaprotereno1   Nifurprazine

Anticholinergic Agents

Atropine   Dihexyverine
Benactizine   Methantheline Bromide
Dicyclomine   Propantheline Bromide

Anticoagulants

Acenocoumarol   Dicoumarol
Anisindione   Diphenadione
Bishydroxycoumarin   Phenindione
Clorindione   Warfarin

Anticonvulsants

Aloxidone   Paramethadione
Diphenylhydantoin   Phenacemide
Ethosuximide   Phensuximide
Ethotoin   Primidone
Mephenitoin   Tetratoin
Methsuximide   Trimethadione

Antidepressants

Amytryptylene   Iproniazide
Butryptylene   Isocarboxazine
Carbamazepine   Methylphenidate
Chloripramine   Nialamide
Desipramine   Nortryptylene
Dibenzepin   Opipramol
Doxepin   Phenelzine
Etryptamine   Pheniprazine
Imipramine   Protriptylene
Iprindol   Tranylcypromine

Antidiarrheal

Diphenoxylate

Antiemetics

Diphenidol   Metopimazine

Antiemetics (cont.)

Oxypendyl   Trimethobenzamide
Pipamazine

Antigout Agents

Allopurinol   Probenecid
Colchicine   Sulfinpyrazone
Oxypurinol

Antihistaminics

Antazoline   Meclastine
Bamipine   Meclizine
Bromodiphenhydramine   Medrylamine
Brompheniramine   Mephenhydramine
Buclizine   Methaphencycline
Chlorocyclizine   Methaphenylene
Chlorothen   Methapyrilene
Chlorpheniramine   Methdilazine
Chlorphenoxamine   Methopromazine
Chlorpyramine   Phenbenzamine
Cinnarizine   Pheniramine
Clemizole   Phenyltoloxamine
Cyclizine   Pirexyl
Cyproheptadine   Promazine
Dexbrompheniramine   Promethazine
Dexchlorpheniramine   Propiomazine
Diethazine   Pyrathiazine
Dimethothiazine   Pyrilamine
Dimethylpyrindene   Pyrindamine
Diphenhydramine   Pyroxamine
Diphenylpyraline   Pyrrobutamine
Doxylamine   Thonzylamine
Fenpiprane   Trimeprazine
Histapyrrodine   Tripelenamine
Isothipendyl   Triprolidine
Mebhydroline   Zolamine
Mebrophenhydramine

Antihypertensives

Bethandine   Clonidine
Bretylium Tosylate   Debrisoquine
Chlorexolone   Deserpidine

Antihypertensives (cont.)

Diazoxide
Dibenamine
Dihydralazine
Guanacline
Guanadrel
Guanethidine
Guanochlor
Guanoxan
Hydralazine
Methyldopa

Minoxidil
Pargyline
Phenoxybenzamine
Phentolamine
Rescinnamine
Reserpine
Syrosingopine
Tolazoline
Tramazoline

Antiinflammatory Steroids

Betamethasone
Cortisone
Flucinolone Acetonide
Fludrocortisone Acetate
Fludroxycortide
Flumethasone
Fluocortolone
Fluorometholone
9α-Fluoroprednisolone Acetate

Fluprednisolone Acetate
Hydrocortisone Acetate
Methylprednisolone
Methylprednisone
16β-Methylprednisone
Prednylidene
Triamcinolone
Triamcinolone Acetonide

Antimalarials

Amidoquine
Amopyroquine
Atabrine®
Chloroguanide
Chloroquine
Chloroguanil
Cycloguanil
Dimethacrine
Hydroxychloroquine
Isopentaquine

Paludrine
Pamaquine
Pentaquine
Primaquine
Proguanil
Pyrimethamine
Quinacrine
Quinine
Sontoquine
Trimethoprim

Antimicrobial Agents - Antibiotics

Acetyl Methoxyprazine
Aminitrazole
Amoxycillin
Ampicillin
Azomycin
Benzylpenicillin

Carbenicillin
Cephalexin
Cephaloglycin
Cephaloridin
Cephalothin
Chloramphenicol

Antimicrobial Agents - Antibiotics (cont.)

Chlormidazole
Chlortetracycline
Cloxacillin
Dapsone
Demethylchlortetracycline
α-6-Deoxytetracycline
Dianithazole
Dicloxacillin
Dimetridazole
Ethambutol
Ethionamide
Flucloxacillin
Furaltadone
Furazolidone
Glucosulfone
Glybuthiazole
Glymidine
Glyprothiazole
Griseofulvin
Hetacillin
INH
Isoniazide
Metampicillin
Methicillin
6-Methylene-5-oxytetracycline
Metronidazole
Minocycline
Morphazineamide
Nafcillin
Nalidixic Acid
Nidroxyzone
Nitrafuratel
Nitrimidazine
Nitrofurantoin
Nitrofurazone
Nitrofuroxime
Oxacillin
Oxytetracycline
Para-Aminosalicylic Acid
Phenbencillin

Phenethicillin
Phenoxymethylpenicillin
Phthaloyl Sulfathiazole
Pivampicillin
Prontosil
Propicillin
Pyrazineamide
Pyrrolidinomethyltetracycline
Salvarsan
Streptomycin
Succinyl Sulfathiazole
Sulfacarbamide
Sulfacetamide
Sulfachlorpyridazine
Sulfadiazine
Sulfadimethoxine
Sulfadimidine
Sulfaethidole
Sulfaguanidine
Sulfaisodimidine
Sulfalene
Sulfamerazine
Sulfameter
Sulfamethizole
Sulfamethoxypyridazine
Sulfamoxole
Sulfanilamide
Sulfaphenazole
Sulfaproxylene
Sulfapyridine
Sulfasomizole
Sulfathiazole
Sulfathiourea
Sulfisoxazole
Sulformethoxine
Sulfoxone
Tetracycline
Thiazosulfone
Thiofuradine

Antimotionsickness Agents

Dramamine®

Diphenhydramine

Antiparasitics

Diethyl Carbamazine
Dithiazanine
Hycanthone

Lucanthone
Thiabendazole

Antiparkinsonism Agents

Biperiden
Cycrimine
Diethazine
Diphepanol
Ethopropazine

Orphenadrine
Phenglutarimide
Procyclidine
Trihexyphenidyl

Antispasmodic Agents

Acephylline
Adiphenine
Ambucetamide
Aminopromazine
Aprophen
Atropine
Chlorbenzoxamine
Chlormidazole
Chlorzoxazone
Cyclandelate
Cyclopyrazate
Dicylomine

Dihexyverine
Dioxyline
Dipiproverine
Fenethylline
Khellin
Methantheline Bromide
Methixen
Oxolamine
Oxybutynin
Papaverine
Piperidolate
Propantheline Bromide

Antithyroid Agents

Carbimazole
Methimazole
Methylthiouracil

PTU
Propylthiouracil
Iodothiouracil

Antitussives

Caramiphen
Carbetapentane
Chlorphendianol
Codeine
Dextromorphan
Dimethoxanate
Eprazinone
Guaiaphenesin

Hydrocodone
Isoaminile
Levopropoxyphene
Methopholine
Oxeladin
Oxolamine
Pentethylcyclanone
Pipazethate

Ataraxic Agent

Fluanisone

Barbiturate Antagonist

Bemegride

CNS Stimulants

Acephylline   Methylphenidate
Aminophenazole   Pentylenetetrazole
Aminophylline   Phendimetrazine
Bamiphylline   Phenmetrazine
Caffeine   Prolintane
Fencamfamine   Theobromine
Fenethylline   Theophylline

Cholinergic Agents

Neostigmine   Physostigmine

Cholesteropenic Agents

Clofibrate   Nicotinic Acid
Dextrothyronine

Coccidiostats

Amprolium   Buquinolate

Coronary Vasodilators

Benziodarone   Oxyfedrine
Chromonar   Prenylamine
Imolamine

Diuretics

Acetazolamide   Caffeine
Altizide   Chloraminophenamide
Amiloride   Chlorazanil
Aminotetradine   Chlorexolone
Amisotetradine   Chlorothiazide
Bendroflumethiazide   Chlorphenamide
Butazolamide   Chlorthalidone

Diuretics (cont.)

Clopamide
Cyclopentathiazide
Cyclothiazide
Dichlorophenamide
Epithiazide
Ethacrynic Acid
Ethiazide
Ethoxysolamide
Flumethazide
Furosemide
Hydrochlorothiazide
Hydroflumethiazide

Meralluride
Mercaptomerine
Merfruside
Methazolamide
Methyclothiazide
Polythiazide
Probenecid
Quinethazone
Thiabutazide
Triamterene
Trichlormethiazide

Estrogens

Benzestrol
Chlorotranisene
Dienestrol
Diethylstilbesterol
Estradiol
Estradiol Benzoate
Estradiol Cypionate
Estradiol Dipropionate

Estradiol Hexahydrobenzoate
Estradiol Valerate
Estrone
Ethynylestradiol
Hexestrol
Mestranol
Methallenestril

Estrogen Antagonists

Clomiphene

Nafoxidine

Glucocorticoids

Bethamethasone
Cortisone
Hydrocortisone

Hydrocortisone Acetate
Prednisolone
Prednisone

Laxative

Phenolphthalein

Local Anesthetics

Ambucaine
Benzocaine
Bupiracaine
Butacaine

Chloroprocaine
Cocaine
Cyclomethycaine
Dibucaine

Local Anesthetics (cont.)

Dimethisoquine
Diperodon
α-Eucaine
β-Eucaine
Hexylcaine
Hydroxyprocaine
Imolamine
Isobucaine
Lidocaine
Lidoflazine
Mepiracaine
Metabutoxycaine
Oxoethazine
Paraethoxycaine

Phenacaine
Piperocaine
Piridocaine
Pramoxine
Prilocaine
Procainamide
Procaine
Proparacaine
Propoxycaine
Pyrrocaine
Tetracaine
Tolycaine
Tropacocaine

MAO Inhibitors

Iproniazide
Isocarboxazine

Nialamide
Tranylcypromine

Midriatics

Atropine
Cyclopentolate

Hydroxyamphetamine

Miotics

Neostigmine

Physostigmine

Mineralcorticoid

Aldosterone

Muscle Relaxants

Carisoprodol
Chlordiazepoxide
Chlormezanone
Chlorphenesin Carbamate
Dipyridamole
Mephenesin

Mephenesin Carbamate
Mephenoxolone
Meprobamate
Metaxolone
Methocarbamol
Phenyramidol

Narcotic Antagonists

Anileridine   Meperidine
Cyclazocine   Nalorphine
Levallorphan   Pethidine
Levophenacylmorphan   Phenomorphan

Narcotics

Bemidone   Methyldihydromorphinone
Codeine   Morphine
Dextromoramide   Naloxone
Dihydrocodeine   Normethadone
Dipipanone   Oxycodone
Ethylmorphine   Oxymorphone
Heroin   Pentazocine
Hydrocodone   Phenadoxone
Hydromorphone   Pholcodine
Isomethadone   Piminodine
Levorphanol   Racemorphan
Methadone   Thebacon

Nasal Decongestion Agents

Cyclopentamine   Propylhexedrine
Naphazoline   Tetrahydrozoline
Oxymetazoline   Xylometazoline
Phenylephrine

Non-Steroidal Antiinflammatory Agents

Aminopyrine   Isopyrine
Antipyrine   Ketasone
Aspirin   Mofebutazone
Benzydamine   Naproxen
Flubiprofen   Nifenazone
Glaphenine   Oxyphenbutazone
Ibufenac   Phenylbutazone
Ibuprofen   Propylphenazone
Indomethacin   Salicylamine

Oral Contraceptives

Chlormadionone Acetate   Lynestrol
Dimethisterone   Medroxyprogesterone Acetate
Ethynodiol Diacetate   Megestrol Acetate

Oral Contraceptives (cont.)

Melengestrol Acetate
Norethindrone
Norethindrone Acetate
Norethinodrel

Norgestatrienone
Norgestrel
Riglovis®

Oral Hypoglycemics

Acetohexamide
Azepinamide
Buformin
1-Butyl-3-metanylurea
Carbutemide
Chlorpropamide

Glyburide
Glyhexamide
Phenformin
Tolazemide
Tolbutamide

Parenteral Anesthetics

Ketamine

Phencyclidine

Peripheral Vasodilators

Acephylline
Cyclandelate
Dihydralazine
Fenethylline
Hydralazine

Isoxsuprine
Minoxidil
Nicotinyl Alcohol
Nylidrin
Tolazoline

Progestational Hormones

Allylestrenol
Chlormadionone Acetate
Dimethisterone
Dydrogesterone
Ethisterone
Ethynodiol Diacetate
Ethynodrel
Hydroxyprogesterone Acetate
Hydroxyprogesterone Caproate

Lynestrol
Medrogestone
Medroxyprogesterone Acetate
Megestrol Acetate
Melengestrol Acetate
Norethindrone
Pregnenolone Acetate
Progesterone

Respiratory Stimulants

Doxapram

Nikethemide

Sedatives - Hypnotics

Allobarbital
Aminoglutethemide
Amobarbital
Aprobarbital
Barbital
Bromisovalum
Butabarbital
Butalbital
Butethal
Butylallonal
Butylvinal
Carbromal
Carbubarbital
Clocental
Cyclobarbital
Cyclopal
Ectylurea
Glutethemide
Heptabarbital
Hexethal

Hydrochlorbenzethylamine
Mecloqualone
Meparfynol
Methaqualone
Methitural
Methohexital
Methyprylon
Pentobarbital
Phenobarbital
Probarbital
Propiomazine
Secobarbital
Sodium Pentothal
Spirothiobarbital
Thalidomide
Thialbarbital
Thiamylal
Thiobarbital
Thiopental
Vinbarbital

Sedatives - Tranquilizers

Acetophenazine
Azacyclonol
Benzquinamide
Bromisovalum
Butaperazine
Captodiamine
Carisoprodol
Carphenazine
Chlofluperidol
Chlordiazepoxide
Chlorimpiphenine
Chlormezanone
Chlorproethazine
Chlorpromazine
Chlorprothixene
Clopenthixal
Clothiapine
Cloxazepam
Diazepam
Dixyrazine
Droperidol

Fluazepam
Fluphenazine
Haloperidol
Hydroxyphenamate
Hydroxyzine
Ketazolam
Lorazepam
Mebutamate
Medazepam
Meprobamate
Mesoridazine
Methoxypromazine
Nitrazepam
Oxanamide
Oxazepam
Oxazolapam
Oxypendyl
Pecazine
Perazine
Perphenazine
Phenaglycodol

Sedatives - Tranquilizers (cont.)

Piperactizine Δ^1-Tetrahydrocannabinol
Pipradol   Thiethylperazine
Prochlorperazine   Thiopropazate
Promazine   Thiordiazine
Promethazine   Thiothixine
Propionylpromazine   Triazolam
Prothipendyl   Trifluoperidol
Spiropiperone   Triflupromazine
Styramate   Trimeprazine

Termination of Pregnancy Agents

Dinoprost   Dinoprostone

Thyroid Hormones

Levothyroxine   Thyroxine
Liothyronine   Triiodothyronine

Vermifuges - Antihelmintics

Methyridine   Pyrantel
Morantel   Tetramisole

Vitamin

Nicotininc Acid

Glossary

Addiction potential. The ability of a compound to elicit compulsive self-administration.

Adrenergic. Relating to epinephrine (adrenaline) or norepinephrine (noradrenaline). Commonly used to describe neurons that utilize norepinephrine as a neurotransmitter and the drugs that interact with these neurons.

Adrenergic blocking agent. A drug that blocks the effects of epinephrine and/or norepinephrine.

Agonist. A compound that elicits a biologic response by mimicking an endogenous substance.

Anabolic activity. The ability of a drug to promote the synthesis of tissue constituents.

Analgetic (analgesic). An agent that causes the loss of response to pain without affecting the general level of consciousness.

Anaphylactic shock. A systemic hypersensitivity response resulting in dramatic decrease in blood pressure.

Androgenic activity. Ability to promote the development of male secondary sex characteristics.

Anesthetic, general. A compound that, when given systemically, causes a reversible loss of consciousness sufficient to allow surgical procedures.

Anesthetic, local. A compound that blocks conduction of nerve impulses, thus rendering insensible the area to which it is

448

applied.

Anorexic. A substance that decreases appetite.

Antagonist. A drug that blocks the biologic effects of an endogenous substance or exogenously applied drug.

Anticholinergic. A drug that blocks the effects of the neurotransmitter, acetylcholine.

Anticoagulant. An agent that interferes with the ability of the blood to clot.

Anticonvulsant. A compound that depresses the central nervous system, thus decreasing frequency and severity of uncontrolled bursts of neuronal activity.

Antidepressant. A drug that elevates the mood of individuals suffering from pathologic sadness.

Antiemetic. A compound that blocks the vomition reflex.

Antihelmintic (Anthelmintic). An agent that is useful in the control of parasitic worms.

Antihistamine. Compound that, by occupying the histamine receptors, antagonizes the effects of histamine.

Antihypertensive. An agent that lowers blood pressure.

Antiinflammatory. A drug that attenuates the swelling and pain induced by tissue damage.

Antimetabolite. A compound that, by competitive blockade of the necessary enzymes, blocks metabolism.

Antinematodal. An anthelmintic effective against round worms (nematodes).

Antiparasitic. A general term for compounds that kill protozoan or metazoan infective organisms.

Antiparkinsoniam. A drug useful in the treatment of the tremors and rigidity associated with Parkinson's disease.

Antipsychotic. A drug that is useful in decreasing the thought

disorders of schizophrenia. Also referred to as major tranquilizer or neuroleptic.

Antipyretic. An agent that normalizes an elevated body temperature.

Antisecretory. An agent that decreases the secretion of digestive
juices in the stomach.

Antispasmodic. A general term for any one of several types of
drugs that block contraction of the gut.

Antithyroid agent. An agent that decreases the synthesis and/or
release of thyroid hormones.

Antitrichomonal. An antiparasitic effective against the proto-
zoan trichomonads.

Antitussive. A drug that blocks the cough reflex.

Anxiety. Mental apprehension frequently accompanied by somatic
signs such as increased heart rate, palpations, and increased
muscle tension.

Anxiolytic. A drug that decreases the mental symptoms and somatic
signs of anxiety.

Asthma. Difficulty breathing due to constriction of the bronchi.

Atherosclerosis. Hardening of the arteries. The formation of
obstructive plaques in the arteries.

Autonomic nervous system. The portion of the nervous system outside of the brain and spinal cord that is responsible for monitor-
ing and controlling the digestive system, cardiovascular system,
and other organs that are not under direct conscious control.

Baroreceptor. Specialized pressure-sensitive tissue located in
carotid arteries. Nerve impulses proportional to arterial blood
pressure are conducted from this tissue to the brain which in
turn exerts control over the blood pressure.

Biogenic amines. A general term usually used to describe endogenous amine-containing compounds such as dopamine, 5-hydroxy-
tryptamine, and norepinephrine that function as neurotransmitters.

Bronchial spasm. Contraction of the smooth muscle of the air passages of the lungs resulting in difficult breathing.

Bronchiodilator. An agent that relaxes the smooth muscle of the air passages of the lungs.

Cardiac arrhythmia. An irregularity of the heart beat.

CNS (Central Nervous System). The brain and the spinal cord.

CNS stimulant. A drug that counteracts fatigue and somnolence.

Cholinergic. An agent that mimics acetylcholine. Also refers to neurons that utilize acetylcholine as a neurotransmitter.

Coccidiosis. Infestation with coccidia, an intestinal parasite.

Coronary vasodilator. A drug that enhances blood flow through the blood vessels of the heart.

Diabetes mellitus. A defect in carbohydrate metabolism leading to the appearance of sugar in the urine.

Diuretic. A drug that increases the volume of urine formed.

Endogenous depression. A serious melancholic state unrelated to the individual's external environment.

Epilepsy, grand mal. A disorder resulting in occasional loss of consciousness and violent uncontrolled contraction of the muscles.

Epilepsy, petit mal. Similar to grand mal except that muscle manifestations are either absent or confined to occasional jerks.

Epinephrine (adrenaline). A biogenic amine released from the adrenal medulla, particularly in moments of stress.

Estrogenic activity. Ability to mimic the female hormone by promoting the development of female secondary sex characteristics and modulating the estrus cycle.

Febrile. Displaying an elevated body temperature.

Ganglionic blocking agent. A drug that blocks neurotransmission at the nicotinic receptors of the sympathetic ganglia, thus blocking vascular reflexes.

G.I. (gastrointestinal). Refers to the digestive system.

Glaucoma. Increased intraocular pressure.

Gram negative. Bacteria that fail to retain Gram stain. This group includes the genera *Salmonella, Pseudmonas, Pasteurella, Escherichia,* and *Brucella.*

Gram positive. Bacteria that retain Gram stain. This group includes the genera *Streptococcus, Staphylococus, Diplococcus,* and *Clostridium.*

Helmintheasis. Infestation with parasitic worms.

Histamine. A diamine found in plant and animal tissues. It is involved in inflammatory responses.

Hormone. A substance produced by a gland and transported by the blood stream to another part of the body where it produces an effect.

Humoral factor. A general term referring to biologically active substances found in the body fluids.

Hydrophilicity. Water soluble.

Hyperlipidemia. Elevated lipid levels in the blood.

Hypertension. Elevated blood pressure.

Hypoglycemic agent. A drug that lowers glucose concentrations in the blood.

Hypnotic. A drug that induces sleep.

Lipophilicity. Soluble in fat or organic solvents.

Major tranquilizer. A drug useful in the control of schizophrenia. Also referred to as neuroleptic or antipsychotic.

Minor tranquilizer. A drug useful in the control of anxiety. Also referred to as anxiolytic.

Myocardial infarction. Blockage of the blood flow to a portion of the heart muscle leading to tissue damage.

MAO (monoamine oxidase) inhibitor. An agent that blocks one of the enzymes that deaminates amines.

Muscle relaxant. A compound that, by either central or peripheral actions, decreases muscle tension.

Mutant culture. Genetically altered growth of microorganisms.

Narcotic analgesic. A drug that alleviates pain by interacting with the morphine receptor.

Narcotic antagonist. A drug that selectively blocks the actions of morphine-like compounds.

Neuroleptic. A drug useful in the control of schizophrenia. Also referred to as an antipsychotic or major tranquilizer.

Neurosis. A general term for mild emotional disorders often associated with anxiety.

Neurotransmitter. A substance that is released from one neuron as a result of depolarization and in turn alters the excitability of adjacent neurons.

Norepinephrine. An endogenous catecholamine that functions as a neurotransmitter.

Parasympathetic nervous system. That portion of the autonomic nervous system that utilizes acetylcholine as the neurotransmitter at the neuro-effector junctions.

Parkinson's disease. A degenerative neurologic condition manifested by tremor and muscular rigidity.

Peripheral sympathetic blocking agent. A drug that disrupts the transmission of nerve impulses to sympathetically innervated structures.

Peripheral vascular disease. An insufficiency of blood flow to the extremities.

Peripheral vasodilitation. Increase in diameter of the vessels in the extremities leading to an enhancement of blood flow.

Pituitary. The primary endocrine gland that controls many of the endocrine tissues of the body. The pituitary is in turn controlled by feedback from those structures and inputs from the brain.

Pharmacophore. The portion of the drug molecule that is responsible for the biologic activity of the drug.

Prodrug. A precursor that, after administration and subsequent transformation in the body, forms the active drug.

Progestational activity. Effects elicited by progestins, principally a cessation of ovulation and other genital changes related to pregnancy.

Prostate gland. One of the male exocrine glands responsible for secreting seminal fluid.

Pulmonary embolism. A blood clot trapped in the blood vessels of the lungs.

Psychoses. Major thought disorders involving distorted perception and hallucinations.

Psychotropic. Affecting the brain in such a way as to alter behavior.

Receptor. A macromolecule with which a drug or endogenous substance interacts to produce its effect.

Respiratory depression. A decrease in the frequency and/or depth of breathing.

Respiratory stimulant. An agent that enhances the frequency and/or depth of respiration.

Schistosome. A genus of blood flukes common to tropical areas.

Schistosomiasis. Infestation with schistosomes.

Sedative. A drug that decreases responsiveness of the central nervous system.

Sedative-hypnotic. A drug that decreases responsiveness of the central nervous system to the point of promoting sleep.

Seminal vesicle. An organ in which a portion of the seminal fluid is retained.

Spasmolytic. A drug that inhibits the contraction of intestinal smooth muscle.

Skeletal muscle relaxant. A drug that decreases the tone of voluntary muscles.

Stroke. A general term commonly used to denote a sudden paralysis resulting from a cerebral hemorrhage.

α-Sympathetic blocking agent. A drug that binds to, but does not stimulate, adrenergic receptors of the α-type.

β-Sympathetic blocking agent. A drug that binds to, but does not stimulate, adrenergic receptors of the β-type.

Sympathetic nervous system. That portion of the autonomic nervous system that utilizes norepinephrine as a neurotransmitter at its neuroeffector junctions.

Sympathomimetic. A drug that produces effects similar to stimulating the sympathetic nervous system, that is, increased blood pressure, dilated bronchi, and mydriasis.

Teratogenic. An agent that alters the normal development of the fetus.

Therapeutic index. Ratio between the median lethal dose (LD_{50}) and the median effective dose (ED_{50}) of a drug.

Thrombophlebitis. Inflammation of the veins involving the formation of blood clots.

Thymoleptic. A mood-elevating drug.

Thyroid gland. An endocrine gland that secretes thyroxin and tri-iodothyronine, hormones that modulate the rate of cellular metabolism.

Uricosuric. An agent that enhances the excretion of uric acid.

Vasoconstrictor. A drug that causes a contraction of the vascular smooth muscle, thus increasing the resistance to blood flow.

Index